Improving Diets and Nutrition

Food-based Approaches

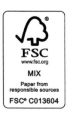

In memoriam
Michael Latham

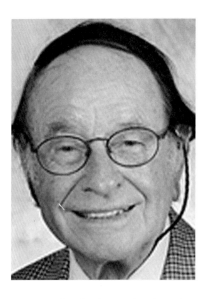

Michael Latham, who died on 1 April 2011 aged 82, was one of the founders of the field of international nutrition that deals with the nutrition problems of low-income countries. Born and raised in Tanganyika of British parents – his father was a colonial doctor in the 1920s and 1930s – he obtained a medical degree from Trinity College Dublin, Ireland, before returning to Tanganyika in 1955 to work first as a 'bush doctor' and later as leader of the Nutrition Unit in the Ministry of Health of the new country of Tanzania. In 1965, he was awarded the Order of the British Empire for these efforts. He then obtained postgraduate degrees from London and Harvard and began teaching at Cornell University in 1969, heading its International Nutrition Department for 25 years and maintaining a substantial workload – even as Emeritus Professor – until his death.

Latham was a lifelong champion of the underprivileged and marginalized and an advocate of the right to food and nutrition, tirelessly calling for measures to redress inequities in global resource allocation and poverty. Generations of the students he both trained and inspired went on to be scientists, academics or technocrats, but also pursued careers dedicated to doing something practical to redress the injustices of this world.

Professor Latham did important research (authoring or co-authoring some 450 articles, including two FAO books (*Human Nutrition in Tropical Africa*, first published in 1965 and revised in 1979; and *Human Nutrition in the Developing World*, published in 1997 and reprinted in 2004) that changed programme and policy orientation related to infant feeding, the control of parasitic diseases in humans, and combating micronutrient malnutrition, particularly food-based approaches. His final articles, including commentaries in *World Nutrition* and his last presentation in this Symposium, focused on the risks associated with 'magic bullet' approaches such as vitamin A capsule distribution (questioning whether in the real world this is actually reducing young child mortality) and the utilization of ready-to-use supplemental foods to prevent malnutrition. In 2008, he received the United Nations System Standing Committee on Nutrition Order of Merit in recognition of his outstanding lifelong contributions and service to nutrition.

He is survived by his life partner, Lani Stephenson, retired Cornell Associate Professor of Nutritional Sciences, and two sons.

Improving Diets and Nutrition

Food-based Approaches

―――――――――――――

Edited by

Brian Thompson

Nutrition Division
Food and Agriculture Organization of the United Nations

and

Leslie Amoroso

Nutrition Division
Food and Agriculture Organization of the United Nations

Published by
The Food and Agriculture Organization of the United Nations
and
CABI

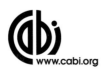

www.cabi.org

fao.org

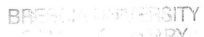

CABI is a trading name of CAB International

CABI	CABI
Nosworthy Way	38 Chauncey Street
Wallingford	Suite 1002
Oxfordshire OX10 8DE	Boston, MA 02111
UK	USA
Tel: +44 (0)1491 832111	Tel: +1 800 552 3083 (toll free)
Fax: +44 (0)1491 833508	Tel: +1 (0)617 395 4051
E-mail: info@cabi.org	E-mail: cabi-nao@cabi.org
Website: www.cabi.org	

A catalogue record for this book is available from the British Library, London, UK.

Library of Congress Cataloging-in-Publication Data

Improving diets and nutrition : food-based approaches/edited by Brian Thompson, Leslie Amoroso.
     p. ; cm.
   Includes bibliographical references and index.
   ISBN 978-1-78064-299-4 (CABI : hbk) -- ISBN 978-9251073193 (FAO)
   I. Thompson, Brian, 1953- editor of compilation. II. Amoroso, Leslie, 1977- editor of compilation.
III. C.A.B. International, issuing body. IV. Food and Agriculture Organization of the United Nations, issuing body.
   [DNLM: 1. Malnutrition--prevention & control. 2. Developing Countries.
   3. Diet. 4. Food. 5. Nutrition Policy. 6. Nutritional Physiological Phenomena. QU 145]

   RA645.N87
   362.1963'9--dc23

                         2013024761

Published jointly by CAB International and FAO
Food and Agriculture Organization of the United Nations (FAO)
Viale delle Terme di Caracalla, 00153 Rome, Italy
Web site: www.fao.org

ISBN: 978 1 78064 299 4 (CABI)
ISBN: 978 92 5 107319 3 (FAO)

Typeset by SPi, Pondicherry, India.
Printed and bound in the UK by CPI Group (UK) Ltd, Croydon, CR0 4YY.

Contents

About the Editors

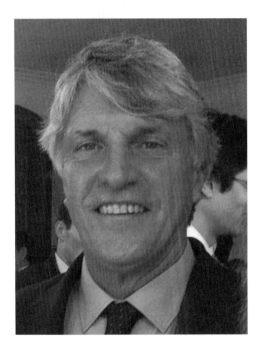

BRIAN THOMPSON
Nutrition Division
Food and Agriculture Organization
of the United Nations (FAO)
Rome, Italy
E-mail: brian.thompson@fao.org

Brian Thompson has a BSc in physiology from the University of London and an MSc in human nutrition from the London School of Hygiene and Tropical Medicine. He is a nutritionist with over 30 years of international development experience. After working in Asia with ICRC (International Committee of the Red Cross), WFP (United Nations (UN) World Food Programme), UNICEF (UN Children's Fund), FAO and the NGO (non-governmental organization) community, he joined FAO at its Headquarters in Rome. He is Senior Nutrition Officer in the Nutrition Division of FAO where he advises Members on the development and implementation of policies, strategies and plans of action for promoting and improving food and nutrition security. Mr Thompson is author/co-editor of a number of peer-reviewed publications, including: Chapter 4 (Sustainable Food and Nutrition Security) of the *Sixth Report on the World Nutrition Situation: Progress in Nutrition* (United Nations System Standing Committee on Nutrition, 2010); the joint FAO/CABI publication *Combating Micronutrient Deficiencies: Food-based Approaches* (2011); and the recently released joint FAO/Springer publication *The Impact of Climate Change and Bioenergy on Nutrition* (2012). Currently, he is responsible for the coordination of FAO's preparations for the Second International Conference on Nutrition.

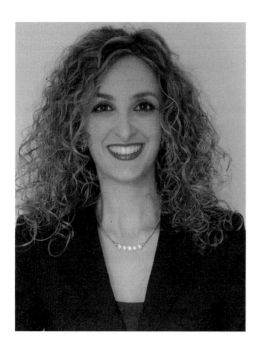

LESLIE AMOROSO
Nutrition Division
Food and Agriculture Organization
of the United Nations (FAO)
Rome, Italy
E-mail: leslie.amoroso@fao.org

Leslie Amoroso has a degree in international relations and diplomatic affairs with a focus on development policies from the Università di Bologna, Italy. She holds a Master's in urban and regional planning for developing countries with emphasis on food and nutrition security and livelihood issues from the Istituto Universitario di Architettura di Venezia (IUAV), Venice, Italy. Ms Amoroso has wide international experience in food and nutrition security policy and programme-related activities, with a focus on childhood, gender and HIV/AIDS in Ethiopia, the Gambia and Nicaragua. She joined FAO Headquarters in Rome in 2007, where she is Programme Officer in the Nutrition Division, working on governance, policy, capacity building, and programme and advocacy activities and initiatives aimed at improving food and nutrition security. Ms Amoroso is currently assisting with the coordination of FAO's preparatory activities for the Second International Conference on Nutrition and is co-editor, along with Brian Thompson, of the joint FAO/CABI publication *Combating Micronutrient Deficiencies: Food-based Approaches* (2011).

Contributor Biographies

Marina Adrianopoli is a food security and nutrition expert at the Ministry of Agriculture and Animal Resources of Rwanda. She previously worked at INRAN (Istituto Nazionale di Ricerca per gli Alimenti e la Nutrizione), Rome and WHO (World Health Organization) in Tajikistan, Uzbekistan and Albania. Her areas of expertise include: food security and nutrition policy, programming and assessments; public health nutrition and emergency nutrition. Recent collaborations are with: WHO, FAO, WFP (UN World Food Programme), UNICEF (UN Children's Fund), European Commission, governmental institutions and international NGOs (non-governmental organizations). Mailing address: Via A Scoppetta 10, 87029 Scalea CS, Italy. E-mail: marina.adrianopoli@gmail.com

Margarita Álvarez Oyarzábal graduated in international relations in Mexico city. She worked in the import/export private sector and was coordinator in Mexico for The Growing Connection Project (TGC), FAO/UN. She is currently developing a project to manufacture and distribute water-efficient containers for vegetable growing to help reduce hunger and malnutrition in Mexico and surrounding countries. Mailing address: Calle Tres no. 86, Colonia Seattle, Zapopan, CP 45150, Jalisco, Mexico. E-mail: maratapatia@yahoo.com.mx

Leslie Amoroso holds a Master's in urban and regional planning for developing countries with emphasis on food and nutrition security and livelihood issues from the Istituto Universitario di Architettura di Venezia (IUAV), Venice, Italy. She has wide international experience in food and nutrition security policy and programme-related activities, with a focus on childhood, gender and HIV/AIDS in Ethiopia, The Gambia and Nicaragua. Ms Amoroso joined FAO Headquarters in Rome in 2007, where she is Programme Officer in the Nutrition Division. She works on governance, policy, programme and advocacy activities and initiatives aimed at improving food and nutrition security. She is currently assisting with the coordination of FAO's preparatory activities for the Second International Conference on Nutrition and is co-editor of the FAO/CABI publication *Combating Micronutrient Deficiencies: Food-based Approaches*. Mailing address: Nutrition Division, Food and Agriculture Organization of the United Nations (FAO), Viale delle Terme di Caracalla, 00153 Rome, Italy. E-mail: leslie.amoroso@fao.org

Christian Borja-Vega is an economist who specializes in impact evaluations, econometric and statistical analysis and development operations. He has worked at the Inter-American Development Bank (IDB) and the World Bank for almost 10 years. Part of his work has focused on estimating long-term health and education impacts of various interventions in Latin American and African regions. Mailing address: The World Bank, 1818 H Street NW, Washington, DC 20433, USA. E-mail: cborjavega@worldbank.org

Howarth E. Bouis received his BA in economics from Stanford University and his MA and PhD from Stanford University's Food Research Institute. Since 1993, he has sought to promote biofortification within the CGIAR (formerly the Consultative Group on International Agricultural Research), among national agricultural research centres and in the human nutrition community. His past research focused on understanding how economic factors affect food demand and nutrition outcomes, particularly in Asia. He holds a joint appointment at the International Food Policy Research Institute (IFPRI, Washington, DC) and the International Center for Tropical Agriculture (CIAT) (Cali, Colombia). Mailing address: International Food Policy Research Institute (IFPRI), 2033 K Street NW, Washington, DC 20006, USA. E-mail: h.bouis@cgiar.org

Khadichamo Boymatova is currently working as National Professional Officer on Nutrition and Food Safety in the World Health Organization (WHO) Country Office in Tajikistan. Her professional experience includes working with the International NGO *Action Against Hunger*, in Nutrition and Mother and Child Health Projects and as a paediatrician and neonatologist in the Emergency Care Unit of hospitals in the country. Her main areas of expertise include the following areas of nutrition: healthy and safe diets, surveillance, policy development, prevention and treatment of micronutrient deficiencies and malnutrition. Mailing address: VEFA Center, Bokhtar Str. 37/1, 734018, Dushanbe, Tajikistan. E-mail: bkh@euro.who.int

Luciene Burlandy is a nutritionist with a PhD in Public Health. She is Professor of the Undergraduate Programme of Nutrition and the Graduate Programme of Social Policy at the Universidade Federal Fluminense (Fluminense Federal University, UFF) of Rio de Janeiro, and coordinates the Centro de Referência em Segurança, Alimentar e Nutricional (Reference Centre on Food and Nutrition Security, CERESAN). She is also a member of the Brazilian Forum on Food and Nutrition Security (FBSAN) and the National Council for Food and Nutrition Security (CONSEA). Mailing address: Faculdade de Nutrição, Universidade Federal Fluminense, Rua Mário Santos, Braga 30 – 4° Andar, Niterói/Rio de Janeiro, CEP 24020-140, Brazil. E-mail: burlandy@uol.com.br

Nimrod O. Bwibo, Professor Emeritus of Paediatrics, has served as Dean and Principal of the University of Nairobi School of Medicine as well as Vice Chancellor of the University of Nairobi. He served as the Kenyan Principal Investigator for the *Role of Animal Source Foods to Improve Diet Quality and Growth and Development in Kenyan SchoolChildren* study and has been a collaborator on three other nutrition studies in Kenyan adults and children. Mailing address: Department of Pediatrics, University of Nairobi, PO Box 19676, Ngong Road, Nairobi, Kenya. E-mail: thebwibos@yahoo.com

Chunming Chen was the founding president of the Chinese Academy of Preventive Medicine (now the Chinese Center for Disease Control and Prevention) during 1983–1992. She has been Professor of Nutrition at the Center since 1985 and Senior Advisor since 1992, focusing on nutrition policy studies and engaging in research on obesity, early child nutrition, nutrition problems in poor areas and nutrition-related chronic diseases in the past 30 years. She designed the National Food and Nutrition Surveillance System in China and has carried out eight rounds of surveillance over the past 20 years (1990–2010), so providing a clear picture of nutritional status in China during its rapid economic development. Mailing address: International Life Science Institute Focal Point in China, Chinese Center for Disease Control and Prevention, Rm903 #27 Nanwei Road, Beijing, China. E-mail: chencm@ilsichina.org

Paola D'Acapito is currently working as Scientific Project Officer for the European Commission's Executive Agency for Health and Consumers (EAHC). Her previous professional experiences include work at the Istituto per l'Infanzia IRCCS (Istituto di Ricovero e Cura a Carattere Scientifico) Burlo Garofolo, World Health Organization (WHO) and UN World Food Programme (WFP). She holds an MSc in human nutrition science. Her main areas of research include nutritional epidemiology and public health. Mailing address: 22, rue due Couvent, L-1363 Howald, Luxembourg. E-mail: dacapito@inran.it

Ian Darnton-Hill has over 40 years of work experience with the UN at WHO (World Health Organization) and UNICEF (UN Children's Fund), most recently as Special Adviser to the UNICEF Executive Director on ending child hunger and undernutrition. He has also worked in USAID (US Agency for International Development)-funded cooperative agreements, for example as Director of the OMNI (Opportunities for Micronutrient Interventions) Project, with the NGO community, e.g. at Helen Keller International (HKI). He is presently an Adjunct Professor in Australia (at The Boden Institute of Obesity, Nutrition, Exercise and Eating Disorders of the University of Sydney), and in the USA (at the Friedman School of Nutrition Science and Policy, Tufts University, Boston, Massachusetts). He recently was awarded the Order of Australia for 'distinguished service to the international community, particularly in the areas of public health and nutrition'. Mailing address: 12–13 Dry Creek Road, Donovans Landing, SA 5291, Australia. E-mail: ian.darnton-hill@sydney.edu.au

Natalie Drorbaugh is a public health nutrition consultant, and earned an MA and an MPH from the University of California at Los Angeles. Ms Drorbaugh has conducted literature reviews on the nutritional status of food aid beneficiaries in several African countries and has co-authored several chapters for FAO publications on the nutritional impact of animal source foods. Mailing address: Fielding School of Public Health, University of California, Los Angeles (UCLA), PO Box 951772, Los Angeles, CA 90095-1772, USA. E-mail: ndrorbau@ucla.edu

Mieke Faber is a nutritionist and chief specialist scientist at the Nutritional Intervention Research Unit of the South African Medical Research Council. Her research focus is on community-based nutrition interventions focusing on food-based approaches to address micronutrient malnutrition in infants and young children, particularly in resource-poor rural populations. She also studies the role of traditional leafy vegetables and dietary diversity within the context of food and nutrition security. Mailing address: Medical Research Council, PO Box 19070, Tygerberg, 7505, South Africa. E-mail: mieke.faber@mrc.ac.za

Marika Ferrari PhD is a biologist and is presently a researcher at INRAN (Istituto Nazionale di Ricerca per gli Alimenti e la Nutrizione) in Rome. She has extensive experience in public health nutrition. She has collaborated with WHO (World Health Organization), WFP (UN World Food Programme) and UNICEF (UN Children's Fund) on nutritional surveys and interventions in Algeria, Zimbabwe, Bangladesh, Tajikistan and Kosovo. She has developed research protocols, and trained and supervised international/local staff in the management of blood collection, laboratory assays and anthropometric data. Mailing address: Istituto Nazionale di Ricerca per gli Alimenti e la Nutrizione (INRAN), Via Ardeatina 546, 00178 Rome, Italy. E-mail: ferrari@inran.it

Constance A. Gewa earned an MSc in applied human nutrition from the University of Nairobi and an MPH and PhD in public health at the University of California, Los Angeles (UCLA). She served as field coordinator for the *Role of Animal Source Foods to Improve Diet Quality and Growth and Development in Kenyan SchoolChildren* study and has published numerous papers on food intake methodology and evaluation. Her recent research focuses on nutrition in HIV-positive mothers and their children in Kenya, as well as the impact of intervention feeding on household food intake. She is on the Nutrition Faculty at George Mason University in Virginia, USA. Mailing address: Department of Nutrition and Food Studies, College of Health and Human Services, George Mason University, MS: 1F8, 4400 University Drive, Fairfax, VA 22030-4444, USA. E-mail: cgewa@gmu.edu

Rosalind S. Gibson, a Research Professor in Human Nutrition at the University of Otago, Dunedin, New Zealand, has had a lifelong interest in international nutrition, initially working in the Ethio–Swedish Children's Nutrition Unit in Ethiopia, and subsequently in collaborative research studies on micronutrients in Papua New Guinea, Guatemala, Ghana, Malawi and, more recently, Thailand, Cambodia, Mongolia, Zambia, Ethiopia and north-eastern Brazil. One focus has been on sustainable food-based strategies to combat micronutrient deficiencies. She is the author of a standard reference text, *Principles of Nutritional Assessment*

(Oxford University Press, 2005), is a Fellow of the American Society of Nutrition and the Royal Society of New Zealand, and a member of the International Zinc Nutrition Consultative Group. Mailing address: Department of Human Nutrition, University of Otago, Union Street, PO Box 56, Dunedin, 9015, New Zealand. E-mail: rosalind.gibson@otago.ac.nz

Ted Greiner has been Professor of Nutrition at Hanyang University in Seoul, South Korea for 5 years and is part time Professor of Nutrition at the Natural Resources Institute, Greenwich University. Before that he had spent 4 years with a non-profit organization called PATH in the USA. He directed its rice fortification programme and was involved in research and technical assistance in infant feeding in the context of HIV in three African countries. He worked at Uppsala University in Sweden for 19 years as Associate Professor of International Child Health and advisor to the Swedish International Development Cooperation Agency (SIDA). Since 2007, he has been the Chair of the NGO/Civil Society Constituency of the UN Standing Committee on Nutrition. Mailing address: Food and Nutrition Department, Hanyang University, 222 Wangsimni Ro, Seoul 133-791, South Korea. E-mail: tedgreiner@yahoo.com

Dalia Haroun currently works as an Assistant Professor in Nutrition at Zayed University, UAE, and holds a consultancy post at UNICEF (UN Children's Fund). She previously worked as a Research Associate at the School Food Trust in the UK carrying out analysis on the primary school food survey. Previous experience includes working on research relating to the body composition of children. Mailing address: Department of Natural Science and Public Health, College of Humanities and Sustainability Sciences, Zayed University, PO Box 19282, Academic City, Dubai, United Arab Emirates. E-mail: dalia.haroun@zu.ac.ae

Clare Harper is a company nutritionist for ISS Facility Services in the UK. Previously she was a research nutritionist at the Children's Food Trust, also in the UK, working on school food projects and specializing in survey design and data coding. She worked on both the primary and secondary school food surveys. Before joining the Trust, she worked as a project officer in primary care health research. Mailing address: ISS Facility Services – Education, Unit 11, Belvue Business Centre, Belvue Road, Northolt, UB5 5QQ, UK. E-mail: clare.harper@uk.issworld.com

Nancy J. Haselow obtained her MPH at the University of California, Los Angeles (UCLA) and is Vice President and Regional Director for Asia Pacific of Helen Keller International (HKI). She has spent the past 25 plus years working in international public health in Asia and Africa, with expertise in the design and testing of delivery strategies to improve access to nutrition and eye health services among the poor, including reducing vitamin A deficiency and linking agriculture to improved nutrition. Mailing address: Helen Keller International (HKI), House # 43Z43, Street 466, PO Box 168, Phnom Penh, Cambodia. E-mail: nhaselow@hki.org

Emily P. Hillenbrand is currently Gender and Livelihoods Technical Advisor at CARE USA. She worked for Helen Keller International (HKI) as Program Manager with HKI Bangladesh from 2008 to 2011, and was Regional Gender Coordinator for HKI, Asia-Pacific Regional Office, Cambodia, in 2012. At HKI, she focused particularly on the gender equity outcomes of HKI projects and the engagement of men in nutrition programming. Emily holds an MA in Women, Gender and Development from the Institute of Social Studies, The Hague. Mailing address: 151 Ellis Street NW, Atlanta, GA 30303, USA. E-mail: ehillenbrand@care.org

Christine Hotz is a nutritionist currently working as a research and programme consultant in her own consulting business, Nutridemics. From the laboratory to remote field locations, her research has always focused on food-based interventions for improved micronutrient status in poor and rural populations. She has served as the founding Executive Officer and Steering Committee member of the International Zinc Nutrition Consultative Group, was a research faculty member of the National Institute of Public Health of Mexico, and the Nutrition Coordinator of HarvestPlus based at the International Food Policy Research Institute (IFPRI) in Washington, DC. She was affiliated with IFPRI at the time of submission of the publication. Mailing address: Nutridemics, 231 Fort York Blvd, Unit 1711, Toronto, Ontario, M5V 1B2, Canada. E-mail: christinehotz.to@gmail.com

Suraiya J. Ismail is a public health nutritionist with extensive international experience. She spent 23 years in academic institutions in the USA, Jamaica and the UK, and 5 years at FAO.

For the last 9 years she has directed a consultancy firm in Guyana that specializes in impact evaluations of large-scale programmes and pilot research studies for the Ministries of Health and Education. Mailing address: Social Development Inc., 4 Ogle Public Road, Georgetown, Guyana. E-mail: sjismail@yahoo.co.uk

Cheryl Jackson Lewis is a Senior Nutrition and Health Advisor at the US Agency for International Development (USAID) Bureau for Food Security. Previously, she was a supervisory nutritionist at the US Department of Agriculture's Food and Nutrition Service. She has over 25 years of experience as a nutritionist and has worked throughout Asia and Africa. She is also a licensed and registered dietitian. Mailing address: US Department of Agriculture Food and Nutrition Service, 3101 Park Center Drive Alexandria, VA 22302, USA. E-mail: cheryl.lewis@fns.usda.gov

Edward A. Jarvis was born and raised in the North West District of Guyana (Region 1), and became a teacher at the Santa Rosa Primary School in Moruca. He came to the Ministry of Education as Hinterland Coordinator in 2001, later joining the team of Education for All Fast-track Initiative (EFA-FTI, now the Global Partnership for Education), a partnership of close to 60 developing countries, donor governments, international organizations, the private sector, teachers and civil society/NGO groups to ensure accelerated progress towards the Millennium Development Goal of universal primary education by 2015. In January 2008, he was appointed Coordinator for the EFA-FTI programme of the Ministry of Education in Guyana, a position that he currently holds. Mailing address: Ministry of Education, 109 Barima Avenue, Georgetown, Guyana. E-mail: edwardjarvis@yahoo.com

George Kent has retired from his position as Professor of Political Science at the University of Hawaii, but he continues to teach online courses on food issues for other universities. He works primarily on food, children and human rights. His latest books are *Ending Hunger Worldwide* (Paradigm Publishers, Boulder, Colorado) and *Regulating Infant Formula* (Hale Publishing, Amarillo, Texas). Mailing address: 6303 Paauilo Place, Honolulu, HI 96825, USA. E-mail: kent@hawaii.edu

Hou Kroeun has been working in the field of food security and nutrition over the last 15 years. Before joining Helen Keller International (HKI) in his current position as Program Manager, he was the agriculture specialist involved in the development, implementation and monitoring of a sustainable integrated farming system project in Cambodia with New Zealand Service Abroad (NSA), Quaker Service Australia (QSA), the Mennonite Central Committee (MCC) and the Japan International Volunteer Center (JVC). He has a degree in agriculture and an MPH. Mailing address: Helen Keller International (HKI), House # 43Z43, Street 466, PO Box 168, Phnom Penh, Cambodia. E-mail: hkroeun@hki.org

Michael C. Latham MD, DTM&H, MPH, FFCM (Hon.), OBE was a medical doctor and nutritionist, with degrees also in public health and tropical medicine. He died on 1 April 2011 at the age of 82. He worked extensively overseas, particularly in East Africa, but also in Asia. He had been a Professor at Cornell University since 1968, and published extensively, particularly on the nutritional problems of low-income countries.

Sunette M. Laurie works as a Senior Agricultural Researcher at the Roodeplaat Vegetable and Ornamental Plant Institute in the Plant Breeding Division of the Agricultural Research Council in South Africa. Her research includes the breeding of orange-fleshed sweet potato, the viability of commercialization of this crop, the establishment of nurseries and the food-based approach to address vitamin A deficiency. She is one of the collaborators in Sweetpotato Action for Health and Security in Africa (SASHA), a research team that is at the forefront of biofortification of orange-fleshed sweet potato in sub-Saharan Africa. Mailing address: Agricultural Research Council Vegetable and Ornamental Plant Institute (ARC-VOPI), Private Bag X293, Pretoria, 0001, South Africa. E-mail: slaurie@arc.agric.za

A. Carolyn MacDonald has worked for over 25 years in international nutrition in both programming and research, focusing on integrating multiple sectors to address malnutrition, including health and food-based approaches. She has managed nutrition programmes in

Ethiopia, Democratic Republic of Congo and Sudan, and conducted fortification research in Malawi. She has worked with World Vision since 1996, first as World Vision Canada's Nutrition and Health Team Director, and then since 2008 with World Vision International. Carolyn holds a BSc in biochemistry from McMaster University and an MSc and PhD in nutrition from the University of Guelph. Mailing address: Nutrition Centre of Expertise, World Vision International, c/o 1 World Drive, Mississauga, Ontario, L5T 2Y4, Canada. E-mail: carolyn_macdonald@worldvision.ca

Bonnie McClafferty has over 20 years of experience working in agricultural research and development within CGIAR (formerly the Consultative Group on International Agricultural Research). She is currently the Director of Agriculture and Nutrition at the Global Alliance for Improved Nutrition (GAIN). Before joining GAIN, she was a founding leader of HarvestPlus, where she worked for 12 years heading up the office on Development and Communication. She was affiliated with the International Food Policy Research Institute (IFPRI) at the time of submission of the publication. Mailing address: Global Alliance for Improved Nutrition (GAIN), 1776 Massachusetts Avenue NW, Suite 700, Washington, DC 20036, USA. E-mail: bmcclafferty@gainhealth.org

Giuseppe Maiani is presently Research Director of the Nutrition Science Area at INRAN (Istituto Nazionale di Ricerca per gli Alimenti e la Nutrizione) in Rome. His research activity focuses on nutritional epidemiology and investigates the mechanisms of intestinal absorption and the bioavailability of natural compounds that can act as antioxidants. His research interest includes analyses of the relationship that occurs between dietary habits and antioxidant status in humans and its subsequent impact on human health. Mailing address: Istituto Nazionale di Ricerca per gli Alimenti e la Nutrizione (INRAN), Via Ardeatina 546, 00178 Rome, Italy. E-mail: maiani@inran.it

Renato S. Maluf has a PhD in political economy and is Associate Professor of the Graduate Programme of Social Sciences in Agriculture, Development and Society (Curso de Pós-Graduação de Ciências Sociais em Desenvolvimento, Agricultura e Sociedade, CPDA), at the Federal Rural University of Rio de Janeiro (Universidade Federal Rural do Rio de Janeiro, UFRRJ). He was President of CONSEA (Conselho Nacional de Segurança Alimentar e Nutricional, 2007–2011), coordinates CERESAN (the Reference Centre on Food and Nutrition Security – Centro de Referência em Segurança, Alimentar e Nutricional), integrates the CPDA Observatory on Public Policies for Agriculture (OPPA), FBSAN (Fórum Brasileiro de Segurança Alimentar e Nutricional) and the Steering Committee of the High Level Panel of Experts in Food Security (HLPE), UN Committee on World Food Security (CFS, 2010–2012). Mailing address: Centro de Referência em Segurança, Alimentar e Nutricional (CERESAN), Curso de Pós-Graduação de Ciências Sociais em Desenvolvimento, Agricultura e Sociedade, Universidade Federal Rural do Rio de Janeiro (CPDA/UFRRJ), Av. Presidente Vargas, 417/8, CEP: 20.071-003, Rio de Janeiro, Brazil. E-mail: renato.maluf@terra.com.br

J.V. Meenakshi is currently on the Faculty of the Delhi School of Economics, University of Delhi. She also coordinated the policy and impact analysis research portfolio at HarvestPlus from 2004 to 2008. Her research interests include agriculture–nutrition linkages, the economics of micronutrient malnutrition and food demand and agricultural markets, areas in which she has published widely. She obtained her PhD from Cornell University in agricultural economics. Mailing address: Centre for Development Economics, Delhi School of Economics, University of Delhi, Delhi 110007, India. E-mail: meena@econdse.org

Janice Meerman holds Master's degrees in public health and public policy from the University of California, Berkeley (UCB), and has consulted for FAO, the World Bank and the UN Standing Committee on Nutrition. Her major focus areas include developing innovative solutions to the challenge of building institutional and operational capacity for nutrition programming and nutrition-sensitive agricultural development. Recent publications include: *The Impact of Climate Change and Bioenergy on Nutrition* (Springer/FAO, 2012); *Scaling Up Community Based Maternal and Child Nutrition and Health Interventions in Nigeria* (World Bank, 2011); and Chapter 4 (Sustainable Food and

Nutrition Security) of the *Sixth Report on the World Nutrition Situation: Progress in Nutrition* (United Nations System Standing Committee on Nutrition, 2010). Mailing address: 1127 El Centro Avenue, Oakland, CA 94602, USA. E-mail: janice.meerman@fao.org

Lorenza Mistura is a statistician and is presently a researcher at INRAN (Istituto Nazionale di Ricerca per gli Alimenti e la Nutrizione) and consultant to FAO. He has extensive experience in research fields related to public health, nutrition and food security, both in Italy and elsewhere. He has developed research protocols, coordinated field work and data collection, and trained and supervised international/local health staff. In addition, he has supervised data collection and analysis of nutrition and anthropometric surveys in developing countries. Mailing address: Istituto Nazionale di Ricerca per gli Alimenti e la Nutrizione (INRAN), Via Ardeatina 546, 00178 Rome, Italy. E-mail: mistura@inran.it

Michael Nelson is Director of Public Health Nutrition Research, and is the former Director of Research and Nutrition at the Children's Food Trust. He worked from 1977 to 1985 as a Scientific Officer at the Medical Research Council (Human Nutrition Research, Cambridge and Environmental Epidemiology Unit, Southampton) before joining King's College London in 1985, where he is Emeritus Reader in Public Health Nutrition. From 2006 to 2013, he was seconded to the School (now Children's) Food Trust as Director of Research and Nutrition. He established Public Health Nutrition Research in 2013. Mailing address: PHN Research Ltd, 59 Thurlestone Road, London, SE27 0PE, UK. E-mail: michael.nelson@ phnresearch.org.uk

Charlotte G. Neumann MD, MPH has pioneered and directed research in maternal and child health and development for over five decades in India and Africa. She attended Harvard Medical School and attained an MPH from Harvard School of Public Health, and is in the University of California, Los Angeles (UCLA) School of Public Health and the School of Medicine. Her recent research has documented the role of animal source foods in ameliorating multiple micronutrient deficiencies and improving growth, activity, cognitive development and school performance in schoolchildren. She is actively involved in nutrition research with HIV-positive mothers and their children in Kenya. Mailing address: Fielding School of Public Health, University of California, Los Angeles (UCLA), PO Box 951772, Los Angeles, CA 90095-1772, USA. E-mail: cneumann@ucla.edu

Jo Nicholas is Head of Research and Evaluation at the Children's Food Trust in the UK and has led the monitoring work for the Trust. She was previously employed as a research coordinator at King's College London. At the Trust, she is project manager for the annual surveys, and for the surveys of provision and consumption in primary schoolchildren in 2005 and in secondary schoolchildren in 2010–11. Mailing address: Children's Food Trust, 3rd Floor, 1 East Parade, Sheffield, S1 2ET, UK. E-mail: jo.nicholas@childrensfoodtrust.org.uk

Akoto Kwame Osei has been working as the Asia Pacific Regional Nutrition Adviser for Helen Keller International (HKI) since 2009. After receiving his BSc from the University of Ghana (2000), he completed an MSc (2004) and PhD (2009) in food policy and applied nutrition and nutrition epidemiology at Tufts University in Boston, Massachusetts. During his studies in Boston, he also completed a certificate in humanitarian assistance in complex emergency (2002–2004). Mailing address: Helen Keller International (HKI), House # 43Z43, Street 466, PO Box 168, Phnom Penh, Cambodia. E-mail: aosei@hki.org

Bob (Robert) Patterson now operates EarthBox Mexico, building space and water-efficient vegetable gardens and production sites, having worked for more than 30 years with FAO/ UN in Africa, Latin America and the Caribbean, and at FAO Headquarters in Rome. Mailing address: 11219 Gainsborough Road, Potomac, MD 20854, USA. E-mail: robertpatterson57@ gmail.com

Jo Pearce is Teaching Fellow in Nutrition at Nottingham University and previously worked at the Children's Food Trust on school food projects, specializing in measuring intake in children and young people. She was research coordinator for the studies on school lunch and behaviour in primary and secondary schools. Before this, she worked as a community nutritionist for Sure Start, a UK government initiative. Mailing address: Division of Nutritional Sciences, School of

Biosciences, University of Nottingham, North Laboratory, Sutton Bonington Campus, Sutton Bonington, LE12 5RD, UK. E-mail: jo.pearce@nottingham.ac.uk

Wolfgang H. Pfeiffer obtained his MSc and PhD in agricultural sciences from Stuttgart-Hohenheim University in Germany. Before joining HarvestPlus, he was Head Plant Breeder for the Intensive Agro-ecosystems Program at the International Maize and Wheat Improvement Center (CIMMYT) in Mexico where he was responsible for applied and strategic bread wheat, durum wheat and triticale improvement under CIMMYT's global germplasm development mandate. He has over 20 years of experience working in international agricultural research. Mailing address: International Center for Tropical Agriculture (CIAT), Apartado Aéreo 6173, Cali, Colombia. E-mail: w.pfeiffer@cgiar.org

Per Pinstrup-Andersen is the H.E. Babcock Professor of Food, Nutrition and Public Policy, the J. Thomas Clark Professor of Entrepreneurship and Professor of Applied Economics at Cornell University and Adjunct Professor, Copenhagen University. He is a fellow of the American Association for the Advancement of Science (AAAS) and the Agricultural and Applied Economics Association (AAEA). He is the 2001 World Food Prize Laureate. His recent publications include *Food Policy for Developing Countries* (Cornell University Press, 2011), co-authored with Derrill Watson. Mailing address: Division of Nutritional Sciences, Cornell University, 305 Savage Hall, Ithaca, New York 14853-6301, USA. E-mail: pp94@cornell.edu

Victoria Quinn joined Helen Keller International (HKI) in 2006 as Senior Vice President of Programs, and has more than 30 years of experience in Africa, Asia and Latin America designing and managing complex and large-scale nutrition and maternal child health country and regional programmes. She received her Bachelor's and Master's degrees in nutrition from University of California, Berkeley (UCB) and Cornell University, respectively, and her doctorate from Wageningen University in the Netherlands. Mailing address: Helen Keller International (HKI), 1120 20th Street, NW Suite 500N, Washington, DC 20036, USA. E-mail: vquinn@hki.org

Cecilia Rocha has a PhD in Economics and is the Director of the School of Nutrition, Ryerson University, where she is an Associate Professor of Food Security and Food Policy. She was an associate researcher and past Director (2005–2010) of the Centre for Studies in Food Security; an associate researcher of the Centre for Global Health and Health Equity at Ryerson University and an active member of the Toronto Food Policy Council from 2006 to 2011. Mailing address: School of Nutrition, Ryerson University, 350 Victoria Street, Toronto, Ontario, M5B 2K3, Canada. E-mail: crocha@ryerson.ca

Santino Severoni is currently Regional Coordinator for Strategic Relations with Countries in the Office of the Regional Director of the World Health Organization (WHO) for Europe. His previous working experience included the position of WHO Representative in Tajikistan and Albania. He has been responsible for the health sector of the Italian Cooperation Office for Serbia, Montenegro and Kosovo. His main professional experience includes the management of major health crises in countries in transition. Mailing address: Piazza G Pepe 2, Cittaducale, 02015 Rieti, Italy. E-mail: sev@euro.who.int

Claire Storey is a psychologist who is currently on a career break. She previously worked for the Children's Food Trust as a researcher, and was the project lead on the secondary school lunch and behaviour project. Before joining the Trust she was a researcher at both York and Leeds Universities. Mailing address: Children's Food Trust, 3rd Floor, 1 East Parade, Sheffield, S1 2ET, UK. E-mail: info@childrensfoodtrust.org.uk

Aminuzzaman Talukder is Country Director for Cambodia and Regional Food Security Advisor for Asia Pacific of Helen Keller International (HKI) and is an international expert on food security and nutrition. For over 25 years, he has provided technical support to governments, NGOs and communities across Asia and Africa to improve policies and implement effective programmes to improve the health and nutrition of vulnerable populations. He is an agriculturist, with postgraduate training from Wageningen

University, the Netherlands and MPH from International University, Cambodia. Mailing address: Helen Keller International (HKI), House # 43Z43, Street 466, PO Box 168, Phnom Penh, Cambodia. E-mail: ztalukder@hki.org

Brian Thompson has a BSc in physiology from the University of London and an MSc in human nutrition, from the London School of Hygiene and Tropical Medicine. He is a nutritionist with over 30 years of international development experience. After working in Asia with ICRC, WFP, UNICEF, FAO and the NGO community, he joined FAO at its Headquarters in Rome. He is Senior Nutrition Officer in the Nutrition Division of FAO where he advises Members on the development and implementation of policies, strategies and plans of action for promoting and improving food and nutrition security. Mr Thompson is author/co-editor of a number of peer-reviewed publications, including: Chapter 4 (Sustainable Food and Nutrition Security) of the *Sixth Report on the World Nutrition Situation: Progress in Nutrition* (United Nations System Standing Committee on Nutrition, 2010); the joint FAO/CABI publication *Combating Micronutrient Deficiencies: Food-based Approaches* (2011); and the recently released joint FAO/Springer publication *The Impact of Climate Change and Bioenergy on Nutrition* (2012). Mailing address: Nutrition Division, Food and Agriculture Organization of the United Nations (FAO), Viale delle Terme di Caracalla, 00153 Rome, Italy. E-mail: brian.thompson@fao.org

Elisabetta Toti is a nutritionist and is currently working at the National Research Institute on Food and Nutrition (Istituto Nazionale di Ricerca per gli Alimenti e la Nutrizione, INRAN) in Rome. Her professional experience includes projects funded by IFPRI (International Food Policy Research Institute), FAO, WFP (UN World Food Programme) and the EC (European Commission), and her main areas of research include nutritional epidemiology and micronutrient bioavailability, in both industrialized countries and countries in transition. Mailing address: Istituto Nazionale di Ricerca per gli Alimenti e la Nutrizione (INRAN), Via Ardeatina 546, 00178 Rome, Italy. E-mail: toti@inran.it

Ursula Truebswasser is now working in the WHO (World Health Organization) Intercountry Support Team for Eastern and Southern Africa in Zimbabwe. Previous professional experience includes stints at the WHO Country Office in Tajikistan, the WHO Regional Office for Europe and the General Hospital in Vienna. Her main areas of expertise are nutrition policy analysis and development, prevention of micronutrient deficiencies, infant feeding and nutrition surveillance. Mailing address: Apfelrosenweg 6, 1140 Vienna, Austria. E-mail: truebswasser@gmx.at

Amin Uddin is the Program Manager for Helen Keller International (HKI) in Bangladesh. He has been with HKI for over 15 years. He started his career with BRAC (formerly the Bangladesh Rehabilitation Assistance Committee and the Bangladesh Rural Advancement Committee), a national NGO in Bangladesh. In 2010, he completed an MBA and he has a Bachelor's degree in agriculture (1988) from Bangladesh Agricultural University. Mailing address: Helen Keller International (HKI), House # 10F, Road 82, Gulshan-2, Dhaka, Bangladesh. E-mail: auddin@hki.org

Paul J. van Jaarsveld is a biochemist and senior specialist scientist at the South African Medical Research Council. His research includes, inter alia, lipid analyses in foods and biological specimens, fatty acids in particular, and carotenoid analyses, specifically the quantification of β-carotene in fresh vegetables and fruits to determine their vitamin A value. An example of his multidisciplinary team research is determining the nutrient content, including β-carotene, of African leafy vegetables and sweet potatoes consumed by the rural poor to address vitamin A deficiency through a food-based approach. Mailing address: Medical Research Council, PO Box 19070, Tygerberg, 7505, South Africa. E-mail: paul.van.jaarsveld@mrc.ac.za

Jillian L. Waid is a Manager of Learning, Evaluation, and Research for Helen Keller International, based in Dhaka, Bangladesh. She received an MSW that concentrated on Social and Economic Development from Washington University in 2009, completing her Master's thesis on son preference in South Asia. Before graduate school, Jillian worked in the World Bank's Poverty Research Unit and on reproductive health and women's livelihood issues with

Kutch Mahila Vikas Sangathan in Gujarat, India. Jillian has a BA in Economics and South Asian Studies from Brown University, Rhode Island. Mailing address: Helen Keller International (HKI), House # 10F, Road 82, Gulshan-2, Dhaka 1212, Bangladesh. E-mail: jwaid@hki.org

Aimee Webb Girard is an assistant professor in the Hubert Department of Global Health at Emory University, Georgia. Her research efforts are primarily focused on infant nutrition and health and she has spent extensive time in Africa and Latin America in support of this work. She received her doctorate in nutrition and health sciences from Emory University and then completed postdoctoral fellowships in nutritional epidemiology at the Harvard School of Public Health and in anthropology at the University of Toronto. Mailing address: Rollins School of Public Health, Emory University, 1518 Clifton Road, Claudia Nance Rollins Bldg, 7021, Atlanta, GA 30322, USA. E-mail: awebb3@emory.edu

Lesley Wood has a PhD in medical statistics and epidemiology and is currently a statistician at the University of Bristol's Centre for Exercise, Nutrition and Health Sciences. While at the Children's Food Trust she carried out the data quality assurance and the data analysis for school food projects and was also involved in questionnaire and survey design. Before joining the Children's Food Trust, Lesley lectured on statistics and research methods. Mailing address: Centre for Exercise, Nutrition and Health Sciences, School for Policy Studies, University of Bristol, 8 Woodland Road, Bristol, BS8 1TZ, UK. E-mail: lesley.wood@bristol.ac.uk

Miriam E. Yiannakis is a nutritionist with over 10 years of experience in programme management and technical support. She has experience in several countries in Southern Africa and the Asia and Pacific regions, including 7 years with the Micronutrient and Health Programme in Malawi. Her expertise lies in managing integrated multi-sectoral programmes for results in maternal and child health and nutrition. In Malawi, she worked with a team to develop a sustainable small business providing fortified food to the rural population. She now advises and develops global nutrition capacity-building initiatives. Mailing address: Yiannakis House, Portianou, Limnos 81400, Greece. E-mail: miriam_yiannakis@worldvision.ca

FAO Contributions: FAO's Departments and Divisions may be contacted through the corresponding Department/Division at the following mailing address:
Food and Agriculture Organization of the United Nations (FAO)
Viale delle Terme di Caracalla
00153 Rome
Italy

For sending electronic messages, please find the appropriate contact for each Department/Division at the bottom of the first page of each of FAO's chapters (Chapters 21–35).

Foreword

The *International Symposium on Food and Nutrition Security: Food-based Approaches for Improving Diets and Raising Levels of Nutrition* was organized by the Food and Agriculture Organization of the United Nations (FAO) to better document the contribution that food and agriculture can make to improving nutrition. FAO, a specialized agency of the United Nations (UN), is mandated to raise levels of nutrition and standards of living and to ensure humanity's freedom from hunger by promoting sustainable agricultural development and alleviating poverty. FAO offers direct development assistance and policy and planning advice to governments for improving the efficiency of the production, distribution and consumption of food and agricultural products; it collects, analyses and disseminates information, and acts as an international forum for debate on food, nutrition and agricultural issues.

Food and agriculture are of critical importance for improving diets and raising levels of nutrition. Focusing on the distinctive relationship between agriculture, food and nutrition, FAO works actively to protect, promote and improve nutrition-sensitive agriculture and food-based systems as the sustainable solution to ensure food and nutrition security, combat micronutrient deficiencies, improve diets and raise levels of nutrition. By doing so, it aims to meet the nutrition-related Millennium Development Goals (MDGs).

The symposium was organized by FAO's Nutrition Division. By providing leadership, knowledge, policy advice and technical assistance for improving nutrition and protecting consumers, FAO helps to ensure that increases in food production, together with improved access to such food, translate into improved food consumption, better health and the nutritional well-being of populations. The papers presented at the symposium provide further evidence that food-based approaches are viable, effective, sustainable and long-term solutions for improving diets and raising levels of nutrition and for achieving food and nutrition security.

FAO argues that unless more attention is given to food-based interventions, the goal of ending hunger and undernutrition may not be easily achieved. Food-based strategies (including food production, dietary diversification and food fortification), focus on the necessity of improving diets in both quantity and quality in order to overcome and prevent malnutrition. The approach stresses the multiple benefits derived from enjoying a variety of foods. Further, it recognizes the nutritional value of food for good nutrition, and the importance and social significance of the food and agricultural sector for reducing poverty and strengthening livelihoods in many countries, especially those where a large proportion of the poor continue to depend upon farming and related activities for their livelihoods.

These proceedings are a useful resource for decision and policy makers, programme planners and implementers, and health workers, all of which work to combat hunger and malnutrition. Likewise, they will have appeal for professionals in the field of food security, nutrition, public health, horticulture, agronomy, animal science, food marketing, information, education, communication, food technology and development. They are also designed as a useful complementary source for graduate and postgraduate courses on: public health; human nutrition (including education and communication courses); community nutrition; international nutrition; food and nutrition security policies, interventions and programmes; nutrition considerations in agricultural research; and the integration of nutrition into food and agriculture.

The publication benefits from the contributions of world-renowned international experts as well as FAO's Departments and Divisions on the linkages between nutrition and agriculture and on nutrition-sensitive agriculture and food-based approaches. Sadly, Professor Michael Latham, who was one of the founders of the field of international nutrition that deals with the nutrition problems of developing countries, and one of the promoters of food-based approaches, died about 4 months after the symposium took place; his contribution to this publication, being one of his last works, is a fitting tribute to his memory.

The symposium called for an international movement committed to the implementation of effective, sustainable and long-term nutrition-sensitive, food-based solutions to hunger, malnutrition and poverty. It is hoped that you will find this book relevant, useful and inspiring, given that most of the nutrition issues and challenges that are discussed are of global concern and must be addressed if food and nutrition security is to be achieved in a sustainable manner.

In order to give new impetus to worldwide efforts on behalf of the hungry and malnourished, I am pleased to announce that FAO and the World Health Organization (WHO), together with the UN and other partners, will convene the Second International Conference on Nutrition (ICN2); this will be held in Rome on 19–21 November 2014. This symposium is a part of the preparatory activities leading up to the ICN2 and these proceedings make a substantial contribution to the background materials for that conference.

Jomo Kwame Sundaram
Assistant Director-General, Economic and Social Development Department
Chair, ICN2 Steering Committee
Food and Agriculture Organization of the United Nations
Rome, Italy

Preface

We are very pleased to present the *Proceedings of the International Symposium on Food and Nutrition Security: Food-based Approaches for Improving Diets and Raising Levels of Nutrition*. The symposium, organized by the Nutrition and Consumer Protection Division of the Food and Agriculture Organization of the United Nations (FAO), was held at FAO Headquarters, Rome, Italy from 7 to 9 December 2010. A significant number of authors from different backgrounds and experiences contributed to the 35 papers that were presented and provide a range of views and analyses that form a rich body of knowledge and experience.

The proceedings aim at collecting and better documenting evidence that demonstrates the impact, effectiveness and sustainability of food-based approaches for improving diets and raising levels of nutrition. It assembles a variety of policy, technical and advocacy chapters with the purpose of encouraging and promoting further attention to the importance of and investment in nutrition-sensitive food-based strategies to overcome nutritional problems, thus achieving food and nutrition security.

FAO's role in eliminating hunger, achieving food security and reducing malnutrition is guided by the commitments set forth by the World Declaration and Plan of Action of Nutrition adopted at the 1992 International Conference on Nutrition (ICN) and by the Rome Declaration on World Food Security and the World Food Summit Plan of Action adopted at the 1996 World Food Summit (WFS). At the WFS, governments pledged to work towards eradicating hunger and, as an essential first step, set a target of reducing the number of hungry people by half by 2015. This became the first goal of the Millennium Development Goals (MDGs) that were adopted at the UN Millennium Summit in 2000. More recently, the L'Aquila Joint Statement on Global Food Security in July 2009, and the Declaration of the World Summit on Food Security held at FAO in Rome in 2009, called for a renewed commitment to take action towards the sustainable eradication of hunger and malnutrition at the earliest possible date and to set the world on a path to achieving the progressive realization of the right to adequate food in the context of national food security. Although improvement has been made and some remarkable success stories exist in individual countries and communities, progress has been unacceptably slow and much remains to be done.

Hunger and all forms of malnutrition continue to cause widespread suffering throughout the world, placing an intolerable burden not only on individuals and national health systems, but on the entire cultural, social and economic fabric of nations. After years of steady progress, recent setbacks in the fight against hunger and malnutrition arising from the combined effects of food price instability and the global economic downturn, coupled with the continuing problems of underdevelopment, civil strife, inadequate food supplies, social discrimination and environmental stress, jeopardize the earlier hopes for achieving the poverty, hunger and nutrition-related MDGs.

FAO estimated that a total of 842 million people were undernourished in 2011–2013. About 45% of the 6.9 million child deaths in 2011 were linked to malnutrition. Some 162 million children under five years of age are stunted owing to chronic undernutrition and 99 million children are underweight. Micronutrient malnutrition or 'hidden hunger' affects about 2 billion people worldwide, with serious public health consequences.

Nutrition-sensitive food-based approaches focus on food, whether natural or processed, and including foods that are fortified, for improving the quality of the diet and for overcoming and preventing malnutrition. The approach recognizes the essential role that food has for good nutrition as well as the importance of the food and agriculture sector for supporting rural livelihoods. It also supports the right-to-food approach in preventing hunger and ensuring health and well-being. FAO argues that nutrition-sensitive food-based approaches are effective, sustainable and long-term solutions to hunger and malnutrition; it advocates nutrition-sensitive, food-based approaches, including food fortification, that increase the availability of, access to and consumption of a variety and diversity of safe, good quality foods as a sustainable strategy for improving the nutritional status of populations. In addition to its intrinsic nutritional value, food has a social and economic significance which, for many people, especially those living in developing countries, is commonly mediated through agriculture and agriculture-related activities that provide employment and sustain rural livelihoods. The multiple social, economic and health benefits associated with successful food-based approaches that lead to year-round availability of, access to and consumption of nutritionally adequate amounts and varieties of foods are clear. The nutritional well-being and health of individuals is promoted, incomes and livelihoods are supported, and community and national wealth is created and protected.

Progress in promoting and implementing food-based strategies to achieve sustainable improvements in nutritional status has been slow. Such strategies were overlooked in the past as governments, researchers, the donor community and health-oriented organizations sought approaches for overcoming malnutrition that had rapid start-up times and produced quick and measurable results. More recently, many developing countries, international agencies, non-governmental organizations (NGOs) and donors have begun to realize that food-based strategies are viable, cost-effective, long-term and sustainable solutions for improving diets and raising levels of nutrition. The symposium was held to focus greater attention on the important role of food and agriculture in improving nutrition.

Abstracts were invited from leading international experts and organizations involved in policy making, research and field programmes from all regions of the world. An 'invitation to submit abstracts' was circulated by e-mail and through different Internet sites and web fora in September 2010. Abstracts were welcomed from relevant disciplines, such as: nutrition; agricultural sciences (horticulture, agronomy, animal science and food marketing); information, education and communication; food technology (preservation, processing and fortification); and development. Abstracts were also invited from FAO's Departments and Divisions to showcase what they do and how they contribute to improving diets and raising levels of nutrition towards achieving food and nutrition security. A Scientific Advisory Committee, coordinated by a Secretariat set within the Nutrition and Consumer Protection Division, was established to select abstracts and provide technical inputs, comments and suggestions to improve their quality. Once selected, the abstracts were developed into the papers that were presented at the symposium. Constant correspondence and communication between the Scientific Advisory Committee, the Secretariat and the presenters/authors, as well as FAO's Departments and Divisions was maintained throughout the preparation process of the abstracts and papers. On the basis of the discussions carried out during the symposium and issues raised in the papers/presentations, the authors and FAO's Departments and Divisions improved, refined and finalized the papers.

The papers: discuss the policy, strategic, methodological, technical and programmatic issues associated with nutrition-sensitive food-based approaches; propose 'best practices' for the design, targeting, implementation and evaluation of specific nutrition-sensitive, food-based interventions, and for improved methodologies for evaluating their efficacy and cost-effectiveness; and provide practical lessons for advancing nutrition-sensitive food-based approaches for improving nutrition at policy and programme level. The papers are arranged around the following topics: (i) initiatives to expand the availability and accessibility of plant and animal food in adequate quality and quantity; (ii) changes of food habits and choices towards more diverse and nutritious diets; (iii) food processing, preservation and storage at household and community level; (iv) improved nutrition education and health service delivery; and (v) capacity building at community, national and regional levels for improving food and nutrition security and addressing specific nutrient deficiencies.

The clearly demonstrated nutritional benefits of food-based approaches as the only sustainable way that the MDGs can be reached calls for nutrition objectives to be incorporated into agriculture, food security, economic and other development policies and programmes. Opportunities and challenges are identified for promoting such approaches and for enhancing and monitoring their impacts on food and nutrition in terms of food quality and safety, food consumption and diets, and nutritional outcomes.

The proceedings of this international symposium will be used to provide practical guidance to FAO, its members and other stakeholders for future work utilizing nutrition-sensitive food-based approaches for improving food and nutrition security and for overcoming specific nutrient deficiencies in the medium- and long term.

We trust that the information, knowledge, experience and insights presented here will encourage further dialogue, debate and information exchange to support, promote and implement effective, sustainable and long-term nutrition-sensitive food-based solutions to hunger and malnutrition. Furthermore, we hope that this book will enable you, the reader, to become a part of the solution by applying nutrition-sensitive food-based strategies and actively engaging in advocacy, policy, programming or ongoing research to make a difference in improving the quality of diets, raising levels of nutrition and achieving food and nutrition security.

Brian Thompson and Leslie Amoroso

Acknowledgements

The editors wish to thank all of those who contributed to the organization of the symposium and to the preparation of these proceedings. We would like to acknowledge with gratitude all of the authors for their expertise and hard work in preparing their papers as well as for their dedication and invaluable cooperation, commitment and patience in meeting our various requests. We also would like to recognize the valuable contributions made by those Technical Departments and Divisions of FAO who presented papers on the way that nutrition issues and considerations are being mainstreamed into their activities.

We would like to give a very special thanks to Sharon Lee Cowan, Nicholas Rubery and Alice Lloyd of FAO's Office for Communication, Partnership and Advocacy, for their support on the design of the logo, banners, letterhead and for the design of the symposium's web page.

A special acknowledgement is due to William D. Clay for his valuable comments and technical guidance. Our warm thanks are extended to Jayne Beaney for her support in checking the final submissions and proofreading the manuscript and to Francesca Matteini, Valeria Scorza, Milica Beokovic and Tatiana Lebedeva from the Nutrition and Consumer Protection Division, FAO, for secretarial support.

Special thanks are due to Rachel Tucker, Office of Knowledge, Exchange, Research and Extension, FAO, for her continuing support in liaising between FAO and CABI throughout the co-publishing process of this work.

Welcome Address

ICN2 Secretariat

Distinguished guests, dear colleagues, ladies and gentlemen, welcome.

It is our great pleasure to welcome you to Rome and to the Headquarters of the Food and Agriculture Organization (FAO). It is also our pleasure to welcome you to this important event, the *International Symposium on Food and Nutrition Security: Food-Based Approaches for Improving Diets and Raising Levels of Nutrition*. The presence of so many eminent scholars and world-renowned experts testifies to the high level of importance you give to this topic.

FAO's Mandate

This international symposium is the first to be held on the contribution that food and agriculture make to diet, food consumption and nutrition. We believe agriculture is of crucial importance for improving diets and raising levels of nutrition and therefore FAO has a major part to play in improving nutrition. FAO is pleased to host this symposium as it is the UN specialized agency with the mandate for raising levels of nutrition and standards of living and ensuring humanity's freedom from hunger by promoting sustainable agricultural development and alleviating poverty. The Organization offers direct development assistance and policy and planning advice to governments for improving the efficiency of the production, distribution and consumption of food and agricultural products; collects, analyses and disseminates information; and acts as an international forum for debate on food, nutrition and agriculture issues.

Food Production Matters

The primary importance of the food and agriculture sector in improving household food security and alleviating and preventing malnutrition is clear. Agriculture is the major source of food, employment and income upon which the majority of mankind relies to provide for and support their livelihood. Large numbers of people, especially the poor, are involved directly or indirectly in agricultural activities and derive multiple benefits from its multifunctional character. When agricultural development falters or fails in countries where no other fast-growing sectors exist to employ people, the chance of the poor rising above the poverty level to play a full part in the economic development of their country is diminished. Given the high level of dependency of many of the world's poor and nutritionally vulnerable on the fruits of the earth, this sector offers the greatest potential for achieving sustained improvements in the nutritional status of the rural poor.

At the national level, boosting agricultural production stimulates overall economic growth and development, particularly in those countries that have a high economic dependence on agriculture. Thus, agricultural and rural development acts as an engine for sustainable economic development making an effective contribution to national economic growth.

At the community level, developments in agriculture lead to increased farm productivity, which reduce food deficits, increase food surpluses and raise incomes. With adequate market access, diversification into higher value products or more capital-intensive forms of agriculture (cash crops, livestock and aquaculture) provide opportunities to generate cash income and can free up labour for other productive activities, for meeting social obligations or for leisure. Improved agriculture production thus provides opportunities to sustainably reduce poverty, food insecurity and malnutrition and thereby improve the quality of life.

Consumption Is Key

Since the purpose of economic growth and agricultural development is to improve living conditions, developments in agriculture must provide sustainable benefits for society as a whole and especially to those communities that depend on the land for their survival and who are resource poor, marginalized, food-insecure and malnourished. Consequently, focus needs to be given not only to increasing the production of and access to food but also its consumption, ensuring that the poor have access to adequate quantities of safe, good quality food for a nutritionally adequate diet. This includes not only energy, protein and fats but also micronutrients – the vitamins and minerals and other trace elements so necessary for normal growth and development.

Agricultural policies influence the quantity and quality of foods farmers produce, as well as the range of crops grown and the production methods used. Therefore, agricultural policies can affect human health and nutrition. In turn, health and nutrition policies can affect agriculture by influencing whether farming families are physically able to work their farms. An undernourished workforce is less able to work, absenteeism and sickness are more frequent and thus poor nutrition acts as a brake to agricultural and economic development. Although they may share goals, professionals in agriculture, nutrition and health rarely have opportunities to discuss areas of mutual interest, exploit synergies and pursue outcomes that are beneficial to society. This we can do over the next 3 days.

Create an Enabling Environment and Increase Investments in Agriculture

Creating an enabling environment to fight hunger includes good governance, the absence of conflict and political, economic and social stability, combined with an enabling macroeconomic and sector policy environment if hunger and malnutrition are to be eradicated. Resources must be made available for agricultural and rural development at a level that reflects the key role agriculture has in building sustainable livelihoods for the world's poorest people. It is also necessary for slowing down the rate of rural-to-urban migration and for preventing a further widening of the rural–urban income gap.

Vital Role of Women in Agriculture and Rural Development

Economic growth and development are reduced if gender inequalities are not addressed. Gender inequality in education and employment reduces rates of economic growth; similarly, gender inequality in access to productive resources and inputs in agriculture reduces efficiency and rural development. Consequently, it is imperative to enhance the status of women in the rural production system, family and society to attain food security and sustainable agricultural development.

Promote Nutrition-sensitive Agriculture and Food-based Strategies

Food- and agriculture-based strategies focus on food as the primary tool for improving the quality of the diet and for overcoming and preventing malnutrition and nutritional deficiencies. The approach stresses the multiple benefits derived from enjoying a variety of foods, and recognizing the nutritional value of food for good nutrition and the importance and social significance of the food and agricultural sector for supporting rural livelihoods. The approach encourages and equips people to consider their total diet in relation to their preferences, individual lifestyle factors, physiological requirements and physical activity levels. Started early, this approach can contribute to physiological, mental and social development, enhance learning potential, reduce nutritional disorders and contribute to the prevention of diet-related diseases later in life. The fact that malnutrition continues to be experienced in countries that apparently have adequate food supplies highlights the need to overcome poverty, marginalization and neglect. We need to increase the production and availability of food, while at the same time ensuring that the poor, the marginalized and the neglected have access to good quality, safe and nutritionally adequate food.

Second International Conference on Nutrition (ICN2)

In order to give new impetus to worldwide efforts on behalf of hungry and malnourished people, the Directors-General of FAO and the World Health Organization (WHO) have decided to convene a Second International Conference on Nutrition (ICN2) at FAO Headquarters in Rome from 19 to 21 November 2014. The purpose is to raise both the political will and the financial resources to fight hunger and malnutrition.

Final Remarks

We are confident that this international symposium will serve as the basis for future dialogue, debate and information exchange and facilitate wider support for an international movement committed to the implementation of effective, sustainable and long-term nutrition-sensitive, food-based solutions to hunger and malnutrition.

We wish you fruitful deliberations and trust that the outcomes of this symposium will be widely shared to guide the way forward for putting an end to hunger and malnutrition.

Thank you.

Opening Address

Brian Thompson

On behalf of the Director, Nutrition and Consumer Protection Division, Food and Agriculture Organization of the United Nations, Rome, Italy

Distinguished guests, dear colleagues, ladies and gentlemen, welcome.

I wish first of all to express my appreciation to you all for coming to join us here in Rome this week to participate in the *International Symposium on Food and Nutrition Security: Food-Based Approaches for Improving Diets and Raising Levels of Nutrition*.

Role of FAO in Food and Nutrition Security

The symposium has been organized by the Nutrition and Consumer Protection Division, one of the five Technical Divisions of the Agriculture Department of FAO. The Nutrition Division provides leadership, knowledge, policy advice and technical assistance for improving nutrition and protecting consumers, thus helping to ensure that agricultural development is accompanied by enhanced access to food and that improved food availability translates into better health and the nutritional well-being of populations.

FAO's role in achieving food security and alleviating and preventing malnutrition is guided by the commitments set forth by the International Conference on Nutrition (ICN, 1992), the Rome Declaration on World Food Security and the World Food Summit Plan of Action, which were adopted at the World Food Summit (WFS) in 1996. At the World Food Summit, governments pledged to work towards eradicating hunger. As an essential first step, they set a target of reducing the number of hungry people by half by 2015, which was amended to become the Millennium Development Goal (MDG) 1 at the UN Millennium Summit in 2000.

More recently, the L'Aquila Joint Statement on Global Food Security in July 2009 and the Declaration adopted by the Heads of State and Government at the World Summit on Food Security held in Rome in November 2009, called for a renewed commitment to take action towards the sustainable eradication of hunger and malnutrition at the earliest possible date and to set the world on a path to achieving the progressive realization of the right to adequate food in the context of national food security. Although headway has been made and some striking success stories exist in individual countries and communities, current data indicate that progress is too slow and much remains to be done.

Magnitude of Hunger and Undernutrition

The combined effects of prolonged underinvestment in food, agriculture and nutrition, the recent food price crisis and the economic downturn have led to increased hunger and poverty, jeopardizing the progress achieved so far in meeting the MDGs. FAO estimates that the number of hungry people fell slightly over the previous year to 925 million people. However, this is higher than before the food and economic crises of 2008–2009 and higher than at the World Food Summit in 1996. Asia and the Pacific is the region with the most undernourished people (578 million people), while the proportion of undernourished people remains highest in sub-Saharan Africa, at 30%.

International Governance of Nutrition

It is partly a consequence of the recent food crisis and the impact of the economic downturn that led to/prompted the increased attention now being given to nutrition. National governments and the international community have repeatedly called for actions to be taken to improve the governance of efforts to end hunger and for nutrition to be better integrated into food security policies and programmes. In response to this call, a number of initiatives have been taken.

The Committee on World Food Security (CFS), the body that serves as the UN forum for review and follow-up of policies concerning world food security, has been undergoing reform to make it an inclusive international platform for policy convergence and the coordination of expertise and action in the fight against hunger in the world. As part of the revitalization of the CFS, a High-Level Panel of Experts on Food Security and Nutrition (HLPE-FSN) is being established that will provide scientific and knowledge-based analysis and advice on specific policy-relevant issues. Active reforms are also underway in the United Nations Standing Committee on Nutrition (UN SCN), the UN forum for harmonizing food and nutrition policy and for promoting cooperation among UN agencies and partner organizations for ending malnutrition. The SCN has recently been included in the Advisory Group and the Joint Secretariat of the CFS.

FAO is fully involved in the international governance of nutrition, particularly through the SCN, and is engaged in a number of initiatives as an active partner, including the REACH (FAO/WHO/WFP/UNICEF Renewed Efforts Against Child Hunger) initiative, which seeks to join forces at country level and scale up proven and effective interventions addressing child undernutrition, the Comprehensive Framework for Action (CFA) of the UN Secretary-General's High-Level Task Force on the Global Food Security Crisis as well as the Scaling-Up Nutrition (SUN) initiative. FAO has strengthened the Joint FAO/WHO Expert Committee on Nutrition that provides scientific guidance to Codex; and for improving response in emergencies, FAO is an active member of the Inter-Agency Standing Committee (IASC) Global Nutrition Cluster. All these initiatives and renewed attention give us hope that the reduction of malnutrition and the elimination of extreme hunger and malnutrition are close at hand.

Food-based Approaches

However, in all these initiatives, FAO is advocating that unless more attention is given to food-based interventions that promote dietary diversity and the consumption of nutritionally enhanced foods, the goal of ending hunger may not be achieved. We see food-based approaches, which include food production, dietary diversification and food fortification, as sustainable strategies for improving nutrition. Increasing access to and availability and consumption of a variety of foods not only has a positive effect on nutrition but, in addition to its intrinsic nutritional value, food has social and economic significance which, for those living in developing countries, is commonly mediated through agriculture and agriculture-related activities that sustain rural livelihoods. The multiple social, economic and health benefits associated with successful food-based approaches that lead to year-round availability of, access to and consumption of nutritionally adequate amounts and varieties of foods are clear. The nutritional well-being and health of individuals is promoted, incomes and livelihoods supported, and community and national wealth created and protected. If, and here I borrow from Professor Latham, if there is any 'fiasco', it is the fact that food-based strategies to prevent malnutrition have not yet properly been developed, tested, implemented, taken to scale and proven adequately to solve the dietary deficits of the world's poorest populations.

Narrowing the Nutrition Gap

Improving food security may be achieved through narrowing the gap between current and potential production yields. Similarly, improving the food-based aspects of nutrition security can be thought of in terms of narrowing the 'nutrition gap' – the gap between current food intake patterns and intake patterns that are optimal in terms of macro- and micronutrient content. Narrowing the nutrition gap means improving the quality and diversity of the diet through increasing availability and access to the foods necessary for a healthy diet, and increasing the actual intake of those foods. There are multiple pathways through which agricultural interventions can contribute to narrowing the nutrition gap and these will be discussed over the next 3 days.

Purpose and Overview of the Symposium

This symposium is being held at a time when much increased attention is being given to nutrition and to the role of food for improving nutrition. Indeed holding this symposium is a reflection of this increased attention and an effort to maintain it and build upon it.

The purpose of the symposium is to increase awareness of policy makers and programmers of the benefits nutrition-sensitive, food-based approaches have for improving diets and raising levels of nutrition. Papers will be presented by leading international experts that clearly demonstrate the nutritional benefits of food-based approaches and which strongly call for nutrition objectives to be incorporated into agriculture, food security, economic and other development policies and programmes as the only sustainable way the MDGs can be reached. Opportunities and challenges will be identified for promoting nutrition-sensitive, food-based approaches and for enhancing and monitoring their impact on food and nutrition in terms of food quality and safety, food consumption and diets, and nutritional outcomes.

This symposium is a part of the preparatory activities leading up to the joint FAO/WHO Second International Conference on Nutrition (ICN2) which is planned to be held at FAO Headquarters, in Rome on 19–21 November 2014, The ICN2 will be an opportunity for nutrition scientists, policy makers and other concerned stakeholders to assess progress made since 1992 and make recommendations for further concerted actions to address all forms of malnutrition.

We will start the symposium with keynote addresses from two distinguished Professors who for many years have been the principle movers and thinkers in the areas of nutrition and agricultural development. They also deserve much of the credit for raising the profile of food and nutrition security within international circles and need no further introduction from me. They are Michael Latham, Graduate School Professor, Division of Nutritional Sciences, Cornell University, USA and Per Pinstrup-Andersen, former Director-General of IFPRI and currently Professor of Food, Nutrition and Public Policy, Division of Nutritional Sciences, also from Cornell.

Ladies and gentlemen, I give you Professor Michael Latham.

Introduction

Brian Thompson and Leslie Amoroso*

Nutrition and Consumer Protection Division (AGN), Agriculture and Consumer Protection Department (AG), Food and Agriculture Organization of the United Nations, Rome, Italy

Malnutrition in all its forms (undernutrition, micronutrient deficiencies and overnutrition) is commonly recognized as being among the most widespread and pernicious causes of human suffering throughout the world. Malnutrition is also recognized as a serious and intractable impediment to economic growth and social progress with far-reaching consequences for both individual welfare and community and national development. However, despite well-meaning declarations by governments and their development partners, progress in overcoming hunger, food insecurity and malnutrition remain unacceptably slow. One reason for this slow progress is that specific responsibility for securing improvements in the nutritional well-being of people 'falls between the cracks' of various disciplines. Agriculturalists often assume that expanding food supplies will automatically lead to such improvements. Economists often assume that raising the gross domestic product (GDP) or household incomes is what is required. Medical nutritionists and those working within the health sector commonly focus on nutrients and pharmacological interventions to improve nutritional status. Children's advocates also often target specific nutrients and what is an ever-shrinking 'window of opportunity' within a child's life as the keys to health and good nutrition. Some see population control as the solution, some hold that nutrition education is the key, some see feeding programmes as the way ahead and others focus solely on food security in its various guises. The list of assumptions about how to improve nutrition, and the corresponding list of approaches for doing so, is dishearteningly extensive.

In reality, each of these approaches may be important, but not equally so in every circumstance. There are significant differences in the factors that lead to various forms of malnutrition among different population groups at different times, and efforts to develop, target and implement effective policies, strategies, plans and programmes to improve nutrition must be based on a clear understanding of the relevant factors that affect the ability of particular households or population groups to acquire and utilize the food they need to be healthy and productive. Without such understanding, any ensuing interventions and strategies are likely to be ineffective and unnecessarily costly.

Unfortunately, costly, ineffectual and unsustainable interventions are all too common in many countries struggling to cope

---

*Contact: leslie.amoroso@fao.org

with problems of widespread malnutrition. Such situations are particularly common in countries where the primary responsibility for nutrition falls within a single sector or is overly influenced by narrowly focused development agencies or advocates. In these instances, there is often a tendency to disregard the underlying and basic causes of malnutrition while attempting to focus more narrowly on specific nutrients or on physiologically vulnerable age groups. The result is that issues related to agriculture, economic development, employment, poverty, food supplies, food security, social injustice, environmental conditions and the inability of households to meet their members' needs are often dismissed as being of secondary importance in the fight against malnutrition. The consequence is often that short-term, quick-fix interventions push out more sustainable longer term food-based strategies as the priority path to better nutrition.

Conversely, in other situations, responses may focus on expanding and diversifying food supplies or on alleviating poverty, but without addressing the social, environmental, health, education, gender or other concerns facing many disadvantaged households. In either case, the result is often the implementation of unsustainable, top-down projects that fail to address the basic and underlying factors that affect a household's ability to acquire and utilize effectively an adequate amount and variety of good quality and safe food that is sufficient to meet the nutritional needs of each family member. This often leaves the fundamental problems of inadequate availability, access to and consumption of nutritionally adequate and safe foods by low-income, resource-poor, food-insecure, socially excluded, economically marginalized and nutritionally vulnerable households unaltered. In such circumstances, the ability of these groups to become more self-reliant is not enhanced, their capacity to secure and utilize food is not improved and neither is their right to food or their nutritional health realized.

Given this situation, the Nutrition and Consumer Protection Division of FAO convened the *International Symposium on Food and Nutrition Security: Food-Based Approaches for Improving Diets and Raising Levels of Nutrition* from 7 to 9

December 2010 at FAO Headquarters in Rome, Italy, to collect and better document evidence that demonstrates the impact, effectiveness, viability and sustainability of food-based approaches for improving diets and raising levels of nutrition.

The papers presented to the symposium are presented in four main parts, each of which – with a diverse and distinctive focus, emphasis and perspective – shows the importance of nutrition-sensitive food and agriculture-based approaches for achieving food and nutrition security. Many authors with different backgrounds contributed to the publication, which is designed to bring together the available information, knowledge and experience – including policy, strategic, methodological, technical, programmatic and advocacy issues, success stories and lessons learned and best practices – to demonstrate that improving diets and raising levels of nutrition through food-based approaches is a viable, sustainable and long-term solution for overcoming nutritional deficiencies. Many different views, reviews and analyses are presented, creating a rich combination of knowledge and experience.

To further encourage and promote attention to the importance of and investment in food-based approaches for improving diets and raising levels of nutrition, a special section of the proceedings was dedicated to the presentation of the FAO/CABI book *Combating Micronutrient Deficiencies: Food-based Approaches*, which was launched during the symposium prior to its official publication in 2011. This brings together available knowledge and case studies on country-level activities as well as lessons learned and best practices that document the benefits of food-based approaches, particularly of dietary improvement and diversification interventions. It provides information that policy makers and others need to better understand, promote, support and implement food-based strategies for preventing and controlling micronutrient deficiencies at country level. This presentation is included in the *Appendix* at the end of the book.

After the *Foreword, Preface* and *Acknowledgements*, this volume includes the *Welcome* and *Opening Addresses* delivered by FAO.

The *Welcome Address*, by ICN2 Secretariat, emphasized that agriculture is of crucial importance for improving diets and raising levels of nutrition, and that FAO has a major part to play in improving nutrition. The address stressed the benefits of food- and agriculture-based strategies for overcoming and preventing malnutrition and nutritional deficiencies. Focus needs to be given not only to increasing the production of and access to a variety of food but also to its consumption, ensuring that the poor have access to adequate quantities of safe, good quality food for a nutritionally adequate diet.

The *Opening Address*, by Brian Thompson, on behalf of the Director, Nutrition Division, highlighted that unless more attention is given to agriculture and food-based interventions that promote dietary diversity and the consumption of nutritionally enhanced foods, the goal of ending hunger may not be achieved. Reference was made to 'narrowing the nutrition gap' the gap between what foods are grown and available and what foods are needed for a healthy diet. Narrowing the nutrition gaps means improving the quality and diversity of the diet through increasing availability and access to the foods necessary for a healthy diet, and increasing the actual intake of those foods. There are multiple pathways through which agricultural interventions can contribute to narrowing the nutrition gap and these are widely discussed in the papers included in this volume.

Following this introduction, and in the main section of the volume, *Part I: Overview*, includes keynote addresses from two distinguished professors, Michael C. Latham and Per Pinstrup-Andersen who, for many years, have been the principle movers and thinkers in the areas of nutrition and agricultural development.

Chapter 1, *Perspective on Nutritional Problems in Developing Countries: Nutrition Security through Community Agriculture*, is an edited transcription of the presentation delivered by Michael C. Latham. His keynote address reasserts that social and economic inequity are the basis for widespread hunger and malnutrition and underscores the fundamental importance of addressing nutritional problems through multifaceted solutions and interdisciplinary approaches, including community agriculture and food-based approaches. Professor Latham argues against the current wide advocacy for, and use of, high-tech commercial products to reduce malnutrition. In particular, his chapter highlights the fallacy and danger of massive vitamin A supplementation programmes to reduce the risk of vitamin A deficiency. He also expresses alarm on the increasing use of commercialized and imported ready-to-use therapeutic foods (RUTFs) as top-down 'magic-bullet' foods to address and even prevent malnutrition, claiming that they are only effective in the treatment of children with severe acute malnutrition. Preferable solutions, he argues, lie in improved local agriculture and affordable home-based nutritious diets. He points to the huge advantages that food-based approaches have over medicinal strategies and reaffirms that food-based approaches are viable, affordable, sustainable and long term, have social, cultural, economic and environmental benefits, and are local and not top-down. Professor Latham passed away a few months after the symposium.

Chapter 2, *Food Systems and Human Nutrition: Relationships and Policy Interventions*, by Per Pinstrup-Andersen, highlights that solutions to nutrition problems are not found in narrowly defined, single agricultural projects, but rather in large changes to food systems that are not necessarily suitable for evaluation through experimental designs with randomized treatment and control groups. Programmes and policies aimed at changing food systems in particular need to do more than pursue curative approaches that do little to affect the underlying determinants of nutrition problems. Several characteristics of contemporary food systems that are likely to influence the nutrition of current and future generations are identified and discussed. While food systems affect human nutrition, human nutrition also affects food systems. Pinstrup-Andersen notes that there are multiple pathways through which the food system affects human nutrition. Understanding these pathways and how they operate is essential to designing agricultural and other food system policies to achieve nutrition goals. The author remarks that a better understanding of the relationships between food systems and human nutrition will offer opportunities for improving nutrition that are currently overlooked. Whether such opportunities are captured will depend on possible trade-offs with the achievement of other development goals, as well as on policy goals and political factors.

Part II of the volume, *Policy and Programme Experiences*, contains Chapters 3 to 20. They have been prepared by leading international experts involved in policy making, research and field programmes from around the world. They demonstrate the nutritional benefits of nutrition-sensitive food-based approaches; explore opportunities and challenges for developing, implementing and monitoring more effective policies and programmes aiming to improve food and nutrition security, dietary intakes and nutritional outcomes; and identify opportunities for incorporating nutrition objectives into national and sectoral development policies and programmes.

Chapter 3, *Enhancing the Performance of Food-based Strategies to Improve Micronutrient Status and Associated Health Outcomes in Young Children from Poor-resource Households in Low-income Countries: Challenges and Solutions*, by Rosalind S. Gibson, provides a critical review of interventions employing dietary diversification and modification (DDM) strategies at community or household level that have the potential to increase the intake of total and/or bioavailable micronutrients. DDM has the potential to prevent coexisting micronutrient deficiencies simultaneously for the entire household and across generations without risk of antagonistic interactions. DDM strategies include: increasing the production and consumption of micronutrient-dense foods through agriculture, small animal production or aquaculture using effective nutrition education and behaviour change and biofortification; incorporating enhancers of micronutrient absorption; and reducing absorption inhibitors. The author emphasizes that, in order to maximize the impact of DDM, especially among children in poor resource settings, DDM should be integrated

with public health interventions designed to reduce the risk of infections. The need for effective communication strategies aimed at changing eating and feeding behaviour is also acknowledged. The chapter stresses that the impact of such integrated programmes needs to be strengthened by enhancing their design, and their monitoring and evaluation components. The author concludes that future targeted DDM and public health interventions should be combined with those that address the underlying causes of malnutrition, such as poverty alleviation, food security enhancement and income generation to ensure more sustainable improvements in micronutrient status, growth and development.

Chapter 4, *Food-based Approaches for Combating Malnutrition – Lessons Lost?*, by Ted Greiner, reviews several large-scale food-based nutrition projects in Tanzania, Zimbabwe and Bangladesh, bringing to light lessons learned from both failures and successes. It reports on research that shows why food-based approaches often do not seem to work well to improve human nutrient status and what can be done to improve this. Ongoing activities and the continuing nutritional benefits arising from these programmes (notably improvements in vitamin A and iron status) are still very much in evidence, and demonstrate the efficacy, cost-effectiveness and sustainability of food-based, community-focused approaches. The author concludes that food-based programmes take time to establish and show impact. In addition, research on their impact is scarce because it is time-consuming and complex. Indeed, research on projects and field work, and even on the operations of ministries, has low status, and few research donors prioritize it. However, such research increasingly suggests that food-based approaches that are adequately funded and given time to mature do work.

Chapter 5, *Critical Issues to Consider in the Selection of Crops in a Food-based Approach to Improve Vitamin A Status – Based on a South African Experience*, by Mieke Faber *et al.*, describes experience in South Africa of dealing with extensive problems of vitamin A deficiency, using published and unpublished case studies as examples. The chapter illustrates many of the considerations for designing a successful intervention. Household food production of β-carotene-rich vegetables and fruit, through home gardening, is a long-term strategy that can contribute to combating vitamin A deficiency. The author shows that issues to consider in the crop-based approach, which has two distinct components – a nutrition component and an agriculture component – are the nutrient content of the crop (focusing on β-carotene-rich crops), diversifying the crop mix to overcome seasonality, promoting the consumption of wild dark-green leafy vegetables to complement the home-grown β-carotene-rich foods, and consumer acceptance of newly introduced crops (orange-fleshed sweet potato). Home gardens focusing on these crops are shown to be successful in: (i) improving year-round dietary intake of vitamin A and a range of other micronutrients; and (ii) sustaining increased dietary vitamin A intake after withdrawal of the research team. It should be noted that, although the crop-based approach described in this chapter focuses on β-carotene-rich vegetables and fruit: (i) households are encouraged to plant these crops in addition to existing crops; (ii) consumption of vitamin A-rich foods of animal origin is promoted in the education part of the nutrition component; and (iii) breastfeeding for infants and small children is promoted. The chapter focuses on crop selection mostly from a nutritional perspective. The success of any gardening project, though, depends not only on the nutritional characteristics of the crops promoted, but also on their agronomic characteristics. The author concludes that partnership between the nutritional and agricultural sectors is, therefore, critical for the success of home garden projects aiming to improve the nutritional status of vulnerable populations.

Chapter 6, *Contribution of Homestead Food Production to Improved Household Food Security and Nutrition Status – Lessons Learned from Bangladesh, Cambodia, Nepal and the Philippines*, by Aminuzzaman Talukder *et al.*, reviews the impact of homestead food production (HFP) programmes and identifies lessons learned for adaptation, replication and potential scale up. Since 2003, Helen Keller International (HKI) has been implementing HFP programmes to increase and ensure the year-round availability and intake of micronutrient-rich foods in poor households of Asia. The HFP programmes in Bangladesh, Cambodia, Nepal and the Philippines have improved household garden practices and dietary diversity both in terms of production and consumption of vegetables, fruits and animal source foods (such as eggs and chicken liver) among beneficiary households (particularly children and women), improved income as well as reducing anaemia among preschoolchildren. HFP programmes also had a positive effect on vitamin A status. The authors note that the strengths of the HFP model include its potential sustainability because it is community based and its focus on women from poor households as the primary beneficiaries. The nutrition education component of the programme has also promoted nutritionally informed food purchasing and consumption choices. The HFP model is 'flexible' in that it can be integrated into or serve as a platform for delivering other public health programmes. The chapter concludes that in the face of factors affecting food availability in developing countries – such as the global food and economic crisis, the increase in biofuel production, negative trade issues and climate change – programmes such as HFP can have a positive effect in poor households by decreasing their dependence on outside food sources and increasing their own production, thereby improving household food security and resilience to unforeseen events. For these reasons, it is important that the HFP programme be expanded to other areas in these poor Asian countries and implemented in more countries where micronutrient deficiencies are a public health problem.

Chapter 7, *The Underestimated Impact of Food-based Interventions*, by Ian Darnton-Hill, shows that food-based approaches to address micronutrient deficiencies have long experience and documented success, but have often been inadequately evaluated and have thus failed to gain scientific acceptance, adequate funding and scale up globally. However, these approaches have acquired more urgency for adoption and proper evaluation in recent years as a result of environmental considerations, increasing disparities, global financial crises and rises in food prices. Evidence of food-based approaches is reviewed from four perspectives. The author notes that measuring effectiveness of food-based programmes should expand indicators of outcomes beyond biological levels of micronutrients to include both clinical outcomes (e.g. reduction in night blindness) and social outcomes (e.g. women's empowerment and local capacity building). Any evaluation of interventions and their cost-effectiveness should attempt to capture these outcomes. An important need is for more research on impact. Evaluations need to be an intrinsic part of the process, and should be factored in earlier in the process and be provided for by governments and funding agencies. Because food-based approaches are harder to quantify, involve social change and are less easily evaluated than, say, number of capsules delivered, they have not received donor support to the same extent as other interventions. The author calls, unequivocally, for greater use of food-based approaches and provides a list of specific conclusions and recommendations, including increasing and improving the dialogue between the agriculture, health and nutrition sectors, to help guide their development.

Chapter 8, *The Current Nutritional Status in China*, by Chunming Chen, describes the dramatic nutrition improvement in under 5-year-old children and the growth of school-aged children and adolescents during the rapid economic growth that has occurred in China. The chapter discusses the improvement of the nutritional status of various population groups, the factors contributing to such improvement and the existing challenges. It reports that the prevalence of stunting in the countryside has declined and there is no longer undernutrition in urban parts of the country. Also, the medians of height-for-age groups of school-aged children and adolescents in cities are close to the World Health Organization (WHO) reference. The diets in rural areas have improved but the trend in urban areas is towards an imbalance in nutrition status. The author notes that anaemia is still a public health problem in China and

that the trend among children shows that rapid economic growth has not significantly improved micronutrient intake. Dietary and lifestyle changes show benefits but also make nutrition factors important risks in relation to the rapidly increasing prevalence of chronic diseases such as obesity, hypertension, diabetes and dislipidaemia. An analysis of the factors contributing to nutrition improvement and challenges is provided, including agriculture policies. With reference to the role of agriculture, the author stresses that better nutrition is the outcome of concerted efforts, especially in agricultural development, by the government. Agriculture is considered not only as production or yield, but also as the integration of rural development and farmers' well-being, which is extremely important in relation to improvements in nutrition.

By the end of 2009, Brazil had met the first Millennium Development Goal (MDG) of reducing poverty and malnutrition by half. Chapter 9, *Integrating Nutrition into Agricultural and Rural Development Policies: The Brazilian Experience of Building an Innovative Food and Nutrition Security Approach*, by Luciene Burlandy *et al.*, shows that innovative programmes have emerged as a consequence of Brazil's National System of Food and Nutrition Security, established in 2006. The chapter analyses how the country is creating connections between programmes and targeting them to the most vulnerable groups through key institutions. It also highlights advances and challenges and discusses some evidence of the integrative approach for improving the quality of diets and raising the level of nutrition. Different assessments are analysed of the Family Grant Program (*Programa Bolsa Familia* – PBF), the Food Acquisition Program (*Programa de Aquisição de Alimentos* – PAA) and the National School Meals Program (*Programa Nacional de Alimentação Escolar* – PNAE). Results indicate that PBF promotes greater access to food, improves the variety of food consumed, reduces food insecurity levels and, in some cases, has contributed to the nutritional recovery of children with severe deficits in weight for height and height for age. Although the prevalence of stunting and wasting is decreasing, the prevalence of over-weight and obesity is increasing, particularly in urban areas, even among the poorest groups. Therefore, PBF is being implemented in an integrative and complementary way with PAA and PNAE programmes so as to improve the availability and consumption of fresh and diversified food, especially fruits and vegetables, in public schools and promote purchases directly from family farmers. These programmes have been designed following a comprehensive approach, establishing joint actions among agriculture, health, nutrition and social sectors, thereby creating closer links between food production and healthy eating.

The authors of Chapter 9 note that it is also important to expand and strengthen other social measures that are essential to promote healthy eating practices, such as greater access to drinkable water, the implementation of infrastructure programmes, food advertising regulations and a culturally based approach guiding the design and the implementation of nutrition programmes. They emphasize that connections among nutrition, agriculture and social protection policies can have an impact on the nutritional well-being of the population in a broader sense. Effective connections that generate nutritional impact require a combination of factors. such as a political process and an institutional framework that have sectorial interactions and social participation as underlying principles. The integration of different institutional mechanisms at the federal level in devising a comprehensive and integrative systemic approach has led, for example, to the formation of CONSEA (National Council for Food and Nutrition Security), which is made up of different sectors of the government (including the ministries of agriculture, health, education and social development) and civil society organizations, and linked to the presidency. Other aspects include political support by the presidency and the inclusion of food and nutrition security in the government's agenda; they also include the formation of inter-ministerial management groups linked to programmes (such as PAA and PBF) that promote sectorial interactions at the technical and political levels. Social

participation in all phases of programme design and implementation, and by all levels of the government (national, state and municipal) has been crucial to promote these political processes.

Chapter 10, *The Gender Informed Nutrition and Agriculture (GINA) Alliance and the Nutrition Collaborative Research Support Program (NCRSP)*, by Cheryl Jackson Lewis, shows how the GINA Alliance of the US Agency for International Development (USAID), which has been piloted in Uganda, Mozambique and Nigeria, has proven effective in reducing hunger and poverty. GINA promoted improved agriculture and nutrition practices, increased agricultural productivity and addressed traditional gender inequities that were detrimental to maternal and child nutrition. The programme employed a gender-focused, community-based approach to improving household food and nutrition security, with a particular emphasis on the nutritional status of children under 5 years. GINA's success is based on recognizing that women have a unique role as primary caregivers and as producers and processors of food at the household level, and that they are central to improving household food and nutrition security.

Overall, the GINA programmes in Uganda, Mozambique and Nigeria were able to improve weight-for-age of 3000 children under 5 years old during the period from the programme baseline to follow-up evaluation. Additionally, GINA resulted in: increased availability of nutritious foods in participating households; increased awareness and understanding of the basic causes of malnutrition; increased food production, leading to greater consumption of nutritious foods and increases in income; a link between markets and GINA farmer groups; and the development of gender-diverse farmer groups complete with a well-functioning organizational structure. GINA's focus on gender roles led to an upgrading in the status of women and their recognition as producers and processors of food. As a result, women's control over their assets and the size of their assets has increased. Lessons learned from the project show that GINA was based on a multi-sectoral programme design, and combined multiple interventions from a number of sectors (agriculture, marketing, nutrition education, hygiene and health care) to address undernutrition. GINA interventions were linked to ongoing activities in other sectors to ensure integration at both the national and district level, where planning and coordination with other partners was critical. Among the recommendations for future programme design there is the need for a more reliable monitoring and evaluation framework, and better communication of lessons learned. USAID is now scaling up the GINA model through a new Nutrition Collaborative Research Support Program to build the evidence base to demonstrate how agricultural interventions implemented and co-located with health activities may lead to improvements in the nutritional status of women and children.

School feeding activities have long been a part of many governments' education policies. Experiences in some countries have revealed that school feeding programmes can achieve improvements in attendance, drop-out rates, academic achievement and nutritional status. Other benefits include the relief of short-term hunger, improved classroom behaviour and better food consumption patterns. In addition to these possible benefits and objectives, school feeding programmes are often seen as safety nets, achieving a transfer to households of the value of the meal or snack provided. The next two chapters (Chapters 11 and 12) report experiences in school feeding programmes by a developing country (Guyana) and a developed country (England). Clearly, the case of England differs greatly from that of Guyana but it shows that school feeding programmes are also important for a developed country.

Chapter 11, *Guyana's Hinterland Community-based School Feeding Program (SFP)*, by Suraiya J. Ismail *et al.*, describes the Hinterland Community-Based School Feeding Programme established by the Ministry of Education and implemented in four administrative regions inhabited by indigenous people, often in remote communities where poverty, food insecurity, malnutrition and lack of diet diversity are common and school attendance is poor. The impact evaluation of the programme, which covered intervention schools and control schools, demonstrated that stunting fell, school attendance increased and participation in learning activities improved in intervention schools and that children also performed better in national academic assessment tests. Parents participated fully in food production and meal delivery activities. Households benefited through increased employment and a more varied food supply. The programme contributed to preserving food security through a period of food price volatility, had a low cost per child in relation to other programmes and had reduced dependence on imports. Outstanding challenges as well as issues of sustainability are discussed.

In England, school meals have been provided to pupils for many decades. From the mid-1970s, however, both the number of meals provided and the quality of food supplied declined. Legislation was introduced in 2001 to ensure that school catering services provided healthy options, but surveys showed that the improved availability of healthy options in school had little or no impact on children's eating habits. Chapter 12, *The Impact of School Food Standards on Children's Eating Habits in England*, by Michael Nelson *et al.*, reports clear evidence of the improvements in the provision, choice and consumption of food in schools following the introduction of legislation and a national programme of work to change catering practices and the attitudes of pupils, parents and others to school meals. It provides evidence of the impact of food choices on children's learning behaviour in the classroom, and of the overall costs and benefits. In 2005, the School Food Trust, a non-departmental public body (NDPB) that promotes the education and health of children and young people by improving the quality of food supplied and consumed in schools was created. School food standards were introduced in 2006–2008 that set out what caterers could and could not provide for children in schools. At the same time, the Trust worked with caterers, schools, pupils, parents, manufacturers, food distributors, institutions providing further education for catering staff and others, in a coordinated programme of change. This approach provides a model for intervention that can be applied at local, regional and national levels. It also provides a platform for transforming children's eating habits, using schools as the centre for both learning and practice relating to healthy lifestyles, and engaging pupils and parents in the development of cooking skills that support healthier eating. These strategies not only improve the nutrition provided to children at school, but are expected to have an impact on their choice of diet, both outside school and as adults. Evidence relating to this wider impact is being generated.

The inclusion of animal source foods (ASFs) in the diet is an important food-based strategy for improving nutrition outcomes globally. ASFs not only supply high-quality and readily digested protein and energy, but also readily absorbable and bioavailable micronutrients. ASFs are inherently richer sources of specific micronutrients, particularly iron, zinc, riboflavin, vitamin A, vitamin B_{12} and calcium, than plant foods. Their inclusion in the diet promotes growth, cognitive function, physical activity and health, and they are particularly important for children and pregnant women. The addition of modest amounts of meat and other ASFs in the diet from a variety of sources can greatly improve the overall energy, protein, micronutrient status, health and function of populations.

Chapter 13, *Animal Source Foods as a Food-based Approach to Improve Diet and Nutrition Outcomes*, by Charlotte G. Neumann *et al.*, reviews the evidence on the impact of ASF consumption. It presents recent studies that document the benefits of food-based approaches that integrate meat and other ASFs. Even a modest amount of meat in the diet of schoolchildren improves cognitive function and school performance, physical activity, growth (increased lean body mass), micronutrient status and morbidity. Outcomes from several nutrition interventions promoting ASF production and consumption also demonstrate improvements in nutrition. The chapter provides examples of the activities of several non-governmental organizations (NGOs) operating in Africa that play a key role in promoting ASFs. It highlights important issues and constraints to raising livestock in Africa. In addition to

current strategies, small freshwater fish and rabbits are two ASF sources with great potential for addressing nutritional deficiencies that have not received sufficient attention. The authors emphasize that food-based approaches using ASFs in rural areas are more likely to be sustainable in improving diet quality and energy density than 'pill-based' approaches. While food-based solutions are more complex and interdisciplinary in nature and require long-term commitments, they are more likely to address malnutrition at its source, leading to long-term sustainable improvements. The authors conclude that interventions that promote ASF consumption need to include more rigorous evaluation to document strategies, problems and outcomes. Investing in diet improvement for children and women of reproductive age would maximize the chances of improving growth, cognitive development and school performance of children and the health of pregnant women. ASFs would also improve adult work performance and productivity by improving iron and overall nutrition status.

As described in Chapter 6, HKI's HFP model is a food-based strategy for increasing the micronutrient intake of individuals, improving household food security and advancing women's empowerment. The standard HFP intervention includes gardening, poultry production, group marketing and nutrition behaviour change communication (BCC). The model has historically been implemented in smallholder households that have a minimal amount of land. However, individuals in ultra-poor households with minimal access to land are among the most food-insecure and malnourished and they require food-based interventions targeted to their unique capabilities.

Chapter 14, *Adapting Food-based Strategies to Improve the Nutrition of the Landless: A Review of HKI's Homestead Food Production Program in Bangladesh*, by Emily P. Hillenbrand and Jillian L. Waid, highlights the urgent nutritional needs of the ultra-poor households and the growing number of landless households in Bangladesh. HKI has been adapting its HFP model to reach this marginalized population. Better nutrition and fewer nutrition-related health complications can translate into sustainable livelihood gains for the ultra-poor, for whom physical labour capacity is often their most important livelihood resource. The chapter looks closely at the problem of landlessness in Bangladesh, and specifically at how landlessness is linked to extreme poverty and nutrition insecurity. It presents the design and evolution of the HFP model in Bangladesh and shows the outcomes that can be attributed to this model. Finally, the chapter discusses the specific challenges and proposed tools for developing a successful food-based HFP model for the landless. It draws on published and unpublished quantitative and qualitative data from a number of HFP projects that have been undertaken by HKI-Bangladesh. The conditions and approaches presented are highly specific to the context of Bangladesh, where land scarcity is extreme and constitutes a defining characteristic of food insecurity and malnutrition. Nevertheless, the authors emphasize that the challenge of extending tried-and-tested food-based, nutrition-sensitive approaches to reach more marginalized populations will be a global imperative in the decades to come, as climate change, urbanization and population pressures limit the availability of resources (including water) for diversified agriculture production.

Chapter 15, *The Growing Connection Project – With a Mexico Case Study*, by Bob Patterson and Margarita Álvarez Oyarzábal, shows that The Growing Connection (TGC), which comprises gardens and vegetable production sites in 12 countries, combines low-cost innovations in intensive horticulture with recent advances in IT and communication technology. TGC's goal is to assist people's access to tools and the information needed for improving nutrition. Project participants – mostly young persons and women – learn how they can directly and positively have an impact on their nutritional status by growing fresh, nutritious vegetables, record their activities and share the lessons learned and best practices in an expanding network of people engaged in solutions to malnutrition, hunger and poverty. TGC project participants have led the way in demonstrating 'how' people with access to tools, information and advice can achieve success.

Biofortification, through conventional plant breeding, can improve the nutritional content of the staple foods that poor people already eat, and provide a comparatively inexpensive, cost-effective, sustainable and long-term means of delivering micronutrients to the poor. This approach not only lowers the number of severely malnourished people, but also helps to maintain improved nutritional status. HarvestPlus seeks to develop and distribute varieties of food staples (rice, wheat, maize, cassava, pearl millet, beans and sweet potato) that are high in iron, zinc and provitamin A through an interdisciplinary, global alliance of scientific institutions and implementing agencies in developing and developed countries.

Chapter 16, *Biofortification: A New Tool to Reduce Micronutrient Malnutrition*, by Howarth E. Bouis *et al.*, explains that the biofortification strategy seeks to take advantage of the regular daily consumption of large amounts of food staples by all family members. Biofortification provides a feasible means of reaching malnourished populations in relatively remote rural areas by delivering naturally fortified foods to people with limited access to commercially marketed fortified foods, which are more readily available in urban areas. The comparative advantages of biofortification are presented, as well as its limitations. Unlike the continued financial outlays that are required for traditional supplementation and fortification programmes, a one-time investment in plant breeding can yield micronutrient-rich plants for farmers around the world to grow for years to come. It is this multiplier aspect of biofortification across time and distance that makes it so cost-effective. The authors conclude that in conceptualizing solutions for a range of nutritional deficiencies, interdisciplinary communication between plant scientists and human nutrition scientists holds great potential. Human nutritionists need to be informed, for example, about the extent to which the vitamin and mineral density of specific foods, as well as the content of the compounds (e.g. prebiotics) that promote and inhibit their bioavailability, can be modified through plant breeding. Plant breeders need to be aware of the influence that agricultural research may

have on nutrient utilization (e.g. the bioavailability of trace minerals in modern varieties
versus bioavailability in traditional varieties)
and the potential of plant breeding for
improvements in nutrition and health.

Food insecurity and malnutrition are
very prevalent in Malawi. Chapter 17,
*Medium-scale Fortification: A Sustainable Food-
based Approach to Improve Diets and Raise
Nutrition Levels*, by Miriam E. Yiannakis *et al.*,
examines the success and sustainability
potential of medium-scale fortification (MSF)
and small-scale fortification (SSF) for increasing rural access to and usage of fortified
flours within the Micronutrient and Health
(MICAH) Programme in Malawi. MICAH
was implemented by World Vision to
address anaemia and micronutrient malnutrition of women and children. It consisted
of a package of community-based multi-
sectoral interventions implemented with
multiple partners. Small- and medium-scale
fortification of maize flour consumed by the
general population, and a specially formulated local complementary food, were part of
an anaemia control package that also included
small animal production and consumption,
backyard gardens, community-based iron
supplementation, deworming of children and
malaria control. Project evaluations provided
strong evidence of impact over the 9 years of
implementation. Anaemia in children under 5
years old and in non-pregnant women
decreased. While these overall improvements
cannot be attributed to fortification alone, it is
likely that the consumption of fortified foods
contributed to the decrease in anaemia. MSF
is an innovative and practical community-
based way of enabling essential nutrients to
reach populations without access to centrally
fortified foods. Including MSF and SSF in
food security and nutrition programmes can
improve the potential impact of the overall
programme and, more importantly, maximize the sustainability of positive micronutrient impact. The authors make a series of
recommendations as priority steps for programmers and policy makers to implement in
order to build on their experience and on the
scaling up of MSF with SSF partnerships for
improved nutrition of the rural poor in
Malawi.

Chapter 18, *Optimized Feeding Recommendations and In-home Fortification to Improve
Iron Status in Infants and Young Children
in the Republic of Tajikistan: A Pilot Project*,
by Marina Adrianopoli *et al.*, evaluates
the efficacy of age-specific Food-Based
Complementary Feeding Recommendations
(FBCFRs), and the long-term effectiveness
and feasibility of in-home fortification using
micronutrient-based powders (Sprinkles), in
order to optimize complementary feeding
and reduce anaemia in infants and young
children in two regions of Tajikistan. There
were two intervention groups: group A of the
study received FBCFRs and group B received
FBCFRs plus Sprinkles. Nutrition education
for caregivers was provided regularly. The
prevalence of anaemia decreased by 30% in
group A and 47% in group B. Improvements
of haemoglobin (Hb) levels were observed at
3 months and at 12 months in both groups.
The chapter discusses how integrated food-
based approaches, supported by behaviour
change communication and by the strengthening of community nutrition knowledge
represent a long-term strategy to improve
complementary feeding patterns and to
address specific micronutrient deficiencies in
early life. This combined intervention represented an integrated strategy aimed at optimizing infant feeding by covering issues such
as nutrition, care and hygiene practices. An
important conclusion is that in-home fortification represents an appropriate intermediate
solution when there is a risk (or occurrence)
of micronutrient deficiencies. However, given
the fact that micronutrient powders are not
food and cannot be consumed without food,
the use of effective and affordable food-based
recommendations, based on feasible combinations of locally available foods, should be
strongly encouraged, taking existing food
patterns and portion sizes into account. This
pilot study confirms the necessity to field test
dietary recommendations, which helps to
evaluate potential difficulties in the implementation, feasibility and sustainability of
feeding recommendations.

A major impediment to securing investments in agriculture and food-based approaches for improving nutrition is providing
proof of efficacy. Developing a credible evidence

base that articulates the links in the chain between agricultural policy, food production, access, intake and nutritional status is essential to meeting this challenge. Chapter 19, *Towards Long-term Nutrition Security: The Role of Agriculture in Dietary Diversity*, by Brian Thompson and Janice Meerman, presents research findings on the links between agriculture, dietary diversity and nutrition that are of particular relevance in poor rural contexts where malnutrition rates are often high. The concept of the 'nutrition gap' – the gap between what foods are grown and available and what foods are needed for a healthy diet – is introduced and discussed. The chapter provides examples of nutrition-sensitive agriculture and food-based strategies and interventions that can be used to improve dietary diversity within specific agro-ecological zones and for particular food types. It concludes by emphasizing the potential that nutrition-sensitive agriculture and food-based approaches have for improving dietary diversity and nutrition. Policy recommendations for increasing political commitment to agriculture's role in reducing malnutrition are presented. The authors note that providing evidence of how agriculture-based interventions can improve nutrition outcomes is essential to increasing the visibility of agriculture on national and international nutrition agendas. Narrowing the nutrition gap can only occur when national policy makers and members of the international development community recognize the essential role that nutrition-sensitive agriculture and food-based approaches can play in reducing malnutrition. In addition to building a strong evidence base, this requires incorporating explicit nutrition objectives and considerations into agricultural research agendas, agriculture development policies and programmes, and also building the capacity of institutions and individuals at country level and promoting nutrition security at regional and global levels. Taken together, the evidence and examples illustrate the crucial role that agriculture can play in improving dietary diversity and nutrition in poor-country contexts. The authors conclude that given that much of the developing world remains agriculture based, and that many of the most malnourished

populations depend upon this sector for their livelihoods, the importance of nutrition-sensitive agriculture and food-based approaches is crucial. Such approaches are viable, cost-effective, long-term and sustainable solutions for improving diets and raising levels of nutrition, so assisting communities and households to feed and nourish themselves adequately is the sustainable way forward.

Nutritional self-reliance refers to the capacity of individuals and communities to make their own good decisions relating to their nutrition. Chapter 20, *Building Nutritional Self-reliance*, by George Kent, discusses matters related to nutritional self-reliance and highlights the importance of this issue. The author explains that some forms of assistance can be disempowering because they only provide short-term relief, make bad situations more tolerable and have outsiders dominate the decision making. In those situations, the gift of assistance tends to stimulate demands for more assistance. In contrast, assistance that is empowering helps people to address their nutrition concerns both individually and together with their neighbours, to build their nutritional self-reliance and to reduce their need for assistance over time. The author asserts that chronic malnutrition in all its forms should be addressed in broad social, political and economic terms, and not only in clinical terms. Treating an issue as a medical problem disempowers people. Similarly, and in support of Professor Latham, he affirms that the suggestion that capsules must be used to treat vitamin A deficiency, without at the same time showing how to make better use of local foods to deal with the problem, is disempowering. The chapter illustrates ways in which agencies could help to build nutritional self-reliance within communities by favouring more empowering approaches. The author concludes that agencies should favour programmes that strengthen people's capacity to define, analyse and act on their own problems, and thus help to build individual and community self-reliance in nutrition.

Part III of this book, *Contributions from FAO Departments and Divisions*, contains Chapters 21 to 35. This part of the proceedings includes chapters from FAO giving examples on how nutrition issues and considerations are being mainstreamed into the work of FAO. More information on these articles is provided on pp. 282–283.

Finally, *Part IV* of the book, *Conclusion*, contains the last chapter of the book and an appendix. Chapter 36, *Selected Findings and Recommendations from the Symposium*, by the editors, lists selected findings that were prepared as a summary of the main conclusions and recommendations of the papers that were presented and the discussions that took place during this international symposium.

These will give practical guidance to FAO, its Members and other stakeholders in their efforts in implementing agriculture and food-based approaches for improving diets and raising levels of nutrition as a viable, sustainable and long-term strategy towards the achievement of food and nutrition security. This is followed by the *Appendix: Presentation of the Publication* 'Combating Micronutrient Deficiencies: Food-based Approaches', which was mentioned at the beginning of this introduction.

1 Perspective on Nutritional Problems in Developing Countries: Nutrition Security through Community Agriculture

Michael C. Latham
Cornell University, Ithaca, New York, USA

Michael C. Latham died only few months after the symposium. What is presented here is an edited transcription of the presentation he made at the symposium – without the slides, for which explanatory information has been added where this would be helpful.

First, I would like to thank Brian Thompson and others at FAO[1] for inviting me to give this talk. I would like to say that in recent years Brian and his colleagues have made a hugely important contribution to the nutrition world by getting agriculture to focus more on its impact on nutrition than has been the practice in the past. Nowadays we talk much more about nutrition security when we talk of food security. Older people like myself, as we enter our dotage, often hark back to what was done three, four, five decades ago, and I will do the same. I also think as we age, some of us become more willing to be controversial and to say things that may not be the majority opinion of the audience.

I have been involved with FAO for a long time, since, I think, before many of you were even born. But for the whole of my 50 year career in nutrition, I have talked about the need for multifaceted solutions and interdisciplinary approaches to tackle the serious nutritional problems of developing countries, or whatever we want to call those poorer countries in the Third World. Malnutrition, especially serious malnutrition, including micronutrient deficiencies, is often presented as a problem of health, but reducing malnutrition requires collaboration from many other disciplines, especially

agriculture. We must therefore strengthen our understanding of the linkages between agriculture and nutrition if we are to tackle malnutrition, which is one of the specific objectives of this symposium. Interdisciplinary approaches are needed in academia and in research but, very importantly, interdisciplinary approaches are also needed on the ground to help solve nutrition problems. Consequently, it is very important that we deal with nutrition security as well as food security.

Let me briefly tell you a little bit of my background. I was first trained as a medical doctor and then in tropical medicine and public health. For 10 years I worked for the Ministry of Health in Dar-es-Salam in Tanzania, the first 7 years of which I was running district hospitals doing mostly curative work – Caesarean sections, orthopaedics, etc. – but I was also responsible for the public health services of a large district. The last 3 of those years I was dragged into the nutrition unit in that same Ministry, but even during my time as a bush doctor, so to speak, I had begun to see the importance of malnutrition. So cases of measles were coming to me and children were dying not because the measles in Tanzania or Africa or anywhere else is a

© FAO 2014. *Improving Diets and Nutrition: Food-based Approaches*
(eds B. Thompson and L. Amoroso)

1

more serious virus than the measles I had treated in the UK, but because the children with measles were malnourished. I realized that to reduce disease and mortality we had to do something about malnutrition, and so I moved more and more into preventive medicine and nutrition.

So much of my talk will be – in what I believe to be a most timely symposium – stressing the crucial importance of strengthening agriculture and nutrition linkages and especially of food-based approaches to improve diets and raise levels of nutrition. So as not to be too general, I have chosen two controversial specific, important, current examples where I believe more emphasis is needed on food-based approaches and less on top-down magic bullet approaches. The first is the Vitamin A Capsule Programme and the second is ready-to-use therapeutic foods (RUTFs).

When I talk about nutrition I have to always mention equity because I think equity is the major cause of hunger and malnutrition; equity not only in incomes but also in food, education, health, water supplies, housing, etc. I am afraid to say, as with all philosophies, worship of what I would call super-capitalism almost all over the world – Russia and China as well as in India – all are becoming super-capitalists while many people remain extremely poor. I believe the situation is getting worse and that is incredibly important in contributing to serious malnutrition around the world. I think there are some rays of hope, but I don't know if any of you have seen the film *South of the Border* by Oliver Stone? That film interviews then-President Lula of Brazil, the first Native American president of a Latin American country, and others, and points out that countries that have been moving away from US hegemony are doing better in some respects with regard to equity. Basic wages are going up, Brazil is doing very well in terms of reducing malnutrition and young child deaths, a trend that I think Bolivia and others will follow, and of course Cuba has always had, or for a long time has had, the lowest mortality rates in the region.

I also can't give a talk on nutrition without mentioning the conceptual framework that is often called the UNICEF Conceptual Framework.[2] Being a Tanzanian, I claim this for Tanzania, when Urban Johnson was working there. The underlying causes are inadequate food, inadequate care and inadequate health. This shows the multidisciplinary nature of the causes of malnutrition. Something should be done about all three of them, not just about any one of them.

There is a child with serious nutritional marasmus: this presents itself as a health problem, but health workers really don't have the power to prevent this from happening. It takes many other disciplines.

Just to cement my support for interdisciplinary approaches, I would like to make reference to three old studies of mine, and I especially want to talk about the first one: 'The district team approach to malnutrition'.[3] That, as you can see, was almost five decades ago. In the remote southern districts in Ruvuma region of Tanzania, we found there was a huge amount of malnutrition presenting itself to us as doctors in the hospital, but to try to do something about it we had to enlist other people. It really was a district team approach, as the article in reference is in fact a compilation of five articles by five different specialists – a physician, agriculturist, social scientist, administrator and educationist – showing that to reduce malnutrition a multidisciplinary approach was needed. A few years later I published *Human Nutrition in Tropical Africa*,[4] which has had a number of editions, and throughout that book, the focus is on community-based multidisciplinary nutrition activity. I followed up with a book for FAO called *Planning and Evaluation of Applied Nutrition Programmes*,[5] which was a compilation of community-based nutrition programmes similar to what was later called the JNSP.[6] I have been involved in this kind of activity for a long time.

I think it is important always to remember how vital malnutrition is in terms of child deaths. This slide illustrates that very few child deaths are due to acute malnutrition and could have been prevented had the children not been malnourished. Around 54% of child deaths would not have occurred if it was not for malnutrition.

I want to now move to 'Vitamin A Supplements and Morbidity – A Conundrum Unanswered', as I have put it.[7] This is the first of two examples that I want to give where we are using a top-down medical approach instead of food-based approaches at the local level, which I think would be more preferable. This worldwide Vitamin A programme consists of providing very high doses of vitamin A every 6 months to some 200 million children in about 100 targeted countries. The dose is so high, so unphysiological, that these doses would not be permissible in the USA and probably not permissible in Italy. In the early days, this was a short-term measure to prevent blindness due to keratomalacia, but now keratomalacia is extremely rare in almost all of these countries where the programme is in operation. The Vitamin A capsule programme is currently being promoted mainly to reduce child mortality. As UNICEF states, dragging on your heartstrings, we have to have this programme to meet the MDGs.[8] However, no evaluation has been conducted in any of these 100 countries to show that it is reducing mortality and almost certainly it is not. There is good reason why the World Vitamin A Capsule programme, I believe, should be phased out and discontinued. It is not doing what it claims to do and, very importantly, it undermines food-based approaches, which are the preferred option. We need to ensure that sustainable food-based approaches favouring locally available foods rich in provitamin carotenoids and other micronutrients are given first priority.

There have been many successful horticulture and home gardening projects and some will be discussed at this symposium. Vitamin A-rich red palm oil is widely used in West Africa, there are new biofortified foods being developed, such as high carotene bananas from the Pacific and elsewhere, high carotene African orange flesh sweet potatoes are tried in Mozambique and Uganda quite successfully, and some countries are fortifying foods with vitamin A. These food-based approaches are socially, culturally, economically and environmentally appropriate. They can be affordable and sustainable and, unlike vitamin A capsules, they provide further important nutritional, health and other benefits.

People forget that vitamin A deficiency seldom occurs in isolation. When I saw children with vitamin A deficiency, I would say 90%, maybe 99%, were anaemic, they were iron deficient, but if we measured their zinc status they would also be zinc deficient. Why do we give only one nutrient to deal with one problem when children have multiple micronutrient and macronutrient problems? Is this sensible?

In the time we have today I will not show the research data on the vitamin A capsules. In the first issue of the Journal on *World Nutrition* published in May 2010,[9] I wrote a paper entitled 'The great vitamin A fiasco', which reviews the scientific data and lays out my own arguments. I will not go into the data now but rather I would like to show you a few slides that illustrate my long-held views stemming from my earlier research. In the early 1970s, I was working with Dr Solan and colleagues from the Philippines. We had a project to improve the production of carotene-rich vegetables which was highly successful and the right kind of approach. There was a child who was blind because of xerophthalmia, 6 or 7 years old, a terrible situation, and obviously we needed to do something about preventing this. The major source of vitamin A for most people in developing countries is from provitamin carotenoids, and for those in the richer countries it is more from animal sources.

This is a slide from 2010. This is by Anna Herforth, who was a student of Per Pinstrup-Andersen, now working for the World Bank. I really like this, which shows that 100 g of amaranth, what we call 'chicha' in Tanzania, and cowpeas provide far more than the total RDAs[10] for a child. Amaranth grows wild in Tanzania and, together with chickpeas, these are good African leafy vegetables that provide adequate carotene.

In the Philippines with Dr Solan at the Cebu Institute of Medicine, we did the only study ever carried out to look at the efficacy of three different interventions, and these are the same three interventions we use today. We haven't changed much over the last 30 years. There are only three main ways to do something about vitamin A deficiency – public health and horticulture interventions,

high-dose capsule intervention and fortification. We selected 12 regions, which were
randomly assigned to one of these three
interventions.

These are the capsules that provide those
massive doses of vitamin A. As they actually
only keep serum vitamin A level raised for
6 to 8 weeks, distributed twice a year, for
4 months out of the 6, the children were back
to the low levels they had at the beginning.
This is the result of those three interventions.
All three interventions significantly reduced
signs of xerophthalmia. Fortification was
judged to be the most economic; this is actually work done by Barry Popkin when he was
PhD student at Cornell. However, the public
health horticulture intervention, in addition
to reducing xerophthalmia, also improved
health and nutrition in general and provided
a broad range of benefits to families. High-
dose vitamin A supplements and vitamin A
fortification can only improve vitamin A and
so there can be no comparison as to which is
the preferred intervention. However, this
does not seem to be recognized and accepted
around the world.

Another point of India's leading nutritionist, Dr Gopalan, to remember is that keratomalacia which used to be fairly prevalent in
India, is no longer considered to be a serious
public health problem there. There has been
similar improvement around the world;
I have talked to people in Indonesia and in
other places where it used to be a serious
problem and it seems that keratomalacia is no
longer a major problem.

In the 1980s and up to 1990 there were
eight major mortality studies where high-dose
vitamin A was given and which looked at its
effect on mortality. In two countries there was
no difference observed, in six of the countries
there was a significant difference in mortality.
George Beaton of Toronto University reviewed
these results and stated that, in contrast to the
very clear effect on mortality, it was concluded
that vitamin A supplements have no impact
on incidence, duration or prevalence of diarrhoeal or respiratory infections. There have
been many studies, including two very
impressive studies, one in Tanzania and one
in South Africa, which have shown very
clearly that vitamin A supplements reduce

measles morbidity, complications of measles
such as pneumonia and case fatality rate,
death rates of measles. So it has been proved
that measles, its complications and mortality
rates, can be reduced by giving vitamin A.

For those who believe that vitamin A
supplements are having such a large impact
on reducing mortality there is a conundrum.
Can most mortality occur without morbidity?
As a doctor, I didn't see many cases arriving
at the hospital and dying without being ill
first. However, we can't seem to show that
there is any impact of vitamin A on morbidity.
I don't think that people who are in favour of
vitamin A capsules are willing to face this or
argue this in any kind of scientific way.

Following these mortality studies, more
were undertaken because we thought if the
children die, we wouldn't be able to observe
the effect on diarrhoeal and respiratory infections. Cornell conducted two studies. Unlike
the mortality studies, these were double-
blind placebo-controlled clinical trials. All
children were immunized, including against
measles; all had access to reasonable health
care. These children were seen frequently to
monitor their illnesses and we saw what
they died of. One study was carried out in
Tanzania, the other in India. There was absolutely no difference in diarrhoeal or respiratory infections in either of these two
well-done studies. There are at least 20 other
studies that also observed no difference in
morbidity from diarrhoeal or respiratory
infections. A few studies, including a particularly impressive one by Dr Diblish in
Indonesia, showed that vitamin A supplements actually increased the respiratory
morbidity in well-nursed children.

I did not think that there would ever
be another large vitamin A mortality study
undertaken, but about 5 years ago a large
study in India began with almost 1 million
children. Of these, half received high dose
supplements and the other half no supplement. There was no significant difference in
death rates of those receiving vitamin A supplements compared with those not receiving.
That, unfortunately, did not provide data on
measles immunization, but by the year 2000
most Indian children were receiving measles
immunization so there should not be a big

difference in measles deaths. In many studies, the causes of death either are not given or are unclear – cause of death is fever, measles causes fever; children died because they were coughing, measles causes coughing; they died because of diarrhoea, measles causes diarrhoea. There is no proof that deaths were not due to measles. Therefore, I honestly believe that vitamin A is reducing measles deaths and not other deaths.

I believe that food-based approaches have huge advantages over medicinal strategies. Food-based approaches provide several micronutrients at once, they are viable, affordable and sustainable, they have social, cultural, economic and environmental benefits and they are local and not top-down. I have this question: why are vitamin A supplement programmes made a part of nutrition interventions and supported by the organizations and the countries themselves? That is a very difficult question to answer. I think some of the countries get cajoled into taking these programmes. It's really quite difficult to get rid of established programmes. I think these organizations find it much easier to have top-down approaches than to improve local consumption and have food-based projects at field level. I think and am very sad to say that there is a small group of people, what I call 'The Vitamin A lobby', that have controlled this agenda for 30 years. I have acted in both the International Vitamin A Consultants Group and the Micronutrient Forum, and the leaders in these organizations have been the same for 30 years; they replace each other, they are never elected and I honestly think they control the vitamin A agenda, and as a nutritionist I think our profession should be ashamed if we allow that to continue.

Why can we not make sure that children all over the world are immunized against measles? We are making progress, but I think children have a right to be immunized against measles. We can eradicate measles from planet earth, which would be a huge saving to countries like Italy and Great Britain and the USA because children would no longer have to be immunized against measles, but we will not put the money into doing it. We did it with smallpox, and we are close to doing it with polio, for which WHO is getting

a lot of credit. I think FAO didn't get enough credit earlier this year when the world eradicated rinderpest. Few people knew about it because it was only on page 10 of FAO's journal. When rinderpest was eradicated the world was rid of one of the most serious of all virus diseases, one I would say that had more negative impact on nutrition than either smallpox or polio, even though these are most awful diseases.

Now I would like to move to my second example, which is the readiness to use therapeutic foods and similar products. I believe this is a new threat to breastfeeding of infants aged 6 to 24 months. The breastfeeding community has managed to get the paediatric associations to accept the norm of 6 months' exclusive breastfeeding. Now our task is to encourage the wider practice and longer duration of breastfeeding from 6 to 24 months, where breast milk becomes the main, basically supplementary food to wheat, maize or other staples in developing countries.

Over recent years, RUTFs have leaped on the stage and their availability and use is expanding exponentially. My first concern was that they could be a threat to breastfeeding, but with the distribution of these products expanding enormously, my main concern is that they could seriously distort family diets, undermine local agriculture and undermine proven nutrition interventions. The claims that have been made for them, I think, are outrageous. Is it not extremely worrying to see this headline in *The New York Times*? Let me quote: 'Could a Peanut Paste Called Plumpy'nut End Malnutrition?'.[11] *Could* a peanut paste called Plumpy'nut end malnutrition? No, no, no, it could not end malnutrition. There are many other exaggerated claims.

RUTF stands for ready-to-use therapeutic foods, but the therapy is being forgotten. Therapy should be provided through the health services and RUTF is good for the treatment of severe acute malnutrition. But now it is being made available well beyond that to reduce malnutrition as a new top-down magic bullet. I see great danger when I hear or see statements suggesting that these products provide for the first time an answer to the world's serious nutrition problem.

Jeffery Sachs of MDG fame has come out equally strongly against the idea that these could help reach the MDGs. These claims have been made not only by the manufacturers but also by agencies and academics. As I have stated, these products are one of a number of good ways to treat severe acute malnutrition, but they are not the only way and we did have success in treating malnutrition before we had RUTFs. I do not believe that they are appropriate for dealing with more chronic mild malnutrition, which is very prevalent, and they should not be used without health supervision and under strict guidelines, and there are no such guidelines. There is an attempt to produce marketing guidelines, but we need strict guidelines for their use. For chronic hunger and mild malnutrition we have proven approaches, including actions to access adequate food, health and care. Here at this symposium we wish to stress actions to improve agriculture and dietary diversity. More attention needs to be given to better local agriculture, including high yields and more nutritious crops. More publicity and more education on topics such as agriculture, health and nutrition linkages should inform a wide range of people on how they may obtain and consume nutritious diets most feasibly, cheaply and easily. RUTFs are not the answer.

This is therefore the definition of RUTFs. It is a strange definition, but it is almost certainly based on Plumpy'nut made by Nutriset. Plumpy'nut is the father and mother of all RUTFs. Plumpy'nut was invented by André Briend, who at one stage was working for WHO, and made by Nutriset in France, but there are many varieties and disputes. RUTFs are usually a product in a plastic sachet, and it looks and tastes like peanut butter. In Tanzania 40 to 50 years ago, we had posters all over saying that if Tanzanians and other Africans eat a handful of groundnuts, which was what Tanzanians called peanuts, a day in addition to their normal foods, malnutrition would disappear from the country. However, these peanuts were grown in Tanzania and eaten by Tanzanians; they were not peanuts from West Africa shipped to France, pushed around, put in packets, shipped back to Africa at 50 times the cost of the original peanuts; and yet that is what seems to be a popular thing to do.

Again, it is important to separate wasted from undernourished children, as there are far fewer wasted children – only 9% in Africa. It is important here to show that sub-Saharan Africa does better nutritionally than South Asia, despite South Asia's greater economic advancement.

The three largest users of RUTFs are UNICEF, Médecins sans Frontières (MSF) and the Clinton Foundation. 'Ready-to-use-food' seems a ridiculous term in English. I would say a banana is a ready-to-use-food, but not in this context. I have been a great supporter of MSF for many years. I have worked in difficult conditions, but I haven't gone to work in foreign places where I could probably get shot at and possibly killed. MSF has done a marvellous job and it deserves the Nobel Peace Prize. About 5 or 10 years ago, MSF seems suddenly to have discovered that there was a huge problem of malnutrition in the world, and it took it upon itself to do something about it. I got upset when I heard the head of MSF on the BBC about a year ago stating: 'There is a huge problem of malnutrition in the world. We in MSF are doctors and have to feed these children'. Again I say 'No, no, no', MSF does not have to feed the world's children and it can't feed the world's children. I do not believe that RUTFs are an effective way to treat severe acute malnutrition. 'The product does provide all the nutrients necessary for good nutrition. It does not contain water, which is stressed as an advantage, although I'm not sure it is a huge advantage because it actually means that the child has to drink other water that may be contaminated. I just think that RUTFs and RUSFs[12] are inappropriate for the prevention of malnutrition. They may threaten and undermine breastfeeding, may distort home-based diets, are culturally inappropriate, and they are extremely expensive. Who is going to pay for them and how much dependency is going to be developed? I think we really should oppose the use of RUTFs other than for treatment that should be under medical supervision. Medicine that replaces family foods sometimes threatens breastfeeding.

I think we have no disagreement that we have a huge crisis of child malnutrition and malnutrition around the world. I also think there is no disagreement about 6 months of exclusive breastfeeding or that from 6 months onwards other foods need to be introduced. The debate is therefore how much of that food is family foods, including breastfeeding, and how much might be RUTFs? I do think that longer and more breastfeeding from 6 to 24 months of age is what we should be doing much more about than is being done, and UNICEF has been a great supporter of breastfeeding. It worries me that they seem to be devoting much more attention to RUTFs than they are to breastfeeding.

Let me come to my overall conclusion. I believe just as we ended the protein fiasco, we now need to end the Vitamin A fiasco and put strong brakes on the wider use of RUTFs. I am not sure it is quite a fiasco yet. In my view, the main and most important approach to ensuring better growth and good nutrition in children, including adequate intakes of micronutrients, such as vitamin A and zinc, should be to ensure food and nutrition security through improving family diets, including local foods and improved agriculture. This approach, I believe, is feasible and economically and environmentally sustainable. It also has huge multiple advantages over top-down magic bullet approaches, including the use of high-tech foods and the pharmaceutical-led prevention of malnutrition. I am not against big business when it can be for the good. I am against big business when it can do harm. We have to accept that there is a very limited amount of funding for nutrition, much too little funding for nutrition for all the organizations. So I believe, for example, that when UNICEF or large NGOs[13] put major funding into either the Vitamin A capsule programme or into RUTFs and similar products, then there is less funding for proven food-based approaches like breastfeeding, home gardens or local agriculture, and even for immunization or bed nets or other really good interventions that we know improve nutrition or health.

Thank you.

Notes

[1]Food and Agriculture Organization of the United Nations.

[2]UNICEF Conceptual Framework for Malnutrition.

[3]Robson, J.R., Carpenter, G.A., Latham, M.C., Wise, R. and Lewis, P.G. (1963) The district team approach to malnutrition: Maposeni Nutrition Scheme. *Journal of Tropical Pediatrics* 8, 60–75.

[4]1st edn (1965), FAO, Rome.

[5]Date of publication 1972.

[6]The WHO (World Health Organization)/UNICEF (UN Children's Fund) Joint Nutrition Support Pogramme.

[7]Latham, M.C. (2011) Vitamin A supplements and morbidity in children – a conundrum unanswered. *Bulletin of the Nutrition Foundation of India* 32(1), 5–7.

[8]Millennium Development Goals.

[9]Journal of the World Public Health Nutrition Association: Latham, M.C. (2010) The great vitamin A fiasco. *World Nutrition* 1, 12–45.

[10]Recommended daily allowances.

[11]Rice, A. (2010) Could a Peanut Paste Called Plumpy'nut End Malnutrition? The Peanut Solution. *The New York Times*, 2 September 2010. Available at: http://www.nytimes.com/2010/09/05/magazine/05Plumpy-t.html?src=tptw (accessed 21 June 2013).

[12]Ready to use supplemental foods.

[13]Non-governmental organizations.

2 Food Systems and Human Nutrition: Relationships and Policy Interventions

Per Pinstrup-Andersen*
Cornell University, Ithaca, New York, USA

Recent dramatic fluctuations in international food prices have drawn much attention to the global food situation and what the future will bring. Can the world feed future generations? Can it do so sustainably, i.e. without reducing the productive capacity of natural resources for future generations? What price will future generations have to pay for food and will food prices continue to be as volatile as they have been during the last few years? What proportion of the future population will have access to sufficient food to be healthy and productive and who will be food-insecure and malnourished? What action is needed to assure food security and good nutrition for all for the foreseeable future? Are there ways to improve the impact of existing food systems on food security and nutrition? Without in any way downplaying the importance of providing answers to the other questions posed here, this chapter is focused on the last one. This focus is justified by the belief that a better understanding of the relationships between food systems and human nutrition will offer opportunities for improving nutrition that are currently overlooked. Whether such opportunities are captured will depend on possible trade-offs with the achievement of other goals as well as on policy goals and political factors.

Contemporary Food Systems Issues Affecting Nutrition

Recent attempts (Ruel, 2001; Berti *et al.*, 2004; Leroy and Fongrillo, 2007; World Bank, 2007; Kawarazuka, 2010; Masset *et al.*, 2011) to evaluate the nutrition effects of agricultural projects have found very little or no impact. There are several plausible explanations for such findings, including the following. First, the projects may in fact not have had any impact on nutrition, either because the projects were poorly designed or implemented, because the projects were too small to have any measurable impact (there is a tendency to limit such evaluations to projects designed as controlled experiments) or because the most limiting constraint to improved nutrition in the particular households or cohort was not food but rather unclean water, poor sanitation, inappropriate childcare or infectious disease. Secondly, the nutrition goal of the project may have conflicted with the household or individual preferences, resulting in behaviour that pursued other goals at the expense

*Contact: pp94@cornell.edu

of potential nutrition effects. Thirdly, the evaluation methodology may have been inappropriate and, lastly, the time between the project intervention and the measurement of nutrition status may have been too short to identify an impact.

It would be grossly misleading to conclude, on the basis of these findings, that projects, policies and other changes in the food system generally do not influence nutrition. Solutions to nutrition problems are not found in narrowly defined, single agricultural projects, but rather in large changes to food systems that are not necessarily suitable for evaluation through experimental designs with randomized treatment and control groups. Programmes and policies aimed at changing food systems in particular need to do more than pursue curative approaches that do little to have an impact on the underlying determinants of nutrition problems. These large changes offer opportunities for very significant improvements. Unfortunately, they also present risks for nutritional deteriorations. Their impact may be very difficult to separate from the impact of other nutrition-related factors. There are several key contemporary issues for food systems of that nature, including the nine that are listed below. These must be taken into account in efforts to improve the impact of food systems on food security and nutrition.

1. Large fluctuations in food production and dramatic food price volatility lead to increases in transitory food insecurity and malnutrition, particularly among the poorest rural and urban populations, many of whom are already suffering from chronic food insecurity and high rates of child morbidity and mortality. These production fluctuations, which will cause fluctuations in food prices, are caused in large part by changing weather patterns, such as irregular rainfall and extreme weather events leading to droughts, floods, wind damage and resulting crop and animal losses. There is some evidence to support the notion that these changes in weather patterns are linked to long-term climate change. The impact on food price volatility is amplified by several factors: irrational or poorly informed expectations by speculators, traders and farmers; volatility in oil prices; the close relationship between food and oil prices through biofuel production and agricultural production costs; and government interventions in international food trade to protect government legitimacy, keep domestic food prices low to benefit domestic consumers and reduce producer incentives to expand production. This situation calls for improved risk management instruments. These include: more appropriate food trade rules; the discontinuation of subsidies and blending mandates for biofuel production that compete with food production for resources; investments in productivity-increasing and risk-reducing research and technology, rural infrastructure and domestic markets; and access to credit and social safety nets.

2. Large variations in the transmission of international food price changes to domestic markets make the estimation of the nutrition effects of international food price volatility difficult. The nutrition effects of volatility in international food prices depend on the extent to which international price changes are transmitted to the markets where the actual or potentially malnourished people buy or sell food. The food price transmission varies greatly among countries and over time. Two groups of countries are likely to have a relatively low food price transmission: the poorest countries, many of which are only weakly integrated with the international food markets; and large, middle-income countries, such as China and India. The latter may use trade policy, such as export restrictions or import subsidies, to reduce price transmission when international prices are high, e.g. the food price spikes during 2007–2008 and 2010–2011, so that domestic consumers are protected from large price fluctuations, while incentives and incomes for domestic farmers are reduced. Therefore, international food price changes may be a poor indicator of country-specific price changes. National and local factors may play a much bigger role than world market prices. The net nutrition effect of government intervention to avoid the transmission of international price spikes to the national market will depend on how many of the actual or potentially malnourished people consume more of the food for which the prices fluctuate and how many are net sellers of such food. In most developing countries, the majority of the actual and potentially malnourished people[1] are found among net buyers of food; they will gain from policies to avoid price spikes. These individuals are largely found in rural areas and most of them belong to farm families. Thus, it might be expected that trade policy to reduce the transmission of increasing international food prices would have a negative nutrition impact. However, many low-income farmers are net buyers of the main food staples that are traded internationally. So unless a higher food price permits them to expand production beyond their own needs, they would be affected negatively by increasing food prices. Actual or potentially malnourished people in countries that are significantly integrated with the international food markets, but are without the necessary political and economic power or desire to use trade policy to influence the price transmission, are likely to be more exposed to international price volatility than the two groups of countries mentioned above.

3. Although lower rates of population growth reduce the rate of increase in food demand, increasing demand for food resulting from higher incomes and the related desire for dietary changes will continue to put pressures on food markets. As such increasing demand is likely to be reflected in an increasing trend, with relatively little year-to-year fluctuation, it is not expected to contribute to price volatility. Demand for food commodities for biofuel may be an exception. Government policies and volatility in oil prices may, in fact, cause large disruptions in overall demand, as occurred during 2007–2008. Furthermore, blending mandates in the USA and the European Union (EU) remove a mandated amount of maize and other food commodities from the food market irrespective of the price, thereby amplifying price fluctuations in the food market. Rapidly increasing demand for foods of animal origin leads to increasing demand for feed, in addition to more obesity and chronic diseases, while at the same time increasing diet diversity and reducing micronutrient deficiencies. Increasing investments in rural infrastructure, research and technology are needed to reduce the unit costs of production, processing and marketing to meet deficiencies in dietary energy and nutrients, as well as reducing overweight, obesity and related chronic diseases. Fiscal policies may be needed to adjust the relative prices of various foods, if the expected dietary transition does not correspond to society's wishes.

4. Failure to pursue the sustainable management of natural resources and policies to mitigate and adapt to climate change is contributing to high levels of rural malnutrition because it undermines the production foundation for smallholder families, many of whom are at risk of malnutrition. A full costing approach, in which the costs associated with unsustainable use of natural resources and negative contributions to climate change are fully added to production costs, is warranted to reduce the risks of food production and income shortfalls among the rural poor. In some cases, this full costing will increase food prices in the short run, but many opportunities exist for triple wins, i.e. achieving nutrition and sustainability goals while lowering food prices (Pinstrup-Andersen and Watson, 2011). In the longer run, full costing will result in lower food prices because natural resource degradation will be reduced or avoided.

5. Complacency in developing country governments with respect to the meeting of future food needs and the associated failure to prioritize investments in sustainable, productivity-increasing research and technology, rural infrastructure and domestic rural markets has contributed to the continued large prevalence of malnutrition. A strong decreasing trend in food prices during the period 1974–2000 led to complacency and to a low priority allocated to investments in agriculture and rural areas. As mentioned above, large food price fluctuations during the last few years have caught the attention of policy makers in both developing and developed countries. International commitments to increased investments in agricultural development and improved food security culminated with commitments by G8 and other countries at the G8 Summit in L'Aquila, Italy, in 2009, to the amount of US$20 billion. A relatively small share of the commitment has been released bilaterally or through the Global

Agriculture and Food Security Program (GAFSP) and other vehicles. However, the follow-up to the L'Aquila meeting by the countries that made the commitments has been disappointing, although initiatives by the Gates Foundation, the US Agency for International Development (USAID), the UK Department for International Development (DFID), The World Bank and several other organizations have made significant contributions. Some developing country governments, e.g. China and Ethiopia, have also expanded investments in agriculture, rural development and improved food security, though many developing countries appear not to have made significant increases in such investments, and only a few of the African countries have achieved the agricultural investment goals agreed to within the NEPAD/CAADP (New Partnership for Africa's Development/Comprehensive Africa Agriculture Development Programme) framework.

6. The prioritization of expanded global and national food production instead of improved food security and nutrition may bypass opportunities to improve nutrition. Food production is a means to an end and not an end in itself. According to FAO (Food and Agriculture Organization of the United Nations), between 800 million and 1 billion people suffer from undernourishment, meaning that these people lack sufficient access to the dietary energy needed for a healthy and productive life. Many more suffer from insufficient intake of nutrients. The consequences of food price volatility are particularly severe for these people because they are close to or below long-term subsistence levels and they have few or no effective risk management tools. Making such tools available, including those mentioned above, must go hand in hand with investments and policies aimed at the expansion of global food supplies. Merely expanding food supplies may be of very limited benefit to these population groups unless their access to food with the required nutrients is enhanced. Pursuing the goal of expanded food production rather than food security or nutrition goals may in some cases result in a worsening of food security and nutrition. Recent and ongoing international land acquisition in low-income countries is an illustration of such a situation: capital-intensive agricultural production for export to middle-income countries displaces smallholder families from land that they cultivate but to which they have no legal title. Both food production and food insecurity are likely to increase in such situations.

7. Failure to explicitly incorporate gender-specific labour demand and power structures and the human health situation into the design and implementation of agricultural policies and projects overlooks potential nutrition benefits. On the assumption that rural areas in most developing countries contain many unemployed and underemployed workers, policies and technologies should be labour using rather that labour saving. Increasing rural employment would be expected to reduce poverty and improve food security and nutrition. However, from a food security and nutrition perspective, it is critically important to understand how these policies and technologies would affect women's labour demand and how increasing demand for women's time will affect other nutrition-related activities traditionally performed by women such as childcare, agricultural work, cooking and the fetching of water and firewood. Programmes and policies that provide new employment opportunities for women should be sensitive to women's need to provide childcare (e.g. by allowing for breastfeeding breaks and childcare assistance during working hours), and be combined with interventions that reduce women's labour demand in other activities without negative nutrition effects – such as improved access to water and fuel and childcare, and increased labour productivity in agricultural activities. Furthermore, the impact on women's control of household incomes and gender-specific decision making may be an important pathway between agricultural development and nutrition. The standard prescription of labour-using technology may also need revision in cases where illnesses such as HIV/AIDS, malaria and TB have reduced labour availability and labour productivity.

8. To enhance the nutrition effect, food systems activities should be designed and implemented with the target groups and the relevant pathways in mind. The characteristics of the specific target group may vary across countries, communities and time, but would generally be low-income households with pregnant and lactating women, children below the age of 2 years, and children and adults at risk of overweight, obesity and related chronic diseases. In many countries, poor rural households and households headed by women tend to show the highest prevalence of malnutrition. Efforts to reduce micronutrient deficiencies may extend beyond those target groups. The slogan 'the first 1000 days' has recently gained ground in the debate; it refers to the importance of assuring good nutrition for a fetus and the first 2 years of a child's life.

9. An integrated policy and investment approach for the food system, natural resource management, climate change and human health and nutrition is essential to achieve sustainable food security and good nutrition for all. Whether in policy making, training or research, the continuation of past and current separation of activities within disciplinary or sectorial compartments is no longer viable and must be replaced by a holistic problem-solving approach (Pinstrup-Andersen, 2010).

Food Systems and Nutrition: The Pathways and Policies

The section above identified a set of key contemporary food system-related issues that are likely to influence the nutrition of current and future generations. This section will address the pathways through which such influence may take place and how government interventions may guide the nutrition outcome. As mentioned above, food systems are a means to an end rather than ends in themselves. They exist to help people and societies meet a variety of goals, including but not limited to, food security and good nutrition.

A conceptual framework of a food system is presented in Fig. 2.1. The environment within which a food system operates may be divided into a human health environment, as well as biophysical, socio-economic, political and demographic environments. Each of these environments may embody goals such as

improved health and nutrition, higher incomes, the production of biofuel and the protection of natural resources, for example, land, water and biodiversity. The environments also present constraints and opportunities for a food system, which include poor health and nutrition of food system workers, inappropriate governance and policies, and agricultural technologies to expand productivity. The environments and the food system are connected by a set of two-way causal links. The environments have an influence on and are influenced by food systems. So, although food systems affect human nutrition, human nutrition affects food systems. The nutritional status of people affects their productivity and income earnings. A large percentage of poor and malnourished people work in the food system, and these people contribute to the low productivity of the system. Therefore, it can be argued that a productive food system begins with a well-nourished labour force interacting with natural resources, such as land, water and biodiversity, and food system inputs such as energy, plant nutrients and capital. A productive food system will, in turn, contribute to a well-nourished population, thus forming a virtuous cycle. A vicious cycle is created when the labour force is malnourished, leading to a low-productivity food system, poverty and poor nutrition.

There are multiple pathways through which the food system affects human nutrition. Understanding these pathways and how they operate is essential to designing agricultural and other food system policies to achieve nutrition goals. While much is said about the link between agriculture and nutrition, the fact is that each of the components of a food system – natural resource management and input use, primary production (agriculture), transport, storage and exchange, secondary production (food processing), and consumption, as shown in Fig. 2.1 – may influence nutrition. Irrespective of their starting point in the food system, most pathways work through the following five entry points: food availability, incomes, prices, knowledge and time allocation. The behaviour of food system agents, including consumers, farmers and traders, mitigate

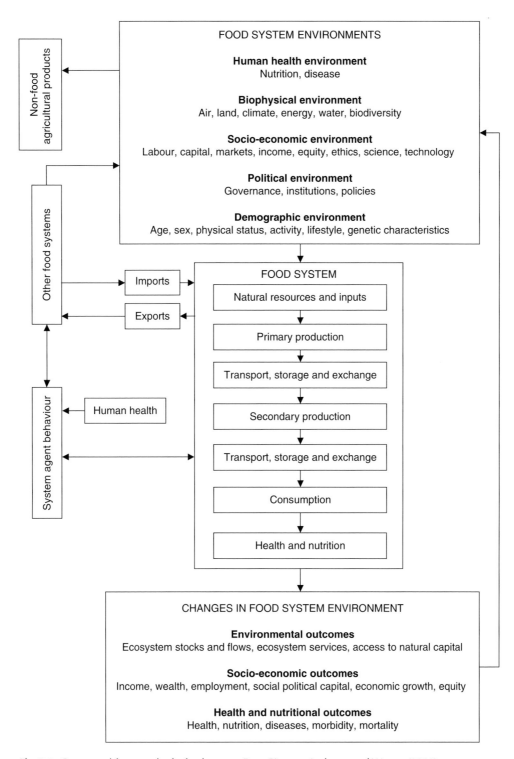

Fig. 2.1. Conceptual framework of a food system. From Pinstrup-Andersen and Watson (2011).

the nutrition effects linked to all five pathways. By being the entry points, these factors are key components of the pathways through which food systems may affect nutrition. However, as shown in Fig. 2.2, the nutrition effect of changes in any of these factors will depend on several other components of the pathways. Consequently, merely pursuing changes in food availability, incomes, food prices, knowledge, time allocation or

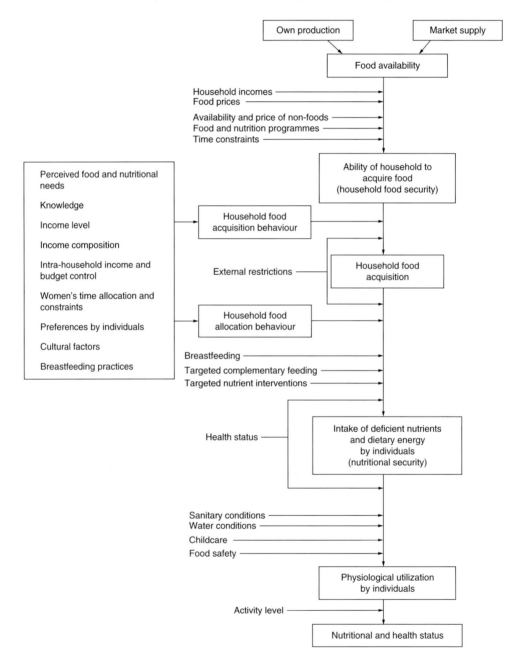

Fig. 2.2. A simplified conceptual framework linking food availability, food security and nutrition. From Pinstrup-Andersen and Watson (2011).

behaviour will not assure the desired nutrition effects. The complete pathway must be understood to help guide the food system for nutritional benefits. Each of the pathways associated with the five entry points is discussed below.

Food Availability

The availability of food is necessary but not sufficient to assure good nutrition. Although the scarcity of particular foods relative to demand would be expected to be reflected in relative prices, the private sector and government policies may remove or make available certain foods in the market. For example, trade liberalization may increase the availability of imported foods with undesirable characteristics, such as processed foods with a high content of fats and sweeteners. Investments in research and processing may develop new products beneficial or harmful to nutrition. Public and private investments in the food marketing sector may also improve food safety and quality. The availability of meat, dairy products, fruits and vegetables may reduce micronutrient deficiencies, while the availability of fats, oils, sugar, sweeteners and energy-dense, nutrient-poor foods may contribute to overweight, obesity and chronic diseases. A high degree of diversity in the food supply, whether from own production or the market, may facilitate consumption diversity and better nutrition.

Opportunities for enhancing consumption diversity, and in that way reducing micronutrient deficiencies, are particularly likely on semi-subsistence farms and isolated local wet markets where the diet may consist of one or two basic staples. Research and policy interventions to promote the production, marketing and consumption of so-called 'orphan crops', i.e. food crops to which little or no attention has been paid by researchers and policy makers, offer such an opportunity. The support of home gardens would be another initiative to be considered, as would promotion of the production, marketing and consumption of animal products such as beef, poultry, pork, goat and sheep meat, and milk.

In locations where water resources are available, the promotion of aquaculture may help to improve diet diversity and nutrition, through both fish and seafood consumption and income-generating sales.

The nutrition value of foods may also be improved by industrial fortification and biofortification. Industrial fortification may increase the price of food and make it less affordable. To be successful, biofortification depends on farmers' adoption of the fortified seed, and consumers' acceptance, ability and willingness to pay a higher price, if necessary. In addition to processing and fortification, the nutritional quality and safety of foods may be improved or reduced by action or lack of action in storage, transportation and other food system activities. Finally, waste and losses in the food supply and consumption chain are large. A recent assessment found that about one third of the food supply is wasted or lost (Gustavsson *et al.*, 2011); add to this the production lost to plant and animal diseases and pest attacks in farmers' fields, and the large opportunities for expanding the food available for actual consumption become obvious.

So, even though food availability is necessary for good nutrition, changes in food availability will not have any impact on nutrition unless the actual or potentially malnourished people have access to that food. As shown in Fig. 2.2, access, or the ability of households to acquire the food that is available, is influenced by income, own production, food prices, the availability and price of non-foods and social safety nets. These factors and the related behavioural aspects are discussed below.

Income

Changes in the food system may affect incomes of the actual or potentially malnourished people in several ways. First, research and technology may generate an economic surplus by improving the productivity of land, water or labour, not only in agriculture but in other parts of the food system. Depending on supply and demand, relative demand and supply elasticities, and market structure, conduct and performance, the surplus may result in higher incomes (in cash or kind) for farmers, traders and other food system agents, lower prices for consumers or, most likely, a combination of the two. This is exemplified by the effects of the Green Revolution, which lowered the unit costs of production of wheat and rice, increased farmers' incomes and lowered consumer prices. Research and technology may also improve the nutritional quality of foods, as exemplified by the above-mentioned biofortification. A second pathway through income that will change access to food relates to changes in labour demand, wages and access to productive resources, e.g. land and water, through labour-using technology, investments in rural infrastructure, changes in land tenure and water policies, and other fiscal and monetary policies. Thirdly, changes in the food system may change gender-specific income control as well as the composition of household incomes (cash or production for own consumption) and cash flow over time. Those changes will, in turn, influence household food acquisition behaviour and the extent to which access is converted to acquisition; they are also likely to influence the allocation of food within the household. Any increase in income and budget control by women is likely to increase the portion of household incomes dedicated to food, particularly as it relates to child feeding.

Prices

As mentioned above, changes in food and non-food prices will influence a household's purchasing power and, as such, its access to food. Changes in relative prices are also important. Lower prices for one food commodity relative to the price of another will usually increase consumption of the former and reduce the consumption of the latter. Technological changes in food production, processing and marketing that reduce unit costs, as well as commodity-specific taxes and subsidies and trade restrictions such as export restrictions and import duties, are examples of policy interventions that may change relative prices. Before such commodity-specific policies are proposed, it is important to clearly specify the nutrition problem to be solved: is it dietary energy deficiencies, micronutrient deficiencies or obesity-related chronic diseases?

Most developing countries experience all three of these problems. This makes the choice of price-related policies difficult. For example, taxes on meat, vegetable oil, sugar and sweeteners may reduce the risks of chronic disease among low-and high-income people, while increasing the deficiency of iron, essential fatty acids and dietary energy in low-income population groups. If these foods are highly preferred by low-income households, such taxes may also reduce purchasing power and the consumption of other foods that are beneficial for nutrition, such as fruits and vegetables. Subsidies on fruits and vegetables may release purchasing power that could be used to acquire foods of lesser or negative nutrient value, for example, drinks high in sweeteners. Increasing productivity and lower unit costs of production and marketing in addition to price subsidies for foods such as fruits, vegetables and animal source foods may reduce micronutrient deficiencies.

As already mentioned, food price fluctuations may be harmful to nutrition. Policies to strengthen price information for all food system agents would reduce fluctuations caused by poor market information. Farmer, consumer and trader associations may be useful for facilitating sound competition and avoiding hoarding in the food supply chain. Social safety nets are needed to protect the nutritional status and general well-being of low-income people.

Knowledge

Improved knowledge of nutrition and its relationship to the food system is needed for all food system agents, including consumers, farmers, traders and policy makers. Nutrition education for consumers has been a commonly used tool to improve nutrition, but with limited success. On the one hand, as might be expected, free-standing nutrition education programmes will only be successful where lack of knowledge is the most limiting factor for good nutrition. Educational efforts with all the right messages may be of no value if the new knowledge cannot be implemented because of time or income constraints. On the other hand, increased incomes, improved production diversity or reduced pressures on time may be of little or no nutrition value in the absence of the relevant knowledge. Therefore, nutrition education should, in most cases, be combined with other efforts to remove constraints to good nutrition. Improved knowledge of food storage, processing and transportation may be effective in improving nutrition and food safety.

In some cases, the achievement of nutrition goals may imply trade-offs with other goals, but win–wins are common and often overlooked. Examples of win–wins include investments in rural infrastructure (e.g. feeder roads and irrigation facilities), agricultural research, food processing technology and market information; these may increase food production, reduce unit costs of production and marketing, reduce consumer prices, increase farmer incomes and improve nutrition. Having nutritional improvements as one of the goals of interventions in the food system is preferable to the relegation of nutrition improvements to narrowly focused food system interventions with the sole objective of nutrition improvement. Nutrition should be mainstreamed in food system interventions instead of relegated to a set of small projects. This point relates back to the earlier point that the ability to use a controlled experimental design should not be a condition directing efforts to improve and assess the nutrition impact of food system interventions.

Time Allocation

Opportunities in the food system for improving – and potentially harming – the nutritional status of pregnant and lactating women and children during the first 2 years of life are often related to how the food system affects women's time allocation. Projects and policies often seek to empower women and improve their well-being, as well as that of

children, by attempting to generate employment. However, some food-system practices make breastfeeding, which is critically important during the first 6 months of life and beyond, very difficult, either because employment takes the lactating mother away from the baby for long periods or because the employment activities are otherwise incompatible with breastfeeding. Furthermore, employment creation by women may harm nutrition by reducing their time available for other important nutrition-related activities such as care, cooking, fetching water and firewood and agricultural work.

Thus, changes in the food system should consider the net effect of changes in women's time before introducing new demands for women's work. Ideally, *ex ante* estimates would be based on total household time, and efforts should be made to facilitate substitution among adults, e.g. between women and men. There is a general perception that women in poor households are overworked while men have time to spare. Although this may be so in many (most?) cases, it is important that it is assessed, along with the substitution possibilities in each specific situation, before making assumptions or introducing policies aimed at increasing gender-specific labour demand.

Introduction of labour-saving and productivity-enhancing technologies for the work traditionally done by women, such as herbicides to replace weeding, improved equipment for food processing, better access to water and fuel and rural infrastructure to improve food marketing and the time needed to bring food to the market as well as childcare facilities appropriate for the particular situation, are examples of actions that could be considered.

Conclusion

Neither the availability of sufficient food, nor household access to it, assures good nutrition. The extent to which food access is translated into actual food acquisition and improved nutrition is determined by household behaviour and the allocation of food within the household. In addition to the nutritional content of the food allocated to the individual and the extent to which it matches with needs, the nutrition effect of the allocated food depends on the quality of available water, on sanitation, on the prevalence of infectious diseases and on other nutrition-related factors. Therefore, the impact of changes in the food system on household food security (access) alone may not be a good indicator of nutrition impact. Poverty reduction, or changes in income, women's time allocation, prices and knowledge may likewise be poor nutrition indicators. These factors serve as entry points to the food system – to nutrition pathways, but do not themselves serve as proxies for nutrition impact.

While narrowly focused nutrition projects and food systems projects with the overriding goals of improved nutrition may contribute to good nutrition, the really important contributions offered by food systems are to be found in the way that they are managed by the private and public sectors. Nutritional improvements should be mainstreamed and integrated with other food system goals. Trade-offs between achieving nutrition goals and other goals should be identified and considered in both private and public policy priorities, as should win–wins. Governments, consumers, farmers and other food system agents should be informed about these potential win–wins as they appear locally, nationally and internationally, and governments should aim to move private goals closer to social goals through incentives, regulation and knowledge.

Note

[1]The term 'malnourished people' is used here to mean people who are deficient in dietary energy and/or nutrients. The prevalence of overweight, obesity and related chronic diseases – another kind of malnourishment – may also be affected by food price fluctuations and policy interventions through changes in relative prices among the various foods.

References

Berti, P., Krasevec, J. and FitzGerald, S. (2004) A review of the effectiveness of agricultural interventions in improving nutrition outcomes. *Public Health Nutrition* 7, 599–609.

Gustavsson, J., Cederberg, C., Sonesson, U., van Otterdijk, R. and Meybeck, A. (2011) *Global Food Losses and Food Waste: Extent, Causes and Prevention Study Conducted for the International Congress SAVE FOOD! at Interpack2011, Düsseldorf, Germany.* Food and Agriculture Organization of the United Nations, Rome.

Kawarazuka, N. (2010) *The Contribution of Fish Intake, Aquaculture, and Small-scale Fisheries to Improving Food and Nutrition Security: A Literature Review.* Working Paper No 2106, The WorldFish Center, Penang, Malaysia.

Leroy, J.L. and Frongillo, E.A. (2007) Can interventions to promote animal production ameliorate undernutrition? *Journal of Nutrition* 137, 2311–2316.

Masset, E., Cornelius, A., Haddad, L. and Isaza-Castro, J. (2011) *What is the Impact of Interventions to Increase Agricultural Production on Children's Nutritional Status? A Systematic Review of Interventions Aiming at Increasing Income and Improving the Diet of the Rural Poor.* Department for International Development, London.

Pinstrup-Andersen, P. (ed.) (2010) *The African Food System and its Interaction with Human Health and Nutrition.* Cornell University Press, Ithaca, New York.

Pinstrup-Andersen, P. and Watson, D. (2011) *Food Policy in Developing Countries: The Role of Government in Global, National, and Local Food Systems.* Cornell University Press, Ithaca, New York.

Ruel, M.T. (2001) *Can Food-based Strategies Help Reduce Vitamin A and Iron Deficiencies? A Review of Recent Evidence.* International Food Policy Research Institute (IFPRI), Washington, DC.

World Bank (2007) *From Agriculture to Nutrition: Pathways, Synergies and Outcomes.* Report No. 40196-GLB, Agriculture and Rural Development Department, The World Bank, Washington, DC.

3 Enhancing the Performance of Food-based Strategies to Improve Micronutrient Status and Associated Health Outcomes in Young Children from Poor-resource Households in Low-income Countries: Challenges and Solutions

Rosalind S. Gibson*

University of Otago, Dunedin, New Zealand

Summary

Sustainable food-based micronutrient interventions are needed in poor-resource settings, where the prevalence of coexisting micronutrient deficiencies and infection is high, especially during childhood. Food-based interventions include fortification, dietary diversification and modification (DDM) and biofortification. This review focuses on DDM strategies that aim to improve the availability, access and utilization of foods with a high content and bioavailability of micronutrients throughout the year. The strategies include: increasing the production and consumption of micronutrient-dense foods through agriculture, small animal production or aquaculture and, in the future, biofortification; incorporating enhancers of micronutrient absorption; and reducing absorption inhibitors. Such strategies must be designed using formative research to ensure that they are culturally acceptable, economically feasible and sustainable. DDM has the potential to prevent coexisting micronutrient deficiencies simultaneously for the entire household and across generations without risk of antagonistic interactions. To maximize the impact of DDM, especially among children in poor-resource settings, DDM should be integrated with public health interventions designed to reduce the risk of infections. Evidence of the impact of such integrated programmes needs to be strengthened by enhancing the design and monitoring and evaluation components. This can be achieved by applying a programme theory framework to identify pathways through which the programme is expected to exert its impact, and selecting the appropriate process, output and outcome indicators. To ensure sustainable impact on micronutrient status, growth and development, the DDM and public health strategies need to be combined with strategies that address the underlying causes of malnutrition, such as poverty alleviation, food security and income generation.

Introduction

More attention is needed to develop sustainable micronutrient interventions in poor-resource settings, where the prevalence of coexisting micronutrient deficiencies and infection is high, especially during childhood. Micronutrient deficiencies at this time can have

---

*Contact: rosalind.gibson@stonebow.otago.ac.nz

major adverse health consequences, contributing to impairments in growth, immune competence and mental and physical development (Viteri and Gonzalez, 2002), which cannot always be reversed by nutrition interventions.

The aetiology of micronutrient malnutrition is multifactorial, stemming initially from poverty and its many sequelae, such as household food insecurity, poor childcare and sanitation, and inadequate provision of health services. These lead to poor dietary intake and disease, which together result in micronutrient malnutrition (UNICEF, 1990). As a result, increasingly, integrated approaches that combine micronutrient interventions with public health strategies are used to combat micronutrient malnutrition, with the overall goal of enhancing child micronutrient status, growth and development. The micronutrient interventions that are commonly used are supplementation, fortification and dietary diversification and modification (DDM). In the future, the biofortification of staple crops – involving strategies to enhance both their micronutrient content and bioavailability – may become a feasible option for improving the micronutrient status of the entire household and across generations in poor-resource settings. For more details of this approach, the reader is referred to Hotz and McClafferty (2007).

Of these four approaches, fortification and DDM are food-based strategies that are widely used at the present time. Fortification can be a cost-effective method, with the potential to improve micronutrient status without any change in existing dietary patterns. Programmes can be implemented at the national level to improve the micronutrient status of the population, or targeted for specific population subgroups, such as the fortification of complementary foods for infants and young children. Complementary foods can be fortified centrally, or in the household, using complementary food supplements such as micronutrient powders – termed Sprinkles – and lipid-based micronutrient fortified spreads. Unlike Sprinkles, the lipid-based spreads provide a source of energy, protein and essential fatty acids as well as micronutrients (Nestel et al., 2003). The benefits of using either centrally processed micronutrient fortified foods or complementary food supplements in the home for enhancing micronutrient status and micronutrient-related functional outcomes have been assessed by Dewey and Adu-Afarwuah (2008) and Dewey et al. (2009), respectively.

In poor-resource settings, fortification may have limited lasting benefits because of problems with accessibility, affordability and reliance on continuing donor support. In such settings, DDM strategies developed by formative research and implemented using a participatory research process may be the preferred option. This chapter provides a critical review of interventions employing DDM strategies at the community or household level that have the potential to increase the intake of total and/or bioavailable micronutrients. The interventions that are included were identified from earlier reviews (Ruel, 2001; Berti et al., 2004; Leroy and Frongillo, 2007; Gibson and Anderson, 2009); details of the keywords used for the literature search are given in Gibson and Anderson (2009). Only those studies that included an indicator of consumption are included.

Dietary Diversification and Modification (DDM) Strategies

DDM is defined as changes in food production and food selection patterns, as well as traditional household methods for preparing and processing indigenous foods. The overall goal is to enhance the availability of, access to and utilization of foods with a high content and bioavailability of micronutrients throughout the year. Several studies have confirmed that the consumption of diets with a higher dietary diversity enhances food intake and, in turn, micronutrient intakes (WHO, 1998; Brown et al., 2002); such diets are accompanied by less negative height-for-age Z-scores, after controlling for household socio-economic status (Arimond and Ruel, 2004). Promoting dietary diversity also provides an important opportunity for infants and young children to appreciate different tastes and textures of foods, both critical attributes for developing good eating habits in the future (WHO, 1998).

The use of DDM has several other advantages. It has the potential to prevent coexisting micronutrient deficiencies simultaneously, without risk of antagonistic interactions, while at the same time being culturally acceptable, economically feasible and sustainable, even in poor-resource settings – provided that a participatory research process that focuses on building relationships with the community and involving them in their design and implementation is used. Additionally, DDM can enhance the micronutrient adequacy of diets for the entire household and across generations.

Several additional non-nutritional benefits may also be achieved through the community-based nature of DDM. These may include the empowerment of women in the community, training and income generation. To be successful, however, the approach requires major changes in attitudes, food-related behaviours and practices, and thus necessitates effective behaviour change and communication. Further, a multidisciplinary team of specialists in agriculture, nutrition epidemiology, rural extension, adult education, psychology and community health are required to assist with the design, implementation, monitoring and evaluation of DDM strategies. In the past, the design and the monitoring, and the evaluation protocols – when used – have often been limited and lacking in scientific rigour. Hence, despite apparent increases in the consumption of micronutrient-rich foods through promotional activities using nutrition education, social marketing and mass media campaigns, evidence for the impact of such interventions on biochemical and micronutrient-related functional outcomes has been limited, with the notable exception of vitamin A (Ruel, 2001). Table 3.1 summarizes the DDM strategies that can be used to combat micronutrient deficiencies among infants from 6 months of age and young children in low-income households. These are discussed below under various headings.

Increasing production, accessibility and consumption of micronutrient-rich foods through agricultural interventions

Of the ten agricultural interventions that were reviewed, all included an indicator of consumption, as well as indicators of production and accessibility in some cases; none were randomized controlled trials (RCTs). Of the ten interventions, eight were based on home gardening with a focus on vitamin A-rich fruits and vegetables; only one study (in Egypt) assessed the impact of increasing the consumption of staple cereals and legumes (Galal et al., 1987). Details of these studies are available in Ruel (2001), Berti et al. (2004), and Gibson and Anderson (2009). Intakes of vitamin A-rich fruits and vegetables were measured in most of the studies. In contrast, only four of them assessed intakes of vitamin A per se, and very few measured serum retinol ($n = 3$), or functional indicators of vitamin A status such as night blindness ($n = 3$).

It is of interest that all of the eight home gardening interventions that included a nutrition education component reported an increase in or greater intakes of vitamin A-rich foods, and sometimes of vitamin A intakes per se (if measured), depending on the intervention design. Although only one of these eight studies examined differences in intakes of vitamin A-rich foods (i.e. β-carotene-rich sweet potatoes) with and without nutrition education, the results clearly indicated a benefit of including nutrition education in the interventions (Hagenimana et al., 1999). The home gardening projects all involved women, and hence had the potential to generate income, and to be more readily integrated with nutrition education and behaviour change strategies, all of which are attributes that have been associated with positive nutrition outcomes.

However, several additional benefits arise when agricultural interventions include cereals and legumes as well as vitamin-A-rich fruits and vegetables. For example, substantial increases in the intakes of other important micronutrients besides provitamin A carotenoids, such as non-haem iron, zinc, copper, vitamin C (an enhancer of non-haem iron absorption), folate, thiamine, niacin, dietary fibre and phytochemicals will result, although the bioavailability of iron and zinc from plant-based foods will be poor, especially from cereals and legumes, owing to their high phytate content. In the future, more emphasis should be given to more comprehensive agricultural interventions that include cereal and

Table 3.1. Dietary diversification and modification (DDM) strategies to combat micronutrient deficiencies among infants from 6 months and young children in low-income households. Modified from Gibson *et al.* (1998a).

Strategy	Technical influence and impact
1. To increase production and consumption of micronutrient-rich foods via:	
Agriculture	Can increase intake of provitamin A-rich fruits and vegetables, as well as folic acid, ascorbic acid, dietary fibre and phytochemicals
Small livestock production or aquaculture	Can increase micronutrient density of foods, especially readily available haem Fe, Zn, B_{12}, B_6, B_2 (dairy), preformed vitamin A (liver), Ca (fish with bones and dairy). Animal source foods are a good source of high-quality protein
Biofortification	Can increase Fe and Zn content of cereals and β-carotene content of sweet potato, cassava, maize
2. To reduce intakes of absorption inhibitors:	
Phytate	Germination and fermentation induce phytase hydrolysis of phytic acid (myo-inositol hexaphosphate). Soaking results in passive diffusion of water-soluble Na and K phytates. Phytate binds Fe, Zn and Ca to form insoluble complexes in the gut which are poorly absorbed. Hence, reducing phytate enhances Zn, Fe and Ca absorption
Polyphenols	During germination, polyphenols complex with proteins. Soaking results in passive diffusion. Polyphenols form insoluble complexes with Fe Hence, reducing polyphenols enhances Fe absorption
3. To increase intakes of absorption enhancers:	
Cellular animal protein	Enhances non-haem Fe and Zn absorption. Mechanism is uncertain
Ascorbic acid	Enhances non-haem Fe absorption by forming an Fe-ascorbate, although its effect in a complete diet is less than from a single meal. May also enhance Se absorption
Low molecular weight organic acids	Have potential to enhance non-haem Fe and Zn absorption by forming soluble ligands with Fe and Zn in the gut, but there are no data from *in vivo* isotope studies
Fat	Enhances absorption of fat-soluble vitamins and provitamin A carotenoids
4. To promote exclusive breastfeeding to 6 months:	
	Breast milk is only dietary source of bioavailable Fe and Zn and other essential nutrients for exclusively breastfed young infants. Breastfeeding also protects against diarrhoea and respiratory infections
5. To promote safe and appropriate complementary foods (CFs) at 6 months + breastfeeding to at least 2 years:	
	At about 6 months of age, breast milk is no longer adequate to meet an infant's needs, so CFs with a high energy and micronutrient density must also be provided until the child is ready to consume family foods

legume staples as well as vitamin A-rich fruits and vegetables, with a design and indicators that permit them to be more rigorously monitored and evaluated. Only in this way can the evidence for their impact on micronutrient intakes, biomarkers and functional health outcomes be strengthened.

Enhancing micronutrient intakes and status by promoting animal production

Fifteen studies were reviewed, and these have been reported in detail elsewhere (Berti *et al.*, 2004; Leroy and Frongillo, 2007; Gibson and Anderson, 2009). Of these studies, four included aquaculture, five dairy production and three poultry production. The remaining three were integrated projects that also included nutrition education. The available evidence suggested that increasing the production of animal source foods through animal husbandry and/or aquaculture can increase the consumption of animal source foods in the household, particularly when nutrition education and/or behaviour change is a component of the intervention. This finding is important because animal source foods have the potential to contribute important and varying amounts (per 100 g; per MJ) of vitamin B_{12}, B_2, readily available haem iron and zinc, calcium and preformed retinol, depending on the type of animal source food consumed.

In most of the 15 studies reviewed, however, only a restricted range of micronutrient intakes were quantified, most notably protein, iron and vitamin A, and sometimes at the household and not at the individual level, so that intra-household allocation preferences could not be taken into account. Further, only four of the studies evaluated the impact of promoting animal production on biomarkers and/or functional indicators of micronutrient status. Of these, haemoglobin and anthropometry were measured most frequently, although in one study, serum ferritin and serum retinol were also measured (Smitasiri and Dhanamitta, 1999). Consistent increases in the incomes of households (but not caregivers), and/or expenditure were also noted when measured (6/6). Some increases in caregiver time and workload were also observed (2/4). Data at baseline or from a control group were not always collected in these studies, or even if they were collected, no details on the selection of a control or comparison group and its comparability to the intervention group at baseline were provided. Further, confounding factors and intermediary outcomes were often not appropriately checked. Hence, limitations in both the design and outcomes measured in these studies make it difficult to conclude that the production of animal source foods has an impact on micronutrient status and health-related outcomes, despite improvements in micronutrient intakes.

Enhancing micronutrient intakes, status and health in young children by promoting or supplying animal source foods in the diets

Eight studies were reviewed, of which five were non-blinded RCTs; details of these studies are given elsewhere (Gibson and Anderson, 2009). In six of these studies, consumption but not production of a range of animal source foods (e.g. chicken livers, eggs, meat or fish) was promoted through nutrition

education and behaviour change, whereas for the remaining two, animal source foods were supplied by the investigators. Results of the five RCTs provide strong evidence that the consumption of animal source foods based on red meat can enhance intakes of bioavailable haem iron and zinc and, in some cases, intakes of vitamin B_{12} and vitamin A. For example, in the RCT where a milk snack, and not meat, was supplied as the intervention, significant improvements in intakes of calcium, riboflavin, vitamin B_{12} and vitamin A were reported (Murphy et al., 2003); these were accompanied by an improvement in height in those Kenyan children with lower baseline height-for-age Z-scores (~1.4) compared with the control group. In contrast, improvements in weight (but not height), muscle mass and certain domains of cognitive functioning (Whaley et al., 2003) were reported in the children receiving the meat-based snack compared with the control group. Additional functional health outcomes that have been investigated include developmental outcomes (Krebs et al., 2006) and morbidity (Englemann et al., 1998).

Hence, it appears that promoting animal source foods can have positive impacts on lean body mass (based on arm muscle area), growth (weight, height or head circumference), cognitive functioning and, in some cases, behaviour (but not morbidity), depending on the source of the animal foods, even though these changes were not always accompanied by improvements in micronutrient biomarkers. The results of two studies in which stunting was significantly reduced (Guldan et al., 2000; Penny et al., 2005), emphasized the beneficial effects of including key educational messages to promote the consumption of animal source foods together with enhanced feeding and caring practices.

Enhancing micronutrient absorption by reducing intakes of absorption inhibitors

There is abundant evidence based on *in vivo* isotope studies that high levels of dietary phytate inhibit the absorption of iron, zinc and calcium to varying degrees, and that by reducing the phytate content of cereal-based diets, the absorption of zinc (Egli et al., 2004), and to a lesser extent of iron (Hurrell *et al.*, 2003) and calcium (Hambidge *et al.*, 2005), can be enhanced. Whether absorption of these minerals can also be enhanced through household strategies designed to reduce the phytate content of cereal-based diets is less certain. Phytate reductions of ~50% have been achieved through soaking pounded maize or maize flour or fermenting maize porridges (Hotz and Gibson, 2001). Moreover, increases in zinc, iron and calcium absorption have been achieved in men fed maize-based meals prepared from maize with a 60% reduction in phytate content compared with meals prepared with the wild-type maize, although the magnitude of the increase for iron and calcium is much less marked than that for zinc (Mendoza *et al.*, 1998; Hambidge *et al.*, 2004, 2005). Hence, these results suggest that some improvement in absorption, at least for zinc, is likely with a 50% phytate reduction, depending on the habitual diet and the study group (Gibson and Anderson, 2009).

Polyphenols, like phytate, form insoluble complexes with certain metal cations, and isotope studies have confirmed the inhibitory effect of polyphenols in tea on iron absorption (Brune *et al.*, 1989). Whether polyphenols inhibit the absorption of zinc and copper is less certain. The content of polyphenols in some cereals and legumes is said to be reduced through soaking (Chang *et al.*, 1977) or germination (Camacho *et al.*, 1992), but whether these polyphenol-reducing strategies have a positive impact on non-haem iron absorption *in vivo* has not been quantified. The inhibitory effect of polyphenols is independent of that of phytate (Hurrell *et al.*, 2003), and can be partly counteracted by consuming ascorbic acid in the same meal (Siegenberg *et al.*, 1991). Therefore, young children should be advised to avoid the consumption of polyphenol-containing beverages such as tea, coffee and cocoa with meals and replace them with vitamin C-rich drinks, fruits or vegetables.

Enhancing micronutrient absorption by increasing intakes of absorption enhancers

Several *in vivo* stable isotope studies have confirmed that flesh foods such as meat, fish or poultry enhance the absorption of non-haem iron (Cook and Monsen, 1976) and zinc (Jalla *et al.*, 2002) from plant-based foods, although the precise mechanism is uncertain. The relative enhancing effect of animal muscle proteins on non-haem iron absorption varies: beef apparently has the highest effect, followed by lamb, pork, liver, chicken and fish (Cook and Monsen, 1976). This enhancing effect is evident even in the presence of phytic acid, but its magnitude appears less when a meal is already high in ascorbic acid (Hallberg *et al.*, 1986).

Studies with cow's milk have not shown an enhancing effect on zinc absorption, attributed by some (Sandström *et al.*, 1983) to its high casein content. However, early radioactive studies based on single meals (Sandström and Cederblad, 1980) suggested that the addition of cellular animal protein counteracted the inhibitory effect of phytate on zinc absorption. In these early studies, the phytate content of the meals supplied varied, limiting the interpretation of these results. In a more recent radioactive isotope study in which phytate levels were controlled so that they were equal in both vegetarian and meat diets, no difference was observed in the fractional absorption of zinc in the two whole-day diets (Kristensen *et al.*, 2006). Nevertheless, the total amount of absorbed zinc was lower in the vegetarian diet, because, as expected, it had a lower content of total zinc than did the meat diet.

Ascorbic acid also enhances non-haem iron absorption from single meals, but the effect is much less pronounced from a complete diet (Cook and Reddy, 2001), and may explain why prolonged supplementation with vitamin C in community-based trials has not shown significant positive effects on iron status (Garcia *et al.*, 2003). The enhancing effect is attributed largely to the formation of an iron-ascorbate chelate in the acid milieu of the stomach, which prevents it from forming a complex with phytate or tannin; Teucher *et al.* (2004) have presented a detailed review. Ascorbic acid may also enhance the absorption of selenium (Mutanen *et al.*, 1985), but whether it affects the absorption of zinc or copper is less certain.

Based on *in vitro* data, other low molecular weight organic acids (e.g. citric and lactic acids) produced during fermentation have the potential to enhance non-haem iron and zinc absorption by forming soluble ligands with iron and zinc in the gut, thereby making them unavailable for binding with phytate to produce a complex. Moreover, the organic acids generate an optimal pH for the activity of any endogenous phytases in cereal or legume flours (Porres *et al.*, 2001). Based on the results of a study in human Caco-2 cells, the effect of organic acids on iron absorption depends on the type of organic acid, the molar ratio of organic acid to iron and the iron source (Salovaara *et al.*, 2002), and is less consistent than that of ascorbic acid. To date, however, evidence from *in vivo* isotope studies is lacking.

The available evidence then, suggests that the addition of even small amounts of red meat consumed with plant-based meals can lead to intakes of bioavailable iron and zinc that are likely to be much higher than the improvements that are likely to occur with non-haem iron or zinc absorption through the consumption of ascorbic acid-rich foods or fermented foods.

Enhancing micronutrient intakes, status and health-related outcomes by integrating dietary diversification and modification (DDM) strategies

The preferred approach to maximize the impact of DDM and overcome the dietary deficits of micronutrients likely to be present is to combine the DDM strategies listed in Table 3.1. This approach has been used in two studies involving infants and young children in rural Malawi (9–23 months old and 3–7 years old), in which the DDM strategies were promoted through nutrition education and social marketing, and employed a quasi-experimental design with a non-experimental control group; details are given elsewhere (Yeudall *et al.*, 2002, 2005; Hotz and Gibson, 2005). In the study on children aged 3 to 7 years, a comprehensive set of process, output and outcome indicators was used to monitor and evaluate the impact of DDM strategies implemented for 12 months. Post intervention, intakes of protein, zinc (but not iron), calcium and

vitamin B_{12} were significantly higher in the intervention than in the control group; this was attributed to increases in intakes of animal source foods (mainly small, whole, soft-boned fish), phytate reduction strategies and the use of germinated cereals to enhance the energy and nutrient density of maize-based porridges. The absence of any effect on iron intakes was attributed to the consumption of fish rather than meat as the major source of cellular animal food, and to the failure to account for the impact of the phytate reduction strategies on the estimates of iron bioavailability (Yeudall *et al.*, 2005). These dietary findings were also accompanied by a significantly enhanced anthropometric index of lean body mass (but not growth) and a lower incidence of both anaemia and common illnesses in the intervention than in the control group (Yeudall *et al.*, 2002).

These data suggest that a combination of DDM strategies can be designed to be feasible and acceptable to caregivers of infants and children in poor-resource households, provided that ongoing nutrition education and social marketing efforts are included to enhance their adoption and to empower the community to sustain them. Nevertheless, in the DDM study on infants and young children aged 9 to 23 months, despite higher intakes of zinc, iron and calcium post intervention (Hotz and Gibson, 2005), median intakes of these micronutrients did not meet the needs estimated by WHO (1998). These findings highlight the need for additional strategies in this age group to meet their high micronutrient requirements, such as the fortification of plant-based complementary foods in developing countries with calcium, iron and zinc; in this context, Gibson *et al.* (1998b) assessed the micronutrient densities of various complementary foods based on recipes from Africa, India, Papua New Guinea, the Philippines and Thailand.

Intervention programmes based on dietary diversification or modification

An integrated food-based approach has been adopted by Helen Keller International (HKI) and World Vision (WV) Malawi, although strategies to reduce phytate intakes were not included. The Homestead Food Production (HFP) Program of HKI integrates animal husbandry with home gardening and nutrition education to increase and ensure year-round availability and intake of micronutrient foods in poor households. The programme is focused on women and children, and was implemented first in Bangladesh, but has now been expanded into Nepal, Cambodia and the Philippines. Evaluation in all four countries has shown improved intakes of animal source foods in programme households, specifically of liver and eggs (Talukder *et al.*, 2010). In addition, more of the programme households earned income from the sale of HFP products. The prevalence of anaemia declined among children aged 6 to 59 months from both HFP and control households in all four countries at end line, but the magnitude of change was higher in households in the programme compared with those of the controls (Talukder *et al.*, 2010).

The Micronutrient and Health Programme (MICAH) of WV Malawi is another example of an integrated programme that also included public health interventions (e.g. the promotion and support of breastfeeding, and the control of infectious diseases, malaria and parasites), vitamin A and iron supplementation for young children, the consumption of iodized salt and nutrition and health education, along with dietary diversification strategies. The latter focused particularly on the production and consumption of dark-green leafy vegetables and orange-yellow fruits, and iron-rich animal source foods. Consumption of the latter was facilitated by a small animal revolving fund set up by WV which resulted in increases in both the production and consumption of guinea fowl, chickens, rabbits, eggs and goat's milk in the MICAH intervention households compared to the comparison group (Radford, 2005). Modest but significant reductions in both stunting (between 1996 and 2000), and anaemia among the children and women from the MICAH households were also achieved compared to the trends observed in the comparison group households (Kalimbira *et al.*, 2010a,b). Indeed, according to the recent

adequacy evaluation of the MICAH programme by Berti *et al.* (2010), the reduction in the prevalence of stunting (approximately 15%) approached the theoretical maximum reduction that would be predicted with the given interventions (Bhutta *et al.*, 2008). The contribution of the DDM strategies alone could not be evaluated in the WV MICAH programme. However, the findings suggest that the combined activities of the MICAH programme have the potential to reduce the prevalence of iodine deficiency among school-aged children, to reduce malaria and anaemia among women and preschoolchildren, and to improve growth among preschoolchildren (Berti *et al.*, 2010). Future improvements in the evaluation design of the HKI and WV programmes should strive for a 'plausibility' evaluation so that a more confident assessment of the impact of the programmes can be achieved.

Challenges of DDM Programmes and Possible Solutions to Maximize their Impact

Based on the studies included in this review, a combination of culturally appropriate DDM strategies that include agricultural interventions with animal husbandry or aquaculture, and implemented using a participatory research process, have the potential to increase intakes of absorbable iron and zinc, along with intakes of other limiting micronutrients such as vitamin B_{12}, vitamin A, vitamin C, folate, calcium and riboflavin, depending on the type of animal source food consumed. The magnitude of the increases, however, depends on many factors, including the age of the participants, their baseline nutritional status, the setting, the duration and type of interventions employed and their adoption rate, how well the individual components of the programme have been integrated, and whether the behaviour change communication has been effective. Whether the interventions also have a long-term impact on micronutrient biomarkers, and on micronutrient-related functional health outcomes, is less clear, because many of the studies reviewed did not evaluate these outcomes over the long term.

It is questionable whether the improvements in micronutrient intakes arising from a combination of DDM strategies will be sufficient to meet the micronutrient needs of infants, given their small gastric capacity, especially for the problem micronutrients – iron, zinc, calcium and vitamin A (WHO, 1998). This is an important consideration because improving nutrition during the first 2 years of life provides an opportunity to secure lasting and lifelong benefits (Ruel et al., 2008). Hence, for infants, ensuring an adequate energy intake and fortifying complementary foods with micronutrients are also necessary, provided that the effectiveness and sustainability of the strategies employed have been confirmed and that they are readily accessible to poor-resource households (Gibson et al., 1998b).

In resource-poor settings, the coexistence of chronic and acute infections can be of special concern. Infection may modify the response to an intervention through several mechanisms. These include impaired appetite, and thus reduced dietary intakes, and alterations in the integrity of the intestinal mucosa, causing increases in intestinal permeability and reductions in nutrient absorption (Bjarnason et al., 1995). Hence, to ensure maximum impact on micronutrient status and health-related outcomes in these settings, the interventions should always be combined with public health strategies, such as immunization, improvements in hygiene conditions, promotion of exclusive breastfeeding up to 6 months old, followed by the use of safe and appropriate complementary foods along with continued breastfeeding to at least 2 years.

In order to enhance the evidence base for interventions based on a combination of DDM and public health strategies, the design of the programmes, and their monitoring and evaluation components, need to be strengthened. In the past, RCTs have seldom been conducted, and control or comparison groups have often been omitted, or have not been comparable to the intervention group at baseline; furthermore, self-selection bias has been ignored, and few micronutrient-related functional responses have been measured.

It is recognized that in large-scale programmes of this type, logistical and ethical considerations often preclude the use of the optimal design – an RCT – to assess impact, so that a probability evaluation cannot always be made (Habicht et al., 1999). However, an alternative design involving two cross-sectional surveys that utilize a control group could be used to provide a plausible evaluation, and thus relatively strong evidence of impact, as long as care is taken to ensure the comparability of the control and intervention groups at baseline, and issues such as self-selection bias and seasonal variation are avoided; further details can be found in Habicht et al. (1999), Des Jarlais et al. (2004) and Victora et al. (2004).

To enhance the plausibility that the programme had its desired impact, a programme theory framework can be used. This framework will identify potential pathways through which a DDM programme is expected to exert its impact; an example based on the HKI HFP programme is given in Olney et al. (2009). The adoption of such a framework will ensure that the programme as designed has the potential to achieve the desired outcomes, and that the appropriate process, output and outcome indicators are included to monitor the provision of inputs, their utilization and coverage, and to evaluate exposure and impact. Attention must also be given to potential mediating and confounding variables to ensure that the necessary information is collected during the evaluation of the programme. Use of this approach can strengthen the evidence base of the impact of the integrated DDM programme on micronutrient status and show how that impact has been achieved, while at the same time providing valuable information for replicating the programme in other contexts.

Whether such integrated DDM programmes will be associated with a sustainable impact in the long term is uncertain. It is becoming increasingly clear that this goal will probably not be achievable unless the underlying causes of malnutrition highlighted in the UNICEF Conceptual Framework are also addressed at the same time. Hence, increasingly, multi-sectoral programmes are being implemented that combine targeted nutrition interventions such as DDM and public health strategies with those that address the underlying causes of malnutrition, such as poverty alleviation, food security enhancement and income generation.

Conclusion

Dietary diversification and modification has the potential to prevent coexisting micronutrient deficiencies, as long as the strategies include promoting the consumption of animal source foods using effective behaviour change and communication. Future DDM strategies, however, should be integrated with public health interventions to reduce the risk of infections and enhance the likelihood of impact. Nevertheless, even integrated DDM and public health interventions may not be sufficient to meet the high energy and nutrient needs of infants and young children because of their small gastric capacities. Hence, for these age groups, strategies to increase the energy density as well as

micronutrient density through micronutrient fortification of complementary foods may also be needed.

Integrated DDM and public health programmes should be designed to include appropriate indicators to monitor inputs, outputs, outcomes and confounders, identified through a programme theory framework. The design of these programmes should be more rigorous and ensure that a probability evaluation can be achieved. Such an approach will provide stronger evidence of their impact, together with an understanding of how the impact was achieved. Impact should be evaluated by measuring micronutrient intakes as indicators of exposure, along with micronutrient biomarkers and associated functional health outcomes. Future targeted DDM and public health interventions should be combined with those that address the underlying causes of malnutrition, such as poverty alleviation, food security enhancement and income generation so as to ensure more sustainable improvements in micronutrient malnutrition (Leroy *et al.*, 2008).

References

Arimond, M. and Ruel, M.T. (2004) Dietary diversity is associated with child nutritional status: evidence from 11 demographic and health surveys. *Journal of Nutrition* 134, 2579–2585.

Berti, P.R., Krasevec, J. and FitzGerald, S. (2004) A review of the effectiveness of agriculture interventions in improving nutrition outcomes. *Public Health Nutrition* 7, 599–609.

Berti, P.R., Mildon, A., Siekmans, K., Main, B. and MacDonald, C. (2010) An adequacy evaluation of a 10-year, four-country nutrition and health programme. *International Journal of Epidemiology* 39, 613–629.

Bhutta, Z.A., Ahmed, T., Black, R.E., Cousens, S., Dewey, K., Giugliani, E., Haider, B.A., Kirkwood, B., Morris, S.S., Sachdev, H.P.S. and Shekar, M. for the Maternal and Child Undernutrition Study Group (2008) What works? Interventions for maternal and child undernutrition and survival. *The Lancet* 371, 417–440.

Bjarnason, I., Macpherson, A. and Hollander, D. (1995) Intestinal permeability: An overview. *Gastroenterology* 108, 1566–1581.

Brown, K.H., Peerson, J.M., Kimmons, J.E. and Hotz, C. (2002) Options for achieving adequate intake from home-prepared complementary foods in low income countries. In: Black, R.E. and Fliescher Michaelson, K. (eds) *Public Health Issues in Infant and Child Nutrition*, Nestlé Nutrition Workshop Series, Pediatric Program Volume 48, Lippincott Williams and Wilkins, Philadelphia, Pennsylvania/Nestec Ltd, Vevey, Switzerland, pp. 239–256.

Brune, M.L., Rossander, L. and Hallberg, L. (1989) Iron absorption and phenolic compounds: importance of different phenolic structures. *European Journal of Clinical Nutrition* 43, 547–557.

Camacho, L., Sierra, C., Campos, R., Guzman, E. and Marcus, D. (1992) Nutritional changes caused by germination of legumes commonly eaten in Chile. *Archivos Latinoamericanos de Nutrición* 42, 283–290.

Chang, R., Schwimmer, S. and Burr, H.K. (1977) Phytate: removal from whole dry beans by enzymatic hydrolysis and diffusion. *Journal of Food Science* 42, 1098–1101.

Cook, J.D. and Monsen, E.R. (1976) Food iron absorption in human subjects. III. Comparison of the effect of animal proteins on nonheme iron absorption. *The American Journal of Clinical Nutrition* 29, 859–867.

Cook, J.D. and Reddy, M.B. (2001) Effect of ascorbic acid intake on nonheme-iron absorption from a complete diet. *The American Journal of Clinical Nutrition* 73, 93–98.

Des Jarlais D.C., Lyles, C., Crepaz, N. and the TREND Group (2004) Improving the reporting quality of nonrandomized evaluations of behavioral and public health interventions: the TREND statement. *American Journal of Public Health* 94, 361–366.

Dewey, K.G. and Adu-Afarwuah, S. (2008) Systematic review of the efficacy and effectiveness of complementary feeding interventions in developing countries. *Maternal and Child Nutrition* 4(Suppl. 1), 24–85.

Dewey, K.G., Yang, Z. and Boy, E. (2009) Systematic review and meta-analysis of home fortification of complementary foods. *Maternal and Child Nutrition* 5, 283–321.

Egli, I., Davidsson, L., Zeder, C., Walczyk, T. and Hurrell, R. (2004) Dephytinization of a complementary food based on wheat and soy increases zinc, but not copper, apparent absorption in adults. *Journal of Nutrition* 134, 1077–1080.

Engelmann, M.D.M., Sandström, B. and Michaelsen, K.F. (1998) Meat intake and iron status in late infancy: an intervention study. *Journal of Pediatric Gastroenterology and Nutrition* 26, 26–33.

Galal, O.M., Harrison, G.G., Abdou, A.I. and Zein el Abedin, A. (1987) The impact of a small-scale agricultural intervention on socio-economic and health status. *Food and Nutrition Bulletin* 13, 35–43.

Garcia, O.P., Diaz, M., Rosado, J.L. and Allen, L.H. (2003) Ascorbic acid from lime juice does not improve the iron status of iron-deficient women in rural Mexico. *The American Journal of Clinical Nutrition* 78, 267–273.

Gibson, R.S. and Anderson, V.P. (2009) A review of interventions based on dietary diversification/modification strategies with the potential to enhance intakes of total and absorbable zinc. *Food and Nutrition Bulletin* 30, S108–S143.

Gibson, R.S., Yeudall, F., Drost, N., Mtitimuni, B. and Cullinan, T. (1998a) Dietary interventions to prevent zinc deficiency. *The American Journal of Clinical Nutrition* 68, 484S–487S.

Gibson, R.S., Ferguson, E.L. and Lehrfeld, J. (1998b) Complementary foods for infant feeding in developing countries: their nutrient adequacy and improvements. *European Journal of Clinical Nutrition* 52, 764–770.

Guldan, G.S., Fan, H., Ma, X., Ni, Z., Xiang, X. and Tang, M. (2000) Culturally appropriate nutrition education improves infant feeding and growth in rural Sichuan China. *Journal of Nutrition* 130, 1204–1211.

Habicht, J.P., Victora, C.G. and Vaughan, J.P. (1999) Evaluation designs for adequacy, plausibility and probability of public health programme performance and impact. *International Journal of Epidemiology* 28, 10–18.

Hagenimana, V., Oyunga, M.A., Lo, J., Njoge, S.M., Gichuki, S.T. and Kabira, J. (1999) *The Effects of Women Farmer's Adoption of Orange-fleshed Sweet Potatoes: Raising Vitamin A Intake in Kenya.* Research Reports Series No. 3, International Center for Research on Women, Washington, DC.

Hallberg, L., Brune, M. and Rossander, L. (1986) Effect of ascorbic acid on iron absorption from different types of meals. Studies with ascorbic acid-rich foods and synthetic ascorbic acid given in different amounts with different meals. *Human Nutrition: Applied Nutrition* 40, 97–113.

Hambidge, K.M., Huffer, J.W., Raboy, V., Grunwald, G.K., Westcott, J.L., Miller, L.V., Dorsch, J.A. and Krebs, N.F. (2004) Zinc absorption from low-phytate hybrid of maize and their wild-type isohybrids. *The American Journal of Clinical Nutrition* 79, 1053–1059.

Hambidge, K.M., Krebs, N.F., Westocott, J.L., Sian, L., Miller, L.V., Peterson, K.L. and Raboy, V. (2005) Absorption of calcium from tortilla meals prepared from low-phytate maize. *The American Journal of Clinical Nutrition* 82, 84–87.

Hotz, C. and Gibson, R.S. (2001) Assessment of home-based processing methods to reduce phytate content and phytate/zinc molar ratios of white maize (*Zea mays*). *Journal of Agricultural and Food Chemistry* 49, 692–698.

Hotz, C. and Gibson, R.S. (2005) A participatory nutrition education intervention improves the adequacy of complementary diets of rural Malawian children: a pilot study. *European Journal of Clinical Nutrition* 59, 226–237.

Hotz, C. and McClafferty, B. (2007) From harvest to health: challenges for developing biofortified staple foods and determining their impact on micronutrient status. *Food and Nutrition Bulletin* 28(2, Suppl.), S271–S279.

Hurrell, R.F., Reddy, M.B., Juillerat, M-A. and Cook, J.D. (2003) Degradation of phytic acid in cereal porridges improves iron absorption by human subjects. *The American Journal of Clinical Nutrition* 77, 1213–1219.

Jalla, S., Westcott, J., Steirn, M., Miller, L.V., Bell, M. and Krebs, N.F. (2002) Zinc absorption and exchangeable zinc pool size in breast-fed infants fed meat or cereal as first complementary food. *Journal of Pediatric Gastroenterology and Nutrition* 34, 35–41.

Kalimbira, A., MacDonald, C. and Randall Simpson, J. (2010a) The impact of an integrated community-based micronutrient and health programme on stunting in Malawian preschool children. *Public Health Nutrition* 13, 720–729.

Kalimbira, A., MacDonald, C. and Randall Simpson, J. (2010b) The impact of an integrated community-based micronutrient and health programme on anaemia in non-pregnant Malawian women. *Public Health Nutrition* 13, 1445–1452.

Krebs, N.F., Westcott, J.E., Butler, N., Robinson, C., Bell, M. and Hambidge, K.M. (2006) Meat as a first complementary food for breastfed infants: feasibility and impact on zinc intake and status. *Journal of Pediatric Gastroenterology and Nutrition* 42, 207–214.

Kristensen, M.B., Heks, O., Morberg, C.M., Marving, J., Bügel, S. and Tetens, I. (2006) Total zinc absorption in young women, but not fractional zinc absorption, differs between vegetarian and meat-based diets with equal phytic acid content. *British Journal of Nutrition* 95, 963–967.

Leroy, J.L. and Frongillo, E.A. (2007) Can interventions to promote animal production ameliorate undernutrition? *Journal of Nutrition* 137, 2311–2316.

Leroy, J.L., Ruel, M., Verhofstadt, E. and Olney, D. (2008) *The Micronutrient Impact of Multisectoral Programs Focusing on Nutrition: Examples from Conditional Cash Transfer, Microcredit with Education, and Agricultural Programs,* October 25, 2008. Report prepared for the Innocenti Review, 5 November 2008. Micronutrient Forum, Washington, DC. Available at: http://www.micronutrientforum.org/innocenti/Leroy-et-al-MNF-Indirect-Selected-Review_FINAL.PDF (accessed 29 May 2013).

Mendoza, C., Viteri, F.E., Lonnerdal, B., Young, K.A., Raboy, V. and Brown, K.H. (1998) Effect of genetically modified, low-phytic acid maize on absorption of iron from tortilla. *The American Journal of Clinical Nutrition* 68, 1123–1127. Erratum in *The American Journal of Clinical Nutrition* (1999) 69, 743.

Murphy, S.P., Gewa, C., Liang, L.L., Grillenberger, M., Bwibo, N.O. and Neumann, C. (2003) School snacks containing animal source foods improve dietary quality for children in rural Kenya. *Journal of Nutrition* 133, 3950S–3957S.

Mutanen, M. and Mykkanen, H.M. (1985) Effect of ascorbic acid supplementation on selenium bioavailability in humans. *Human Nutrition: Clinical Nutrition* 39, 221–226.

Nestel, P., Briend, A., de Benoist, B., Decker, E., Ferguson, E., Fontaine, O., Micardi, A. and Nalubola, R. (2003) Complementary food supplements to achieve micronutrient adequacy for infants and young children. *Journal of Pediatric Gastroenterology and Nutrition* 36, 316–328.

Olney, D.K., Talukder, A., Iannotti, L.L., Ruel, M.T. and Quinn, V. (2009) Assessing impact and impact pathways of a homestead food production program on household and child nutrition in Cambodia. *Food and Nutrition Bulletin* 30, 355–369.

Penny, M.E., Creed-Kanashiro, H.M., Robert, R.C., Narrow, M.R., Caulfield, L.E. and Black, R.E. (2005) Effectiveness of an educational intervention delivered through health services to improve nutrition in young children: a cluster-randomised controlled trial. *The Lancet* 365, 1863–1872.

Porres, J.M., Etcheverry, P. and Miller, D.D. (2001) Phytate and citric acid supplementation in whole-wheat bread improves phytate-phosphorus release and iron dialyzability. *Journal of Food Science* 66, 614–619.

Radford, K.B. (2005) *World Vision Malawi's Micronutrient and Health (MICAH) Program. Small animal revolving fund.* World Vision Canada, Mississauga, Ontario.

Ruel, M.T. (2001) *Can Food-based Strategies Help Reduce Vitamin A and Iron Deficiencies? A Review of Recent Evidence.* International Food Policy Research Institute (IFPRI), Washington, DC.

Ruel, M.T., Menon, P., Habicht, J.P., Loechl, C., Bergeron, G., Pelto, G., Arimond, M., Maluccio, J., Michaud, L. and Hankebo, B. (2008) Age-based preventive targeting of food assistant and behaviour change and communication for reduction of childhood undernutrition in Haiti: a cluster randomized trial. *The Lancet* 371, 588–595.

Salovaara, S., Sandberg, A.-S. and Andlid, T. (2002) Organic acids influence iron uptake in the human epithelial cell line Caco-2. *Journal of Agricultural and Food Chemistry* 50, 6233–6238.

Sandström, B. and Cederblad, Å. (1980) Zinc absorption from composite meals. II. Influence of the main protein source. *The American Journal of Clinical Nutrition* 33, 1778–1783.

Sandström, B., Cederblad, Å. and Lönnerdal, B. (1983) Zinc absorption from human milk, cow's milk and infant formulas. II. Influence of the main protein source. *The American Journal of Diseases of Children* 137, 726–729.

Siegenberg, D., Baynes, R.D., Bothwell, T.H., Marfarlane, B.J., Lamparelli, R.D., Car, N.G., MacPhail, P., Schmidt, U., Tal, A. and Mayet, F. (1991) Ascorbic acid prevents the dose-dependent inhibitory effects of polyphenols and phytates on nonheme iron absorption. *The American Journal of Clinical Nutrition* 53, 537–541.

Smitasiri, S. and Dhanamitta, S. (1999) *Sustaining Behaviour Change to Enhance Micronutrient Status: Community and Women-based Interventions in Thailand.* Research Report No. 2, International Center for Research on Women/Opportunities for Micronutrient interventions, Washington, DC.

Talukder, A., Haselow, N.J., Osei, A.K., Villate, E., Reario, D., Kroeun, H., SokHoing, L., Uddin, A., Dhungel, S. and Quinn, V. (2010) Homestead food production model contributes to improved household food security and nutrition status of young children and women in poor populations – lessons learned from scaling-up programs in Asia (Bangladesh, Cambodia, Nepal and Philippines). In: Duchemin, M. (ed.) *Field Actions Science Reports (FACTS Reports), Special Issue 1, 2010: Urban Agriculture.* Institut Veolia Environnement, Paris. Available online at: http://factsreports.revues.org/index404.html (accessed November 2010).

Teucher, B., Olivares, M. and Cori, H. (2004) Enhancers of iron absorption: ascorbic acid and other organic acids. *International Journal of Vitamin Nutrition Research* 74, 403–419.

UNICEF (1990) *Strategy for Improved Nutrition of Children and Women in Developing Countries.* United Nations Children's Fund, New York.

Victora, C.G., Habicht, J.-P. and Bryce, J. (2004) Evidence-based public health: moving beyond randomized trials. *American Journal of Public Health* 94, 400–405.

Viteri, F.E. and Gonzalez, H. (2002) Adverse outcomes of poor micronutrient status in childhood and adolescence. *Nutrition Reviews* 60, S77–S83.

Whaley, S.E., Sigman, M., Neumann, C., Bwibo, N., Guthrie, D., Weiss, R.E., Alber, S. and Murphy, S.P. (2003) The impact of dietary intervention on the cognitive development of Kenyan school children. *Journal of Nutrition* 133, 3965S–3971S.

WHO (1998) *Complementary Feeding of Young Children in Developing Countries: A Review of Current Scientific Knowledge.* World Health Organization, Geneva, Switzerland.

Yeudall, F., Gibson, R.S., Kayira, C. and Umar, E. (2002) Efficacy of a multi-micronutrient dietary intervention based on haemoglobin, hair zinc concentrations, and selected functional outcomes in rural Malawian children. *European Journal of Clinical Nutrition* 56, 1176–1185.

Yeudall, F., Gibson, R.S., Cullinan, T.R. and Mtimuni, B. (2005) Efficacy of a community-based dietary intervention to enhance micronutrient adequacy of high-phytate maize-based diets of rural Malawian children. *Public Health Nutrition* 8, 826–836.

4 Food-based Approaches for Combating Malnutrition – Lessons Lost?

Ted Greiner*

Hanyang University, Seoul, Republic of South Korea

Summary

This chapter describes programmes that focused on dietary quality in Tanzania, Zimbabwe and Bangladesh, a crucial but neglected part of food and nutrition security. These programmes utilized various approaches and were all in some way successful though, as usual, valuable lessons often come from dealing with unexpected difficulties that frequently arise, especially in such large-scale programmes as most of these were. Although some of these programmes are no longer in operation, the lessons they taught are still valuable and are reported here because they are generally not among the better known projects that have been repeatedly reported at international meetings. The chapter also reports on research illuminating why food-based approaches commonly do not seem to work well to improve human nutrient status and what can be done to improve such projects. Carotenes, by far the main source of vitamin A in low-income diets, tend to be poorly absorbed, but adding small amounts of fat and doing routine deworming will correct much of this problem; both of these options are very low in cost and convey additional benefits. Similarly, consuming vitamin C-rich foods at or close to meal times is a feasible way to improve iron absorption from plant foods. Early studies have shown little impact of this approach, but a recent trial using a fruit like guava with a higher vitamin C content has shown potential. One hopes that further research in real-life settings will further elucidate how such findings can best be incorporated into future food-based programming.

Introduction

Food-based approaches not only work to improve nutritional status, they can achieve a number of other objectives, including an increase in incomes. This makes such approaches among the most attractive and sustainable nutrition interventions available, yet they have been widely neglected for decades, especially by the health sector, which often considers them to belong to the agricultural domain, rather than as something that can improve long-term health and nutritional outcomes. Another reason for this neglect is the widely promoted (and often exaggerated) evidence from a few research trials that have found disappointing short-term impacts of food-based studies on nutrient status. This chapter provides details from unpublished and/or poorly publicized large-scale food-based programmes in Tanzania, Zimbabwe and Bangladesh, as well as from research suggesting that food-based approaches can work, including their use for improving micronutrient status. The chapter

*Contact: tedgreiner@yahoo.com

focuses on hard-won practical lessons learned that need to be highlighted to prevent them from being lost. Some of these efforts ended years ago; others may still continue in some form but have not been reported upon recently. However, the lessons learned in the past are still largely valid today.

Tanzania

In my experience, when governments can choose (i.e. when spending their own money or donor money that is not too tightly earmarked), they choose food-based approaches for nutrition interventions. The preference is usually to improve diets sustainably in the long run, focusing as much as possible on the lowest income or most nutritionally vulnerable populations. This is particularly true in a country such as Tanzania where local resources are especially scarce, and the use of donor funds can be valuable in the long term (mainly) when it generates permanent improvements in people's lives.

Brief discussions are presented here of three food-based pilot trials. The district level proved to be the smallest scale likely to provide realistic information on costs as well as on management and training needs for scale up. When pilot projects are smaller in scale than this, costs may be so much higher that scale up seems too expensive; management quality also tends to be so much higher per participant that scaling up can result in disappointingly poor-quality programme outcomes.

While funded by other donors, the three programmes discussed benefited indirectly from substantial support from the Swedish International Development Cooperation Agency (Sida) to the Tanzania Food and Nutrition Centre (TFNC), a parastatal to the Ministry of Health (MOH). The Sida funding was relatively non-earmarked, with the overall aim of institution building and capacity building from the time of TFNC's founding in 1973 until 2000. The current increased attention to nutrition, certainly otherwise a positive development, may not be giving enough attention to the kind of slow, patient effort that is required to build countries' capacity, focusing instead on their existing 'readiness' to improve their nutrition situation (Nishida *et al.*, 2009).

School gardening and feeding

In the early 1980s, UNICEF (United Nations Children's Fund) supported a district-wide school feeding programme in one of the dry (and thus more vitamin A deficient) central regions, Dodoma. Each participating school needed to have land allocated adjacent to the school that could be used for a large school garden. UNICEF funds were used to 'sensitize' relevant officials and staff in the three key sectors (health, agriculture and education), train a teacher in each school and provide gardening tools, large-scale cooking utensils and a first allotment of seed and seedlings. Each school's land was divided into four plots, one each for growing maize, beans, vegetables and fruit.

Improvement of the nutritional status of schoolchildren was a major priority of the programme, but two other considerations were also important. First, in a largely rural country such as Tanzania where most children do not study beyond elementary school, schools need to teach what is most likely to improve their families' lives – improved agricultural practices, including the use of appropriate technology for food processing and storage and, where possible, offering practical opportunities to learn and practice agricultural skills under trained supervision. Secondly, when schools do not provide food, children cannot attend for very many hours each day, so the provision of food from the programme at school was important. Even among schools that did not manage to achieve the levels of food production required for daily school feeding, at times of important exams, children were fed and the schools kept open longer hours.

Parents were brought together and the programme explained to them, including the roles they would have to play. Messages would be sent home whenever school lunch was to be provided, and on those days each child was to bring a plate, a spoon and a piece of firewood to school. The village health committees were engaged, asked to give additional attention to providing better sanitation and safe water access for participating schools and also to take responsibility for cooking the food on school feeding days and ensuring that hygiene and food safety received appropriate attention.

A few years after project funding ended, district education sector officials told a TFNC evaluation team (Burgess *et al.*, 1986) that most schools still maintained the gardens, although most could not grow enough to feed the children all year round. Perhaps the greatest constraint to this approach is that someone must tend, protect and maintain these quite large gardens even when school is not in session. In the kinds of areas where the gardens are most needed (i.e. where rain is scarce and soil fertility low), a substantial proportion of the harvest must be used to invest in next year's crops and to pay for the labour that cannot be provided by the teachers and children if the garden is to remain viable year after year.

Vitamin A programmes

In the late 1980s, the World Bank's International Development Association (IDA) offered Tanzania substantial multi-year interest-free loans for two national programmes – one to combat anaemia and the other to combat vitamin A deficiency. The MOH was the collaborating partner. In contrast to the much more common donor approach (offering countries the choice between vitamin A capsules or nothing), when donors avoid tight earmarking they strengthen local decision-making processes.

To plan these programmes, TFNC called national meetings, bringing together all relevant domestic experts and two or three nutritionists or other regional specialists from each of the 20 mainland provinces (called regions) and Zanzibar. TFNC did not view these problems narrowly but brought in all relevant sectors. After technical presentations had been completed and appropriate debates had taken place, it was decided that two of the three vitamin A programmes deserving the highest priority should be food based. The third was to provide a short training programme to one staff member from each health facility on the existing disease-based vitamin A capsule programme, which was linked to the essential drug programme. The first two programmes are briefly described below.

Strengthening the red palm oil industry in one district

Red palm oil has extremely high levels of well-absorbed β-carotene but in much of Tanzania harvests were low, largely owing to a lack of simple equipment. An earlier assessment by FAO (Food and Agriculture Organization of the United Nations) had recommended how the constraints could best be redressed. Kyela, a district with high potential, was chosen, and a needs assessment among palm tree plantation owners and a study of the market were conducted.

It was found that local demand and willingness to pay far outstripped producers' ability to produce and market red palm oil with keeping qualities adequate for the long timespans required to harvest, process, transport and sell the product. Facilities for refining and adequately packaging the oil were rudimentary, if they existed at all. Nuts were often crushed manually and consumers came to sales points with their own bottles, speeding up spoilage when rancid residues had not been adequately removed.

While improved production technology deserved priority, its cost was beyond what the loan could cover. TFNC thus decided to attempt a two-step process. Trucks for transport from the plantation to the processing site were provided and the many small producers were encouraged to form cooperatives that could make optimal use of them. Assuming that this could increase profits, improved processing equipment could then be jointly purchased. However, within the health sector, such an ambitious approach proved not to be feasible in such a short time and with so little funding, in part because of the management skills required to build viable cooperatives among so many small, competing growers.

Exploring how to build the demand and year-round supply of low-cost high-carotene foods

This pilot trial was conducted in two divisions in another dry region of Tanzania – Singida. Some training was provided to all villagers, some to leaders and some to selected women. Training covered the importance of vitamin A, the importance of optimal early breastfeeding practices, which fruits and vegetables were good sources of carotene and how to grow, preserve and cook them. The schools were provided with seeds and trained to grow mango and papaya seedlings and to sell them at prices that would ensure sustainability, but which local farmers were quite willing to pay. Again, local demand for these high-carotene foods was far above supply because growers lacked access to seedlings and the knowledge of how to grow them. The project also provided solar driers to 44 of the villages.

Baseline vitamin A and dietary assessments were done in one division and in a nearby control division of the same size. An evaluation 5 years after project funding ended (Kidala *et al.*, 2000) found that about half of the schools were still growing and selling seedlings. All but one of the solar driers were still in use. Over twice as many households in the project area were still growing the high-carotene crops promoted by TFNC as there were in the control division (67% versus 31%). The consumption of green leaves was associated with increased serum retinol ($P = 0.01$) and nearly twice as many children in the project area consumed green leaves ≥ 7 times a week (65% versus 37%).

Zimbabwe

Sida began supporting nutrition in Zimbabwe at independence in 1980. In the early years, supplemental feeding for young children was implemented on a large scale to bring down the high levels of acute malnutrition that had resulted from the disruption and displacement caused by the fight for independence.

The Government soon requested Sida to support a more long-term, sustainable approach, the nationwide Supplemental Food Production Programme, which later changed its name to the Community Food and Nutrition Programme (CFNP). Each ward (sub-district) had a malaria control officer, but in most districts this person had little to do, so these officers were asked to mobilize villagers to form groups and write proposals to compete for programme funding. At first, winning proposals were simply provided some support to grow groundnuts, on the assumption that adding these to the children's porridge was all that was needed to sustainably support good nutrition.

By 1985, an evaluation showed that many people could not grow groundnuts well and that the programme suffered from numerous other problems as well. In 1987, Sida decided to end its support to the programme, but the national nutrition department (at a high level in the MOH and thus rather powerful) demonstrated that the programme had already greatly improved in the 2 years since the earlier evaluation. In villages with CFNP programmes (there were several hundred by then), the community development workers would, every few months, borrow a scale from the district health office and weigh all children under 5 years old, noting how many children were below the 'road to health' (i.e. below the 3rd percentile in weight-for-age). In numerous villages, it was clear that, at least in the previous year, these numbers were dropping substantially.

Sida was therefore urged to reconsider, in order that the project could demonstrate its achievements and build on the lessons learned, rather than be shut down after years of patient support, when it was finally starting to pay off (Antonsson-Ogle and Greiner, 1987). The result was that another 3 years of funding was agreed, and then this support was renewed once more as well. Pleased at how the CFNP continued to develop, Sida probably would have continued funding beyond that, but in the meantime, the Nutrition Department was 'demoted' to being a unit under the Maternal and Child Health (MCH) Division of the MOH. MCH requested that Sida no longer support CFNP but shift funding to other MCH priorities. However, by then, the programme was so successful and had so much political support around the country that when the Sida funding (which was of the order of US$400,000/year) stopped, the government took over funding (though for a few years it did so via a loan from the World Bank).

Some innovative aspects of projects under the CFNP umbrella are listed below:

1. Communities often proposed to raise small animals, but because costs per recipient

were higher than for other proposals, this resulted in fewer people receiving support. The 1985 evaluation found that, given the lack of veterinarian services, too many animals died and project groups could not afford as easily to replace them as they could, for example, crops that failed. Although small animals continued to predominate in projects in very dry areas of the country, gradually the CFNP evolved into what was largely a community gardening project.

2. Gardening is often attractive where the labour input on a small piece of land has high returns on investment (money and time). These crops are of greater interest in situations/settings where they can be sold with relatively little effort and expense. At the same time, the poorer quality fruits that were harder to sell were used to diversify the variety and taste of the family diet. Nutrition projects work well and are sustainable when they not only focus on behaviour change or health components but are also are linked to ways of increasing family income. (To achieve sustainability, the nutrition component must usually be subservient to the income-generating component.)

3. The most common project proposal involved a request from the village for funding for a metal fence to surround the community garden plot. In return, the villagers were normally expected to provide the poles and the labour required to erect the fence. This overcame what most communities experienced as the greatest constraint to community gardening: the inability to construct fences strong enough to keep out animals that would otherwise destroy or consume too many of the crops. Improved seeds and seedlings were another scarce commodity that was often requested.

4. In the mature project, in order to increase their chances of receiving support, communities often offered the following:

(a) They set aside reasonably good land for the project close enough to a water source so that the crops would not risk failing as a result of drought.

(b) A minimum of a dozen villagers agreed to participate, but projects were often much larger than this, up to 200. Usually, each person received his or her own plot (women were generally more interested in participating) within the fenced-in community garden area.

(c) In the best projects, each participant paid a 'tax' on his or her harvests that would be used to feed children in a nearby day-care facility which was tended by the participants on a rotating basis.

(d) This day care was then open to participants' children, but frequently also to a number of children identified by the community development worker as the most malnourished in the village. It provided both a nutritious meal and day care.

5. Gradually, as the projects became more numerous, they changed what agricultural extension agents were doing. Agents, who mostly were men, were already under pressure to serve women farmers, but doing so on an individual basis was culturally problematic. Being able to serve the needs of a group of women was a less sensitive option and allowed them to more easily fulfil their monthly quotas. Secondly, while the greatest need was for improved methods of planting and caring for horticultural crops, agents were mainly trained to assist with staples and export crops. Hence the project led to a 'bottom-up' demand, and resulted in the strengthening of horticulture in the in-service and basic training of extension agents.

6. At district level, the best community group proposals were chosen and sent to provincial level. Here again, the best were chosen and submitted to the national committee that made the final decisions on allocation of the available funds. At each level, these committees were multi-sectoral and met every 3 months. Thus, multi-sectoral committees *can* work, but only when they actually make decisions they perceive as relevant to their sectors. When decisions affect the allocation of resources, members will take committee meetings seriously to ensure their interests are not neglected, join in debates about priorities and share their relevant expertise.

7. Funding went via the MOH, but health officials perceived the project as largely an agricultural one and gave it little attention in the beginning. So at the inter-sectoral meetings, it was usually the agricultural sector

officials that showed enthusiasm, presented information about project progress, claimed credit for successes, and pushed for effective decision making. Gradually, the health representatives felt pressure to pay more attention and become more involved, with some even gradually learning that there was a connection between agriculture, nutrition and health that was important to their sector's objectives.

8. By the early 1990s, there were some 3000 village-level projects. Sida agreed that the next evaluation could be done internally, but assigned a representative to ensure that it was planned in such a way as to assure maximum learning rather than just to impress the donor. One challenge for an evaluation of such a complex project was to achieve adequate objectivity without being too expensive (outsider experts cost more and require more time to understand basic issues about the project that its participants are already aware of). The method agreed upon resulted in the development of a series of 13 questionnaires designed for each type of functionary involved at each level and for a sample of beneficiaries. In each province, the questionnaires were administered by an inter-sectoral team involved in the programme (and therefore knowledgeable about its goals) from a different province. No two provinces were allowed to study each other, although this meant that language difficulties had to be overcome. This approach avoided the extremes of constantly finding the glass too empty (which unfairly often results in promising projects being prematurely stopped because they are not yet achieving initial, often unrealistic, goals) or largely full (which can result in few lessons being learned that could improve the project and enhance its chances for successful replication).

Here are some general recommendations that emerged from the evaluation of projects carried out under the CFNP (Tagwireyi and Greiner, 1994):

- Offer increased funding and other support to those provinces with higher levels of malnutrition because they also tend to be those with lower staffing levels and poorer infrastructure development.

- Improve reporting and monitoring, with the provincial level (where Zimbabwe had nutritionists stationed at the time) taking major responsibility.
- Integrate better with water and sanitation, functional literacy and preschool activities.
- Ensure more regular growth monitoring of children involved in the project.
- Conduct nutritional screening as part of the project proposal for communities seeking to participate in CFNP.
- Use the Provincial Food and Nutrition Management Teams to analyse what other approaches are needed in addition to CFNP to improve nutrition in each province.

Many of these recommendations were achieved in the following years, at least partially. Levinson (1991) called the CFNP one of 'the two most important African successes in such integrated programmes'. It succeeded in the end in part because the donor: (i) was patient; (ii) allowed budgeting in its bilateral support to be at the broad level of projects and did not require initial notional budget subheadings to be adhered to (Sida just requested explanations after the fact for changes); and (iii) did not force outside technical assistance on to the project (which often tends to exert too much influence and control), but provided access to consultants only on request.

Bangladesh

In 1981, Sida begin providing, via UNICEF, what it thought was about a third of the funds needed to run the national vitamin A supplementation project in Bangladesh. By 1989, coverage rates were still too low to have a public health impact, and Sida explored why this was and what alternative approaches to improving vitamin A status were ongoing and might prove to be more effective. Interviews with the government, the United Nations (UN) and even representatives of non-governmental organizations (NGOs) revealed that virtually no other projects were ongoing or planned, despite widespread recognition that vitamin A deficiency was a serious public health problem in the country. Even if it was 'imper-fect' and failed to reach women and other tar-get groups, the distribution of vitamin A capsules was seen as all that could be justified, given that there were so many competing pri-orities (Greiner and Ekström, 1989).

Among the options available, Sida decided to support a project run by a local communication NGO called Worldview International Foundation (WIF). WIF, with its headquarters in Sri Lanka, was established by a Norwegian NGO to provide developing countries with the capacity for independently producing their own news and exploring how communication technology could further their own development goals (Greiner and Mannan, 1999). The Bangladesh office of WIF reported to the Ministry of Education (MOE), so its projects had little influence in either the health or agriculture sectors and there has been little awareness of its work in the 'nutri-tion community' either there or abroad.

In 1982, when Helen Keller International (HKI) assisted in conducting the first national vitamin A survey in Bangladesh, WIF decided to explore how to use its communication expertise to improve vitamin A status. In dis-cussions with HKI, who provided technical assistance in the early years, as did the MOE, it was decided that WIF should develop pro-ject proposals aiming to increase consumption of key foods available to the poor in the dis-tricts where 4% or more of the young children suffered from night blindness. Funding for these district-level projects was first obtained from NGOs in the Netherlands and Norway.

WIF did not embrace the common approach of going for the 'low hanging fruit' and supporting only existing projects or cen-tres of excellence, i.e. it did not go for rapid, cost-effective impact by neglecting the poor-est, most underserved groups. Rather, it aimed to cover every rural household in entire districts. With HKI's help, messages were designed that were conveyed through a broad range of locally appropriate media. The decision was made to focus on promot-ing affordable carotene-rich foods as a means of avoiding night blindness, which was well known in the communities. Gradually, the approach evolved to include equal emphasis on increasing the demand for and supply of these foods, particularly by promoting school and home gardening, and mobilizing WIF-hired agronomists to assist with this.

WIF did not pursue the rather recidi-vist approach called for in social marketing approaches, where, for example, consump-tion of only a single food might be pro-moted (Smitasiri et al., 1993). As detailed below, WIF either distributed or promoted the consumption of a large range of foods, focusing mainly on dark-green leafy vege-tables (DGLVs). These are not just extremely nutrient dense, but are also the cheapest food available to low-income people, with some widely consumed varieties available wild. That they tend to have low status and so are rarely consumed as often as they could be was one of the reasons that they were given extra attention in nutrition edu-cation messages. WIF chose varieties that had different growing seasons as well as promoting varieties that were sweet and non-fibrous and therefore more acceptable to young children.

The following is an outline of what WIF did during its 3 year project in Gaibandah District, where about half of the population of 1.5 million was effectively landless:

- Sixteen teams of traditional singers were hired and the issues explained to them. Each then wove some relevant messages into songs and chants that they devel-oped and illustrated with flip charts. WIF realized that, when working with artists, one should explain the technical issues to them and let them independently develop the media and methods for con-veying relevant messages. Later research suggested that the free performances pro-vided in hundreds of villages proved to be the most effective way to reach men.
- One hundred and sixty-five 'women vol-unteers' (WVs) were hired and trained from all over the district. Each was assigned several nearby villages to work in. They were provided with a bicycle and taught its basic maintenance; its cost was gradually deducted from the US$20/ month honorarium that each WV received. The WVs were provided with flip charts and supervisors visited regularly to ensure

that they ran through the messages regularly with groups of women in each village. They were also taught how to grow seedlings of papaya and mango to be sold to villagers, and how to buy improved seeds for project-promoted high-carotene crops; they sold the seeds as well. The improved seed, though locally unavailable otherwise, typically doubled the crop yield. The WVs were taught how to teach villagers about mulching and composting and, eventually, how to make live fences. As in Zimbabwe (though for different reasons), fencing was the greatest constraint to gardening among those who had access to some land. Live fencing is the best solution but this requires knowledge of which locally available species best meet a series of criteria such as low cost (usually growing wild nearby), no detrimental effects, durability, effectiveness and provision of benefits other than fencing (Andersson, 1994).

- The WVs were first asked to request landowners to let the landless use land for gardening at a cost of about half of the harvest. However, all too often the landless were removed from the land once fencing, mulching etc., had improved it. So the project then focused on the use of high-carotene vine crops as the best solution. Every rural household in the district was provided with three free seeds each of bean, squash (whose leaves were eaten) and pumpkin. Landless or nearly landless families grew these vines on their roofs, on trellises and even in trees near their huts. The WVs promoted the consumption of ten additional foods that were either high in carotene and were easy to grow, very cheap or grew wild, as well as the use of small amounts of fat in children's diets needed to increase the absorption of carotene but are low in rural Bangladeshi diets.

- The WVs were also trained to identify night blindness, and when a family member was found to be suffering from it, they received follow-up attention

every few weeks and free seeds for nine high-carotene foods. Nearly 1800 such families were identified in the second year of the project alone. These families were repeatedly urged to provide high-carotene foods to the person who was night blind. Months of increased use of these foods were typically required before the night blindness disappeared. WIF requested the district Civil Surgeon to provide vitamin A capsules to these cases or to let their WVs do so, but were usually turned down. Nor could these families afford to visit distant health facilities outside dire emergencies.

- One hundred and sixty schools throughout the district were supported in school gardening and seeds for nine foods were provided to 2400 of the most motivated students to start home gardens.

- To reach other groups, key messages were conveyed through billboards, radio and slide shows in cinemas. WIF hired the most famous film director in Bangladesh to make a feature film, and used drama and comedy to highlight the project messages. Sixteen film projectors and generators were purchased, and outdoor night-time showings of the film took place in hundreds of villages – with a typical attendance of thousands for each showing.

In Rangpur District, a follow-up study was carried out to determine how much of the project outcome was sustained 3 years after donor funding ended (Hussain *et al.*, 1993). Its results were mixed, but qualitative research done in some of the same areas (Greiner, 1997) found that vegetable and seed vendors were still enjoying increased sales of carotene-rich as compared with carotene-poor foods. Most of them guessed that the 'government propaganda' using the traditional singers was responsible for this increase.

Sida funding that is normally available for evaluations was only a small proportion of what was spent on the project. To justify a more rigorous evaluation, a rapid appraisal needed to be done; otherwise, an expensive impact evaluation may have arrived at a conclusion of 'no impact' in a situation where a simple process evaluation would have indicated that no impact was possible. This study was carried out by visiting well-established vegetable and seed vendors in markets in five towns – four of them in project areas. The study indicated that sales of the vegetables and seeds promoted by WIF were increasing compared with others (Greiner, 1997).

These results were considered to be adequate evidence for moving forward with a large-scale quasi-experimental evaluation of the impact of the third year of the 3 year project (Greiner and Mitra, 1995). The diets of a probability sample of children in the entire district of Gaibandah were compared with those of children in equally large portions of two nearby non-project districts; the assessments were repeated on two new probability samples of the same areas taken exactly a year later (thereby controlling for the effect of season); the total sample size was 10,000. Flooding did not occur in either year. Children's intakes of all but the low-carotene vegetables increased significantly in Gaibandah. While there were many increases in the non-project area as well, their consumption of DGLVs significantly decreased. The price of rice had also decreased significantly during that year, leading many to shift away from 'poor man's food' – such as DGLVs – to more expensive foods. Thus, at end line, 52% of young children in the project area ate DGLVs the day before the survey, compared with 26% in the non-project areas.

WIF conducted similar projects in five other districts in Bangladesh, covering a total population of about 9 million rural people. It learned that people in cities did not see sufficient benefit in a project like this to make them willing to participate wholeheartedly. The first project district, Rangpur, received support for 7 years, because much of this time was devoted to developing an efficient and effective project model. Otherwise, the approach required only 3 years per district. Remarkably, its cost in Gaibandah was calculated to be only about US$0.15/year per capita.

Research on Whether Food-based Approaches Actually Work

The efficacy of carotene-rich foods

Food-based programmes take time to establish and time to show impact. Much research claiming that such programmes do not work has simply not given them enough time or resources. Nascent interest in food-based approaches began to decline further when international meetings throughout the mid-to-late 1990s began to give great attention to a study suggesting that carotene was absorbed more poorly from green leaves and other vegetables than was previously thought (de Pee et al., 1995). Indeed, as part of an agenda to promote a single approach – universal semi-annual distribution of massive dose vitamin A capsules (VAC) to young children – research on the poor bioavailability of carotene often comprised the only 'food-based' research presented at such meetings during this period. The fact that other vitamin A deficient groups apart from young children would be ignored by this total focus on VAC distribution never received attention. This particularly applied to women, for whom VAC is actually inappropriate except in the early weeks after delivery. Meanwhile, studies such as the one in Zimbabwe described next showed that women were desperately in need of vitamin A and that food-based approaches could provide this.

In the drier districts of Matebeleland, in Zimbabwe, it was suspected that pregnant and breastfeeding women might be particularly vulnerable to vitamin A deficiency. In one district, a food frequency questionnaire was used to identify the most at-risk area, which consisted of 12 villages. Blood was drawn from 207 of the total of 211 women residing in those villages who had infants between 2 and 12 months old (all breastfeeding). Some 76% were found to have low liver stores of vitamin A (relative dose response >20%) and 40% were found to be vitamin A deficient (serum retinol <20 μg/dl) (Ncube et al., 2001a).

Before it was known how vitamin A deficient these women were, a study was conducted to test whether papaya or carrot might effectively improve vitamin A status in women who had given birth too long ago to be eligible to receive massive-dose VAC. Equal numbers were randomly allocated to one of four groups, each to receive daily a placebo, or about 6 mg of β-carotene, either in a capsule, or in a drink made of 650 g of pureed papaya, or as 100 g of grated carrot. Two hundred and one women completed the trial, but six were excluded from the analysis because they had elevated levels of C-reactive protein. There were significant improvements in serum retinol in all three treatment groups and in serum haemoglobin in the β-carotene capsule and papaya groups (and an almost significant increase in the carrot group), but none in the control (placebo) group (Ncube *et al.*, 2001b). Papaya performed nearly as well as pure β-carotene.

The role of intestinal helminths in carotene absorption

Because even children apparently consuming a large amount of green leaves took so long to recover from night blindness, WIF suspected that the low dietary fat levels seen in Bangladesh (10 g/day per capita) (Government of Bangladesh, 1992) might be responsible. An informal study was performed to see whether WIF should also give them some oil to speed up the recuperation process. It turned out that providing 20 ml of food oil daily shortened the recovery time to an average of 6 weeks, compared with 7 weeks among those who received no oil (Wallén, 1994). What surprised both WIF staff and local villagers was that even the children who received no oil recovered much more rapidly than in the 3–6 months ordinarily required. The most likely explanation for this was the deworming of all children in the study 2 weeks before it commenced.

In the Tanzania study referred to earlier (Kidala *et al.*, 2000), the mean serum retinol levels were actually lower in the project area, where they were 14 µg/dl, compared with 19 µg/dl in the control area. The explanation was that children infected with intestinal helminths had half the serum retinol concentration of those who were uninfected – 12.3 µg/dl

compared with 24 µg/dl, and 79% of children in the experimental area were infected, compared with 49% in the control area. Parasitism had not received attention either in the baseline study or in project activities, which is a reminder for food-based projects that public health issues may also need attention. Indeed, intestinal helminths can eliminate the effects of efforts to improve the diet, as they decrease absorption from the main sources of vitamin A in the diet of low-income populations – the carotenes that are found in green leaves and other vegetables. These are present in a difficult to digest fibrous matrix.

Persson conducted a more in-depth study among Bangladeshi schoolchildren to further elucidate this question (Persson *et al.*, 2001). She picked children at random to receive a daily meal for 6 weeks that contained about 4.4 mg β-carotene from green leaves or 1.5 mg β-carotene from pumpkin (assuming that absorption from this would be better) or vegetables containing virtually no β-carotene. Serum retinol was measured before and after supplementation. All children were dewormed before the trial. The study confirmed that β-carotene is absorbed better from pumpkin than from green leaves, but showed that β-carotene absorption from both sources was better than had been found in the earlier study by de Pee *et al.* (1995), in which subjects had not been dewormed in advance.

Thus, the findings of these studies strengthened those of earlier studies (Marinho *et al.*, 1991; Jalal *et al.*, 1998; Takyi, 1999), which all suggested that the poor absorption of β-carotene found from vegetables may to a large extent be overcome by consuming fat at the same time and by deworming children regularly. Over the past decade, this body of evidence has been ignored, thereby ensuring that food-based approaches were considered ineffective and focusing donor attention exclusively on universal VAC distribution.

Can food-based approaches even improve iron status?

Conventional wisdom seems to be that only iron pills can improve iron status, at least in people who are iron deficient. Food fortification is typically acknowledged only to be useful in preventing iron deficiency, though trials with iron-fortified rice have shown that this works well both in iron-deficient women (Hotz *et al.*, 2008) and schoolchildren (Moretti *et al.*, 2006). The consumption of most natural foods by toddlers – even of red meat – is likely to be too low for it to be an effective means of treating iron deficiency. However, iron fortified milk has improved iron deficiency (Szymlek-Gay *et al.*, 2009) and fortified rice was found to do so better than iron drops (Beinner *et al.*, 2010).

In low-income areas, fortified foods and animal foods are often not viable alternatives, while rich sources of vitamin C may often be available and affordable. Although vitamin C is known to improve the absorption of iron (which is actually common in plant foods, but poorly absorbed from them), past human trials have not shown it to be effective in this role. However, the larger dose of vitamin C that is obtainable from certain tropical fruits may be effective in promoting iron absorption, as was recently demonstrated with fresh guava juice provided at 200 mg/meal to children once on each school day (Monárrez-Espino *et al.*, 2011). This had a small but statistically significant effect on the haemoglobin and plasma ferritin concentrations in children consuming high-phytate diets, even though the school meals already contained substantial iron in animal foods. So the consumption of high vitamin C foods such as a fresh guava drink with as many meals as possible is likely to be useful for overall iron status, particularly among low-income groups.

Conclusions

This chapter has reviewed several large-scale food-based nutrition projects in low-income countries, and brought to light lessons learned from both failures and successes. The donors to these food-based programmes shared a willingness to fund large-scale programmes that required a long period to build local capacity and to develop effective methods of implementation. They avoided earmarking funds too tightly, and did not forbid the recipient institution from using them somewhat differently from the way in which they had originally been budgeted in response to developments in the field. Nor did they demand that only the latest, proven methods of project implementation be used, which would have required excessive outside technical assistance.

The most successful projects were actually rarely planned and budgeted in great detail in advance. Many factors are unpredictable in large projects that run over a long period of time. Part of the reason for the effectiveness of these projects was that they were given opportunities for learning and replanning as they went along. Not only were the donors patient, but they recognized and accepted that people, communities and governments in low-income countries need to take the lead, making their own decisions even if what they decide to do may not seem to the donor or its experts to be the 'best' or 'most modern' way forward. In particular, donors whose aim is not to achieve rapid impact but to build the capacity of countries to independently solve their own problems do not always consider negative evaluations to be a signal for withdrawal, but rather as a means of finding ways to make more intensive and effective efforts, often through building a wider range of practical technical and managerial capacities.

Research on the impact of food-based approaches is scarce because it is time-consuming and complex. Indeed, research on projects, field work and even on the operations of ministries has low status, and few research donors prioritize it. However, increasingly, such research suggests that food-based approaches that are adequately funded and given time to mature do work.

References

Andersson, A. (1994) *A Study on Small-scale Vegetable Gardening with Special Focus on Live Fences*. Working Paper 267, International Rural Development Centre, Swedish University of Agricultural Sciences, Uppsala, Sweden.

Antonsson-Ogle, B. and Greiner, T. (1987) *Report on technical consultations on nutrition between Sida's nutrition consultants and the Department of Nutrition, Ministry of Health, Zimbabwe*. Sida Consultant Report, Swedish International Development Cooperation Agency, Stockholm.

Beinner, M.A., Velasquez-Melendez, G., Pessoa, M.C. and Greiner, T. (2010) Iron-fortified rice is as efficacious as supplemental iron drops in infants and young children. *Journal of Nutrition* 140, 49–53.

Burgess, L., Greiner, T., Mrisho, F., Antonsson-Ogle, B., Sarakikya, E., Tobisson, E. and Wagara, A. (1986) *The Tanzania Food and Nutrition Centre, a Joint TFNC/Sida Evaluation*. Sida Consultant Report, Swedish International Development Cooperation Agency, Stockholm.

de Pee, S., West, C.E., Hautvast, J.G.A.J., Mulihal, Karyadi, D. and West, C.E. (1995) Lack of improvement in vitamin A status with increased consumption of dark-green leafy vegetables. *The Lancet* 346, 75–81.

Government of Bangladesh (1992) *Bangladesh Country Paper*. Dhaka.

Greiner, T. (1997) Rapid appraisal before impact evaluation studies. *World Health Forum* 18, 66–67.

Greiner, T. and Ekström, C.-E. (1989) *Report to Sida on a Nutritional Blindness Prevention Programme Review Mission in Bangladesh*. International Child Health Unit, Uppsala University, Uppsala, Sweden.

Greiner, T. and Mannan, M.A. (1999) Increasing micronutrient intakes in rural Bangladesh: an NGO's search for sustainability. In: Marchione, T. (ed.) *Scaling Up and Scaling Down: Overcoming Malnutrition in Developing Countries*. Gordon and Breach, London, pp. 157–177.

Greiner, T. and Mitra, S.N. (1995) Evaluation of the impact of a food-based approach to solving vitamin A deficiency in Bangladesh. *Food and Nutrition Bulletin* 16, 193–205.

Hotz, C., Porcayo, M. Onofre, G., Garcia-Guerra, A., Elliott, T., Jankowski, S. and Greiner, T. (2008) Efficacy of iron-fortified Ultra Rice in improving the iron status of women in Mexico. *Food and Nutrition Bulletin* 29, 140–149.

Hussain, A., Kvaale, G., Ali, K. and Bhuyan, A.H. (1993) Determinants of night blindness in Bangladesh. *International Journal of Epidemiology* 22, 1119–1126.

Jalal, F., Nesheim, M.C., Zulkarnain, A., Diva, S. and Habicht, J.P. (1998) Serum retinol concentrations in children are affected by food sources of beta-carotene, fat intake, and anthelmintic drug treatment. *The American Journal of Clinical Nutrition* 68, 623–629.

Kidala, D., Greiner, T. and Gebre-Medhin, M. (2000) Five-year follow-up of a food-based vitamin A intervention in Tanzania. *Public Health Nutrition* 3, 425–431.

Levinson, F.J. (1991) *Addressing Malnutrition in Africa: Low-cost Program Possibilities for Government Agencies and Donors*. SDA Working Paper No. 13, Program Design and Implementation, Social Dimensions of Adjustment in Sub-Saharan Africa, World Bank, Washington, DC.

Marinho, H.A., Shrimpton, R., Giugliano, R. and Burini, R.C. (1991) Influence of enteral parasites on the blood vitamin-A levels in preschool-children orally supplemented with retinol and or zinc. *European Journal of Clinical Nutrition* 45, 539–544.

Monárrez-Espino, J., López-Alarcón, M. and Greiner, T. (2011) Randomized placebo-controlled trial of guava juice as a source of ascorbic acid to reduce iron deficiency in Tarahumara indigenous schoolchildren of northern Mexico. *Journal of the American College of Nutrition* 30, 191–200.

Moretti, D., Zimmermann M.B., Muthayya, S., Thankachan, P., Lee, T.-C., Kurpad, A.V. and Hurrell, R.F. (2006) Extruded rice fortified with micronized ground ferric pyrophosphate reduces iron deficiency in Indian schoolchildren: a double-blind randomized controlled trial. *The American Journal of Clinical Nutrition* 84, 822–829.

Ncube, T.N., Malaba, L., Greiner, T. and Gebre-Medhin, M. (2001a) Evidence of grave vitamin A deficiency among lactating women in the semi-arid rural area of Makhaza in Zimbabwe. A population-based study. *European Journal of Clinical Nutrition* 55, 229–234.

Ncube, T.N., Greiner, T., Malaba, L.C. and Gebre-Medhin, M. (2001b) Supplementing lactating women with pureed papaya and grated carrots improved vitamin A status in a placebo-controlled trial. *Journal of Nutrition* 131, 1497–1502.

Nishida, C., Shrimpton, R. and Darnton-Hill, I. (2009) Landscape analysis on countries' readiness to accelerate action in nutrition. *SCN News* 37, 4–9.

Persson, V., Ahmed, F., Gebre-Medhin, M. and Greiner, T. (2001) Increase in serum beta-carotene following dark green leafy vegetable supplementation in mebendazole-treated school children in Bangladesh. *European Journal of Clinical Nutrition* 55, 1–9.

Smitasiri, S., Attig, G., Valyasevi, A., Dhanamitta, S. and Tontisirin, K. (1993) *Social Marketing Vitamin A-rich Foods in Thailand*. Thailand Institute of Nutrition, Mahidol University, Nakhon Pathom, Thailand in cooperation with UNICEF (United Nations Children's Fund), East Asia and Pacific Regional Office (EAPRO), Bangkok.

Szymlek-Gay, E.A., Ferguson, E.L., Health, A.L., Gray, A.R. and Gibson, R.S. (2009) Food-based strategies improve iron status in toddlers: a randomized controlled trial. *The American Journal of Clinical Nutrition* 90, 1541–1551.

Tagwireyi, J. and Greiner, T. (1994) *Nutrition in Zimbabwe*. World Bank, Washington, DC.

Takyi, E.E.K. (1999) Children's consumption of dark green, leafy vegetables with added fat enhances serum retinol. *Journal of Nutrition* 129, 1549–1554.

Wallén, A. (1994) *A Field Trial to Reduce the Time Required to Cure Night Blindness due To Vitamin A Deficiency*. Minor Field Study No. 68, Unit for International Child Health, Uppsala University, Uppsala, Sweden.

5 Critical Issues to Consider in the Selection of Crops in a Food-based Approach to Improve Vitamin A Status – Based on a South African Experience

Mieke Faber,[1]* Sunette M. Laurie[2] and Paul J. van Jaarsveld[1]

[1]*Medical Research Council, Cape Town, South Africa; [2]Agricultural Research Council, Pretoria, South Africa*

Summary

Vitamin A deficiency is of public health significance in the developing world. Household food production of β-carotene-rich vegetables and fruits is a long-term strategy that can contribute to combating vitamin A deficiency. It is, however, important to grow food crops to meet the nutritional needs of vulnerable populations taking into consideration the β-carotene content of these foods and their potential contribution towards the vitamin A requirements of the target population. Although the focus here is on vitamin A, β-carotene-rich vegetables and fruits do have the potential to contribute significantly towards the dietary intake of various micronutrients other than vitamin A. Seasonality affects the availability of vegetables and fruits, and a variety of both warm-weather and cool-weather crops should be planted to ensure year-round availability of β-carotene-rich vegetables and fruits. A focus on both indigenous and exotic vegetables will further help to ensure year-round availability, particularly in terms of dark-green leafy vegetables. When promoting increased consumption of indigenous vegetables, it is important that the promotion campaign is appropriate for the setting. When introducing new crops, such as the orange-fleshed sweet potato, both the nutrient content and the sensory attributes of the food need to be considered so as to ensure consumer acceptance. The chapter discusses the above-mentioned issues, using published and unpublished South African case studies as examples.

Introduction

Globally 190 million (33.3%) children under the age of 5 years old are vitamin A deficient, with Africa having one of the highest prevalences, at 44.4% (WHO, 2009). Vitamin A deficiency impairs the immune system and, as a result, vitamin A-deficient children have a lower resistance against common childhood infections, such as respiratory and diarrhoeal diseases, measles and malaria (Rice *et al.*, 2004).

The great majority of South African children consume a diet that is low in animal foods, vegetables and fruits, which, as a result, is poor in micronutrient density. Approximately half of 1–9 year-old South African children were shown to consume less than 50% of the required amount of

---

*Contact: mieke.faber@mrc.ac.za

various micronutrients, including vitamin A (Labadarios et al., 2000), and in 2005, 63.6% were shown to be vitamin A deficient, with a serum retinol content of <20 μg/dl (Labadarios, 2007). Compared with the results of a national survey that was done in 1994 (Labadarios et al., 1995), the vitamin A status of South African children appears to have deteriorated, despite a national vitamin A supplementation programme that was introduced in 2002 and a national food fortification programme that has been in operation since 2003.

Dietary diversification is a long-term strategy that complements supplementation and food fortification programmes (Tontisirin et al., 2002). Within the dietary diversification strategy, a variety of approaches can be used to improve the vitamin A status of vulnerable populations. These include strategies that aim to increase: (i) the production and availability of and access to vitamin A-rich foods; (ii) the consumption of vitamin A-rich foods; and/or (iii) the bioavailability of vitamin A in the diet (Ruel, 2001). Although preformed retinol from foods of animal origin, for example dairy products, liver and eggs, are the most bioavailable dietary source of vitamin A, regular consumption of these foods is often out of the financial reach of the poor. Foods of plant origin containing provitamin A carotenoids are more affordable. Plant foods that are inherently rich in provitamin A carotenoids (particularly β-carotene) include dark-green leafy vegetables (for example spinach and wild-growing leaves), and dark yellow/ orange vegetables (for example carrot, orange-fleshed sweet potato, butternut squash and pumpkin) and fruits (for example mango and papaya). The consumption of cooked green leafy vegetables (Takyi, 1999; Haskell et al., 2004, 2005), sweet potato (Jalal et al., 1998; Haskell et al., 2004; van Jaarsveld et al., 2005) and carrots (Haskell et al., 2005) has been shown to improve vitamin A status, thus providing evidence to support the use of β-carotene-rich vegetables in the crop-based approach to addressing vitamin A deficiency. These foods may, however, not always be available in local shops, particularly in rural areas (Faber and Laubscher, 2008).

Home gardening has been shown to be an important means of improving the intake of β-carotene-rich vegetables and fruits, particularly for resource-poor households, and in countries where plant foods are the main source of vitamin A (Talukder et al., 2000). West and Mehra (2010) argued that homestead food production is a sustainable approach to increasing dietary diversity, particularly in areas with restricted market access to nutritious foods, and is also an important future element in coping with food price fluctuations. Encouraging home gardening to alleviate vitamin A deficiency is, therefore, particularly important in areas where β-carotene-rich vegetables and fruits are not locally available or are too expensive.

There is a large body of evidence from the Asia-Pacific region supporting the role of homestead food production in improving dietary intake, decreasing micronutrient deficiencies, increasing household earnings and improving women's involvement in household decision making, as reported from a study by Helen Keller International (HKI Asia-Pacific, 2010) in Asia. The homestead gardens in the HKI project focused on year-round supply of a large variety of vegetables and fruits. In a rural village in South Africa, another home garden project that focused on the production and consumption of β-carotene-rich vegetables and fruits – together with nutrition education – proved to be successful in improving the vitamin A status of children of 2–5 years old. The prevalence of vitamin A deficiency decreased from 58% at baseline to 34% (Faber et al., 2002b), and there were indications that children in the intervention village suffered less from diarrhoea than children in the control village (10% versus 22% during the 2 weeks before the follow-up survey) (Faber et al., 2001). This project forms the foundation of a crop-based approach that was developed by the South African Medical and Agricultural Research Councils over the past decade (Faber et al., 2006).

Figure 5.1 gives a schematic overview of the crop-based approach. The approach has two distinct components, namely, a nutrition component and an agricultural component. The aim of the nutrition component is to increase the awareness and knowledge of vitamin A nutrition, food choices and food preparation methods so as to maximize bioavailability of β-carotene through health education and promotion. The aim of the agricultural component is to increase the household's access to and availability of vitamin A-rich foods through: (i) the establishment of demonstration gardens, which are used for the training of community members in gardening activities; (ii) the establishment of a community-based nursery for the propagation and distribution of sweet potato cuttings, spinach seedlings and seeds for carrot, butternut squash and spinach; and (iii) household production of β-carotene-rich crops in people's own home gardens. The combination of the increased awareness, access to and availability of β-carotene-rich vegetables will lead to increased consumption of these vegetables, which leads to an increased dietary vitamin A intake and, ultimately, an improved vitamin A status (Faber *et al.*, 2002a,b). This approach has also been shown to reduce the prevalence of child morbidity as reported by their caregivers (Faber *et al.*, 2001a; Laurie and Faber, 2008).

Home gardens are small plots within close proximity to the homes, so the mothers do not have to travel long distances or spend several hours away from home to work in the planting fields, and the time available for care for their children is minimally affected. The main focus of the home gardens is to produce β-carotene-rich vegetables for household consumption, and secondarily, only if there is surplus produce, for income generation. In theory, a well-planned home garden of approximately 15 × 10 m can supply a sufficient amount of β-carotene-rich vegetables to fulfil the vitamin A requirements of a household of six throughout the year (Faber *et al.*, 2006). This size of garden makes provision for space to follow a proper crop rotation cycle. Home gardens may progress towards larger production and income generation, particularly as a demand is created through education and promotion activities (Laurie and Faber, 2008).

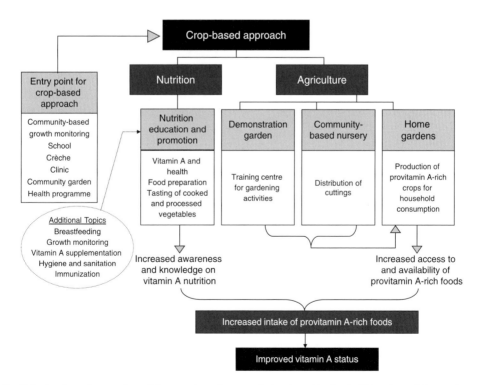

Fig. 5.1. A schematic overview of the crop-based approach developed in South Africa. From Faber and Laurie (2011).

All household members are potential beneficiaries of the home garden, whereas vitamin A
supplementation programmes, for example,
only target children younger than 5 years.
Home gardens have the further benefit that
the β-carotene-rich foods produced provide
additional nutrients other than vitamin A. The
carotenoids in β-carotene-rich vegetables and
fruits also have other health benefits, independent of their vitamin A activity, such as the
reduction of the risk of degenerative diseases,
certain types of cancer and cardiovascular disease (Krinsky and Johnson, 2005). Increasing
the intake of vegetables and fruits in general
could then have a large impact on reducing
non-communicable diseases (Lock *et al.*, 2005).
This is a major benefit considering the high
prevalence of chronic diseases in South Africa
(Steyn *et al.*, 2006).

Selection of Crops

When selecting crops to be promoted in home
garden projects, it is important to consider the
nutrient content of the crop, seasonal availability of vegetables and fruits, indigenous
foods and the consumer acceptance of new
crops. These topics are discussed below.

Nutrient content of the crop

Monocrop production of crops with low nutrient content does not translate into food and
nutrition security. Hence, it is important to
diversify the crops, taking into consideration
the nutrients that are limited in the diet of the
target population. Against the backdrop of a
low dietary vitamin A intake and the high
prevalence of vitamin A deficiency among
South African children (Labadarios *et al.*, 2000;
Labadarios, 2007), the focus of the crop-based
approach is predominantly on improving the
vitamin A intake of the nutritionally at-risk
populations. The β-carotene content of the
crop and its potential contribution towards
the vitamin A requirements of the target population therefore needs to be considered.

The potential effect of home gardens that
focus on β-carotene-rich crops for improving

dietary vitamin A intake is illustrated by data
from a home garden project that was carried
out in a rural village in South Africa (Faber
and Laurie, 2011). The change in dietary vitamin A intake over time in this village is shown
in Fig. 5.2. This shows the median dietary
vitamin A intake at baseline (February 1999),
1 year after implementation of the garden
project (February–March 2000), at the end of
the formal intervention (November 2000),
and during a period of low-intensity promotion (February, May, August, November
2005). The values shown in Fig. 5.2, and in
all dietary intake data presented hereafter, are
expressed as retinol equivalents (RE; preformed retinol plus the corresponding retinol
equivalent of the provitamin) as this is the
unit used in the South African food composition database, and in most other food composition tables. Current guidelines recommend
that provitamin A activity is expressed in retinol activity equivalents (RAE), using a conversion factor of 12 μg β-carotene to form 1 μg
RAE (Institute of Medicine, 2001), versus a
conversion factor of 6 μg β-carotene to form
1 μg RE.

Before implementation of the home
garden project (February 1999), the dietary
intake of vitamin A-rich foods was low,
resulting in a median vitamin A intake of 35%
of the required amount for 2–5 year old children (Faber *et al.*, 2001b). During the intervention period, children from households
with a project garden had significantly higher
dietary vitamin A intakes than children from
households without a project garden, as
shown by the results of the two surveys that
were done during February and November
2000 (Faber *et al.*, 2001c).

Results from the February 2000 survey
showed that dietary vitamin A intake had
increased significantly, not only in children
from households with a project garden, but
also in children from households without a
project garden (though to a lesser extent). The
β-carotene-rich vegetables and fruits contributed more than 85% of total dietary vitamin A
intake, regardless of whether the household
had a project garden or not. The increased
intake of vitamin A in children from households without a project garden was a result of
an increased awareness in the village – created

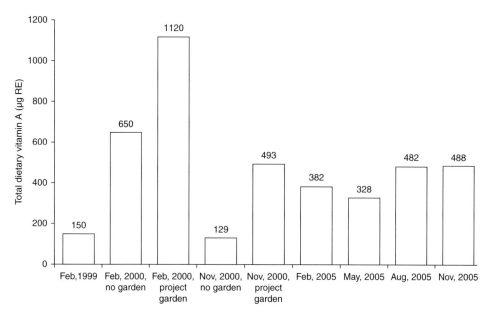

Fig. 5.2. Median dietary vitamin A intake in µg RE (retinol equivalents – preformed retinol plus the corresponding retinol equivalent of the provitamin) for 2 to 5 year-old children over time in a rural village in South Africa. February 1999 – before implementation of a home garden project; February 2000–1 year after implementation of a home garden project; November 2000 – follow-up survey of home garden project and end of formal intervention; February–November 2005 – consumption promoted but at a much lower intensity than during the formal intervention. From Faber *et al.* (2001b,c; 2002b), Faber and Laubscher (2008).

by the visibility of the gardens and by the nutrition education and promotion activities that were done at community-based growth monitoring sites. Some households opted not to grow their own β-carotene-rich vegetables and fruits, although many of them realized the nutritional benefits of these foods and negotiated with family, friends or neighbours to obtain some of the vegetables and fruits grown. Following the awareness that was created, the shop owner saw an opportunity, and butternut squash became available in the local shops (Faber *et al.*, 2002a). At the time, the availability of butternut squash in the local shops was seen as a significant outcome of the project. However, this was not sustained, as results of a study that recorded year-round availability of vegetables and fruits in the local shops during 2004 showed that butternut squash was available only for 2% of the records made in February (Faber and Laubscher, 2008).

After the November 2000 survey, the research team withdrew gradually from the area. During this period, a community-based nursery for orange-fleshed sweet potato and a seed distribution system were put in place to ensure that the community had easy access to seeds and sweet potato cuttings. Although at a much lower intensity than during the formal intervention, the consumption of β-carotene-rich vegetables and fruits was promoted until the beginning of 2006, when the community-based growth monitoring activities, which had served as a platform for the promotion, was terminated. The results of a dietary survey that was done during February, May, August and November 2005 (the final year of low-intensity promotion) showed higher vitamin A intakes than the baseline figures, with β-carotene-rich vegetables and fruits contributing 49–74% of total dietary vitamin A intake (Faber and Laubscher, 2008). The median dietary vitamin A intake for 2–5 year-old children has thus stabilized at about a three-fold increase, to 328–488 µg RE, from 150 µg RE at baseline.

Papaya trees were growing in the area naturally before the garden project, but this was not viewed as a food for human consumption. During the February 1999 and 2000 and the November 2000 surveys, the consumption of papaya was very low: it was consumed by 2% or less of the children during the 24 h recall period (Faber *et al.*, 2001c). In the November 2005 survey, 36% of the children consumed papaya over the 5 day recall period (Faber and Laubscher, 2008). Even though the November 2005 survey used a 5 day repeated dietary recall versus a single dietary recall as in the other studies, the finding that at least a third of the children consumed papaya indicates a significant change. The consumption of papaya was confirmed by the results of a survey that was done in 2007, which showed that the fruit was consumed by 43% of the children at least once a week; and in 98% of the cases, the papaya was locally grown (unpublished data). Changing people's perception on the use of papaya was a slow process: the change was observed 5 years after the formal intervention ended, during the period of continuous but low-intensity promotion.

In March 2007, a year after complete withdrawal of the research team, the results of a dietary survey showed that the median (interquartile range 25th–75th percentile) vitamin A intake for primary schoolchildren was 561 (406–797) µg RE, and for caregivers 662 (444–886) µg RE (Faber and Laurie, 2011). This is substantially higher than both the median vitamin A intake of 352 (415–517) µg RE reported for primary schoolchildren (Faber *et al.*, 1999) and the 177 (97–644) µg RE reported for caregivers (Faber *et al.*, 2001b) before implementation of the home-garden project. The consumption of fortified staple foods (maize meal and bread) contributed partly towards the higher vitamin A intake in the 2007 survey. The sustainability of the gardening activities is further illustrated by the findings that in 2007 more than 40% of the households planted β-carotene-rich vegetables in their own gardens and approximately a third of the households obtained β-carotene-rich vegetables from a community or group garden (Faber and Laurie, 2011).

Micronutrients other than vitamin A

Vegetables and fruits, including those rich in β-carotene, generally contain a wide range of micronutrients. Garden projects focusing primarily on β-carotene-rich crops may, therefore, result in an improvement of the overall nutritional quality of the diet, and address multiple nutrient deficiencies simultaneously. One year after the implementation of the home garden project (February 2000 in Fig. 5.2) described above, children from households with a project garden were shown to have significantly higher dietary intakes for riboflavin, vitamin B_6 and vitamin C, and a tendency towards a higher calcium intake; β-carotene-rich vegetables and fruits contributed more than 50% of the total dietary intake for calcium and iron, and 25–50% of total intake for magnesium, riboflavin and vitamin C (Faber *et al.*, 2002a). The contribution of β-carotene-rich vegetables and fruits towards the dietary intake of these nutrients (calcium and iron, and to a lesser extent magnesium, riboflavin and vitamin C) was confirmed in a series of dietary surveys that were done in 2005 (Faber and Laubscher, 2008). This is a significant additional benefit of the home gardening project, the more so as these nutrients were all shown to be deficient in the diets of 1–9 year-old South African children (Labadarios *et al.*, 2000).

Seasonality of crops

The production of vegetables is generally affected by climatic and seasonal patterns. In the project discussed above, the availability of β-carotene-rich vegetables over seasons and the impact thereof on dietary intake was reflected in the results of the data collected from February to December 2003, and during February, May, August and November in 2004 and 2005. These data showed that butternut squash, pumpkin and orange-fleshed sweet potato were consumed mostly during the first quarter/half of the year, while spinach and carrot were consumed mostly during the second half of the year (Faber and Laubscher, 2008). Consequently, planting a variety of both warm-weather (e.g. butternut squash, pumpkin, orange-fleshed sweet potato) and cool-weather crops (e.g. carrot, spinach) is needed to ensure the year-round availability of β-carotene-rich foods. From an agronomic point of view, planting a variety of β-carotene-rich crops will also help to maintain soil health and protect against plant pests and diseases – especially soil-borne diseases (Agrios, 2005), and thereby reduce the risk of crop failure.

The seasonal availability of certain β-carotene-rich vegetables can be prolonged by manipulating agricultural practices. Du Plooy et al. (2008) showed, for example, that the availability of orange-fleshed sweet potato can be extended to at least 9 months of the year in areas with a moderate winter climate by using various planting and harvesting dates, plant spacings and soil storage. Freshly harvested orange-fleshed sweet potato roots can be stored at room temperature for a maximum of approximately 12 weeks. The roots can also be stored in a simple pit structure for 12 weeks without any effect on their acceptability from a consumer and sensory perspective (Tomlins et al., 2007). The β-carotene content of orange-fleshed sweet potato was shown to be still substantial after 22 weeks of in-ground storage (van Jaarsveld, 2008). Through application of compost or chicken manure as top dressing, one planting of spinach can be grown for more than 7 months of the year – weather permitting – and allows for a constant supply of fresh leaves (Neluheni and Zulu, 2009). The period of availability can also be lengthened through staggered planting, i.e. small, regular plantings at intervals during the planting season.

Promoting the use of wild-growing leafy vegetables can further help to overcome seasonal shortages and ensure year-round availability of β-carotene-rich vegetables, as described in the next section.

Wild-growing leafy vegetables

Generally, in South Africa wild-growing green leafy vegetables are available during the summer months (Steyn et al., 2001; Vorster, 2007; Faber et al., 2010), while spinach is available during the cooler winter months. This is reflected in the results of a dietary survey that was done in February, May, August and November of 2005, which showed that traditional leafy vegetables were consumed mostly during the first and last quarter of the year (summer), and spinach (mostly Swiss chard) was consumed during the third quarter (winter). For children consuming dark-green leafy vegetables (spinach and traditional vegetables combined), these vegetables contributed 42–68% of total dietary vitamin A intake. Further, these green leafy vegetables contributed significantly to the dietary intake of calcium, iron and riboflavin (Faber et al., 2007).

Amaranth is among the most popular species of wild-growing leafy vegetables consumed in South Africa (Vorster, 2007; Faber et al., 2010). The mean vitamin A values (μg RAE) per 100 g boiled and fried amaranth were reported as 429 μg RAE and 627 μg RAE, respectively (Faber et al., 2010). A portion of 100 g boiled or fried amaranth will, therefore, provide more than 100% of the recommended dietary allowance (RDA) of 4–8 year-old children (400 μg RAE/day; Trumbo et al., 2001) and more than half of the RDA for vitamin A of adult females (700 μg RAE/day; Trumbo et al., 2001), suggesting that amaranth (and probably many of the other wild-growing leafy vegetables) can potentially contribute significantly to the vitamin A requirements of nutritionally vulnerable communities.

Promotion of the consumption of wild-growing leafy vegetables to complement the β-carotene-rich vegetables planted in the home gardens is an integral part of the crop-based approach. Although not planted in the project gardens, an increase in the consumption of traditional leafy vegetables was observed 1 year after the implementation of the garden project described in this chapter (Faber et al., 2002a).

Strategies used to promote the consumption of wild-growing green leafy vegetables need to be appropriate for the setting, taking into consideration differences between provinces, as well as rural/urban differences within a province in terms of dietary practices for these leafy vegetables (Faber et al., 2010). In certain areas in South Africa, the leaves are often dried, either in the sun or in the shade, for consumption during the winter

(Faber *et al.*, 2010). As sun drying may reduce the concentration of carotenoids (Mosha *et al.*, 1997; Mulokozi and Svanberg, 2003), optimal drying and storage conditions are needed to minimize such nutrient loss. Also, wild-growing leafy vegetables are often regarded as a poor person's food (Vorster, 2007; Faber *et al.*, 2010), so the aspect of affordability should be avoided or used carefully during promotion. Rather, the emphasis should be on the potential nutritional and hence the health benefits that the consumption of these vegetables could offer (Faber *et al.*, 2010).

The benefit of including indigenous vegetables in the crop-based approach, even though they were not planted in the project gardens, is that the households are familiar with these vegetables, and this probably helps with the adoption of some of the more unfamiliar ones that were planted. The potential value for food security and rural development of gathering wild foods is recognized by an international initiative (under the umbrella of the Convention on Biological Diversity) led by the Food and Agriculture Organization of the United Nations (FAO), together with the Bioversity International (formerly IPGRI – International Plant Genetic Resources Institute), with the overall aim of promoting the sustainable use of biodiversity in programmes contributing to food security and human nutrition (Toledo and Burlingame, 2006).

Consumer acceptance of a new crop

The white-fleshed sweet potato that is generally grown and consumed in South Africa contains virtually no β-carotene. A number of promising orange-fleshed sweet potato varieties with varying flesh colour and taste are available for possible use in the crop-based approach for addressing vitamin A deficiency (Laurie, 2010). The orange-fleshed sweet potato is an example of a biofortified crop in which the β-carotene content has been enhanced through conventional plant breeding. When sweet potato is used in crop-based intervention programmes as a strategy for addressing vitamin A deficiency, a target breeding level of 7500 µg β-carotene/100 g

raw weight has been proposed for populations where sweet potato is the sole source of β-carotene; if a mixed diet is eaten, the target is 3700 µg β-carotene/100 g raw weight (Nestel *et al.*, 2006). The intensity of the orange colour generally reflects the amount of β-carotene in the sweet potato.

The majority of South Africans are not familiar with the orange-fleshed sweet potato. As it is a newly introduced crop, the success of its use in the crop-based approach will depend on its acceptability to consumers in terms of its sensory characteristics, in addition to its agronomic characteristics. It should be noted that sweet potato is not eaten as a staple food in South Africa, and the strategy used to promote the production and consumption of orange-fleshed sweet potato will therefore differ from strategies used in countries where sweet potato is consumed as a staple or secondary staple food.

The contents of β-carotene and moisture, and consumer acceptance, were determined for nine orange-fleshed sweet potato varieties that were cultivated under controlled conditions and harvested 5 months after planting (Faber *et al.*, 2008). Five of the varieties exceeded 7500 µg β-carotene/100 g raw weight (the upper target breeding level), while four varieties had less than the upper target level, but exceeded 3700 µg β-carotene/100 g raw weight (a medium target breeding level). The retention of β-carotene after cooking varied from 78% to 94%. This is similar to the findings of a previous study, which reported that 70–92% of the β-carotene in orange-fleshed sweet potato is retained during cooking (van Jaarsveld *et al.*, 2006). For all nine varieties, an average portion of 100 g boiled sweet potato will provide at least 100% of the RDA for vitamin A of 4–8 year-old children (400 µg RAE/ day; Trumbo *et al.*, 2001), while four of the varieties will provide 100% of the RDA for vitamin A of 19–30 year-old women (700 µg RAE/day; Trumbo *et al.*, 2001).

The colour and taste acceptance of boiled sweet potato was evaluated by 168 children and 48 adults using a 5-point hedonic scale. Mean consumer acceptability scores for the nine varieties differed significantly for taste, but not colour. For three of the varieties, taste acceptability was low, probably because of low dry matter content. Although the variety Khano was shown to have the highest β-carotene content, consumer acceptance was low, so it is not a suitable variety to be included in the crop-based approach. The variety Resisto had the second highest β-carotene content. In a randomized controlled trial done in South Africa, 5–10 year-old children were randomly allocated to receive either 125 g (½ cup) boiled and mashed orange-fleshed sweet potato (Resisto variety) or an equal amount of white-fleshed sweet potato as part of the school meal for 53 school days. The orange-fleshed sweet potato was well accepted by the children. The study also showed an improvement in the vitamin A liver stores of children consuming the orange-fleshed sweet potato relative to children consuming the white-fleshed sweet potato (van Jaarsveld et al., 2005). The Resisto variety was successfully introduced in the home garden project described earlier (Faber et al., 2002b).

Postharvest products

As already noted, orange-fleshed sweet potato is a new crop in South Africa. Using a variety of postharvest products could potentially lead to a more frequent use and larger demand for the orange-fleshed sweet potato, which, in turn, could potentially enhance the sustainability of local production thereof. For example, a variety of preparation and processing methods for orange-fleshed sweet potato, with emphasis on sweet potato bread, soup, chutney, juice, sweet potato leaves as green vegetables and a sweet potato curry dish, was introduced in a gardening project in the Eastern Cape Province in South Africa (Laurie and Faber, 2008). When using orange-fleshed sweet potato in, for example, baking bread, part of the wheat flour is substituted with boiled orange-fleshed sweet potato. It is also important that the dark orange varieties are used in order to ensure that the baked bread provides adequate amounts of vitamin A (Low and van Jaarsveld, 2008). It is also important that the nutrients are retained during processing to ensure that the consumer enjoys the maximum nutritional benefit from the locally produced β-carotene-rich foods. Fat, sugar and salt should be used in moderation in postharvest products, particularly against the backdrop of a high prevalence of overweight/obesity (56% of adult females are either overweight or obese; Department of Health, 2007) and chronic diseases (Steyn et al., 2006) in South Africa.

Not all orange-fleshed sweet potato postharvest products will have a significant nutritional benefit in terms of vitamin A. For example, through a partnership between the Provincial Department of Agriculture, the Msinga Community and the Agricultural Research Council, orange-fleshed sweet potato jam was produced and marketed successfully in a local supermarket (Ngubane, 2008). However, because of its high sugar content, this jam should be consumed sparingly, and in any case, an average portion size of jam is relatively small and will not make a significant contribution towards dietary vitamin A intake. Orange-fleshed sweet potato jam is, therefore, an example of a postharvest product that should not be promoted as a means of addressing vitamin A deficiency, but rather as a value-added product for income generation.

Concluding Remarks

Issues to consider in the crop-based approach to improving micronutrient status are the nutrient content of the crop (focusing on β-carotene-rich crops), diversifying the crops to overcome seasonality, promoting the consumption of wild-growing dark-green leafy vegetables to complement home-grown β-carotene-rich foods, and consumer acceptance of newly introduced crops. In the projects described in this chapter, home gardens focusing on these crops were shown to be successful in: (i) improving the year-round dietary intake of vitamin A and a range of other micronutrients; and (ii) sustaining the increased dietary vitamin A intake after withdrawal of the research team.

Factors that contributed towards the sustained increase in dietary vitamin A intake include the following:

1. The households had easy access to a continuous supply of affordable and high quality planting material through the

community-based nursery. The nursery for the distribution of vines for the orange-fleshed sweet potato can be either an open-field nursery or in an enclosed netted structure. For a nursery to be successful, fertile soil, water for irrigation, fencing (or a netted structure) and access to virus-indexed mother plants are required. For sustainability, the nursery needs to be financially feasible, so there must be a demand for the planting material within its supply area.

2. During the intervention phase, the project had a strong nutrition education component and there are indications that the increased nutritional knowledge was sustained (unpublished data).

3. During the intervention phase, there was a focus on capacity building through training of the community members in gardening activities in the demonstration gardens.

4. A variety of both warm and cool weather β-carotene-rich crops was planted, which helped to reduce seasonal shortages. This also allows for crop rotation, which is needed to maintain soil health and to reduce the risk of plant pests and diseases.

5. Wild-growing green leafy vegetables were promoted to complement the β-carotene rich vegetables grown in the garden. The households were familiar with these vegetables, and had easy access to them.

6. Papaya trees were growing naturally in the area, so the community had easy access to these at no cost. Changing people's perception on the use of papaya for human consumption was, however, a slow process.

It should be noted that, although the crop-based approach described in the chapter focuses on β-carotene-rich vegetables and fruits: (i) households are encouraged to plant these crops in addition to existing crops; (ii) the consumption of vitamin A-rich foods of animal origin is also promoted in the education part of the nutrition component of the crop-based approach; and (iii) breastfeeding for infants and small children is promoted.

The chapter has focused on crop selection mostly from a nutritional perspective. The success of any gardening project will depend though not only on the nutritional characteristics of the crops promoted, but also on their agronomic characteristics. Limiting factors for successful home gardens need to be addressed, particularly the lack of water for irrigation and a lack of fencing, which resulted in roaming animals destroying the crops. A partnership between the nutritional and agricultural sectors of a crop-based approach is therefore critical for the success of home garden projects aiming to improve the nutritional status of vulnerable populations.

References

Agrios, G.N. (2005) Plant Pathology, 5th edn. Elsevier Academic Press San Diego, California, pp. 300–301.

Department of Health (2007) *South Africa Demographic and Health Survey 2003: Full Report*. Pretoria, South Africa. Available at: http://www.measuredhs.com/pubs/pdf/FR206/FR206.pdf (accessed 2 June 2010).

Du Plooy, C.P., van den Berg, A.A. and Laurie, S.M. (2008) Production systems for orange-flesh sweetpotato. In: Faber, M., Laurie, S. and van Jaarsveld, P. (eds) *Proceedings Orange-Fleshed Sweetpotato Symposium, Pretoria, 3 October 2007*. South African Medical Research Council, Cape Town, pp. 25–28.

Faber, M. and Laubscher, R. (2008) Seasonal availability and dietary intake of β-carotene-rich vegetables and fruit of 2-year-old to 5-year-old children in a rural South African setting growing these crops at household level. *International Journal of Food Sciences and Nutrition* 59, 46–60.

Faber, M. and Laurie, S.M. (2011) A home gardening approach developed in South Africa to address vitamin A deficiency. In: Thompson, B. and Amoroso, L. (eds) *Combating Micronutrient Deficiencies: Food-based Approaches*. Food and Agriculture Organization, Rome and CAB International, Wallingford, UK, pp. 163–182.

Faber, M., Smuts, C.M. and Benadé, A.J.S. (1999) Dietary intake of primary school children in relation to food production in a rural area in KwaZulu-Natal, South Africa. *International Journal of Food Sciences and Nutrition* 50, 57–64.

Faber, M., Phungula, M., Venter, S., Dhansay, M. and Benadé, A.J.S. (2001a) A home-gardening programme focussing on yellow and dark-green leafy vegetables to improve household food security and under-nutrition with special reference to vitamin A status of preschool children. South African Medical Research Council, Cape Town.

Faber, M., Jogessar, V.B. and Benadé, A.J.S. (2001b) Nutritional status and dietary intakes of children aged 2–5 years and their caregivers in a rural South African community. *International Journal of Food Sciences and Nutrition* 52, 401–411.

Faber, M., Venter, S., Phungula, M.A.S. and Benadé, A.J.S. (2001c) An integrated primary health-care and provitamin A household food production program: impact on food consumption patterns. *Food and Nutrition Bulletin* 22, 370–375.

Faber, M., Venter, S. and Benadé, A.J.S. (2002a) Increased vitamin A intake in children aged 2–5 years through targeted home-gardens in a rural South African community. *Public Health Nutrition* 5, 11–16.

Faber, M., Phungula, M.A.S., Venter, S.L., Dhansay, M.A. and Benadé, A.J.S. (2002b) Home gardens focussing on the production of yellow and dark-green leafy vegetables increase the serum retinol concentrations of 2–5-y old children in South Africa. *The American Journal of Clinical Nutrition* 76, 1048–1054.

Faber, M., Laurie, S. and Venter, S. (2006) Home-gardens to address vitamin A deficiency in South Africa: a food-based approach. Agricultural Research Council, Pretoria.

Faber, M., van Jaarsveld, P.J. and Laubscher, R. (2007) The contribution of dark-green leafy vegetables to total micronutrient intake of two- to five-year-old children in a rural setting. *Water SA* 33, 407–412.

Faber, M., Laurie, S. and van Jaarsveld, P. (2008) *Nutrient Content and Consumer Acceptability for Different Cultivars of Orange-fleshed Sweetpotato. Project 202, Report to South African Sugar Association.* South African Medical Research Council, Cape Town.

Faber, M., Oelofse, A., van Jaarsveld, P.J., Wenhold, F.A.M. and Jansen van Rensburg, W.S. (2010) African leafy vegetables consumed by households in the Limpopo and KwaZulu-Natal provinces in South Africa. *South African Journal of Clinical Nutrition* 23, 30–38.

Haskell, M.J., Jamil, K.M., Hassan, F., Peerson, J.M., Hossain, M.I., Fuchs, G.J. and Brown, K.H. (2004) Daily consumption of Indian spinach (*Basella alba*) or sweet potatoes has a positive effect on total-body vitamin A stores in Bangladeshi men. *The American Journal of Clinical Nutrition* 80, 705–714.

Haskell, M.J., Pandey, P., Graham, J.M., Peerson, J.M., Shrestha, R.K. and Brown, K.H. (2005) Recovery from impaired dark adaptation in nightblind pregnant Nepali women who receive small daily doses of vitamin A as amaranth leaves, carrots, goat liver, vitamin A-fortified rice, or retinyl palmitate. *The American Journal of Clinical Nutrition* 81, 461–471.

HKI Asia-Pacific (2010) Homestead food production model contributes to improved household food security, nutrition and female empowerment – experience from scaling-up programs in Asia (Bangladesh, Cambodia, Nepal and Philippines). *Nutrition Bulletin* 8(1), Helen Keller International, Asia-Pacific Regional Office, Phnom Penh. Available at: http://www.hki.org/research/APRO%20Bulletin_HFP%20and%20Food%20Security.pdf (accessed 12 November 2010).

Institute of Medicine (2001) *Dietary Reference Intakes: Vitamin A, Vitamin K, Arsenic, Boron, Chromium, Copper, Iodine, Iron, Manganese, Molybdenum, Nickel, Silicon, Vanadium, and Zinc.* National Academy Press, Washington DC.

Jalal, F., Nesheim, M.C., Agus, Z., Sanjur, D. and Habicht, J.P. (1998) Serum retinol concentrations in children are affected by food sources of β-carotene, fat intake, and anthelmintic drug treatment. *The American Journal of Clinical Nutrition* 68, 623–629.

Krinsky, N.I. and Johnson, E.J. (2005) Carotenoid actions and their relation to health and disease. Review. *Molecular Aspects of Medicine* 26, 459–516.

Labadarios, D. (ed.) (2007) *National Food Consumption Survey – Fortification Baseline (NFCS-FB): South Africa, 2005.* South African Department of Health, Pretoria.

Labadarios, D., van Middelkoop, A., Coutsoudis, A., Eggers, R.R., Hussey, G., Ijsselmuiden, C. and Kotze, J.P. (1995) *Children Aged 6 to 71 Months in South Africa, 1994: Their Anthropometric, Vitamin A, Iron and Immunisation Coverage Status.* South African Vitamin A Consultative Group (SAVACG), Johannesburg.

Labadarios, D., Steyn, N.P., Maunder, E., MacIntyre, U., Swart, R., Gericke, G., Huskisson, J., Dannhauser, A., Vorster, H.H. and Nesamvuni, A.E. (2000) *National Food Consumption Survey of 1–9 year old children in South Africa, 1999.* Directorate of Nutrition, South African Department of Health, Pretoria.

Laurie, S.M. (2010) Agronomic performance, consumer acceptability and nutrient content of new sweet potato varieties in South Africa. PhD thesis, University of the Free State, South Africa.

Laurie, S. and Faber, M. (2008) Integrated community-based growth monitoring and vegetable gardens focusing on crops rich in β-carotene: project evaluation in a rural community in the Eastern Cape. *Journal of the Science of Food and Agriculture* 88, 2093–2101.

Lock, K., Pomerleau, J., Cause, L., Altmann, D.R. and McKee, M. (2005) The global burden of disease attributable to low consumption of fruit and vegetables: implications for the global strategy on diet. *Bulletin of the World Health Organization* 83, 100–108.

Low, J.W. and van Jaarsveld, P.J. (2008) The potential contribution of bread buns fortified with β-carotene-rich sweet potato in Central Mozambique. *Food and Nutrition Bulletin* 29, 98–107.

Mosha, T.C., Pace, R.D., Adeyeye, S., Laswai, H.S. and Mtebe, K. (1997) Effect of traditional processing on the total carotenoid, β-carotene, α-carotene and vitamin A activity of selected Tanzanian vegetables. *Plant Foods for Human Nutrition* 50, 189–201.

Mulokozi, G. and Svanberg, U. (2003) Effect of traditional sun-drying and solar cabinet drying on carotene content and vitamin A activity of green leafy vegetables. *Plant Foods for Human Nutrition* 58, 1–15.

Neluheni, K.O. and Zulu, S. (2009) Spinach cultivation practices. *Farming SA*, Supplement, January 2009, p. 13.

Nestel, P., Bouis, H.E., Meenakshi, J.V. and Pfeiffer, W. (2006) Biofortification of staple food crops. *Journal of Nutrition* 136, 1064–1067.

Ngubane, H.T. (2008) Msinga orange-fleshed sweetpotato jam project based on market research. In: Faber, M., Laurie, S. and van Jaarsveld, P. (eds) *Proceedings Orange-fleshed Sweetpotato Symposium, Pretoria, 3 October 2007*. South African Medical Research Council, Cape Town, pp. 57–60.

Rice, A.L., West, K.P. Jr and Black, R.E. (2004) Vitamin A deficiency. In: Ezzati, M., Lopez, A.D., Rodgers, A. and Murray, C.J.L. (eds) *Comparative Quantification of Health Risks. Global and Regional Burden of Disease Attributable to Selected Major Risk Factors*. World Health Organization, Geneva, Switzerland.

Ruel, M.T. (2001) *Can Food-based Strategies Help Reduce Vitamin A and Iron Deficiencies? A Review of Recent Evidence*. International Food Policy Research Institute, Washington, DC.

Steyn, K., Fourie, J. and Temple, N. (eds) (2006) Chronic Diseases of Lifestyle in South Africa: 1995–2005. Technical Report, South African Medical Research Council, Cape Town. Available at: http://www.mrc.ac.za/chronic/cdl1995-2005.htm (accessed 16 January 2011).

Steyn, N.P., Burger, S., Monyeki, K.D., Alberts, M. and Nthangeni, G. (2001) Seasonal variation in dietary intake of the adult population of Dikgale. *South African Journal of Clinical Nutrition* 14, 140–145.

Takyi, E.E.K. (1999) Children's consumption of dark green, leafy vegetables with added fat enhances serum retinol. *Journal of Nutrition* 129, 1549–1554.

Talukder, A., Kiess, L., Huq, N., de Pee, S., Darnton-Hill, I. and Bloem, M.W. (2000) Increasing the production and consumption of vitamin A-rich fruits and vegetables: lessons learned in taking the Bangladesh homestead gardening programme to a national scale. *Food and Nutrition Bulletin* 21, 165–172.

Toledo, A. and Burlingame, A. (2006) Biodiversity and nutrition: a common path toward global food security and sustainable development. *Journal of Food Composition and Analysis* 19, 477–483.

Tomlins, K., Ndunguru, G., Stambul, K., Joshus, N., Ngendello, T., Rwiza, E., Amour, R., Ramadhani, B., Kapanda, A. and Westby, A. (2007) Sensory evaluation and consumer acceptability of pale-fleshed and orange-fleshed sweetpotato by school children and mothers of preschool children. *Journal of the Science of Food and Agriculture* 87, 2436–2446.

Tontisirin, K., Nantel, G. and Bhattacharjee, L. (2002) Food-based strategies to meet the challenges of micronutrient malnutrition in the developing world. *The Proceedings of the Nutrition Society* 61, 243–250.

Trumbo, P., Yates, A.A., Schlicker, S. and Poos, M. (2001) Dietary reference intakes: vitamin A, vitamin K, arsenic, boron, chromium, copper, iodine, iron, manganese, molybdenum, nickel, silicon, vanadium, and zinc. *Journal of the American Dietetic Association* 101, 294–301.

van Jaarsveld, P. (2008) Retention of β-carotene in boiled orange-fleshed sweetpotato and during storage: importance of nutrient content for nutritional impact. In: Faber, M., Laurie, S. and van Jaarsveld, P. (eds) *Proceedings Orange-fleshed Sweetpotato Symposium, Pretoria, 3 October 2007*. South African Medical Research Council, Cape Town, pp. 63–68.

van Jaarsveld, P.J., Faber, M., Tanumihardjo, S.A., Nestel, P., Lombard, C.J. and Benadé, A.J.S. (2005) β-carotene-rich orange-fleshed sweet potato improves the vitamin A status of primary school children assessed with the modified-relative-dose-response test. *The American Journal of Clinical Nutrition* 81, 1080–1087.

van Jaarsveld, P.J., Marais, DeW., Harmse, E., Nestel, P. and Rodriguez-Amaya, D.B. (2006) Retention of β-carotene in boiled, mashed orange-fleshed sweet potato. *Journal of Food Composition and Analysis* 19, 321–329.

Vorster, H.J. (2007) The role and production of traditional leafy vegetables in three rural communities in South Africa. M.Sc. thesis, University of Pretoria, Pretoria. Available at: http://upetd.up.ac.za/thesis/available/etd-02122009-115129/ (accessed 08 July 2009).

West, K.P. and Mehra, S. (2010) Vitamin A intake and status in populations facing economic stress. *Journal of Nutrition* 140, 201S–207S.

WHO (2009) Global prevalence of vitamin A deficiency in populations at risk 1995–2005. WHO global database on vitamin A deficiency. World Health Organization, Geneva, Switzerland. Available at: http://whqlibdoc.who.int/publications/2009/9789241598019_eng.pdf (accessed 26 July 2009).

6 Contribution of Homestead Food Production to Improved Household Food Security and Nutrition Status – Lessons Learned from Bangladesh, Cambodia, Nepal and the Philippines

Aminuzzaman Talukder,[1]* Akoto K. Osei,[1] Nancy J. Haselow,[1] Hou Kroeun,[1] Amin Uddin[2] and Victoria Quinn[3]
[1]*Helen Keller International (HKI), Phnom Penh, Cambodia;*
[2]*Helen Keller International (HKI), Dhaka, Bangladesh;*
[3]*Helen Keller International (HKI), Washington, DC, USA*

Summary

Malnutrition is a serious public health problem in Asia. Since 2003, Helen Keller International (HKI) has been implementing homestead food production (HFP) programmes to increase and ensure year-round availability and intake of micronutrient-rich foods in the poor households of Asia. The aim of this chapter is to review the impact of HFP programmes and identify lessons learned for adaptation, replication and potential scale up. Impact evaluation data were reviewed that had been collected from a representative sample (10–20% of ~30,000 households) in HFP programme villages, and from similar numbers of comparison non-HFP programme villages, in Bangladesh, Cambodia, Nepal and the Philippines. The information assessed included household garden practices, dietary intake, income and prevalence of anaemia and night blindness among children (6–59 months) and non-pregnant women. A review of the implementation process was also undertaken. The HFP programme improved household garden practices, food production and consumption, and dietary diversity. The number of crop varieties consumed was significantly increased from a range of 2–3 to 8–9 between baseline and end line among programme households. The change in proportion of households consuming eggs and/or liver was higher among programme (24–46%) than comparison (12–18%) households. The median income earned from selling surplus HFP produce in the month before the assessment increased from US$1 to US$7 in all programmes. Anaemia prevalence was lower among children in the programme households at end line compared with baseline, although the decrease was only significant in Bangladesh (from 63.9% to 45.2%), and the Philippines (from 42.9% to 16.6%). Overall, the HFP programme improved household garden practices, food consumption, dietary diversity and income, as well as reducing anaemia among preschoolchildren.

*Contact: ztalukder@hki.org

Introduction

Protein energy malnutrition and micronutrient deficiencies are major contributing factors to the high mortality in children and women in developing countries (Black *et al.*, 2008). An estimated 35% of the disease burden in children, and 3.5 million deaths in children and women annually, have been associated with malnutrition (World Bank, 2010). About 171 million children under 5 years of age in developing countries are stunted (low height for age), 55 million are wasted (low weight for height) (MOHP *et al.*, 2007; NIPORT *et al.*, 2009) and approximately10–19% of women of reproductive age are undernourished, with a body mass index (BMI) of less than 18.5 kg/m^2 (World Bank, 2010). At least a third of the children under 5 years of age in Bangladesh, Cambodia, Nepal and the Philippines are stunted or underweight, and about half are affected by anaemia (Martorell *et al*, 1995; NIPH *et al.*, 2006; MOHP *et al.*, 2007; FNRI, 2009; NIPORT *et al.*, 2009). As in most developing countries, nutritional deficiencies in these countries are partly due to limited dietary intake and infections, which, in turn, results from food insecurity, inadequate care practices and limited access to proper sanitation, clean drinking water and quality health services. The typical diet consists mainly of cereals and lacks the optimal diversity and quality to meet the nutrient needs of most people. Infants, young children and pregnant/lactating women are particularly at risk because of their high nutritional needs relative to energy intake, and also to the frequent episodes of infection, which often result in reduced appetite, decreased nutrient absorption and increased loss of nutrients from the body. Beside its effect on childhood mortality and growth, malnutrition during early life often impairs cognitive and psychological development, which then affects productive potential in adult life (MOHP *et al.*, 2007; Ivanic and Martin, 2008; NIPORT *et al.*, 2009).

Recent global issues, including the 2008 food and economic crisis, climate change, increased biofuel production and negative trade issues, have resulted in substantial increases in food prices, raised overall poverty and pushed more people into malnutrition.

The food price crisis alone is thought to have moved over 100 million people back into poverty and erased some of the global progress towards the achievement of the Millennium Development Goals (MDG) (FAO, 2010). In 2010, the Food and Agriculture Organization of the United Nations (FAO) estimated the number of hungry people in the world to be 925 million (Klotz *et al.*, 2008). To cope with the recent crises, many hungry households have been forced to adopt harmful strategies for survival, such as cutting back on food consumption, replacing nutrient-rich foods with staple foods, selling household and agricultural assets, and increased borrowing; these actions further exacerbate food insecurity, malnutrition and the health situation (Kiess *et al.*, 2001).

As inadequate dietary intake and proper care and health are some of the main causes of nutritional deficiencies, it seems logical that community-based agriculture interventions that ensure adequate access to and consumption of diversified diet, in conjunction with education for improved knowledge of, attitude and practices related to dietary intake, care and health, could contribute substantially to better nutrition in developing countries (Cerqueira and Olson, 1995; Victora *et al.*, 2008). An integrated agriculture–nutrition intervention can also contribute to poverty reduction in a variety of ways, and this, in turn, adds to the improvement of nutritional status (de Pee *et al.*, 2000; Ruel and Levin, 2000; Bloem *et al.*, 2001). Increasing the availability and consumption of nutrient-rich foods through a household's own production is considered to be a sustainable approach because the process empowers household members, particularly women, to take ultimate responsibility for the quality of the diet of the household through their own production and improved nutritional knowledge. The nutrition education component of this approach also ensures that household members make informed consumption choices (West *et al.*, 2002). For this reason, Helen Keller International (HKI) initiated projects in Bangladesh, Cambodia, Nepal and the Philippines that integrate homestead food production (HFP) – consisting of home gardening with small animal husbandry, with behavioural change communication to enhance adequate dietary intake and optimal care for household members, particularly infants, young children and pregnant and lactating women.

This chapter describes HKI's HFP model, presents findings from the programmes for which impact evaluations have been completed and provides an overview of ongoing HFP programmes and innovations incorporated into the current programmes in Asia.

Helen Keller International's Homestead Food Production Model

HKI has been implementing HFP programmes in several countries in Asia for the past two decades. The programme – which was initiated as a pilot home gardening project in Bangladesh – has focused on improving vitamin A status by encouraging households to produce and consume vitamin A-rich fruits and vegetables. However, during the 1990s, evidence from research showed that the bioavailability of micronutrients such as vitamin A from plant foods was lower than had been originally thought (Talukder *et al.*, 2000). The model was therefore revised by HKI to include both home gardens and small animal husbandry, together with nutrition education. This integrated model is currently one of the major HKI interventions in Bangladesh, Cambodia, Nepal and the Philippines.

The main objectives of the HFP programme are to encourage participating households to: (i) increase the diversity and year-round production of micronutrient-rich fruits and vegetables; (ii) increase the year-round production of poultry and eggs; (iii) improve and encourage consistent consumption of fruits and vegetables and animal source foods by households, through increased production and nutrition-related education; and (iv) improve health and nutrition outcomes of women and children through behavioural change communication to ensure optimal care, feeding, hygiene and disease prevention practices and to stimulate demand for primary health services. All of these aims are believed to ultimately improve food and nutritional security of household members.

The HFP model achieves these objectives by encouraging households to establish home gardens and small animal husbandry (mainly poultry), and by conducting education for behaviour change to inform optimal intra-household nutrition and feeding and care practices, as well as to improve health-seeking behaviour. HFP also generates additional income for households through the sale of surplus food products from the home gardens and/or animal husbandry. This income can be used to purchase other nutrient-rich foods and pay for household expenses such as health care and children's education needs (Spielman and Pandya-Lorch, 2009).

In most poor households in rural areas of Asia, home gardening is already a common practice; however, the gardens and gardening practices are suboptimal and do not offer adequate nutritious year-round products. Under the HFP model, household gardens are classified into three categories: 'traditional', 'improved' and 'developed'. Traditional gardens are seasonal and are often maintained on scattered plots with a few traditional fruits and vegetables, such as pumpkins and gourds. This type of home gardening is usually practised by most households in Asia, especially when there is no external assistance for improved agricultural practices. Improved gardens are gardens maintained on fixed plots that produce more varieties of fruits and vegetables than the traditional gardens, but only during certain times of the year. Developed gardens are maintained on fixed plots and produce a diversified variety of fruits and vegetables that are available throughout the year (i.e. year round).

HKI's HFP model encourages both the improved and developed gardens, but promotes and assists households to ultimately establish the developed type of garden together with animal husbandry. The model works by providing technical assistance, training, agricultural supplies and management support through local non-governmental organization (NGO) partners to support primarily women farmers from poor households. In establishing the HFP model, HKI first works with the local NGO partners to provide initial inputs, such as seeds, seedlings, saplings and chicks, to participating households and also to establish village model farms (VMFs) in the target communities. The VMFs serve as a continuous community-based resource for the supply of seeds, seedlings, saplings and chicks to participating households for their year-round food production after the external assistance by HKI is withdrawn; they also serve as a focal point for community support, demonstrating agricultural methods and providing practical training and inputs for production by targeted households. The owner of the VMF also coordinates and supports women's groups of household producers/farmers in the programme, and helps to link them to additional health and agriculture services, as well as to markets.

The strengths of the HFP model include its potential sustainability because it is community based and focuses on women from poor households as the primary beneficiaries, placing farming inputs, knowledge and skills in their hands. This gives poor women access to and control over the resources provided by the programme and therefore partly addresses the gender constraints within these societies. The HFP model is also 'flexible' in that it can be integrated with or serve as a platform for delivering other public health programmes. One such programme was in Bangladesh, where the HFP programme was implemented as part of a Title II Development Assistance Program funded by the US Agency for International Development (USAID) with the combined objective of addressing household food insecurity, maternal and child health, the livelihood of flood-affected victims and their communities, and local preparedness for such emergencies. Similarly, in Nepal the HFP model is being explored as a platform for delivering micronutrient powders (MNPs) to preschoolchildren. Other innovations in Nepal include setting up the HFP at household level as one of the conditions for cash transfer and food for work programmes, so to ensure sustainable improvements in household food and nutrition security.

Altogether, the HFP programme has reached over a million households, representing about 5.5 million beneficiaries, particularly women and children, in Bangladesh,

Cambodia, Nepal and the Philippines. The number of beneficiaries is continuously increasing as the programme is currently being expanded to other districts in these countries, and in some cases with added operational research components to identify innovative ways for further refining the model. To date, the majority of the HFP programmes are implemented with HKI support for about 3–4 four years, after which such support is withdrawn and the community takes over. The success of the HFP programme has been recognized by several high-profile documents, including the *2010 Bread for the World's Annual Hunger Report* (Bread for the World Institute, 2010) and *The Millions Fed*, a report by the International Food Policy Research Institute in 2009 (Spielman and Pandya-Lorch, 2009). The programme was also selected as one of the innovative programmes at the World Bank Development Market place forum in Bangladesh in 2009.

Methodology

Reports on evaluations of the HFP programmes in Bangladesh, Cambodia, Nepal and the Philippines were reviewed to assess the combined impact of the programme on process indicators such as household garden practices, vegetable, fruit and poultry production, food consumption and household income, and outcome indicators such as impact on anaemia among children and women. Since 2003, the HFP programme has been implemented in more than 30,000 households in various project sites in these countries. Data collected from representative samples of about 10–20% of households in HFP programme villages, and from a similar number of comparison (control) households in non-HFP programme villages, were reviewed to illustrate the benefit of the programme. The households in HFP programme villages received training and inputs for homestead food production, as well as nutrition education from HKI through trained personnel of local NGO partners.

In all the countries involved in this review, cross-sectional data were collected from households in the programme and comparison villages before the start of the HFP programme (baseline) and after a certain period of programme implementation (end line). The dates during which baseline and end-line surveys were conducted in the respective countries are given in Table 6.1. In each country (except Cambodia), baseline and end-line surveys were conducted at around the same time of the year to reduce the influences of normal variations in production resulting from seasonality. The changes in outcome variables of interest between baseline and end-line surveys were compared between the programme and control communities in each country in order to determine the impact of the HFP projects.

In all four countries, data were collected through interviews with beneficiary (and control sample) women on household garden practices and food production. The data included: (i) type of home garden, quantity and variety of vegetables and fruits produced in the home garden and the number of eggs produced by the poultry; (ii) household food consumption, including the number of different varieties of fruits and vegetables consumed by household members and the consumption of animal foods such as eggs and liver by household members in the week before the survey; (iii) household income generated from the sale of HFP products in the month preceding the survey and the utilization of such income; and (iv) household socio-economic indicators, including women's involvement in household decision making. It is worth noting that other information on household characteristics was also collected during these surveys, but only the data relevant to this review are mentioned here.

Table 6.1. Dates of baseline and end-line data collection for homestead food production (HFP) programme evaluations in Bangladesh, Cambodia, Nepal and the Philippines.

	Date of baseline survey	Date of end-line survey
Bangladesh	July 2003	June 2005
Cambodia	October 2005	May 2007
Nepal	May 2003	May 2006
Philippines	April 2005	July 2007

The weight and height of children were also measured in all four countries, and in a subsample of households, a finger prick of blood was collected by trained staff from ~1000 children aged 6–59 months and ~1200 non-pregnant women, before and after programme implementation, for measurement of haemoglobin using a HemoCue analyser. The subsample included ~125 children aged 6–59 months and ~200 non-pregnant women from each of the programme and control households in each country. Blood samples were collected only for children and not for mothers in the Philippines survey, because children were considered the primary focus of anaemia assessment for the impact evaluation in this country. Anaemia was defined as haemoglobin <110 g/l for children aged 6–59 months, and <120 g/l for non-pregnant women (HKI, 2004). All the respondents were informed about the purpose of the survey, and verbal and written consent was received from all of them before their participation. The confidentiality of all information released by respondents was assured. Ethical approval for the studies was granted by the National Ethics Committee in all four countries. In addition to the impact evaluation surveys presented in this review for the HFP programmes, secondary data from the second national vitamin A survey conducted in Bangladesh in 1999 was also used to assess the impact of home gardening and poultry production on the prevalence of night blindness in children.

Country-specific data was analysed separately using the Statistical Package for Social Science (SPSS). For each of the four countries, proportions, means and medians of key outcome variables of interest were used to describe the data collected from the baseline and end-line surveys. Comparisons were made on each outcome indicator between baseline and end-line surveys to assess whether these parameters had changed over time. The changes in the programme and comparison households were then compared to assess the impact of the programme. Country-specific programme evaluation results have been presented in various reports, bulletins and other publications (Kiess *et al.*, 1998; HKI, 2007, 2008; Olney *et al.*, 2009). For most of the results presented in this review, the raw data were not pooled and reanalysed, but rather the findings presented in the various reports and bulletins were reviewed and presented to illustrate the impact of the HFP programmes. However, in cases where the raw data from the different countries were available for a particular indicator, they were reanalysed separately for each country, and also pooled together and reanalysed, to verify and clarify the findings obtained from the already published reports and bulletins.

Results

Changes in home garden practices

In all the countries, there was evidence of the HFP programme households exhibiting the use of the improved and developed garden and poultry techniques promoted by the HFP model. As shown in Fig. 6.1, the type of gardens cultivated in the programme changed significantly between baseline and end-line surveys for both the programme and comparison households in Cambodia. The number of developed gardens, with diverse varieties of vegetables, was very low in both programme and control areas at baseline, although at the end-line evaluation, a significantly greater

proportion of households in the programme had developed gardening than the control households.

In one of the HFP programmes in Bangladesh, the percentage of households that had developed gardens increased from 13% at baseline to 30% at end line, and even among a subsample of households that had graduated from the programme, 45% were still practising the improved and developed garden techniques promoted by the programme. These increases in the use of garden techniques suggest that the HFP programme had a positive impact on household food production practices.

Changes in vegetable production and consumption

Figure 6.2 presents the consolidated findings from the end-line evaluation surveys in Bangladesh and Cambodia HFP programmes. It shows the number of vegetable varieties produced, the production (by weight) in the 2 months before the survey and the frequency of vegetable consumption by children in the week before the survey for the different types of home gardens (traditional, improved and developed garden types) in these communities. The data indicate that the total number of varieties of vegetables and the amount being

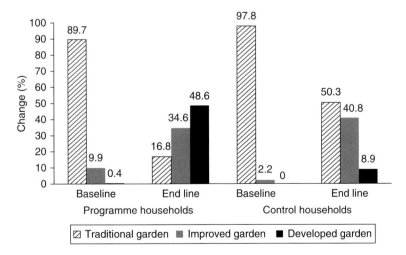

Fig. 6.1. Changes in type of household (home) gardens practised by households between baseline and end line surveys of the homestead food production (HFP) programme in Cambodia (2005–2007).

produced was highest among households that practised the developed and improved gardening techniques, compared with households that kept the traditional types of garden. Compared with traditional gardens, there were twice the number of vegetable varieties and the quantity of vegetables in home gardens in households cultivating improved gardens and, in turn, three to four times the amount in households with developed gardens (Fig. 6.2). Consequently, the production of nutrient-rich fruits and vegetables such as dark-green leafy vegetables, orange and yellow vegetables and fruits increased among households in the HFP programme in all countries (data not shown).

Vegetable consumption by young children followed a similar trend to the data for production, so that children from households with developed gardens consumed the highest amount and diversity of vegetables, followed by children from households with improved gardens, and with the least consumption of vegetables occurring among households with traditional gardens. Only four types of vegetables were eaten by children when households practised traditional gardening compared with eight and 13 types

of vegetables eaten when households practised the improved and developed gardening, respectively. Frequency of consumption of vegetables by children was also 1.6 times higher among children in households that had developed gardens and 1.3 times higher among children in households with improved gardens compared with those in households with traditional gardens (Fig. 6.2). The high diversity and frequency of vegetable consumption among children from households that had improved and developed gardens was also associated with an increased consumption of vitamin A-rich foods. More children in households with developed gardens consumed vitamin A-rich foods, such as green leafy vegetables and yellow fruits, than did children in households without a garden or with a traditional garden (data not shown).

Changes in animal food consumption

The findings from pooled data of the surveys in Bangladesh and Cambodia showed that consumption of chicken liver increased from 24% to 46% from baseline to end line in programme households. Egg consumption by household members, as well as by mothers

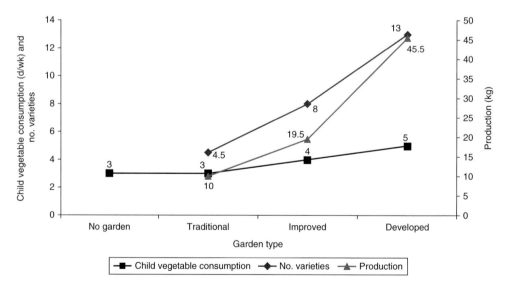

Fig. 6.2. Type of household (home) garden related to production and consumption (by children) of vegetables (days/week), and number of vegetable varieties grown, at the end-line surveys of the homestead food production (HFP) programmes in Bangladesh (2003–2005) and Cambodia (2005–2007).

and children, also increased in the pro-gramme households ($P < 0.05$) (Table 6.2).

These findings suggest that the HFP pro-gramme improved overall household access to a wide variety of foods. In one of the pro-grammes in Bangladesh, household dietary consumption as measured by a dietary diversity score was higher among the HFP programme households (average score of 5.8) than among comparison households (average score of 5.4). Besides vegetables, fruits and eggs, a higher consumption of other nutritious foods such as legumes/pulses, meat and fish was also reported by the programme households.

Income earned from homestead food production and its utilization

One of the benefits of the HFP programme is the increase in household income from the sale of surplus produce from homestead food production. This is critical for poor families, mainly subsistent farmers, who are net buy-ers and spend an average of more than 50% of their incomes on food. Impact evaluations of the HFP programmes in Bangladesh showed that the household's bimonthly earnings from the sale of vegetables and fruits from the home gardens increased from an average of US$0.62 at baseline to US$1.25 at end line. The average income from the sale of eggs and poultry also increased from US$1.62 to US$2.16 between these surveys. An increase in the income earned by house-holds from the sale of HFP garden products was also observed in Cambodia. On average,

Cambodian households earned US$3.75 at the baseline, which increased to US$17.50 at end line, from the sale of vegetables and fruits from home gardens. There was only a small increase of income in households in Cambodia from the sale of poultry products (US$9 at baseline to US$9.75 at end line).

Up to 92% of households in Cambodia and 70% of households in Bangladesh used the income earned from the sale of home garden produce to purchase additional food. Over 80% of households in Cambodia and almost half in Bangladesh (46%) spent the income obtained from selling animal prod-ucts obtained from homestead food produc-tion to purchase other foods (Table 6.3). Some of the HFP programme households in Bangladesh also used the income earned from the sale of HFP products on other important household expenditure, such as education (including materials and clothing for school) and investing in income-generating activities of the household – for example, reinvesting in the HFP to purchase seeds, seedlings, sap-lings and chicks, or investing in other income-generating activities.

Evidence of improvement in gender roles

As stated above, HFP programmes target women in poor households who are given inputs from the programme. A review of survey results from Bangladesh, Cambodia and Nepal showed that for almost three quarters (73%) of the households in HFP vill-ages, the majority of HFP activities – including

Table 6.2. Consumption of chicken liver and eggs at baseline and end-line surveys of the homestead food production (HFP) programmes in Bangladesh and Cambodia (2003–2007).

Consumption of chicken liver/eggs	Baseline survey		End-line survey	
	%	No.	%	No.
Households that consumed chicken liver in the 7 days before the survey	24	720	46	720
Median number eggs consumed in the 7 days before the survey:				
Household	2	720	5	720
Mothers	1	254	1.5	402
Children	1	266	2	407

Table 6.3. Proportion of homestead food production (HFP) programme households in Bangladesh and Cambodia that spent income earned by selling garden produce, poultry and eggs on various items at end line.

Household commodities invested in using income from HFP products sold (in order of expenditure)	Bangladesh[a] (in last 2 months)		Cambodia (in last 1 month)	
	Household spending income from selling home garden products (%)	Household spending income from selling eggs and poultry (%)	Household spending income from selling home garden products (%)	Household spending income from selling eggs and poultry (%)
Food	70	46	92	82
Education	30	26	1	3
Production/Reinvestment	22	25	1	3
Clothes	14	22	0	3
Saving	11	24	0	0
Medicine	8	0	2	6
Housing	1	3	0	0
Amusement	1	2	0	0
Social activities	0	1	1	2
Other	0	0	3	1

[a]Multiple responses allowed.

deciding what type of garden to have at the homestead – were managed by women. Women were also the major decision makers on the use of the income earned by selling garden produce. In addition, the behavioural change communication and nutrition education component of the programme empowered women beneficiaries through improving their knowledge of dietary intake and primary health care practices. These benefits are in line with one of the core objectives of the programme, which was to address gender inequities by placing resources in the hands of women, encouraging women's participation in household decision making and improving their knowledge.

Impact on prevalence of anaemia among children aged 6–59 months

The prevalence of anaemia among children 6–59 months of age decreased in programme households in all four countries after implementation of the project (Fig. 6.3). However, the decrease in anaemia prevalence among children was significant only in Bangladesh (63.9 at baseline versus 45.2% at end line, $P < 0.001$) and the Philippines (42.9 at baseline versus 16.6% at end line, $P < 0.001$). Among the control households, anaemia prevalence among children remained unchanged in Nepal, decreased slightly in Cambodia, but

showed significant decreases in Bangladesh and the Philippines. In all four countries though, the magnitude of the decrease in anaemia among children was higher in programme households than in control households, although the inter-group difference was not statistically significant.

Impact on anaemia prevalence among non-pregnant mothers of children aged 6–59 months

In communities that were beneficiaries of the HFP programme, anaemia prevalence among non-pregnant mothers of children aged 6–59 months decreased by 26% ($P < 0.05$) and 12% ($P = 0.08$) in Nepal and Bangladesh, respectively. However, anaemia prevalence among non-pregnant mothers of the children in the control communities remained relatively unchanged in both of these countries (Fig. 6.4). There was no significant change in anaemia prevalence among non-pregnant mothers in either the HFP programme or the control communities in Cambodia (Fig. 6.4).

Potential impact on vitamin A deficiency

HKI reasserted the importance of HFP in the control of night blindness based on the findings of the last national vitamin A survey in rural Bangladesh. The study showed that

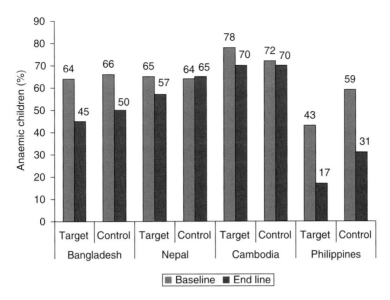

Fig. 6.3. Anaemia prevalence among children aged 6–59 months from homestead food production (HFP) programme and control households at baseline and end line surveys of the programmes in Bangladesh (2003–2005), Cambodia (2005–2007), Nepal (2003–2006) and the Philippines (2005–2007).

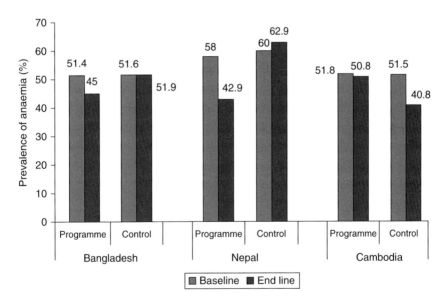

Fig. 6.4. Anaemia prevalence among non-pregnant mothers of children aged 6–59 months in homestead food production (HFP) programme and control households at the baseline and end line of the programmes in Bangladesh (2003–2005), Cambodia (2005–2007) and Nepal (2003–2006).

among children aged 12–59 months who had not received a vitamin A capsule (VAC) in the 6 months before the national survey, the prevalence of night blindness (clinical vitamin A deficiency) was significantly lower in households with a garden and/or poultry than in households without either (Fig. 6.5). Among children who received a VAC, no such

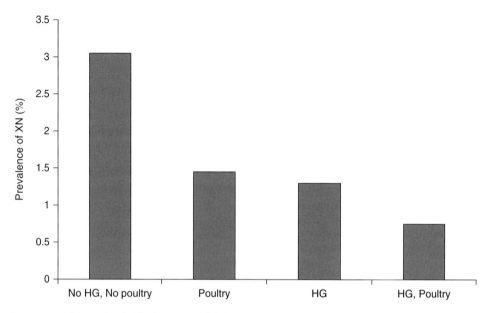

Fig. 6.5. Prevalence of night blindness (xerophthalmia, XN) among children aged 12–59 months who had not received a vitamin A capsule (VAC), by home garden (HG) and poultry ownership (*n* = 4296).

difference was found, which seems to indicate that the large-dose VAC overshadowed any additional impact of the improved diet.

Discussion

This review of the results from the evaluation of HFP programmes in Bangladesh, Cambodia, Nepal and the Philippines has shown that the programme improved household garden practices, increased dietary diversity in terms of both the production and consumption of vegetables, fruits and animal source foods (such as eggs and chicken liver) among beneficiary households, particularly children and women. Thus, the programmes improved household food security by increasing the year-round availability and diversity of micronutrient-rich foods at the household level, by informing optimal nutritional behaviour through nutrition education and by improving the economic resources of the participating families.

The increased diversity in vegetable and animal food consumption was important to ensure adequate intake of essential vitamins and minerals for optimal growth and development; both eggs and liver are good sources of micronutrients, and an increase in dietary diversity has been shown to improve micronutrient intake (Ruel and Levin, 2000). In the HFP programme, this was evident in the reduction of anaemia among children and their non-pregnant mothers, and in the reduction of night blindness among children in some of the countries studied. Insufficient dietary intake of iron is believed to be the main cause of anaemia in most developing countries. Although these evaluations did not study the impact of HFP on dietary iron intake or iron status, improved intake of dietary iron and other micronutrients (such as vitamin A), and improved childcare, health and hygiene practices, as a result of the HFP programme may have contributed to the reduction of anaemia in the intervention communities. The programme's impact on anaemia reduction appears promising, even though results were not consistent across all four countries. The varied results may be due to the slight variation in the design of the impact evaluation and to differences in the aetiology of anaemia among these groups in the different countries. Hence, a more tightly controlled study design may be necessary to evaluate the impact of HFP on anaemia. Further, among young children in particular, additional interventions that are based on sound knowledge of contextual factors associated with anaemia may be needed to adequately reduce anaemia in these populations.

Equally important, the findings from this review showed that surplus HFP produce can be sold, so generating additional income for the family. The nutrition education component of the HFP programme also promoted nutritionally informed food purchasing and consumption choices, and the findings showed that the majority of households used the additional income to buy supplementary food items, such as meat, fish and cooking oil, thereby further increasing the diversity of the family's diet. The income was used to cover other essential household expenses and to invest in productive assets as well – including reinvesting in HFP activities. More recently, HKI has found that this investment in productive assets helped families to cope during times of economic difficulty or natural disaster (Olney *et al.*, 2009).

Through targeting women as HFP managers, HFP programmes empowered women, giving them more control over resources and income generated from the programme. Such control over resources and income enhanced women's participation in household decision making. This also had a positive impact on overall household spending, food preparation, food choices and intra-household food allocation, as well as on the care-seeking behaviour of women. As seen by the reduction of night blindness (a clinical sign of vitamin A deficiency) among children living in households with gardens and/or poultry, HFP programmes also had a positive effect on vitamin A status. HFP has been shown to be an important way to improve the intake of vitamin A-rich and other micronutrient-rich foods, particularly in poor households.

Despite the series of impacts outlined above, no clear impact of the HFP programme

has been demonstrated on child growth indicators (i.e. anthropometry), and aside from the impact on anaemia and night blindness, no clear impact of the HFP programme has been demonstrated on any other micronutrient status indicators (e.g. for iron, folate, or other micronutrients). This is in line with findings from several recent systematic reviews of the impact of agriculture programmes with a nutrition focus, which also found no impact of such interventions on growth indicators. This is partly because the past impact evaluations of the programme were not rigorously designed to capture effects on child growth indicators such as stunting, underweight and wasting, or on other biochemical or functional indicators of micronutrient status. One major constraint was that the programme was implemented for an average period of 3–4 years, which is too short a time to demonstrate significant impact on growth indicators like stunting, without a very large sample size. Large sample sizes and biochemical assessments require substantial funding, which is often beyond the budget allocated for the impact evaluations of previous HFP programmes. To assess most biochemical indicators of micronutrient status also requires the collection, transportation and processing of blood samples, which is sometimes limited by cultural resistance to having blood drawn and the difficulty of maintaining a cold chain in some of the rural areas where the HFP programme was implemented.

None the less, the programme results presented here are encouraging. The contribution of the programme to overall household food consumption and improved micronutrient status, however, can be maximized by implementing it in coordination with other interventions for combating micronutrient deficiencies, such as deworming, vitamin A supplementation and home fortification with micronutrient powders. The integration of HFP into other types of development programmes should be explored and encouraged as a way to scale up the HFP model more quickly. For instance, HFP can complement programmes aimed at improving gender equality through its positive effect on women's empowerment and increased control of household resources. In addition, the HFP model, which promotes developed gardening *with* targeted nutrition education, should be introduced into agriculture programmes that promote home gardening and livestock to better ensure that more available food translates into increased consumption and also into improved nutrition among vulnerable household members. The HFP model can also be used to target specific vulnerable groups, such as households with people living with HIV/AIDS, because such households require additional food and have added healthcare costs, which put further demands on their limited resources.

As shown by the results of this review, homestead food production has the potential to increase micronutrient intake and improve the health and nutritional status of nutritionally at-risk women and children in various ways, including increased household production for the families' own consumption, increased income from the sale of products and improved social status of women through greater control over resources and knowledge.

On-going HFP Projects in Asia

Lessons learned from the evaluations and monitoring results have been used to expand and improve the HFP programme over time. Nevertheless, additional data are needed to better understand its impact on growth and other micronutrient status indicators of children and women. There is also a need for improved documentation of programme activities and for the standardization of tools and procedures for the implementation, monitoring and evaluation of the programme to encourage its effective operation at scale. To address these concerns, HKI is currently undertaking operational research in several countries to look more closely at the HFP programme, including evaluations of its impact pathways to ensure adequate implementation of the model (i.e. proper programme delivery).

Such studies are envisioned to provide answers to some of the questions that remain about the potential impact of the HFP model in order to enhance its wide-scale adoption and scale up. In Nepal, three HFP programmes are currently under way, each with a distinct focus of addressing a particular operations research or implementation question. One of the projects, called *Action Against Malnutrition through Agriculture* (AAMA) is implemented in two districts of the far western region of Nepal. In one of the districts, the focus of the project is to assess the impact of the programme on child growth indicators (stunting, wasting, underweight) and anaemia using a community-based cluster-randomized controlled design in which some communities are randomly assigned to receive the HFP programme for a period of 4 years and other communities (not receiving the programme) serve as controls. This project also entails a substudy to assess whether providing micronutrient powders (MNPs) to young children in households receiving the HFP programme will provide any added benefits to child growth and prevalence of anaemia. In the second district, the HFP programme is implemented as a district-wide model, with all villages focusing on assessing the enablers and constraints for wide-scale implementation of the programme. A third HFP programme, implemented in another district of Nepal, has the objective of assessing approaches for effective governance of the project, thus finding effective ways to enhance collaboration between the ministries of agriculture and health as well as between partners working in these areas to ensure its effective delivery. All of these programmes are funded by USAID.

In Cambodia, HKI has recently completed the end-line surveys of three HFP programmes, including two at a large scale, with funding from the European Commission. One of these is called *Support to Food Security for Women and Rural Poor in Cambodia*, and is being implemented in two provinces. The other, *Facility for Rapid Response to Soaring Food Prices in Developing Countries*, is being implemented in four provinces of Cambodia. A third and recently completed HFP project in Cambodia is called *Improving Micronutrient and Socio-economic Status among People Living with HIV/AIDS*, and has funding from the Neys-Van Hoogstraten Foundation in the Netherlands. All three projects focus on improving household food security and dietary intake of vulnerable household members. However, the third project, in Cambodia, also has an operations research component that focuses on assessing the impact of the HFP programme on anaemia and on serum biochemical indicators such as retinol, ferritin and the soluble transferrin receptor status of children and their mothers. The International Food Policy Research Institute (IFPRI) has also worked with HKI to conduct research to understand the impact pathways of programmes and has developed an enhanced homestead food production (HFP) model for better health and nutrition in Cambodia. There is also another HFP research project under way in collaboration with WorldFish and the University of British Columbia, which is assessing ways of integrating aquaculture into the HFP model (i.e. fish farming in addition to garden and poultry rearing at the household level).

In Indonesia, HKI has implemented the HFP project in the Timur Tengah Selatan District of the country, as part of the *Project Laser Beam*, with funding support from Kraft Foods Inc. and World Food Programme.

Conclusion and Recommendations

HFP is a strategy that has shown positive results in poor countries for improved household food consumption, decreased prevalence of anaemia among children in some countries, increased household income and the potential empowerment of poor women. Due to the multiple benefits of the programme, HFP could conceivably contribute to the achievement of the MDGs, including those for hunger and poverty reduction,

the promotion of gender equity and women's empowerment, the reduction of child mortality and improvement of maternal health. Considering the factors that are affecting food availability in developing countries – such as the global food and economic crisis, the increase in biofuel production, negative trade issues and climate change – programmes such as HFP can have a positive effect among poor households by decreasing their dependence on outside food sources and increasing their own production, thereby improving household food security and resilience to unforeseen events. For these reasons, it is important that the HFP programme be expanded to other areas in these countries and implemented in other countries where micronutrient deficiencies are a public health problem.

Acknowledgements

We gratefully acknowledge the generous financial support for the programmes discussed in this chapter. In Bangladesh, Oxfam Novib provided support, in Nepal, the US Agency for International Development (USAID), in Cambodia, USAID, the Canadian International Development Agency (IRDC/CIDA) and the European Commission, and in the Philippines, Monsanto. We are also thankful to additional donors who are funding HKI's HFP programmes in Asia, including IDRC/CIDA, Kraft Foods and the World Food Programme. We also thank all staff who worked on these projects and, most of all, our sincere appreciation goes to the families who were involved in the programme as well as in the impact evaluations.

References

Black, R.E., Allen, L.H., Bhutta, Z.A., Caulfield, L.E., de Onis, M., Ezzati, M., Mathers, C. and Rivera, A. (2008) Maternal and child undernutrition: global and regional exposures and health consequences. *The Lancet* 371, 243–60.

Bloem, M.W., Moench-Pfanner, R. and Kiess, L. (2001) Combating micronutrient deficiencies: an important component of poverty reduction. Biomedical and Environmental Sciences 14, 92–97.

Bread for the World Institute (2010) *Our Common Interest: Ending Hunger and Malnutrition, 2011 Hunger Report. Twenty-first Annual Report on State of World Hunger.* Bread for the World Institute, Washington, DC.

Cerqueira, M.T. and Olson, C.M. (1995) *Nutrition education in developing countries: an examination of recent successful projects*. In: Pinstrup-Andersen, P., Pelletier, D. and Alderman, H. (eds) *Child Growth and Nutrition in Developing Countries: Priorities for Action*. Cornell University Press, Ithaca, New York, pp. 53–77.

de Pee, S., Bloem, M.W. and Kiess, L. (2000) Evaluating food-based programmes for their reduction of vitamin A deficiency and its consequences. *Food and Nutrition Bulletin* 21, 232–238.

FAO (2010) *The State of Food Insecurity in the World: Addressing Food Insecurity in Protracted Crises*. Food and Agriculture Organization of the United Nations, Rome.

FNRI (2009) *The Sixth National Nutrition Survey Results*. Food and Nutrition Research Institute, Manila.

HKI (2004) *Homestead Food Production Activities in Cambodia – A Mapping Review Report*. Helen Keller International Cambodia, Phnom Penh.

HKI (2007) Homestead Food Production Program improves food and nutrition security by increasing consumption of micronutrient-rich foods and family income in HHs with HIV/AIDS and other chronic diseases. *Nutrition Bulletin* No. 7(1), Helen Keller International Cambodia, Phnom Penh. Available at: http://www.hki.org/research/CmbNutriBul_vol7_iss1.pdf (accessed 3 June 2013).

HKI (2008) *Homestead Food Production Program in Char Area in Bangladesh. Report of the Final Evaluation of the Project*. Helen Keller International Bangladesh, Dhaka.

Ivanic, M. and Martin, W. (2008) *Implications of Higher Global Food Prices for Poverty in Low Income Countries*. Policy Research Working Paper 4594, World Bank, Washington, DC.

Kiess, L., Bloem, M.W., de Pee, S., Hye, A., Khan, T., Talukder, A., Haque, M. and Ali, M. (1998) Bangladesh: xerophthalmia free. Combined effect of vitamin A (VA) capsule distribution and homestead gardening in reducing vitamin A deficiency (VAD). In: *American Public Health Association 126th Annual Meeting Report, November 15–18, 1998*. Washington, DC, p. 361 [abstract]. Reprinted in Appendix 13 of HKI Asia-Pacific (2001) *Homestead Food Production – A Strategy to Combat Malnutrition and Poverty*. Helen Keller International, Jakarta, Indonesia, p. 118.

Kiess, L., Moench-Pfanner, R. and Bloem, M.W. (2001) Food-based strategies: can they play a role in poverty alleviation? *Food and Nutrition Bulletin* 22, 436–442.

Klotz, C., de Pee, S., Thorne-Lyman, A., Kraemer, K. and Bloem, M. (2008) Nutrition in the perfect storm: why micronutrient malnutrition will be a widespread health consequence of high food prices. *Sight and Life Magazine* 2, 6–13.

Martorell, R., Schroeder, D.G., Rivera, J.A. and Kaplowitz, H.J. (1995) Patterns of linear growth in rural Guatemalan adolescents and children. *Journal of Nutrition* 125, 1060S–1067S.

MOHP, New ERA and Macro International (2007) *Nepal Demographic and Health Survey 2006*. Population Division, Ministry of Health and Population and New ERA, Kathmandu with Macro International Inc., Calverton, Maryland. Available at: http://www.measuredhs.com/pubs/pdf/FR191/FR191.pdf (accessed 3 June 2013).

NIPH, NIS and ORC Macro (2006) *Cambodia Demographic and Health Survey 2005*. National Institute of Public Health and National Institute of Statistics, Phnom Penh with ORC Macro, Calverton, Maryland. Available at: http://www.measuredhs.com/pubs/pdf/FR185/FR185%5BApril-27-2011%5D.pdf (accessed 3 June 2013).

NIPORT, Mitra and Associates and Macro International (2009) *Bangladesh Demographic and Health Survey 2007*. National Institute of Population Research and Training and Mitra and Associates, Dhaka with Macro International Inc., Calverton, Maryland. Available at: http://www.measuredhs.com/pubs/pdf/FR207/FR207%5BApril-10-2009%5D.pdf (accessed 3 June 2013).

Olney, D.K., Talukder, A., Iannotti, L.L., Ruel, M.T. and Quinn, V. (2009) Assessing impact and impact pathways of a homestead food production program on household and child nutrition in Cambodia. *Food and Nutrition Bulletin* 30, 355–369.

Ruel, M.T. and Levin, C.E. (2000) *Assessing the Potential for Food-based Strategies to Reduce Vitamin A and Iron Deficiencies: A Review of Recent Evidence*. FCND Discussion Paper No. 92, Food Consumption and Nutrition Division, International Food Policy Research Institute, Washington, DC. Available at: http://www.ifpri.org/sites/default/files/publications/fcndp92.pdf (accessed 3 June 2013). Also available as Discussion Paper Brief in *Food and Nutrition Bulletin* (2001) 22, 94–95.

Spielman, D.J. and Pandya-Lorch, R. (eds) (2009) *Millions Fed: Proven Successes in Agricultural Development*. International Food Policy Research Institute (IFPRI), Washington, DC.

Talukder, A., Kiess, L., Huq, N., de Pee, S., Darnton-Hill, I. and Bloem, M.W. (2000) Increasing the production and consumption of vitamin A-rich fruits and vegetables: Lessons learned in taking the Bangladesh homestead gardening programme to a national scale. *Food and Nutrition Bulletin* 21, 165–172.

Victora, C.G., Adair, L., Fall, C., Hallal, P.C., Martorell, R., Richter, L. and Sachdev, H.S. (2008) Maternal and child undernutrition: consequences for adult health and human capital. *The Lancet* 371, 340–57.

West, C.E., Eilander, A. and van Lieshout, M. (2002) Consequences of revised estimates of carotenoid bioefficacy for dietary control of vitamin A deficiency in developing countries. *Journal of Nutrition* 32, 2920S–2926S.

World Bank (2010) *What Can We Learn from Nutrition Impact Evaluations? Lessons from a Review of Interventions to Reduce Child Malnutrition in Developing Countries.* Independent Evaluation Group, International Finance Corporation and Multilateral Investment Guarantee Agency, The World Bank, Washington, DC.

7 The Underestimated Impact of Food-based Interventions

Ian Darnton-Hill*

*Tufts University, Boston, Massachusetts, USA and
University of Sydney, Sydney, Australia*

Summary

With the exception of iodine in certain ecological settings, micronutrients are found abundantly in plant and animal foods. Nevertheless, the diets of families in low-income environments are frequently of poor micronutrient quality. Foods rich in vitamins and minerals and other health-protecting dietary components are usually both more expensive and less accessible, aggravated by a bioavailability that is often low. Sufficiently diversified diets are adequate for the prevention of micronutrient deficiencies in very young children and in pregnancy, but can be a challenge for correcting some deficiencies, especially in the face of repeated infectious disease or prematurity. Food-based approaches to address micronutrient deficiencies have long experience and documented success, but have often been inadequately evaluated and thus have failed to gain scientific acceptance and adequate funding. They have acquired more urgency for adoption and proper evaluation in recent years due to environmental considerations, increasing disparities, the global financial crises and severe rises in food prices. Programmes such as home gardening in Bangladesh, now scaled up to over 800,000 households, and expanded into African and other Asian countries, have demonstrated successful impact on micronutrient deficiencies, and biofortification is looking promising. However, measuring the effectiveness of food-based programmes should use indicators of outcomes that go beyond biological levels of micronutrients to clinical outcomes (e.g. reduction in night blindness) and social outcomes, and to longer term more indirect benefits, such as likely increased women's empowerment and strengthening of local capacity and non-governmental organizations (NGOs), all of which have been documented. Any evaluation of interventions and their cost-effectiveness needs to attempt to capture these outcomes.

Background

With the exception of iodine and some other minerals in certain ecological settings, vitamins and minerals (micronutrients) are found abundantly in many plant foods and animal products. Nevertheless, the diets of families in low-income environments are frequently of poor quality with low micronutrient bioavail- ability while, at the same time, micronutrient-rich foods are often both more expensive and less accessible. It is poor dietary quality rather than quantity that is the key determinant of impaired micronutrient status. Further, it is likely that an appropriately diversified diet is sufficient for maintaining micronutrient status in most populations, even in young children and in pregnancy, but is more of a

*Contact: ian.darnton-hill@sydney.edu.au

challenge when deficiencies need to be corrected, at least for vitamin A, iron and zinc. There is long experience in the use of food-based approaches to address micronutrient deficiencies, although these have generally been inadequately evaluated, funded and scaled up globally (Darnton-Hill, 2008). The difficulty of cross-sectoral collaboration and communication between nutrition, health and agricultural and horticultural sectors has been a further major constraint (World Bank, 2007).

Food-based approaches will be mainly considered here as integrated small-scale horticulture such as homestead gardening. However, fortification, especially home-based fortification for multi-micronutrient powders to add to complementary foods (Zlotkin and Tondeur, 2007), and biofortification are both likely to play a significant role in contributing to micronutrient-adequate diets in resource-poor settings in the future (Bouis, 2003). Other assumptions, based on good scientific evidence, are: that poor families spend a large proportion (up to 80%) of their resources on food (World Bank, 2007; UN SCN, 2010); that women, compared with men, spend more of the resources over which they have control on food and health care, especially for their children (Quisumbing et al., 1995); and that it is difficult, especially in poor diets consisting largely of one staple, to achieve adequate micronutrient consumption without some animal-derived foods (HKI, 2001; Neumann et al., 2011). Using these assumptions, the size of the micronutrient problem will be briefly considered and the evidence for impact of food-based approaches will be reviewed, with the proposition that, for largely sociocultural reasons, the impact and cost-effectiveness of food-based approaches for improving micronutrient nutrition have both been underestimated, with consequences that are addressed in the conclusions at the end of the chapter.

Size of the Nutrition Problem of Micronutrient Deficiencies

The magnitude of undernutrition has shown stubborn resistance to much improvement at a global level, with some major exceptions, such as East Asia (UN SCN, 2010). While this may reflect generally inadequate attention and insufficient resources being directed to the problem, as well as poor capacity at a national level, the prevention and control of micronutrient deficiency have received the greatest attention and share of nutrition resources globally over the last two decades (Darnton-Hill, 2008). Along with a third of children globally stunted (approximately 171 million), the estimates of around 2 billion remain largely unchanged for micronutrient deficiencies (WHO, 2010).

A recent figure gives the burden of disease caused by micronutrient deficiencies as 7.2% of the total global problem. Nearly 11% of all child deaths under 5 years of age are thought to be due to the four micronutrient deficiencies of vitamin A, zinc, iron and iodine (Bhutta, 2008). Besides the global burden of disease, micronutrient deficiencies have enormous social and economic costs, and these tend to be borne mostly by women and children (Darnton-Hill et al., 2005; Webb et al., 2007). A systematic review, which identified all studies that had been published between 1988 and 2008 reporting on micronutrient intakes in women living in resource-poor environments, showed that, except for vitamin A (29%), vitamin C (34%) and niacin (34%), the reported mean/median intakes in over 50% of the studies were below the estimated average requirements (EAR), demonstrating that inadequate intakes of multiple micronutrients are common among women living in resource-poor settings, including in urban settings (Torheim et al., 2010).

WHO has recently updated estimates of mineral and vitamin (micronutrient) deficiencies based on estimates available in 2008 for anaemia (of which about half is generally attributed to iron deficiency), iodine and vitamin A (WHO, 2010). Globally, anaemia affects 1.62 billion people, or a quarter of the population. Almost half of preschool-age children are anaemic, with the lowest prevalence of anaemia in men. Regional estimates, up to 2008, indicate that the highest proportion of individuals affected are in Africa (47.5–67.6%), while the greatest number, approximately 315 million, are in the World Health Organization (WHO) region of South-east

Asia (WHO, 2010). These are the two regions that are most affected for virtually all micronutrients.

Between 1995 and 2005, 45 and 122 countries had vitamin A deficiency of public health significance based on the prevalence, in pre-school-age children, of night blindness and biochemical vitamin A deficiency, respectively. Regional estimates indicate that the highest proportion of preschool-age children affected by night blindness – 2.0% (2.55 million) – or almost half of the children affected globally, is in Africa, a value that is four times higher than that estimated in South-east Asia (0.5%), which was traditionally seen as the area of greatest concern and has the greatest number of children and pregnant women affected when measured by serum retinol levels (WHO, 2010).

The risk of iodine deficiency disorders (IDDs), based on urinary iodine concentrations, shows a rather more uneven distribution of risk, with a higher risk in Europe than in many parts of the rest of the world (WHO, 2010). There has been a decline in countries with an iodine public health problem due to the great success of the iodization of salt programmes globally (WHO, 2010; UN SCN, 2010). Other micronutrient minerals supplied by the diet may also be at risk of being deficient, and one recent estimate has suggested that a quarter or more of the world's population is likely to be at risk of deficiency of iron, zinc, calcium, magnesium and/or potassium, and that other elements likely to be deficient, depending on the global environment, include selenium and copper (Broadley and White, 2010). Declines in folate deficiency have been documented in more affluent countries that have fortified their wheat flour over the last decade.

Despite the real successes in reducing the prevalence of IDDs and of severe vitamin A and folate deficiencies, though with little if any progress for iron, the overall prevalences and trends suggest that current approaches, despite considerable effort and funding, are insufficient (Mayer et al., 2008; WHO, 2010). Consequently, there may be a need to emphasize more sustainable and localized interventions that work through more sustainable food-based approaches and a scaling up of the associated interventions (World Bank, 2007).

Addressing Micronutrient Deficiencies

The prevention and control of micronutrient deficiencies became higher global priorities partly because the magnitude and distribution of the problem was thought to be not only reasonably easy to demonstrate, but also because interventions were known that would address the problems, and the impact could, at least theoretically, also be relatively easily measured – all of which were particularly attractive to major bilateral donor countries (Darnton-Hill, 2008). Interventions that are being implemented are: (i) food-based approaches, including dietary diversification, nutrition education and the fortification of staple and value-added foods; (ii) supplementation with vitamin A capsules, iron–folic acid tablets and iodized oil, with increasing interest in multi-micronutrient supplements and intermittent weekly lower-dose supplements; (iii) public health interventions, such as immunization, adding vitamin A supplementation to other programmes such as National Immunization Days and Child Health Days, the promotion of breastfeeding, deworming and the treatment of infectious diseases; and (iv) changes in the possibilities that are available to people through modification of the political, socio-economic and physical environment – although as with so much of public health, those that are most vulnerable are those who are poorest.

The important point about these different approaches is that they are complementary, and should be considered as complementary because they may have different time frames and differing feasibilities depending on local circumstances (Darnton-Hill, 2008). However, the majority of funding and effort so far has been on supplementation, and less so, on fortification, with comparatively little attention paid to food-based approaches. The relatively recent report by the World Bank (2007) on nutrition and agricultural links suggested that the food supply chain linking food production with food consumption and human nutrition could be usefully considered in terms of five pathways:

- Subsistence-oriented production for the household's own consumption.
- Income-oriented production for sale in markets.

- Reduction in real food prices associated with increased agricultural production.
- Empowerment of women as agents instrumental to household food security and health outcomes.
- Indirect relationships between increasing agricultural productivity and nutrition outcomes through the agriculture sector's contribution to national income and macroeconomic growth.

Clearly, household production for the household's own consumption is the most fundamental and direct pathway by which increased production translates into greater food availability and food security, while the different types of foods produced determine the impact of the production increase on diet quality (World Bank, 2007). One of the contentions made will be that dietary diversification methods have advantages over extended supplementation programmes for poverty reduction, and for sustainability, social and even biological reasons as well (Gibson, 2011). Food-based strategies have also been advocated as safe methods for controlling and preventing mild micronutrient deficiencies (Szymlek-Gay et al., 2009), especially when the deficiencies are multiple (Torheim et al., 2007).

Evidence for the Impact of Food-based Approaches

There is widespread consensus that there are serious limitations to the indicators currently available for the assessment of micronutrient status, especially for their functional consequences, but also for research, clinical, policy and programmatic needs and applications (Allen, 2009; Raiten et al., 2011). This has led to difficulties in a lack of congruence between cut-offs denoting deficiency and adverse functional consequences, inconsistent methods of evaluating the confounding effects of infections on micronutrient status indicators and for the measurement of cost-effectiveness, and a lack of sensitivity in measuring programmatic impact and for use in developing policy (Allen, 2009; Raiten et al., 2011). When assessing the impact of dietary diversification and modification in food-based

programmes, randomized controlled trials are not feasible, so there need to be process and output indicators; for assessing the actual impact, there also need to be outcome indicators such as exposure and change in biomarkers, and especially indicators of functional outcomes, including growth, morbidity and milestones achieved (Gibson, 2011). Measuring the effectiveness of programmes requires indicators of outcomes that go beyond the biochemical serum and blood levels of micronutrients and clinical outcomes, e.g. reduction in night blindness, to include social outcomes such as women's empowerment (Bushamuka et al., 2005; Webb et al., 2007; Darnton-Hill, 2008).

Consequently, there remains some ongoing scepticism towards food-based approaches to nutrition, with the result that interventions such as home gardening, homestead food production, nutrition education and dietary diversity enhancement have been criticized as being relatively ineffective, unsustainable and difficult to scale up (Ruel and Levin, 2000; Sommer personal communication, 2002). Gibson et al. (2003) and others, however, have demonstrated the potential effectiveness of food-based programmes for improving iron, zinc and vitamin A deficiencies in low-income countries, though they also noted – for zinc and iron especially – the quite intensive effort needed to do this for already overburdened women and impoverished families, given the poor availability, and especially the poor accessibility, of appropriate foods.

There are different types and levels of evidence for food-based approaches. This chapter will briefly review the evidence from four perspectives: (i) biochemical and clinical measures of effect; (ii) dietary and adequacy estimations and modelling; (iii) cost-effectiveness; and (iv) measures of impact on social and cultural indicators - which are not usually seen as health and nutrition indicators. If the fourth category can be shown to be supported by adequate evidence, then it will be argued that these should be more strongly factored into decisions on food-based programmes as a measure of wider positive impact, likely increased sustainability and intergenerational impact, all of which will have an effect on cost-effectiveness. Other major factors that have been infrequently considered in measuring impact are the impact on the environment of the different approaches, and the need to address poverty and the very poor separately, especially in light of the recent, and continuing, high food price increases.

Biochemical and clinical evidence

Most of the studies providing evidence for food-based approaches have used changes in KAP (knowledge, attitudes and practices) or dietary intake. Gibson (2011) has tabulated data from six studies (subsequently expanded to 14, across as many countries) that have provided information on observed and potential health-related outcomes in young children in dietary diversification and modification programmes. The studies using biochemical measures that are cited here usually identified changes in measures of vitamin A (mostly serum retinol, but also night blindness symptoms), although there have been some studies on changes in iron levels with food-based interventions, as well as with zinc levels. Because a study in Indonesia had showed that β-carotene was less available from many foods in the diet, and so the relative contribution to vitamin A status of β-carotene from vegetable foods was far less than previously thought, many in the public health nutrition sector concluded that children in low-income countries could never get enough vitamin A without supplementation (de Pee et al., 1995, 1999). This view generally dominated the discussion until recently (Latham, 2010). Subsequently, it was discovered that while the conversion ratio of β-carotene to retinol equivalents for dark-green leafy vegetables may be a low 1:28, for orange-fleshed vegetables and fruits it was probably around 1:12, which made the viability of a diet-based approach more scientifically feasible, and which led to a reappraisal of the role of vegetables, and especially of fruit, in the diet (de Pee et al., 2000).

A study of Chinese schoolchildren a few years later found they were protected from becoming biochemically vitamin A deficient during seasons when provitamin A sources are limited through the consumption of green–yellow vegetables and over a 10 week period (even though they required about 250 g of vegetables/day) (Tang et al., 1999). Devadas (1987) reported several successful behaviour change interventions to increase intakes in India, at least one of which reported a reduction in corneal xerosis (as a severe manifestation of vitamin A deficiency). In Indonesia, ownership of a home garden indicated increased long-term vitamin A intake from plant foods (de Pee et al., 2000). Also in Indonesia, in central Java, Helen Keller International (HKI) found good evidence for an impact on vitamin A status of a social marketing campaign for the increased consumption of eggs and dark-green leafy vegetables; this found that within a year of the programme starting, the population's consumption of eggs and vegetables had increased, as had vitamin A intake; furthermore, vitamin A status had improved (de Pee et al., 2000). In a national survey on vitamin A status in rural Bangladesh in 1997–1998 (HKI, 1999), young children who had not received a vitamin A supplement were half as likely to be night blind if the family had a home garden (Kiess et al., 1998). Talukder et al. (2000) described significant reductions in rates of night blindness in children in programmes taking place in Bangladesh, Cambodia, Nepal and the Philippines. Home gardens in KwaZulu-Natal showed an increase in dietary intakes, and significant increases in serum retinol and in levels of riboflavin, vitamin B_6 and vitamin C in those with home gardens (Faber et al., 2001). The consumption of β-carotene-rich sweet potato introduced into East Africa was also responsible for both an increased consumption and change in serum retinol levels (Low et al., 2007). Gibson (2011) has itemized changes in serum ferritin and retinol and anthropometric change in Ghana, anthropometric changes in Bangladesh, China, Peru and the USA, and changes in haemoglobin from Denmark in response to nutrition interventions that supplied or promoted the consumption of animal source foods among infants and toddlers; all of these lend support to the increased body of

evidence showing that food-based approaches can demonstrate biochemical and
clinical change when they are looked for
(Gibson, 2011).

Dietary estimations and studies

As a measure of exposure to food-based interventions, changed intakes have been a more
commonly used indicator (Gibson, 2011). An
early evaluation in Thailand of the impact of
consumption of the vitamin A-rich ivy gourd
plant found that the programme markedly
increased the production and consumption of
ivy gourd, although the effects on vitamin A
status were inconclusive (Smitasiri, 1994;
de Pee et al., 2000). The Asian Vegetable
Research and Development Center in Taiwan
reviewed the feasibility of combating micronutrient deficiencies through the use of vegetables, a greater challenge than using fruits
and mixed diets, and concluded that, at the
very least, this was a neglected area in Asia,
while also noting that such efforts to address
micronutrient deficiencies are not targeted at
a single vegetable or a single micronutrient,
but rather to the overall vegetable supply as
an important contributor to diversified diets
(Ali and Tsou, 1997). Successful experience in
providing such integration and increasing the
number of vegetable varieties grown and
consumed has been well documented by
HKI, especially in Bangladesh (Talukder et al.,
2000; HKI, 2001).

The concept of home gardening has been
increasingly broadened to include the rearing of small animals such as poultry, small
animal husbandry and/or fish ponds (HKI,
2001) and increases the intake (and presumably the bioavailability) of vitamin A, iron,
zinc and other micronutrients such as vitamin B_{12}. There is well-documented evidence
that home gardening, and especially homestead gardens, have a direct impact on vitamin A deficiency, and perhaps on the
deficiency of other micronutrients, through
increasing the consumption of micronutrient-
rich foods resulting from the increased access
through production, preservation and/or
distribution between and within households
(Marsh, 1998; de Pee et al., 2000; Talukder et al.,

2000; Arimond et al., 2011; Gibson, 2011).
Increased production and consumption of
micronutrient-rich foods has also been demonstrated in Vietnam after the start of homestead production activities (English et al.,
1997; HKI, 2001).

HKI (2001) has also been able to demonstrate and document both the direct impact of
homestead gardening, such as the production
of food, and indirect impacts due to increased
money being earned by women, a large part
of which is spent on micronutrient-rich foods.
A probable key to the success of homestead
production interventions in the HKI programmes in Bangladesh and Vietnam, and
the subsequent replications in other countries
since, has been suggested to be the community-
level approach and its emphasis on sustainability, which, by collaborating with local
NGOs and encouraging the participation of
women from the communities, has allowed
the programme to expand without having to
receive further input from HKI – other than
technical assistance (programme management and planning (HKI, 2001, 2006)). In addition, village nurseries, created by local NGOs
and community groups, have played a major
role in providing the necessary resources,
teaching healthy nutrition practices and various techniques for year-round gardening,
and increasing the variety of fruits and vegetables. Community members have also been
involved in designing, implementing, and
evaluating the programme. After 1 year of
implementing a large-scale programme in
1997, the percentage of households without
home gardens decreased from 25% to 2%, and
the consumption of green leafy vegetables by
children in households with developed home
gardens was 1.6 times higher than in households that did not participate in the programme (HKI, 2006).

However, iron deficiency is more challenging, and results from a model in Indonesia
showed that theoretical iron requirements
could not be reached using local food sources,
from which the highest iron level achievable
was estimated to be 63% of that recommended; adequate levels of niacin, zinc and
calcium would also have been difficult to
achieve (Santika et al., 2009). Notwithstanding,
work in other countries, e.g. in parts of Africa

by Gibson and colleagues, has shown that in theory, and under applied semi-research conditions, an adequacy of iron and zinc should be possible from food-based approaches (Gibson, 2011). In a community-based dietary diversification/modification intervention that employed a quasi-experimental design in southern Malawi, the content and bioavailability of micronutrients in maize-based diets consumed by stunted children aged 30–90 months were able to be increased (Gibson et al., 2003). After controlling for baseline variables, mean haemoglobin was significantly higher post intervention, and the incidence of anaemia and common infections was lower in the intervention groups than in the control groups, with no change in malaria or hair zinc status. Dietary strategies reduced the prevalence of inadequate intakes of protein, calcium, zinc and vitamin B_{12}, but not of iron, probably because fish was the major source of animal food consumed (Gibson et al., 2003). In urban women of reproductive age in Burkina Faso, low micronutrient intakes, especially of vitamin B_{12} (only 4% of the required intake), folate, riboflavin and niacin were found to be significantly less with higher intakes of offal, flesh foods, vitamin A- and vitamin C-rich fruits and vegetables, and legumes and nuts (Becquey and Martin-Prevel, 2010).

In a review by Ruel and Levin (2000) of the International Food Policy Research Institute (IFPRI), dietary improvement interventions for increasing vitamin A and iron intakes are noted to have used a combination of actions, including: identifying foods with high vitamin A content and promoting their consumption; promoting income-generating activities as an indirect way of improving supply of vitamin A-rich foods; and applying a behaviour change communication strategy to increase the level of knowledge and awareness of beneficiaries. This review noted that whereas vitamin A supplementation emphasizes the *compliance* of beneficiaries as a facilitating factor to achieving high coverage rate, dietary improvement focuses on *empowerment*, especially of women and of populations with a low socio-economic status (Ruel and Levin, 2000; Bushamuka et al., 2005). Nevertheless, neither the evaluation from IFPRI (Ruel and Levin, 2000) nor that from ICDDR,B

(International Centre for the Control of Diarrhoeal Diseases, Bangladesh, at Dhaka) (Fuchs et al., 2001) found home gardening (not homestead production) to have a sufficient impact for this to suggest that a donor should support greater investment.

A subsequent evaluation (Leroy et al., 2008) has also reviewed the impact of various multi-sectoral programmes and of more general approaches such as cash transfers, and so on, on nutritional outcomes. The evaluation included approximately 40 agricultural programmes, including those of HKI. Leroy et al. (2008, p. 71) concluded that 'programs promoting home gardening and animal production are likely to increase production, may increase household consumption and individual intake, but may have little to no effect on children's nutritional outcomes unless nutritional inputs are revisited and strengthened.' None the less, reflecting the diversity of programmes and their implementation, Leroy et al. also concluded that the lack of consistent effects on nutrition could have been due to inadequate programme design and/or weakness in the monitoring and evaluation design. As has been noted by HKI, the scaling up – including to other countries – of homestead production is strongly recommended as a way of contributing to improved micronutrient status of poor rural populations. HKI has subsequently expanded its Homestead Food Production (HFP) Program to Cambodia, Nepal, the Philippines and West Africa. Success with the production and increased consumption of β-carotene-rich yellow-fleshed potato has been documented in East Africa in rural Mozambique (Low et al., 2007; Arimond et al., 2011). There have also been several single-country evaluations – in Cambodia and Mozambique (Low et al., 2007) and in Bangladesh (Ianotti et al., 2009) – that all showed increased production and consumption of vitamin A-rich foods, if not always their impact (Arimond et al., 2011).

The review of activities in Bangladesh by Ianotti et al. of IFPRI in 2009, however, concluded that homestead food production had expanded its reach into half the Bangladesh subdistricts and that the evidence showed that the programme had 'improved food security for nearly 5 million people in diverse agroecological zones' in Bangladesh (Iannotti et al., 2009). An excellent recent review of past and new evidence of agricultural interventions and nutrition by Arimond et al. (2011) using the five pathways described earlier, was considerably more positive on outcomes; it provides some useful lessons for the design and evaluation of food-based (agriculture and nutrition) interventions and identifies the need for further work on investigations of cost-effectiveness, scaling-up processes and sustainability. It then explores in some detail the two successful examples of the yellow-fleshed sweet potato and HKI homestead production models. The overall conclusion, especially from the HKI (2001) review and from the latest three reviews (Ianotti et al., 2009; Arimond et al., 2011; Gibson, 2011) is of a strong evidence base for an impact on micronutrient intake and status by agricultural/horticultural and dietary diversification and modification interventions.

Cost-effectiveness

Besides the proven benefits to health, growth and intellectual development, there are strong economic reasons for addressing micronutrient deficiencies. A figure often quoted is that of the World Bank Development Report 1993 (World Bank, 1993) that not addressing micronutrient malnutrition will cause a country a loss of up to 3% GNP, whereas the cost of addressing the problem is only 0.5%. The way in which these figures came about is not entirely clear, but they have been widely, and effectively, used for advocacy. Both iodine and iron deficiencies negatively affect physical and cognitive function and subsequent educational attainments and economic productivity, while vitamin A and zinc and other micronutrient deficiencies, such as those of folate, have considerable impact on child mortality, morbidity and health care cost burdens. Anaemia increases the risk of maternal deaths and decreases productivity and wages. Overall costs can be very large in countries such as in China, India and Indonesia where micronutrient deficiencies have been estimated to be costing US$5 billion,

US$2.5 million and US$0.75 billion, respectively (Alderman et al., 2003).

Cost-effectiveness has not generally been demonstrated for food-based approaches, although recent evidence has shown that the poorest people in the societies of low- and middle-income countries are not being reached by most programmes, even when the progress in a country, on average, appears to be adequate, e.g. towards the child survival Millennium Development Goal (MDG) target (Gwatkin, 2006). This need to specifically target the poor has recently been further affirmed in a report by UNICEF that demonstrated that the MDGs would not be reached unless the very poor are directly targeted (UNICEF, 2007). Scaling up food-based approaches to the very poor would help to reach many subsistence farmers, most of whom are women. Following the steep food prices rises and economic financial problems from about 2007 onwards, and the ways the poor have to cope (Darnton-Hill and Cogill, 2010), it was found that the urban poor, who now exceed the rural poor in numbers, but often have fewer resources to spend on food –which they cannot grow – are being particularly affected.

Several attempts have also been made to compare different interventions for the same micronutrient (Sanghvi, 1996). In these comparisons, food-based approaches (excluding fortification) appeared to come out worst compared with supplementation and fortification (Sanghvi, 1996). China has also made estimates of cost-effectiveness based on data from the China National Nutrition and Health Survey, 2002 (CNNHS 2002) to help prioritize interventions for micronutrient deficiencies. The costs and cost-effectiveness of supplementation, food diversification and food fortification were estimated using the standard WHO approach of DALYs (disability-adjusted life years) (Ma et al., 2008).

Among the interventions for iron and zinc deficiency, biofortification showed the lowest per capita costs, while dietary diversification through health education represented the highest cost. When iron deficiency alone was examined, the most cost-effective intervention was food fortification, which was about a third to a half more cost-effective than supplementation and dietary diversification.

For zinc deficiency, the corresponding ratio was about 400:150:100 for the cost-effectiveness of supplementation, fortification and dietary diversification, respectively, based on the international dollar figures of Ma *et al.* (2008). However, as has already been noted, each approach to alleviating micronutrient deficiencies has its particular strengths for different time frames and sub-populations, and ideally they should complement one another. These sub-populations are not usually identified in cost-effectiveness estimations, which rely on the assumptions made and the immediacy of the outcomes. Of the two long-term intervention strategies, i.e. dietary diversification and biofortification with improved varieties of plants, the latter is especially feasible and cost-effective for rural populations but is still some way in the future in terms of effectiveness. Supplementation and fortification can be used as short-term strategies for specific groups (Darnton-Hill, 2008; Ma *et al.*, 2008), whereas dietary diversification has the advantage of addressing a range of micronutrient problems and has proved sustainable; it is currently estimated to be reaching more than 950,000 families in rural Bangladesh (Talukder, personal communication).

Social and cultural aspects

Evaluations of food-based approaches have tended, at least until recently, to be narrowly focused on a biomedical/pharmaceutical model whereby the measured outcome is the biochemical levels of a particular micronutrient, or at best the calculated dietary intake, with the latter rarely investigating household food distribution or the effect of gender (Darnton-Hill *et al.*, 2005; Kurz and Johnson-Welch, 2007; Webb *et al.*, 2007).

The potential outcomes can be direct, such as change in the biological or clinical levels of micronutrients already discussed, or more indirect, as in women's empowerment from owning a home garden. The longer term benefits, and the social and cultural aspects, such as women's empowerment from having a small independent income from home gardening,

are generally not captured in cost-effectiveness calculations (Darnton-Hill, 2008). These benefits include those such as increased use of health services by women, increased and earlier taking of sick children for treatment and increased expenditure on children's food and education (Quisumbing *et al.*, 1995; Marsh, 1998; Bloem *et al.*, 2005; Bushamuka *et al.*, 2005; Darnton-Hill *et al.*, 2005; Kurz and Johnson-Welch, 2007; Webb *et al.*, 2007). The additionality of impact has been described as tapping into women's roles as income earners and food producers on the one hand, and their roles as food processors and caregivers on the other (Hagenimana *et al.*, 2001). Increased income for and empowerment of women can also result in increased intakes of micronutrient-rich foods such as eggs and meat, as well as of other foods such as oil, and improved caring practices (de Pee *et al.*, 2000; HKI, 2001; Bushamuka *et al.*, 2005).

Such social and cultural aspects also have an impact on attempts to measure the comparative cost-effectiveness of other interventions, such as supplementation and fortification, both of which generally do not have the added social and communal impact of the presence of home gardens, such as increased social cohesion, and the strengthening of local capacity and of NGOs, all of which have been documented, and which, if they could be more accurately calculated, would give a very much more realistic estimation of the contribution of the sociocultural aspects of home gardening to its cost-effectiveness (Bloem *et al.*, 2005; Darnton-Hill, 2008).

Implications of Food-based Approaches

The ultimate success of a food-based programme is when each household member has access to a dietary intake sufficiently adequate that his or her optimal micronutrient status is maintained. Obviously, where requirements are increased, e.g. in high infectious disease-load environments, this intake may need to be greater than that for a healthy child growing up in a privileged and healthy environment. This is dependent not just on micronutrient delivery, whether through the diet or supplemented in some way, but also on the health and care of the child, and the environment in which he/she is growing. In circumstances where children have repeated episodes of diarrhoea and pneumonia, it is unlikely that a single micronutrient intervention can overcome this effect on health, and subsequently on nutrition and growth and development (World Bank, 2007). Increasingly, even more distal influences, such as the level of women's education in the country, equity and pro-poor policies nationally, and the global trade environment, are all recognized as reaching down to the village and having a potential nutrition and health impacts on rural and urban children.

Because food-based approaches are harder to quantify, involve social change and are less easily evaluated than say, number of capsules delivered, they have also not received donor support to anything like the same extent as other interventions. This is despite the recognized fact that where a very low-income woman's discretionary income is increased, she is more likely than a husband to use it for food for children, take the children to health systems earlier and even use it for increasing female education (Quisumbing et al., 1995; Darnton-Hill et al., 2005; Webb et al., 2007). Other social safety net interventions, such as conditional cash transfers have been demonstrated to work (Lagarde et al., 2007), especially in the Latin American countries, e.g. on anaemia levels in Mexico. A recent reanalysis of the crisis in Indonesia in the late 1990s found that there were significant increases in the income elasticity of both micronutrients and macronutrients during the times of a crisis, so that cash transfer programmes can play an integral role in helping households to protect their consumption of essential nutrients during crises – as the quickest and the cheapest interventions to scale up in order to reach households that are most likely to be adversely affected under such conditions (Skoufias et al., 2011). However, to ensure the protection of the all-important micronutrients, it was noted that relying entirely on cash transfers may not be sufficient (Skoufias et al., 2011), so complementary interventions such as dietary diversification and modification, and increased home availability

and accessibility through such approaches as food-based methods, remain important, especially for the very poor (Ianotti et al., 2009; Arimond et al., 2011; Gibson, 2011).

The reviews from HKI (2001) and the World Bank (2007), the Innocenti Review (Leroy et al., 2008), the review from IFPRI (Ianotti et al., 2009), and the reviews prepared by Arimond et al. (2011) and Gibson et al. (2011), along with this re-examination (prepared for FAO's International Symposium on Food and Nutrition Security: Food-based Approaches for Improving Diets and Raising Levels of Nutrition held in 2010 in Rome), have all found that agricultural and horticultural interventions promoting increased production of fruit and vegetables with the raising of small animals – such as those involving homestead gardens – carry considerable potential to effectively address micronutrient deficiencies.

Effective population-specific, food-based complementary feeding recommendations are needed to complement interventions that are used to combat micronutrient deficiencies (Santika et al., 2009), reinforced by education (especially of females), community action and essential nutrition actions. This review has identified a significant body of evidence documenting the success of food-based approaches in raising production, income, household consumption, and raising the intake of targeted fruit and vegetables by vulnerable population groups. The programmes reviewed also showed significant impacts on dietary and biochemical indicators of micronutrient deficiencies, and especially so when they included components designed to change behaviour through education and to empower women (World Bank, 2007).

One of the consistent factors found is that it appears to be essential to have a very broad coalition, with complementary, and often overlapping roles. The multi-sectoral, multi-intervention approach has gone through several iterations: initially a single micronutrient 'silo' approach, which may well have been appropriate in the initial launching of these interventions, then a very integrated approach, and now a more country-specific approach. While multi-sectoral efforts to address agriculture and nutrition together have often in the past been hindered by institutional barriers and insufficient resources, the strengthening and expansion of these new partnerships should continue, and common, locally agreed goals and responsibilities designated that reflect each partner's comparative advantage (World Bank, 2007).

As also noted by the World Bank (2007), the key lessons learned from the type of accumulated evidence above are that food-based interventions are most likely to affect nutrition outcomes when they 'involve diverse and complementary processes and strategies that redirect the focus beyond agriculture for food production and toward broader consideration of livelihoods, women's empowerment, and optimal intrahousehold uses of resources'. Successful projects are those that invest broadly in improving human capital, sustain and increase the livelihood assets of the poor, and focus on gender equality (World Bank, 2007). Programmes that include an education/behaviour change communications component have been shown to be more effective in improving nutrition than those that focus just on production (Leroy et al., 2008) and what has been called an 'econutrition' approach (Wispelwey and Deckelbaum, 2010).

Conclusions

There is enough evidence to move ahead with scaling up integrated homestead food production when nutrition education and such aspects as essential nutrition actions are included, and would be expected to have an impact on nutrient intakes and probably also on micronutrient levels and clinical signs of deficiency. Properly targeted, such programmes would be expected to have an impact on women's empowerment, and hence on the nutrition and education of children of the poorest households. Questions on cost-effectiveness remain, but given the likely longer term factors not usually factored in, and good evidence of sustainability, the answers are probably often better than usually cited. An important need is for more research on impact, especially on impacts often not looked for or measured. Unintended consequences of integrated homestead food production need to be borne in mind, but ultimately it is a decision of the women themselves, who are

presumably best placed to decide whether to pursue this avenue if they wish – as they seem to have done in the examples evaluated. Evaluations also need to be an intrinsic part of the process, and should be factored in earlier in the process and be provided for by governments and funding agencies.

Below is an outline of the overall conclusions from this review:
- There is enough evidence to move ahead with scaling up integrated homestead food production in resource-poor communities, including:
  ○ integration of small animals such as fish and poultry;
  ○ incorporation of other maternal and child nutrition actions such as the Essential Nutrition Actions approach; and
  ○ scaling up of other proven interventions such as female education and improved antenatal care and nutrition.
- Other food-based approaches should continue to be expanded, including:
  ○ home-based at-point fortification with micronutrients of complementary foods;
  ○ fortification of staples through the private sector, which will probably not reach the bottom of the demographic pyramid; and
  ○ biofortification, which while still needing time could, if successfully adopted widely, reach the poorest farmers.
- Impact can be expected on:
  ○ micronutrient intakes;
  ○ biological levels of some micronutrients;
  ○ probably some clinical signs and symptoms of micronutrient deficiencies;
  ○ women's empowerment and spending resources; and
  ○ children's education and use of health facilities.
- Governments and agencies should invest in the following:
  ○ scaling up integrated homestead interventions as above;
  ○ more and better research on impact;
  ○ more and better research on evaluations, including likely sustainability;

○ more and better research on cost-effectiveness, including the often unmeasured indirect impacts;
○ the relationship with conditional cash transfers;
○ considerations of environmental issues; and
○ increased targeting of the very poor.

More optimistically, improved dialogue between the agricultural sector and the health and nutrition sectors would also improve the chance of successful outcomes. Using the success of food-based approaches might be one vehicle for such increased and improved dialogue between the sectors.

References

Alderman, H., Hoddinott, J. and Kinsey, B. (2003) *Long-term Consequences of Early Childhood Malnutrition*. FCND Discussion Paper No 168, Food Consumption and Nutrition Division, International Food Policy Research Institute, Washington, DC. Available at: http://are.berkeley.edu/courses/ARE251/2004/papers/Alderman_Hoddinott.pdf (accessed 4 June 2013). World Bank, Washington, DC.

Ali, M. and Tsou, S.C.S. (1997) Combating micronutrient deficiencies through vegetables – a neglected food frontier in Asia. *Food Policy* 27, 17–38.

Allen, L.H. (2009) Limitations of current indicators of micronutrient status. *Nutrition Reviews* 67(Suppl. 1), S21–23.

Arimond, M., Hawkes, C., Ruel, M.T., Sifri, Z., Berti, P.R., Leroy, J.L., Low, J.W., Brown, L.R. and Frongillo, E.A. (2011) Agricultural interventions and nutrition: lessons from the past and new evidence. In: Thompson, B. and Amoroso, L. (eds) *Combating Micronutrient Deficiencies: Food-based Approaches*. Food and Agriculture Organization, Rome and CAB International, Wallingford, UK, pp. 41–75.

Becquey, E. and Martin-Prevel, Y. (2010) Micronutrient adequacy of women's diet in urban Burkina Faso is low. *Journal of Nutrition* 140, 2079S–2085S.

Bhutta, Z.A. (2008) Micronutrient needs of malnourished children. *Current Opinion in Clinical Nutrition and Metabolic Care* 11, 309–314.

Bloem, M.W., de Pee, S. and Darnton-Hill, I. (2005) Micronutrient deficiencies and maternal thinness. First chain in the sequence of nutritional and health events in economic crises. In: Bendich, A. and Deckelbaum, R.J. (eds) *Preventive Nutrition. The Comprehensive Guide for Health Professionals*, 3rd edn. Humana Press, Totowa, New Jersey, pp. 689–710.

Bouis, H.E. (2003) Micronutrient fortification of plants through plant breeding: can it improve nutrition in man at low cost? *The Proceedings of the Nutrition Society* 62, 403–411.

Broadly, M.R. and White, P.J. (2010) Eats roots and leaves. Can edible horticultural crops address dietary calcium, magnesium and potassium deficiencies? *The Proceedings of the Nutrition Society* 69, 601–612.

Bushamuka, V.N., de Pee, S., Talukder, A., Kiess, L., Panagides, D., Taher, A. and Bloem, M. (2005) Impact of a homestead gardening program on household food security and empowerment of women in Bangladesh. *Food and Nutrition Bulletin* 26, 17–25.

Darnton-Hill, I. (2008) Global micronutrient goals (1990–2005). PhD thesis, University of Tasmania, Australia.

Darnton-Hill. I. and Cogill, B. (2010) Maternal and young child nutrition adversely affected by external shocks such as increasing global food prices. *Journal of Nutrition* 140, 162S–169S.

Darnton-Hill, I., Webb, P., Harvey, P.W.J., Hunt, J.M., Dalmiya, N., Chopra, M., Ball, M.J., Bloem, M.W. and de Benoist, B. (2005) Micronutrient deficiencies and gender: social and economic costs. *The American Journal of Clinical Nutrition* 81, 1198S–1205S.

de Pee, S., West, C.E., Muhilal, Karyadi, D. and Hautvast, J.G.A.J. (1995) Lack of improvement in vitamin A status with increased consumption of dark-green leafy vegetables. *The Lancet* 346, 75–81.

de Pee, S., Bloem, M.W., Tjiong, R., Martini, E., Satoto, Gorstein, J., Shrimpton, R. and Muhilal (1999) Who has a vitamin A intake from plant foods, but a low serum retinal concentration? Data from women in Indonesia. *European Journal of Clinical Nutrition* 53, 288–297.

de Pee, S., Bloem, M.W. and Kiess, L. (2000) Evaluating food-based programmes for their reduction of vitamin A deficiency and its consequences. *Food and Nutrition Bulletin* 21, 232–238.

Devadas, R.P. (1987) Currently available technologies in India to control vitamin A malnutrition. In: West, K.P. Jr and Sommer, A.(eds) *Delivery of Oral Doses of Vitamin A to Prevent Vitamin A Deficiency and*

Nutritional Blindness. A State-of-the-art Review. Nutrition Policy Discussion Paper No. 2, ACC/SCN State-of-the-Art Series, United Nations Administrative Committee on Coordination/Subcommittee on Nutrition, Rome, pp. 97–104.

English, R., Badcock, J., Tu Giay, Tu Ngu, Waters, A.-M. and Bennett, S.A. (1997) Effect of nutrition improvement project on morbidity from infectious diseases in preschool children in Vietnam: comparison with control commune. *British Medical Journal* 315, 1122–1125.

Faber, M., Jogessar, V.B. and Benade, A.J. (2001) Nutritional status and dietary intakes of children 2–5 years and their caregivers in a rural South African community. *International Journal of Food Sciences and Nutrition* 52, 401–411.

Fuchs, G., Faruque, A.S.G. and Khan, M. (2001) Impact of the Helen Keller International Home Gardening Programme in rural Bangladesh. International Centre for the Control of Diarrhoeal Diseases, Dhaka, Bangladesh (ICDDR,B) for US Agency for International Development (USAID), Washington, DC.

Gibson, R.S. (2011) Strategies for preventing multi-micronutrient deficiencies: a review of experiences with food-based approaches in developing countries. In: *Combating Micronutrient Deficiencies: Food-based Approaches.* Food and Agriculture Organization, Rome and CAB International, Wallingford, UK, pp. 7–27.

Gibson, R.S., Yeudall, F., Drost, N., Mtitimuni, B.M. and Cullinan, T.R. (2003) Experiences of a community-based dietary intervention to enhance micronutrient adequacy of diets low in animal source foods and high in phytate: a case study in rural Malawian children. *Journal of Nutrition* 133, 3992S–3999S.

Gwatkin, D.R. (2006) IMCI: what can we learn from an innovation that didn't reach the poor? *Bulletin of the World Health Organization* 84, 768.

Hagenimana, V., Low, J., Anyano, M., Kurz, K., Gichuki, S.T. and Kabira, J. (2001) Enhancing vitamin A intake in young children in Western Kenya: orange-fleshed sweet potatoes and women farmers can serve as key entry points. *Food and Nutrition Bulletin* 22, 370–387.

HKI (1999) *Vitamin A Status Throughout the Lifecycle in Rural Bangladesh: National Vitamin A Survey, 1997–98.* Helen Keller International Bangladesh, Dhaka.

HKI (2001) The strength of linking surveillance and programs: historical perspective of HKI's experience in homestead food production in Bangladesh, 1982–2001. In: Bloem, M.W., de Pee, S., Graciano, F., Kiess, L., Moench-Pfanner, R. and Talukder, A. (eds) *Homestead Food Production – A Strategy to Combat Malnutrition and Poverty.* Helen Keller International, Asia-Pacific Region Office, Phnom Penh, pp. 119–121 (Appendix 14).

HKI (2006) *Homestead Food Production for Improving Micronutrient Status of Women and Children, Poverty Reduction and Promotion of Gender Equality.* Report, Helen Keller International, New York.

Ianotti, L., Cunningham, K. and Ruel, M. (2009) *Improving Diet Quality and Micronutrient Nutrition: Homestead Food Production in Bangladesh.* IFPRI Discussion Paper 00928, International Food Policy Research Institute, Washington, DC (accessed 22 November 2010). Available at: http://www.ifpri.org/sites/default/files/publications/ifpridp00928.pdf (accessed 4 June 2013).

Kiess, L., Bloem, M.W., de Pee, S., Hye, A., Khan, T., Talukder, A., Haque, M. and Ali, M. (1998) Bangladesh: xerophthalmia free. Combined effect of vitamin A (VA) capsule distribution and homestead gardening in reducing vitamin A deficiency (VAD). In: *American Public Health Association 126th Annual Meeting Report, November 15–18, 1998.* Washington, DC, p. 361 [abstract]. Reprinted in Appendix 13 of HKI Asia-Pacific (2001) *Homestead Food Production – A Strategy to Combat Malnutrition and Poverty.* Helen Keller International, Jakarta, Indonesia, p. 118.

Kurz, K. and Johnson-Welch, C. (2007) Enhancing women's contributions to improving family food consumption and nutrition. *Food and Nutrition Bulletin* 22, 443–53.

Largarde, M., Haines, A. and Palmer, N. (2007) Conditional cash transfers for improving uptake of health interventions in low- and middle-income countries. *Journal of the American Medical Association* 298, 1900–1910.

Latham, M. (2010) The great vitamin A fiasco. *Journal of Nutrition* 1, 12–45. Available at: http://www.wphna.org/downloads/WPHNA_web_commentary_may2010.pdf (accessed 4 June 2013).

Leroy, J.L., Ruel, M., Verhofstadt, E. and Olney, D. (2008) *The Micronutrient Impact of Multisectoral Programs Focusing on Nutrition: Examples from Conditional Cash Transfer, Microcredit with Education, and Agricultural Programs,* October 25, 2008. Report prepared for the Innocenti Review, 5 November 2008. Micronutrient Forum, Washington, DC. Available at: http://www.micronutrientforum.org/innocenti/Leroy-et-al-MNF-Indirect-Selected-Review_FINAL.PDF (accessed 29 May 2013).

Low, J.W., Arimond, M., Osman, N., Cunguara, B., Zano, P. and Tschirley, D. (2007) A food-based approach introducing orange-fleshed sweet potatoes increased vitamin A intake and serum retinol concentrations in rural Mozambique. *Journal of Nutrition* 137, 1320–1327.

Ma, G., Jin, Y., Li, Y., Zhai, F., Kok, F.J., Jacobsen, E. and Yang, X. (2008) Iron and zinc deficiencies in China: what is a feasible and cost-effective strategy? *Public Health Nutrition* 11, 632–638.

Marsh, R. (1998) Building on traditional gardening to improve household food security. *Food, Nutrition and Agriculture Journal* 22, 4–9.

Mayer, J.E., Pfeiffer, W.H. and Beyer, P. (2008) Biofortified crops to alleviate micronutrient malnutrition. *Current Opinion in Plant Biology* 11, 166–170.

Neumann, C.G., Bwibo, N.O., Gewa, C.A. and Drorbaugh, N. (2011) Animal-source foods as a food-based approach to address nutrient deficiencies and functional outcomes: a study among Kenyan school-children. In: *Combating Micronutrient Deficiencies: Food-based Approaches*. Food and Agriculture Organization, Rome and CAB International, Wallingford, UK, pp. 117–136.

Quisumbing, A.R., Brown, L.R., Feldstein, H.S., Haddad, L. and Peña, C. (1995) *Women: The Key to Food Security*. Food Policy Report, International Food Policy Research Institute, Washington, DC.

Raiten, D.J., Namasté, S., Brabin, B., Combs, G. Jr, L'Abbe, M.R., Wasantwisut, E. and Darnton-Hill, I. (2011) Executive Summary: Biomarkers of Nutrition for Development (BOND): building a consensus. *The American Journal of Clinical Nutrition* 94, 633S–650S.

Ruel, M.T. and Levin, C.E. (2000) *Assessing the Potential for Food-based Strategies to Reduce Vitamin A and Iron Deficiencies: A Review of Recent Evidence*. FCND Discussion Paper No. 92, Food Consumption and Nutrition Division, International Food Policy Research Institute, Washington, DC. Available at: http://www.ifpri.org/sites/default/files/publications/fcndp92.pdf (accessed 3 June 2013). Also available as Discussion Paper Brief in *Food and Nutrition Bulletin* (2001) 22, 94–95.

Sanghvi, T.G. (1996) *Economic Rationale for Investing in Micronutrient Programs. A Policy Brief Based on New Analyses*. Office of Nutrition, Bureau for Research and Development, US Agency for International Development, Washington, DC.

Santika, O., Fahmida, U. and Ferguson, E.L. (2009) Development of food-based complementary feeding recommendations for 9- to 11-month peri-urban Indonesian infants using linear programming. *Journal of Nutrition* 139, 135–141.

Skoufias, E., Tiwari, S. and Zaman, H. (2011) *Can We Rely on Cash Transfers to Protect Dietary Diversity During Food Crises? Estimates from Indonesia*. Policy Research Working Paper 5548, Poverty Reduction and Economic Management Network, Poverty Reduction Unit, The World Bank, Washington, DC. Available at: http://elibrary.worldbank.org/docserver/download/5548.pdf?expires=1370369449&id=id&accname=guest&checksum=1819C35A3E5EA9EECFA84CAD78871AAC (accessed 4 June 2013).

Smitasiri, S. (1994) *Nutri-action Analysis. Going Beyond Good People and Adequate Resources*. Amarin Printing and Publishing Public Company, Bangkok.

Szymlek-Gay, E.A., Ferguson, E.L., Heath, A.L., Gray, A.R. and Gibson, R.S. (2009) Food-based strategies improve iron status in toddlers: a randomized controlled trial. *The American Journal of Clinical Nutrition* 90, 1541–1551.

Talukder, A., Kiess, L., Huq, N., de Pee, S., Darnton-Hill, I. and Bloem, M.W. (2000) Increasing the production and consumption of vitamin A-rich fruits and vegetables: lessons learned in taking the Bangladesh homestead gardening programme to a national scale. *Food and Nutrition Bulletin* 21, 165–172.

Tang, G., Gu, X., Hu, S., Xu, G., Qin, J., Dolnikowski, G.G., Fjeld, C.R., Gao, X., Russell, R.M. and Yin, S. (1999) Green and yellow vegetables can maintain body stores of vitamin A in Chinese children. *The American Journal of Clinical Nutrition* 70, 1069–1076.

Torheim, L.E., Ferguson, E.L., Penrose, K. and Arimond, M. (2010) Women in resource-poor settings are at risk of inadequate intakes of multiple micronutrients. *Journal of Nutrition* 140, 2051S–2058S.

UN SCN (2010) *Sixth Report on the World Nutrition Situation: Progress in Nutrition*. United Nations System Standing Committee on Nutrition, c/o World Health Organization, Geneva, Switzerland Available at: http://www.unscn.org/files/Publications/RWNS6/report/SCN_report.pdf (accessed 13 February 2011).

UNICEF (2007) *Report on the State of the World's Children*. United Nations Children's Fund, New York.

Webb, P., Nishida, C. and Darnton-Hill, I. (2007) Age and gender as factors in the distribution of global micronutrient deficiencies. *Nutrition Reviews* 65, 233–245.

WHO (2010) Vitamin and Mineral Nutrition Information System (VMNIS): Micronutrients Database. World Health Organization, Geneva, Switzerland. Available at: http://www.who.int/vmnis/database/en/ (accessed 16 November 2010).

Wispelwey, B.P. and Deckelbaum, R.J. (2010) Econutrition: preventing malnutrition with agrodiversity interventions. In: Bendich, A. and Deckelbaum, R.J. (eds) *Preventive Nutrition*, 4th edn. Humana Press, Totowa, New Jersey, pp. 51–78.

World Bank (1993) *World Development Report 1993: Investing in Health*. Published by Oxford University Press, New York for the World Bank, Washington, DC.

World Bank (2007) *From Agriculture to Nutrition: Pathways, Synergies and Outcomes*. Agriculture and Rural Development Department, The World Bank, Washington, DC.

Zlotkin, S. and Tondeur, M.C. (2007) Chapter 17: Successful approaches – Sprinkles. In: Kraemer, K. and Zimmermann, M.B. (eds) *Nutritional Anaemia*. Sight and Life Press, Basel, Switzerland, pp. 269–284.

8 The Current Nutritional Status in China

Chunming Chen*

*International Life Science Institute Focal Point in China, Chinese
Center for Disease Control and Prevention, Beijing, China*

Summary

Based on data collected in China by the Food and Nutrition Surveillance System in 1990–2010, the National Survey on Fitness of Students in 1985, 2000 and 2005, and the 2002 National Nutrition And Health Survey, this chapter demonstrates the dramatic improvement in the nutrition of children under 5 and the growth of school-aged children and adolescents during the period of rapid economic growth in China. Now, there is no longer undernutrition in urban areas and the prevalence of stunting in the countryside has declined from 40.3% in 1990 to 12.6% in 2009. The median height of various age groups of school-aged children and adolescents in cities are close to the reference used by the World Health Organization (WHO). Overall, the study showed an evident reduction in undernutrition in line with the rapid economic development in China, although the prevalence of and trends in anaemia among children illustrated that rapid economic growth has not meaningfully improved micronutrient (iron) intake and that anaemia prevalence has not significantly reduced during recent years. Dietary and lifestyle changes have demonstrated benefits but have also demonstrated that nutritional factors are important risks in relation to the rapidly increasing prevalence of chronic diseases such as obesity, hypertension, diabetes and dislipidaemia. An analysis of the factors and challenges contributing to nutritional improvement is made with special reference to agricultural policies, together with a strategic consideration of nutritional improvements in China.

Introduction

Tracking changes in a target population's nutritional status during economic development not only helps to measure the achievements of economic development, but also to identify timely interventions for nutrition-related problems, and to ensure optimal development for a better future. Regular nutrition surveillance of the population is an integral part of the framework for achieving the Millennium Development Goals (MDGs).

China launched its first National Nutrition Survey (later the China National Nutrition and Health Survey) in 1959. In 1982, the country decided to conduct the survey every 10 years, and surveys were carried out in 1982, 1992 and 2002. Abundant data have been obtained since then, and this provides important scientific evidence for policy making. The nutritional status of children is the most sensitive indicator reflecting changes in socio-economic development. However, the current 10 year time interval is too long to

*Contact: chencm@ilsichina.org

identify problems in a timely fashion for children, and opportunities for interventions would be missed if only these data were used. In this connection, the Chinese Academy of Preventive Medicine (now called the Chinese Center for Disease Control and Prevention) established a team in 1989 to set up a Food and Nutrition Surveillance System in China, which aimed to conduct nutrition surveillance among children every 2–3 years. With the support of the Department of Disease Control and Prevention, of the Ministry of Health (MOH) of China and of the United Nations Children's Fund (UNICEF), as well as the unremitting efforts of the team, seven rounds of surveillance were carried out in 1990, 1995, 1998, 2000, 2005, 2008 and 2009. Coupled with the data from two National Nutrition Surveys in 1992 and 2002, data on the nutritional status of children under 5 years old has been collected in nine sets of consecutive surveillance data over 20 years. The Ministry of Education, in collaboration with the MOH, has also been conducting National Surveys on Fitness of Students every 5 years since 1985, which outlines the changes among schoolchildren aged 7–18 years old.

This chapter uses data from three of these surveys (1985, 2000 and 2005), to demonstrate reports on the nutritional status of the Chinese population during the past 30 years – since the adoption of the reform and the opening-up policy in the late 1980s. It also presents a preliminary analysis on the factors favourable to improvement in nutrition and some strategic considerations.

Data Sources

The information presented in this chapter was from the following sources:

1. The China Food and Nutrition Surveillance System (CFNSS) with seven rounds of surveillance in 1990, 1995, 1998, 2000, 2005, 2008 and 2009. The system covered 40 sites (14 urban sites and 26 rural sites, including nine poor rural sites) that had been randomly cluster sampled, and included around 16,000 children under 5 years of age (Chang et al., 2006; Chen et al., 2011).
2. The China National Survey on Fitness of Students (CNSFS) in 1985, 2000 and 2005.

This covered 30 provinces with randomly cluster-sampled sites, and included around 240,000 young people aged between 7 and 18 years (Chen et al., 2009).
3. The 2002 National Nutrition and Health Survey (CNNHS 2002) that covered 31 provinces with random cluster samples of 250,000 people of all ages (Yang and Zhai, 2006).

The WHO 2006 Child Growth Standards are used for assessment of the physical development of children under 5 years old (WHO, 2006) and the WHO Growth Reference for Schoolchildren and Adolescents is applied for the physical development assessment of older children (de Onis et al., 2007). The cut-offs for overweight and obesity in adults and children/adolescents are those of the Chinese guidelines (Bureau of Disease Control, Ministry of Health, 2003, 2007).

Results and Discussion

Along with the rapid economic growth of China, the nutritional status of the population improved dramatically. Below is a discussion on the improvement of the nutritional status of various population groups, the factors that are attributed to this improvement and the existing challenges.

Nutritional improvements

Reduction in undernutrition

Undernutrition among children under 5 years old has reduced rapidly since 1995. From 1990 onwards, the prevalence of underweight and stunting of children of this age in China has declined (Table 8.1). By 2009, the prevalence of underweight in rural areas had dropped to close to normal, although the stunting rate remained at 12.6% in rural China. There was little progress before 1995, but the situation has improved remarkably since then.

The analysis on undernutrition in different age groups in the past two decades has demonstrated a greater reduction among children aged 0–5 months and 6–11 months; however, the reduction in children older than 1 year has been slowing down (Figs 8.1 and 8.2).

Table 8.1. Prevalence of underweight, and stunting of, children under 5 years old in China during 1990–2009. There was no surveillance in urban sites during 2008 and 2009. From China Food and Nutrition Surveillance System (CFNSS); China National Survey on Fitness of Students (CNSFS).

Year	Underweight (%)			Stunting (%)		
	National	Urban	Rural	National	Urban	Rural
1990	13.7	5.3	16.5	33.1	11.4	40.3
2000	8.2	2.0	10.3	20.0	4.1	25.3
1992[a]	16.2	6.5	19.4	32.1	9.2	39.7
1995	11.4	3.4	14.1	33.2	10.4	40.8
1998	7.8	1.8	9.8	22.3	5.3	27.9
2002[a]	7.8	3.1	9.2	14.3	4.9	17.3
2005	4.9	1.4	6.1	13.0	3.1	16.3
2008			5.1			13.7
2009			4.6			12.6

[a]Data from CNSFS.

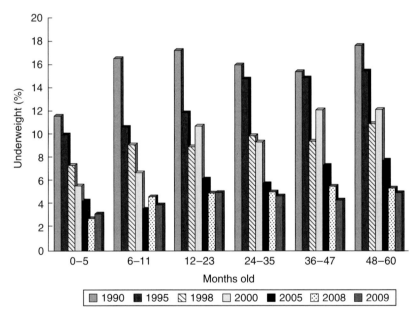

Fig. 8.1. Prevalence of underweight children by age groups from 1990 to 2009 in rural China (average for rural children under 5 years old in 2009, 4.6%).

Overall nutritional status

The overall nutritional status of children in China has been stable except for that of infants under 12 months during the global economic crisis. The data from the surveillance in 2009 was designed for tracking the changes in nutritional status that have occurred since 2008 during the global economic crisis. Comparison of the prevalence of undernutrition in 2008 and 2009 gave the impression that the overall nutritional condition had not worsened in terms of undernutrition among children under 5 years. This is illustrated by the prevalence of stunting in rural China, which was stable (i.e. not worse) even in the poor rural areas (Fig. 8.3): stunting was around 9–10% in the general rural areas (excluding the poor rural areas) and around 18% in the poor rural areas.

However, from 2008 to 2009, there was an increase in the prevalence of stunting

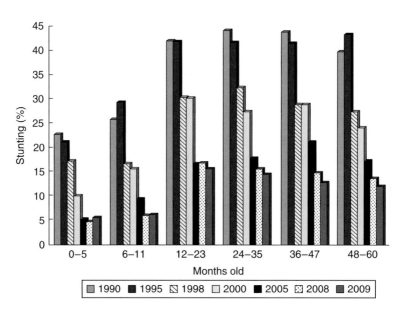

Fig. 8.2. Prevalence of stunting in children by age groups from 1990 to 2009 in rural China (average for rural children under 5 years old in 2009, 12.6%).

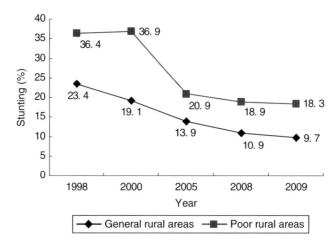

Fig. 8.3. Prevalence of stunting in children under 5 years old in China in general rural and poor rural areas from 1998 to 2009.

in children under 12 months old in poor rural areas. This increased from 5.7% to 9.1% in children aged 0–5 months and from 6.7% to 12.5% in those aged 6–11 months, in contrast with the prevalence of stunting in the same age groups in the general rural areas, which remained the same or decreased from 4.9% to 4.2% and from 6.2% to 3.8% respectively (Table 8.2). The immediate negative impact of the economic crisis on infants could be integrated into the average figure of the children under 5 years old as a whole.

Increases in height of schoolchildren

The increase in height of schoolchildren is speeding up. The mean height increase of Chinese schoolchildren aged 6–19 years during 1992–2002 was 3.8 cm and 3.1 cm in urban and rural boys, and 3.3 cm and 2.9 cm for girls, respectively. Figure 8.4 illustrates the medians of height for boys at different ages in 2005 compared with the World Health Organization (WHO) standards and those of the US Centers for Disease Control and Prevention (US-CDC). The height of urban children is the same as international standards per age group, but the heights of boys more than 15 years old and girls more than 13 years old were a little lower than the USA-CDC standards. The medians were close to the standards in urban areas of China, but the growth in height of rural boys still lagged behind the standards.

Diets in rural areas

Diets in rural areas of China have improved but the trend in the urban areas is towards an imbalance in nutritional status. In the past two decades, the dietary pattern of rural people has become more balanced. From 1992 to 2002, energy obtained from carbohydrates shifted from 73.7% to 61.5%, that from fats from 18.6% to 27.5% and that from proteins from 6.2% to 10.3%. During the same time period, the dietary pattern of urban people worsened, in that energy obtained from fats shifted from 28.4% to 35%, with carbohydrate use reducing from 57.4% to 48.5%. The oil and fat consumption of urban and rural residents was the same (44 and 41 g/day per person, respectively) in 2002 (Zhai and Yang, 2006). Such a shift in dietary pattern has become the main factor in the increase of chronic disease morbidity (including obesity).

Table 8.2. Prevalence of stunting (as %) in children during 1990–2009 in general rural and poor rural areas in China. From China Food and Nutrition Surveillance System (CFNSS).

Age in months	1998	2000	2005	2008	2009
0–5	17.4 (23.2)[a]	10.3 (13.2)	5.3 (5.2)	4.9 (5.7)	4.2 (9.1)
6–11	17.9 (22.9)	15.8 (23.3)	9.6 (13.1)	6.2 (6.7)	3.8 (12.5)
12–23	30.6 (39.6)	30.0 (44.2)	16.8 (21.8)	17.0 (23.5)	12.3 (22.7)
24–35	32.6 (42.1)	27.7 (40.9)	18.1 (23.6)	15.7 (22.7)	11.8 (20.4)
36–47	29.1 (37.9)	29.2 (42.2)	21.4 (27.5)	14.9 (20.5)	9.6 (18.4)
48–60	27.6 (37.7)	24.3 (36.7)	17.5 (20.3)	13.9 (20.2)	8.9 (17.1)
Total	23.4 (36.4)	19.1 (36.9)	13.9 (20.9)	10.9 (18.9)	9.4 (18.3)

[a]Figures in parentheses indicate % prevalence in poor rural areas.

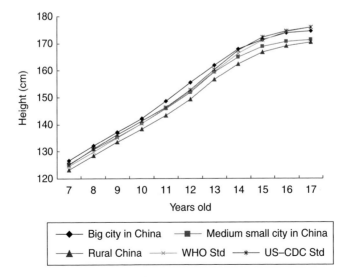

Fig. 8.4. Mean height of Chinese students by age compared with World Health Organization (WHO) and US Centers for Disease Control and Prevention (US-CDC) standards in 2005.

Nutrition challenges and emerging nutrition-related issues

Anaemia

Anaemia is a public health problem in China. Iron deficiency anaemia in particular is widespread owing to the low iron absorption rate (<5% has been reported) from the traditional staple diet of cereal, and it has become an important public health problem. In 2002, the national prevalence of anaemia was 20.1% (male 15.8%, female 23.3%; urban 18.2%, rural 20.8%). It was prevalent among the vulnerable age groups, but the differences between urban and rural China were insignificant (Table 8.3).

The distribution of anaemia by age in the Chinese population in 2000–2008 peaked at 6–11 months of age. Anaemia could be found in 34–53% of children of this age and still remained high (at 25–34%) at 12–23 months of age, as shown in Fig. 8.5.

Table 8.3. Prevalence of anaemia (% population) in China in 2002. From 2002 China National Survey on Fitness of Students (CNSFS).

	Urban	Rural	National
By gender			
Male	13.4	16.7	15.8
Female	21.5	24.0	23.3
Prevalence in different age groups			
Children 6–11 months	40.6	37.5	38.3
Children 12–23 months	29.2	28.9	29.0
Children <5 years	12.7	20.8	18.6
Women 18–44 years	23.7	27.2	
Pregnant women	23.5	30.0	27.9
Lactating mothers	25.3	33.2	30.7
Elderly >60years	21.3	30.4	28.0

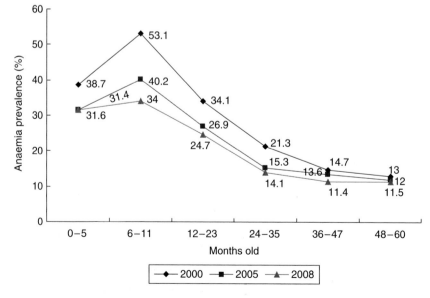

Fig. 8.5. Prevalence of anaemia in children under 5 years old in rural China in 2000–2008 (by age group).

It is worth noticing that the prevalence of anaemia in children under 2 years old has not significantly declined with the rapid economic growth of the country, even though undernutrition has dramatically improved during this time (Table 8.1). During the 2008–2009 global economic crisis, there was no change in the prevalence of anaemia in children under 5 years in general rural areas (measured with the poor rural areas excluded); however, in the poor rural areas, the prevalence of anaemia in all age groups during 2008–2009 increased to the levels in recorded in 2005 (Fig. 8.6).

Child stunting in rural areas

Child stunting is still high in rural areas, and especially in the poor rural areas. During the course of a dramatic drop in undernutrition in children, little change was observed in the prevalence of undernutrition among children in poor rural surveillance sites during 1998 to 2000: the prevalence of stunting stagnated at around 36% (Table 8.2), 1.5–2 times higher than that in general rural areas. This situation remained unchanged until 2002 (data from 2002 CNNHS), but has experienced a significant improvement since 2005. Despite the

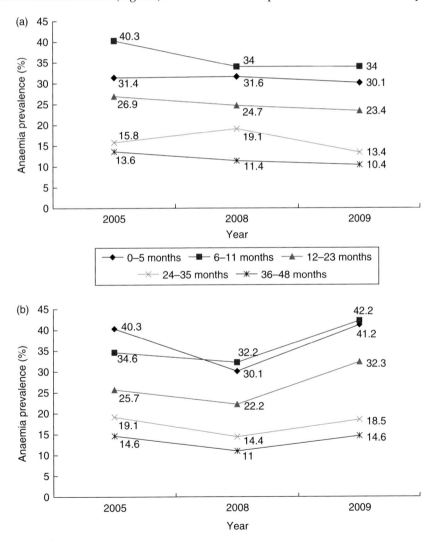

Fig. 8.6. Prevalence of anaemia in children in rural areas of China during the period of the global economic crisis (2008–2009): (a) general rural areas (excluding poor rural areas); and (b) poor rural areas.

improvement, nearly 20% of children under 5 years old were still stunted in 2009.

Stunting and wasting of schoolchildren and adolescents

Despite an improvement (decrease) in the level of stunting among children and adolescents in poor rural areas between 2002 and 2005, the prevalence of stunting still remained relatively high, especially in the poor regions of southwest China (Table 8.4), where stunting occurred in 14–18% of schoolchildren aged 5–18 years in 2005.

Wasting among schoolchildren and adolescents deserves special attention. The occurrence of wasting is a result of severe malnutrition during physical development, which has a long-term impact on the health, learning capacity and physical performance of younger children and adolescents. The prevalence of wasting was only around 3% among children under 5 years old. However,

it was as high as 7.9% and 11.3% among 13–18 year old boys in poor counties of north-west China and south-west China, respectively, in 2002 and 10.3% and 14.7% in 2005 (Chen et al., 2009), thus showing an increasing rather than a decreasing trend. Follow-up monitoring needs to be conducted to find out what are the causes of poor weight gain during school age.

Nutrition-related obesity and other chronic diseases

The prevalence of nutrition-related chronic disease is increasing. Data from the 2002 CNNHS and the surveillance data of the Center for Chronic Disease Prevention and Control of China show that the obesity problem is becoming prevalent among the urban population (Table 8.5). The increase in the number of overweight people (adults) has been faster than that for obesity in adults, and the increases in overweight and in obesity in

Table 8.4. Prevalence of stunting in schoolchildren in poor rural areas. From 2002 China National Nutrition and Health Survey (CNNHS); 2005 China National Survey on Fitness of Students (CNSFS).

	Boys		Girls	
Age and region	2002[a]	2005[b]	2002[a]	2005[b]
5–12 years				
North-west	15.4	7.4	10.9	10.2
South-west	38.0	15.0	38.2	18.0
13–18 years				
North-west	27.4	10.3	11.4	5.5
South-west	40.9	15.8	36.5	13.5

[a]Data from CNNHS; [b]Data from CNSFS.

Table 8.5. Trends in prevalence of overweight, and obesity in, adults in China. From 2002 China National Nutrition and Health Survey (CNNHS); 2004 and 2007 Risk Factor Surveillance Reports by Chinese Center for Disease Control and Prevention (CCDPC/China CDC).

	Overweight (%)			Obese (%)		
Region	2002[a]	2004[b]	2007[b]	2002[a]	2004[b]	2007[b]
National	22.8	23.1	27.3	7.1	7.0	8.0
Urban	28.1	26.6	29.7	9.8	7.8	9.1
Rural	20.6	21.8	25.7	6.6	6.7	7.3

[a]Data from CNNHS; [b]Data from CCDPC (China CDC).

the rural population in the past 5 years have both been greater than in the urban areas (Center for NCD Prevention and Control, 2008). However, the increase has not been as fast as expected, which may reflect the impacts of the nationwide promotion of the *Action on Healthy Lifestyle for All* programme initiated by the MOH in 2007 on lifestyle changes in urban areas.

In children aged 7–18 years old, obesity is now an urgent issue in the field of public health: the prevalence of both overweight and obesity has increased greatly over the past 20 years (Ji, 2007). Based on data from the 2005 CNSFS, the prevalence of overweight/obesity has increased dramatically to around 13.9%, even in inland cities, and to approximately 6% in non-poor rural areas. Among boys aged 7–12 years in Beijing and Shanghai, increases have been by 5–7 times in the 20 years from 1985 to 2005 (Table 8.6). The data in Table 8.6 also show that the increase in (inland) Beijing between 2000 and 2005 was much faster than in (coastal) Shanghai. The prevalence of overweight/obesity in girls was lower than in boys. The factors related to differences in the rate of increase in overweight and obesity need further investigation.

With the rapid economic development that has occurred in China, the population now enjoys a better income and standard of living. Money for food and clothing is basically secure, but the dietary pattern has become unbalanced as a result of changes in food consumption behaviour. Nutrition has turned out to be the most important factor leading to the rapid increase that there has been in the major chronic diseases. The occurrence of hypertension, diabetes and hyperlipidaemia, which have been on the rise over the last 20 years, reached 19%, 2.6% and 18.6%, respectively, in 2002. The trends in these increases as shown in Fig. 8.7 present standardized prevalences for comparison.

Analysis of the relative risks of these diseases for dietary factors such as the percentage of fat consumed and energy obtained from cereals concluded that the risk of hypertension and dislipidaemia increased by 7% and 30% if the energy obtained from cereals was less than 55%. The risk increase of overweight/obesity and hyperlipidaemia rose to 36% and 50%, respectively, if the energy share from fat was higher than 25%; if the share exceeded 35%, the increase in risk of the two diseases would be 46% and 89%, and the risk of diabetes would increase by 21% (Chen *et al.*, 2008).

The total intake of energy has not shown any major changes over the past 20 years, even dropping slightly. However, more and more people are now engaged in sedentary work and do less physical activity.

Table 8.6. Trends in prevalence of overweight/obesity (% overweight + obesity) among children and adolescents aged 7–18 years from 1985 to 2005. From 1985–2005 China National Surveys on Fitness of Students (CNSFS).

	Boys		Girls	
Year and city	7–12 years	13–18 years	7–12 years	13–18 years
1985				
Beijing	5.8	4.8	4.3	5.1
Shanghai	5.4	2.7	2.2	2.8
1995				
Beijing	17.5	18.1	12.0	11.6
Shanghai	20.5	15.7	11.8	8.0
2000				
Beijing	29.0	25.0	17.3	14.6
Shanghai	28.9	17.2	15.3	9.6
2005				
Beijing	40.1	31.5	20.2	20.0
Shanghai	30.0	17.6	11.9	10.6

(a) Hypertension

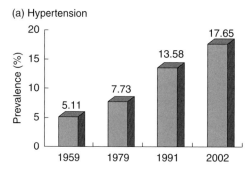

(b) Diabetes

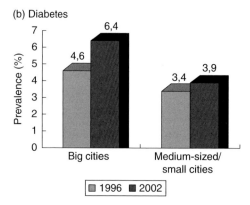

Fig. 8.7. Trends in standardized prevalences of disease in adults in China: (a) trends in hypertension from 1959 to 2002; (b) trends in diabetes by type of urban area in 1996 and 2002. From Report on 2002 CNHS (2006).

According to a cohort study, the energy imbalance of overweight people in China was on average 80 kcal in excess daily (Zhai et al., 2008), so a positive energy imbalance is also a risk factor for obesity and related diseases.

Analysis of factors contributing to nutrition improvement and the current challenges

Government efforts

Any improvement in nutrition is the outcome of the concerted efforts of the government, especially in agricultural development. Agricultural production is the basis for the availability of sufficient food and income in both urban and rural areas of China, and the application of policies

favourable to farmers since 2000 has stimulated the improvement of nutrition of rural poor children. The Chinese government has combined agricultural production with rural development and farmers' livelihoods together as '3 AGRI' in national planning. This covers progress in various aspects, including:

- Tax exemption and subsidies: a tax exemption for agriculture since 2006 (27 Yuan/person income increase); direct subsidies for the growing of grains (80 Yuan/mu, where 1 mu = 666.67 m²); risk funds for grain purchasing at a protected price, etc.
- Increases in income: per capita income increased from 2253 Yuan in 2000 to 5919 Yuan in 2010, the annual real increase was above 7.1%.
- Rural development: construction plans for new townships and villages; subsidies for rural households on electric appliances – purchased with 13% discount; tuition fee waivers and free textbook supplies for rural primary and junior schools.
- Livelihood: subsidies for the poorest households; pensions for the rural elderly; meal subsidies for rural boarding schools; new Rural Collaborative Medical Care and public health services.

Agriculture is, therefore, considered not only in terms of production or yield, but also as the integration of rural development and farmers' wellbeing, which is extremely important in relation to the improvement of nutrition.

The poverty reduction programme

The principles of the poverty reduction programme involved a transfer of funds from relief to local economic development, which contributed greatly to the nutritional improvement of rural children. The number of extremely poor people fell from 94.23 million (10.2% of the rural population) in 2000 to 35.97 million (3.8% of the rural population) in 2009. The government has set the poverty line at 1500 Yuan per capita based on international standards. The number of poor people in China increased to 100 million in 2011, the first year of the 12th Five-Year National Socio-economic Development Plan, but more actions will be taken to alleviate poverty.

Social conditions

The social conditions of mothers, such as education, are directly related to improvement in child nutrition, and the migration of mothers has a negative effect on the nutritional security of children. An analysis of data for 2005 showed that the attributable risk (percentage) of education of mothers and migrant mothers contributed to a total of 34% in child stunting.

Food fortification programmes

Food fortification programmes at the national level and lifestyle adjustment programmes at the community level have not been a component of the Chinese national development plan, which has been a factor in the still high levels of micronutrient deficiencies, especially in iron deficiency anaemia, and the risk of nutrition-related chronic diseases increasing rapidly during the surge in economic development.

Strategic Considerations for Nutrition Improvement in China

Finally, some of the strategic considerations for integrating nutrition improvement into the basic public health services of medical care reform in China are enumerated below.

1. Investments in nutrition security for children under 2 years old in the rural areas and for students in rural boarding schools should be the priority in national development planning.
2. A national food fortification programme for the prevention of micronutrient deficiency should be set up, with special emphasis on iron deficiency.
3. Nutrition education should be included in the basic public health services of medical care reform.
4. There should be promotion of the *Action on Healthy Lifestyle for All* programme and strengthening of the implementation of the community-based chronic disease prevention programme (healthy weight and healthy blood pressure) in terms of guiding public education and management of high-risk populations.
5. Nutrition improvement should be focused on rural areas, on children under 2 years old and on schoolchildren in rural areas.

References

Bureau of Disease Control, Chinese Ministry of Health (2003) *Guidelines for Overweight and Obesity Prevention and Control in Chinese Adults.* People's Medical Publishing House, Beijing.

Bureau of Disease Control, Chinese Ministry of Health (2007) *Guidelines for Overweight and Obesity Prevention and Control in Chinese Children and Adolescents Aged 7–18 Yrs Old.* People's Medical Publishing House, Beijing.

Center for NCD Prevention and Control (2008) *Report on Risk Factor Surveillance 2007.* Center for Non-Communicable Disease Prevention and Control, Ministry of Health, Beijing.

Chang, S., He, W. and Chen, C. (2006) Trend of child nutritional status in 15 years. *Hygiene Research* 35, 768–774 [in Chinese].

Chen, C., Zhao, W., Yang, Z., Zhai, Y., Wu, Y. and Kong, L. (2008) The role of dietary factors in chronic disease control in China. *Obesity Reviews* 9, 100–103.

Chen, C., Ji, C. and Wang, Y. (2009) *Report on the Undernutrition of Children and Adolescents, Mengkui Wang: For the Future of the Country.* Chinese Development Publishing House, Beijing, pp. 30–34 [in Chinese].

Chen, C., He, W., Wang, Y., Jia, F. and Deng, L. (2011) *Nutritional Status During Rapid Economic Development in 2010. Report on Nutrition Policy Research.* Ministry of Health, Beijing [in Chinese].

de Onis, M., Onyago, A.W., Borghi, E., Siyam, A., Nishida, C. and Siekmann, J. (2007) Development of WHO growth reference for school-aged children and adolescents. *Bulletin of the World Health Organization* 85, 660–667.

Ji, C. (2007) Report on childhood obesity in China (4): prevalence and trend of overweight and obesity among school-aged children and adolescents in urban China in 1985–2000. *Biomedical and Environmental Sciences* 20, 1–5.

WHO (2006) *WHO Child Growth Standards: Methods and Development*. Department of Nutrition for Health and Development, World Health Organization, Geneva, Switzerland.

Yang, X. and Zhai, F. (2006) *Report on Nutrition and Health of Chinese Residents, Vol. 3*. Chinese Medical Publishing House, Beijing, pp. 74–77 [in Chinese].

Zhai, F. and Yang, X. (2006) *Report on Dietary Intake of Chinese Residents, Vol. 2*. Chinese Medical Publishing House, Beijing, pp. 21–23 [in Chinese].

Zhai, F., Wang, H. and Wang, Z. (2008) Closing the energy gap to prevent weight gain in China. *Obesity Reviews* 9, 107–112.

9 Integrating Nutrition into Agricultural and Rural Development Policies: The Brazilian Experience of Building an Innovative Food and Nutrition Security Approach

Luciene Burlandy,[1]* Cecilia Rocha[2] and Renato Maluf[3]

[1]*Universidade Federal Fluminense, National Council of Food and Nutrition Security (CONSEA), Rio de Janeiro, Brazil; [2]Ryerson University, Toronto, Ontario, Canada; [3]Universidade Federal Rural do Rio de Janeiro and National Council of Food and Nutrition Security, Rio de Janeiro, Brazil*

Summary

Established in 2006, Brazil's National System of Food and Nutrition Security is made up of representatives of civil society organizations and different governmental sectors. Innovative programmes have emerged as a consequence of this institutional framework. Effective connections made at programme design and implementation level have generated concrete results, such as the convergence of different programmes geared to the poorest groups. This chapter analyses different assessments of the Family Grant Programme (Programa Bolsa Família – PBF), the Food Acquisition Programme (Programa de Aquisição de Alimentos – PAA) and the National School Meals Programme (Programa Nacional de Alimentação Escolar – PNAE). Results indicate that PBF promotes greater access to food, improves the variety of food consumed, reduces food insecurity levels and, in some cases, has contributed to the nutritional recovery of children with severe deficits in weight-for-height and height-for-age measurements. However, families participating in PBF are increasingly choosing industrialized foods, following the food profile that prevails in the country. Although the prevalence of stunting and wasting is decreasing, the prevalence of overweight and obesity is increasing, particularly in urban areas, and especially in lower income groups. Hence, PBF is being implemented in an integrative way with programmes such as PAA and PNAE so as to improve the availability and consumption of fruits and vegetables in public schools and promote purchases directly from family farmers. These programmes have been designed based on a comprehensive, systemic and participatory approach, thus contributing to the establishment of joint actions among agriculture, health, nutrition and social sectors, and forging closer links between food production and healthy eating. Challenges are related to conflicts of interests and institutional capacity in some municipalities.

*Contact: burlandy@uol.com.br

Introduction

Both food policy, as a process of regulating the supply of food for a population, and food security, as a strategy for ensuring secure access to food, have a long history (Coveney, 2003; Maluf, 2007). Similarly, nutrition programmes and actions aimed at overcoming diet-related diseases and promoting public health have been part of social protection systems in different countries for many decades. Despite that, the gap between food policy and health promotion is a key challenge in most countries (Coveney, 2003). In Brazil, the aim has recently emerged to integrate nutrition into agricultural and rural development policies, to build a food system that guarantees the human right to adequate food and to use an innovative approach to policy, all of which link food and nutrition security.

For more than two decades, social mobilization for food and nutrition security (FNS) in Brazil, comprising social movements, civil society organizations and different sectors of the government, has occupied a prominent space in the public agenda. According to national legislation, FNS consists of 'realizing the right of all to regular and permanent access to good quality food, in sufficient quantity, without compromising the access to other essential needs, on the basis of food habits that promote health and respect cultural diversity and that are environmentally, culturally, economically and socially sustainable' (Presidency of the Federative Republic of Brazil, 2006).

In Brazil, hunger, malnutrition, anaemia, hypovitaminosis A, and other diet-related diseases have been joined by obesity as a manifestation of food insecurity and as a major public health problem, in common with many other parts of the world. The growing prevalence of these problems has been affected by significant demographic, economic, social and technological changes in recent decades (Harnack *et al.*, 1999; French *et al.*, 2001; Ludwig *et al.*, 2001; WHO, 2003, 2004; Arkes, 2009). Greater consumption of processed and convenience foods, and more meals outside the home, have all been associated with a lower prevalence of diets that are rich in fruits, vegetables, whole grains and lean meats, and an increased preference for fatty and sweet foods. Economic interests linked to agribusiness and the global food industry have further contributed to the complexity of factors shaping modern dietary patterns (Chopra *et al.*, 2002; Nestle, 2003).

Considering that dietary patterns are affected by multiple factors of a biological, psychological, socio-economic and cultural nature, it is important to promote the convergence of different kinds of actions to influence these factors at both a macro-policy level and within institutions, communities and families. This chapter analyses how Brazil is establishing connections between programmes and targeting them to the most vulnerable groups through key institutions, such as public schools.

Based on the comprehensive approach to FNS, a national institutional framework and some key innovative programmes are being designed and implemented in Brazil aiming at establishing linkages among agriculture, nutrition and social protection, integrating health into the agriculture and social sector, and linking food production, health promotion and social welfare. These programmes, such as the Family Grant Programme (*Programa Bolsa Família* – PBF); the Food Acquisition Programme (*Programa de Aquisição de Alimentos* – PAA) and the National School Meals Programme (*Programa Nacional para Alimentação Escolar* – PNAE), have expanded the availability and accessibility of food, particularly of fruits and vegetables, and given priority to people and institutions with difficult access to food and populations subject to food insecurity situations.

The chapter highlights the advances that have been made, as well as the challenges, and discusses some evidence for the integrative approach in improving the quality of diets and raising the level of nutrition. It is based on a review and analysis of various studies and documents: evaluation studies of federal programmes; documented programme proposals and federal legislation of the Ministries of Health and of Social Development and Fight against Hunger (MDS); technical and evaluation reports of the federal government; and minutes of meetings and official documents of the National

Council and National Conferences of Food and Nutrition Security from 2003 to 2010.

The first section of the chapter presents information on the national social and nutritional profile of Brazilians, analysing it as a consequence of the non-sustainable practices in food production and food processing models that are prevalent in the country and have contributed to reducing food diversity. The second section briefly describes the national institutional framework of FNS, which is composed of different governmental sectors and civil society organizations. This section analyses how existing laws, policies and policy instruments that address FNS, based on a comprehensive and participatory approach, contribute to the effective implementation of inter-sectoral policies for healthy diets. The third section presents details of programmes that were designed as a consequence of this institutional process, highlighting some advances and challenges to the formulation process, and looking at evidence for improvements in diets and nutrition levels.

Social and Nutritional Profile of the Brazilian Population

Brazil is a federal republic with around 190 million inhabitants and a total land area of 8.5 million km^2, divided into 27 states and 5564 municipalities. While recent statistics estimate the gross domestic product (GDP) as US$1.9 trillion in 2010 (which puts Brazil among the world's largest economies), the country is also among the most socially unequal on the planet.

By the end of 2009, Brazil had met the first Millennium Development Goal (MDG) of reducing poverty and malnutrition by half. There had been a sizeable reduction in extreme poverty, from 17.4% in 2001 to less than 9% in 2008 (CONSEA, 2009a). The evolution of poverty, especially in Latin America, generally depends on three elements: the level of inequality, the variation in this level and the economy's rate of growth (Maluf and Burlandy, 2007). The Gini inequality index declined from 0.580 in 1995 to 0.566 in 2001, and then to 0.528 in 2007; recent studies indicate that income

sources not derived from paid employment, including the conditional cash transfer (CCT) programmes, contributed to the reduction of inequality by 24% from 1995 to 2004, particularly because these programmes are directed precisely at the lowest income sectors of the population (Kawani et al., 2006; Néri, 2006; Saboia, 2008; Barros, 2009; CONSEA, 2009a,b; Schutter, 2009).

Major FNS problems in the country include overweight and obesity, undernutrition, micronutrient deficiency (anaemia, hypovitaminosis A), hunger, unequal access to healthy food, water and land, an extensive use of pesticides, and challenges to biodiversity (CONSEA, 2004; 2007; 2009a,b; MS, 2005b).

Although still a problem in some specific regions and for some specific groups – such as indigenous people, and *quilombolas* (descendants of runaway slaves) – the prevalence of child stunting in the poorest region of the country (the north-east) fell by a third between 1986 and 1996 (from 33.9% to 22.2%) and by almost three quarters between 1996 and 2006 (from 22.2% to 5.9%). In the former period, the decline was associated with improvements in maternal schooling and in the coverage of water and sewage services. Increasing purchasing power of the poorest families and, again, maternal schooling, were more relevant in the latter period. Infant mortality rates in the region also declined from 55/1000 in 1996 to 24/1000 in 2007 (Lima et al., 2010). Though the prevalence of stunting and wasting is decreasing, overweight and obesity are growing problems in the country, particularly in urban areas. The latest estimates for Brazil (2009) indicate that 49.9% of adults are overweight and 14.8% are clinically obese. The prevalence of overweight in children from 5 to 9 years old was 34.8% and of obesity 16.6%. For adolescents (10–19 years old) the prevalences of overweight and obesity were 20.5% and 4.9%, respectively. In the north-east, 30.3% of children were overweight in 2009 compared with 8.7% in 1989 (IBGE, 2010).

The food consumption profile of the Brazilian population is characterized by high levels of saturated and hydrogenated fats – the substitution of food products that are rich in nutrients (vegetables and fruits) by industrialized food that is energetically dense and poor in micronutrients. Over the past two decades, the consumption of animal foods, fats, sugar and industrialized food has increased. A low intake of fruits is observed in nationwide surveys. The overall availability of fruits and vegetables is equivalent to 30% of the World Health Organization's recommendation of 400 g/day. The purchase of fruits and vegetables is below the recommended levels in all income groups (Levy-Costa, 2005; MS, 2005b; Claro *et al.*, 2007; CONSEA, 2009a,b).

The Brazilian Food Insecurity Scale (EBIA) is used to evaluate the capacity of families to access food of appropriate quantity and quality.[1] A National Household Sample Survey (Pesquisa Nacional por Amostra de Domicílios –PNAD, Segurança Alimentar) that used EBIA was conducted in 2004 and revealed that food security existed in 65.2% of Brazilian households (33.7 million households of 109.2 million people). The remaining 34.8% of households (18 million households of 72.2 million people) living in food insecurity were distributed as follows: 16% in mild food insecurity (8.3 million), 12.3% in moderate food insecurity (6.4 million) and 6.5% in severe food insecurity (3.4 million). The association between poverty and more intense levels of food insecurity becomes evident in the fact that food security is present in only 17.5% of households in extreme poverty, while 61.2% of them are affected by moderate or severe food insecurity. The incidence of moderate or severe food insecurity was higher among rural households (26.0% compared with 17.4% in urban areas), and three times higher in the north-east and northern regions than in the south of the country (IBGE, 2006).

The same survey conducted in 2009 indicated that the households living in a food insecurity situation fell from 34.8% in 2004 to 30.5% in 2009. These households were distributed as follows: 18% in mild food insecurity, 6.5% in moderate insecurity and 5.0% in severe insecurity (IBGE, 2010). Compared with the 2004 survey, there was an increase of households reporting mild food insecurity, and a decrease of households reporting moderate and severe food insecurity.

Increases in the purchasing power of the poorest families, and decreases in undernutrition and food insecurity rates, have also been associated with social programmes, particularly with cash transfer programmes (PNAD 2004; see IBGE, 2006).

Institutional Framework

The National Law on FNS (2006) established the right to food as a human right and formalized the National System of FNS as composed of: (i) the National Council (Conselho Nacional de Segurança Alimentar e Nutricional – CONSEA) – an advisory body to the country's President, formed by representatives of civil society organizations (two thirds) and different governmental sectors (one third); (ii) National Conferences held every 4 years; and (iii) the inter-ministerial chamber on Food and Nutrition Security (Câmara Interministerial de Segurança Alimentar – CAISAN). Following directives from CONSEA, CAISAN is responsible for designing the National Policy and Plan on Food and Nutrition Security, and coordinating its implementation (Presidency of the Federative Republic of Brazil, 2006; CAISAN, 2009; CONSEA, 2009a,b).

The Institutional Framework and Innovative Programmes

Innovative programmes designed to promote access to healthy food, while strengthening family farmers, have emerged as an outcome of the participatory institutional framework outlined above. These focus on families subject to food insecurity situations that are also entitled to CCT programmes. The political pressure of civil society organizations and of the inter-sectoral decision-making process established by CONSEA were key factors in the designing of these programmes.

The PBF is the main example of CCT in Brazil. This was implemented in 2003 by combining and redirecting four other CCT programmes: School Allowance (Ministry of Education, MEC), Meal Allowance (Ministry of Health, MS), Gas Coupons and Meal Cards (Ministry of Social Development and Fight Against Hunger, MDS) (MDS, 2003). Institutional arrangements integrated by three different governmental sectors (education, health, social development) at the three levels of the government (national, state and municipal) were developed to promote inter-sectoriality.

The PBF is based on the principles of FNS and is part of the 'Zero Hunger' ('Fome Zero') strategy to assure the human right to adequate food, and gives priority to people with difficult access to food (MS, 2005b). Hence, one of its goals was to eradicate hunger and promote FNS by increasing the family's income for food, but also for health, education and social services, and considering the sets of conditions encountered by the participating families. In 2010, the PBF reached more than 12 million families with a monthly per capita income of US$82.00 or less. Under the programme, families receive an amount that varies from US$12.00 to US$118.00/month. Those qualified to be in the programme are families with a per capita monthly income of up to US$41.00, irrespective of their composition, or those with a per capita income of US$41.00–82.00/month with pregnant or breastfeeding women, or children and adolescents between 0 and 15 years old. Families must keep their children at school and ensure that they receive basic preventive healthcare (vaccination schedules for children between 0 and 6 years, and a prenatal and postnatal agenda for pregnant women and breastfeeding mothers).

Evaluations of the Meal Allowance Programme (PBA) and the PBF indicate that dietary diversity and family food expenditures increased, and families tended to give most of the food obtained to children (Morris *et al.*, 2004; MS, 2005a; IBASE, 2008). Furthermore, for improvements in food consumption, there is evidence that the CCT programme has contributed to the nutritional recovery of children with severe weight-for-height and height-for-age deficits (Morris *et al.*, 2004; MS, 2005b).

A national assessment of the impact of the PBF conducted in 2005 (WHO, 2006), using a sample of 15,240 households and groups of PBF beneficiaries and non-beneficiaries,

showed a rate of 19% of chronic infant malnutrition (6–23 months) in beneficiaries of the PBF; acute malnutrition was detected in 10% of these participants. The prevalence of overweight was 11% in children aged 24–60 months, and 15% in children aged 6–23 months. There was no significant difference in the nutritional status of children participating in the PBF compared with those not doing so, with the exception of children aged 12–35 months in the northern and central western regions, where PBF contributed to the decrease of chronic and acute malnutrition (CEDEPLAR, 2006).

Assessment of the impact of the PBF and the PBA in north-east Brazil (MS, 2005a; Assis, 2006) has shown an improvement in children's nutritional conditions, with an increase in weight and height and a lower prevalence of anaemia. However, the impact on children's nutritional status and early childhood growth depends on many factors, such as the availability of public services (healthcare, education, sanitation) and the costs of accessing them, the duration of the programmes, transfer amounts, family sizes and intra-family rules for allocating resources (Burlandy, 2009). CCT programmes alone are not sufficient to ensure a more equitable distribution of public goods and services or for providing these at the necessary quality. Brazil faces serious problems, for example, in relation to access to drinking water and sanitation, adequate housing and high-quality public services. In education, the main problem has been quality, given that school attendance is practically universal up to the age of 14 years, although it decreases substantially among youngsters aged 15 years and older. Hence, public investments are needed for the provision of services and in resolving problems related to their quality (Maluf and Burlandy, 2007). It is crucial to integrate CCT programmes with other projects (access to public services, healthy food, sanitation) in order to ensure their impact on food and nutrition security. CONSEA has been playing a strategic role through integrated policy planning in this field (Burlandy, 2009).

A national survey, aimed at examining the perception of PBF beneficiaries of their food security and nutritional conditions, interviewed 3000 families in 2006. The results indicated improvements in the quality and especially in the variety of food available to the family, as well as an increase in frequency of the number of meals a day. Some 85% of the beneficiaries reported improvement in the quality of food accessed, and 100% reported accessing a greater variety. However, it is also important to note that 85% of the beneficiaries indicated frequent consumption of sugar, sweets and candy, while only 30% reported the consumption of vegetables and greens, and only 15% consumed fruit. In a situation of scarce resources, an increase in the consumption of high energy-density foods is often seen, in detriment to the consumption of sources of vitamins such as fruits, greens and vegetables that have a low cost/calorie ratio (Brandão *et al.*, 2007; Silva *et al.*, 2007).

Research using both qualitative and quantitative methods (5000 families interviewed) in 2008 concluded that 87% of families used PBF benefits for purchasing food and that the programme contributed to increases in both the quantity and diversity of food. In this research, 75% of those interviewed reported a higher consumption of sugar, 55% a higher consumption of fruits and 40% of vegetables. Families favoured foods with a better cost/calories and cost/satiation rate, such as industrialized food, rather than fruits and vegetables. The regularity of payments received through the PBF was highlighted as a positive factor that influenced changes in food pattern (IBASE, 2008).

A comparison of data from the PNAD 2004 survey (IBGE, 2006) and the 2006 Demographic Health Survey (Pesquisa Nacional de Demografia e Saúde da Criança e da Mulher – PNDS 2006; see MS, 2009), by Segall-Corrêa and Marin-León (2008) indicated that the prevalence of food security in low-income households receiving the Family Grant from PBA increased from 32.3% in 2004 to 38.5% in 2006. Segall-Corrêa *et al.* (2008), analysing national data on food and nutrition security, showed a positive association between cash transfer and household food security, regardless of the effects of other explanatory factors, such as income, education, skin colour, rural/urban areas. Monteiro *et al.* (2006), analysing the food and nutrition profile of children in the north-east region of

the country, also noted that the federal income transfer programmes (35.3% of the studied families were receiving federal grants) seem to have led to a reduction of almost 30% in the frequency of malnutrition (from 6.8% without the programme to 4.8% with it); the reduction reached as much as 62.1% in children of 6–11 months old (from 5.3% to 2.0%).

Understanding food practices and all forms of nutrition problems (such as obesity, malnutrition, hunger, micronutrient deficiencies) as a consequence of a multifactorial process is fundamental to the implementation of a comprehensive and integrative FNS approach. With such an approach, it is important to consider nutrition as part of the food system and encompassing policy flows, the use of agricultural land and its impact on the availability and price of food, and how food is produced, processed, marketed, distributed, sold and consumed.

The food and nutrition profile of Brazilian people is the outcome of multiple factors related to the food system, starting from the production and marketing conditions, and extending to the food transformation parameters imposed by industries and the advertising market. Brazil is one of the world leaders in the production and export of various agricultural products, but its export agribusiness sector uses a food production system that is characterized by the prevalence of intensive, mechanized agricultural production and a high use of chemical products, with significant social and environmental impacts. This system tends to reduce biodiversity and also the food diversity that is crucial for healthy food practices (CONSEA, 2004; MS, 2005a, 2009a,b; Schutter, 2009).

The family farming sector can contribute to the promotion of food diversity and healthy eating as it is primarily responsible for the food supply to the domestic market. This sector is also characterized by small-sized holdings (18.37 ha) and its food production is based on regional agriculture (CONSEA, 2009a,b). One of the most important strategies for promoting inter-sectorality in the food system in Brazil rests on the articulation between actions designed to guarantee access to healthy food, especially in schools, and actions for strengthening family farming.

Some 84% of the PBF beneficiary children have access to school meals. However, there is a tendency for the families participating in the programme to choose industrialized food, such as soft drinks, biscuits and snacks (Silva *et al.*, 2007). There is thus an urgent need to implement actions to promote healthy eating, especially in schools, as being a place where children can learn healthy eating habits. Based on the FNS approach, some new programmes were designed (such as the PAA), and old programmes were redesigned (such as the PNAE) that aimed to promote inter-sectoriality by linking different dimensions and sectors of the food system, especially agriculture, health and education. These programmes expand the availability of healthy food, especially fruits and vegetables, to public schools and social institutions that look after people in situations of food insecurity. CONSEA became the locus of action for strengthening these programmes.

The PAA was established in 2003 by the federal government to promote purchases of food products directly from family farmers, including those settled under the land reform programme, as well as from traditional groups and communities (such as indigenous communities). Food purchased through the programme is used for building food stocks (and regulating food prices) and to look after populations in food insecurity situations in programmes such as 'popular restaurants', community kitchens, food banks and schools, thereby facilitating access to healthy food (MDA, 2003). The Management Group for the PAA comprises the different ministries that coordinate the programme – the MDA, MDS, MEC, Ministry of Agriculture, Livestock and Food Supply (Ministério da Agricultura, Pecuária e Abastecimento – MAPA) and Ministry of Finance (Ministério da Fazenda – MF). Hence, the programme is implemented on an inter-sectoral basis (MDA, 2008).

The PAA programme served 5% of the Brazilian population living in food insecurity in 2007–2008, and has been implemented in 2300 municipalities all over the country. Between 2005 and 2009, the number of people in the programme increased fourfold, reaching 15 million in 2009 and covering 25,000 institutions. Since 2003, the government has spent US$ 3.5 billion and bought 3.1 million t of food from family farmers. In 2008, 1,189,000 farmers sold their products to the PAA, and the programme has donated food to 16.8 million people (CONSEA, 2009a,b; 2010). The PAA also helps to increase the purchase and availability of regional food, especially regional fruits and vegetables, at schools and social institutions (MDS, 2010).

A quantitative evaluation of PAA conducted in 2006 in the north-east of the country interviewed 398 family farmers, as well as beneficiary entities and associations. The results indicated a real increase in the average income of the family farmer. The other most evident changes were in food variety and quality (Sparovek, 2007). Another evaluation of the PAA that combined qualitative and quantitative methods and was conducted in the same year in the south and north-east regions indicated that schools and institutions receiving food declared that PAA increased food quality and availability. For these institutions, the programme has some positive points, such as cheaper school meals, the strengthening of family agriculture, the elimination of intermediaries and support to the local economy. The PAA has the potential of reaching target groups that would most benefit from public policies, such as agrarian reform settlers (Curralero and Santana, 2007).

These studies also indicated that there were problems in the direct delivery of food to the end user, such as transportation problems, delays in the disbursement of funds and a lack of or insufficient provision of technical assistance. Agrarian reform settlers suffer the worst production conditions. It was also observed in all the states analysed that civil society organizations, cooperatives and entities play an important role in the operation of the PAA – mobilizing and orienting a large portion of PAA beneficiaries, and helping them to overcome obstacles related to technical assistance, and to production, transport and storage (Curralero and Santana, 2007; Sparovek, 2007).

In 2006, the PAA commercialized 43 different kinds of fruits and 28 different kinds of vegetables (Schmitt and Guimarães, 2008). In 2008, representatives of family farmers and institutions that are beneficiaries of the PAA from all over the country evaluated the programme in a CONSEA meeting. The main advantages of the programme mentioned were:

- its capacity for promoting the organization and integration of local systems of production, commercialization and consumption of food and its provision of incentives for transition and/or adoption of agro-ecological methods;
- its capacity to promote greater integration between rural and urban areas, and between food producers and consumers;
- its capacity to promote diversification in production and a greater value of local products; and
- its capacity to increase access to fruits and vegetables by food-insecure families.

Social institutions that are beneficiaries of the PAA reported that the programme contributed to the increase in quantity and variety of foods based on regional products, thereby reinforcing cultural values. The main challenges are related to limits on financial and human resources (CONSEA, 2008).

Greater access to healthy food was also promoted by the recent remodelling and expansion of the PNAE – a programme originally launched in 1954. Today, the PNAE guarantees 15% of the daily dietary needs of school-aged children, and 30% of the needs of children in public day-care centres, indigenous and *quilombola* schools (MEC, 2006). In 2006, the government released official guidelines on the nutritional profile of school meals together with inter-ministerial legislation from the MEC and MS stating that 'Schools should restrict foods high in fat, saturated fat, trans-fats, free sugars and salt, and develop healthful food options and meals' (MEC/MS, 2006b). In 2009, the new law established a set of new regulations requiring that at least 30% of the foods in school meals be purchased directly from family farms and local rural enterprises. This ensures the commercialization of that production and, at the same time, provides quality meals in schools and makes fresh local products available (MEC, 2009). The PNAE had, up to 2008, provided an average of 35 million daily meals to children between the ages of 0 and 14 years. In 2009, this figure increased to 47 million daily meals, with the inclusion of secondary school students.

Results from a national research on the PNAE conducted in 2950 municipalities indicated that the consumption of fruits and vegetables increased between 2004 and 2006. In 2004, fruits were available in 28% of the schools, and in 2006 in 62%. In 2004, vegetables were included in 57% of schools' menus and by 2006 this had grown to 80% (Campbell, 2007). The legislation introduced in 2009 is expected to further increase the consumption of fruits and vegetables among children.

Conclusions

Different assessments of the programmes that were analysed in this chapter, based on both quantitative and qualitative research, indicate that they promote greater access to food and improve the variety of food available to the most vulnerable populations (low-income groups such as children attending public schools and those who live in food-insecure situations). CCT programmes contribute to a greater diversity and quality in diets, as families tend to spend most of this extra income on food. These programmes are also contributing to the reduction of stunting and wasting. However, the impact on nutritional status depends on many factors, especially the availability of public services and goods, as well as on the quality of these services and the costs of accessing them. Nutrition interventions should be assessed not only in terms of their immediate nutritional impact. Hence, CCT programmes are also important instruments in guaranteeing nutritional well-being when integrated into a broader social policy.

Obesity is a growing problem in the country, even among the poorest groups. The consumption of vegetables and fruits is below the recommended amount for all income brackets at national level, but low-income groups tend to consume fewer vegetables and fruits than their higher income counterparts. It is, therefore, essential to increase the availability of fresh foods, particularly to school-aged children, at a time when food practices are being formed.

The PAA and the PNAE are important strategies for promoting food diversity and improving the availability of fresh foods in schools, food banks and social institutions. At the same time, they strengthen family farmers by guaranteeing the marketing of their products through public programmes. The government, through its institutions (schools, hospitals, etc.), is a strategic actor in the food market, and its criteria for food purchasing, including decisions on the kind of food to purchase and from whom, can affect the position of the different producers in the market and have an impact on local and regional economies.

It is also important to expand and strengthen other social measures that are essential to promoting healthy eating practices, such as greater access to drinkable water, the implementation of infrastructure programmes (transport, national roads), the effective implementation of food advertising regulation and a culturally based approach guiding the design and the implementation of nutrition programmes.

As stressed in this chapter, connections among nutrition, agriculture and social protection policies can have an impact on the nutritional well-being of the population in a broader sense. Effective connections that generate a nutritional impact require a combination of factors, for example, a political process and an institutional framework that have inter-sectoriality and social participation as underlying principles. Once programmes are designed based on a comprehensive, systemic and participatory FNS approach, they contribute to establishing joint actions among agriculture, health, nutrition and social sectors, thus forging closer links between food production and healthy eating.

In Brazil, another factor in FNS has been the integration of different institutional mechanisms at the federal level in devising a comprehensive and integrative systemic approach. This has led, for example, to the formation of CONSEA, which is integrated by different sectors of the government (including ministries of agriculture, health, education and social development) and civil society organizations, and linked to the presidency. Other factors include political support by the presidency and the inclusion of FNS in the government's agenda, and the formation of inter-ministerial management groups linked to programmes (such as the PAA and PBF) that promote inter-sectoriality at the technical and political levels. Social participation in all phases of programme design and implementation, and at all levels of the government (national, state and municipal) has been crucial in promoting these political processes.

Some challenges must be highlighted. Considering that these programmes integrate food production, commercialization and consumption, different actors are involved at different levels (family, school, community; teachers, school administrators, employees, suppliers; government sectors; industry; farmers, traders and producers). Conflict and convergence of interests and ideas of the actors involved in promoting FNS and inter-sectoriality can be identified. Municipal governments, particularly in metropolitan areas, face challenges in purchasing from local family farmers as they consider their capacity to supply the market, and the difficulties faced by small producers in dealing with technical procedures or other issues such as delivery arrangements, budgets, the purchasing process, and also the political resistance of the former suppliers of the school meal programme. Impacts on the preparation of the school meal (time spent, ability to prepare fresh food) and economic interests linked to agribusiness and the food industry should also be considered.

Note

[1]An adaptation developed by Brazilian researchers of the methodology created at Cornell University and adopted by the US Department of Agriculture (USDA). The households are classified into four categories: those with food security (assured access to regular meals of sufficient quantity and quality), mild food insecurity (poorer diet without limits on quantity), moderate food insecurity (quantitative limits on food intake without experiencing hunger) and severe food insecurity (limited access with hunger).

References

Arkes, J. (2009) How the economy affects teenage weight. *Social Science* and *Medicine* 68, 1943–1947.

Assis, A.M.O. (2006) *Avaliação do Impacto Epidemiológico e Social do Programa Nacional de Renda Mínima Vinculado a Saúde – Bolsa Família em Municípios Baianos*. Report presented to National Council for Scientific and Technological Development (CNPq), Ministério da Saúde, Brasília.

Barros, R.P. (2009) *Sucessos e Desafios para a Política Social Brasileira (Apresentação)*. Textos para Discussão n. 985, Instituto de Pesquisa Econômica Aplicada (IPEA), Brasília.

Brandão, A., Dalt, S. Da and Gouvêa, V.H. (2007) Segurança alimentar e nutricional entre os beneficiários do Programa Bolsa Família [Food and nutrition security among beneficiaries of Bolsa Família]. In: Vaitsman, J. and Paes-Sousa, R. (eds) *Avaliação de Políticas de Programas do MDS – Resultados, Volume 2 – Bolsa Família e Assistência Social [Evaluation of MDS Policies and Programmes – Results, Volume 2 – Bolsa Família and Social Assistance]*. Secretaria de Avaliação e Gestão da Informação/Ministério do Desenvolvimento Social e Combate à Fome (SAGI/MDS), Brasilia, pp. 99–115.

Burlandy, L. (2009) A construção da política de segurança alimentar e nutricional no Brasil: estratégias e desafios para a promoção da intersetorialidade no âmbito federal de governo [Construction of the food and nutrition security policy in Brazil: strategies and challenges in the promotion of intersectorality at the federal government level]. *Ciências e Saúde Coletiva* 14, 851–860.

CAISAN (2009) *Subsídio para Balanço das Ações Governamentais de Segurança Alimentar e Nutricional e da Implantação do Sistema Nacional*. Câmara Interministerial de Segurança Alimentar, Brasília.

Campbell, U. (2007) *Aumenta o Consumo de Frutas e Hortaliças na Merenda das Escolas Publicas*. Correio Brasiliense, Brasília.

CEDEPLAR (2006) *Avaliação de Impacto do Programa Bolsa Família em Brasileira* [Impact evaluation of Bolsa Família Program in Brazil]. Centro de Desenvolvimento e Planejamento Regional de Minas Gerais/Universidade Federal de Minas Gerais (UFMG), Belo Horizonte, Brazil.

Chopra, M., Galbraith, S. and Darnton-Hill, I. (2002) A global response to a global problem: the epidemic of overnutrition. *Bulletin of the World Health Organization* 80, 952–958.

Claro, R.M, Carmo, H.C.E, Machado, F.M.S. and Monteiro, C.A. (2007) Renda, preço dos alimentos e participação de frutas e hortaliças na dieta. *Revista de Saúde Pública* 41, 557–564.

CONSEA (2004) *II Conferência Nacional de Segurança Alimentar e Nutricional. Relatório Final*. Conselho Nacional de Segurança Alimentar e Nutricional, Brasília.

CONSEA (2006) *Documento Final do Encontro Nacional de Segurança Alimentar e Nutricional*. Conselho Nacional de Segurança Alimentar e Nutricional, Brasília.

CONSEA (2007) *III Conferência Nacional de Segurança Alimentar e Nutricional. Relatório Final*. Conselho Nacional de Segurança Alimentar e Nutricional, Brasília.

CONSEA (2008) *Programa de Aquisição de Alimentos da Agricultura Familiar. Cinco Anos. Balanços e Perspectivas. Documento Síntese do Seminário de Avaliação do PAA*. Conselho Nacional de Segurança Alimentar e Nutricional, Brasília.

CONSEA (2009a) *Síntese das Contribuições dos Encontros Regionais de Segurança Alimentar e Nutricional*. Conselho Nacional de Segurança Alimentar e Nutricional, Brasília.

CONSEA (2009b) *Building Up the National Policy and System for Food and Nutrition Security*. Food and Agriculture Organization of the United Nations/Instituto Interamericano de Cooperação para a agricultura (FAO/IICA), Brasília.

CONSEA (2010) *Food and Nutritional Security and the Human Right to Adequate Food in Brazil, Indicators and Monitoring, Executive Summary*. Conselho Nacional de Segurança Alimentar e Nutricional, Brasília.

Coveney, J. (2003) Why food policy is critical to public health. *Critical Public Health* 13, 99–105.

Curralero, C.B. and Santana, J.A. (2007) Programa de Aquisição de Alimentos nas regiões sul e nordeste [The food acquisition program in the south and northeast regions]. In: Vaitsman, J. and Paes-Sousa, R. (eds) *Avaliação de Políticas de Programas do MDS, Volume 1 – Segurança Alimentar e Nutricional [Evaluation of MDS Policies and Programmes, Volume 1 – Food and Nutrition Security]*. Secretaria de Avaliação e Gestão da Informação/Ministério do Desenvolvimento Social e Combate à Fome (SAGI/MDS), Brasília, pp. 49–105.

French, S., Story, M. and Jeffery, R. (2001) Environmental influences on eating and physical activity. *Annual Review of Public Health* 22, 309–335.

Harnack, L., Stang, J. and Story, M. (1999) Soft drink consumption among US children and adolescents: nutritional consequences. *Journal of the American Dietetic Association* 99, 436–441.

IBASE (2008) *Repercussões do Programa Bolsa Família na Segurança Alimentar e Nutricional das Famílias Beneficiadas.* Instituto Brasileiro de Analises Socio-Economicas, Rio de Janeiro, Brazil.

IBGE (2006) *Pesquisa Nacional por Amostra de Domicílios. PNAD Segurança Alimentar 2004.* Instituto Brasileiro de Geografia e Estatística, Rio de Janeiro, Brazil.

IBGE (2010) *Pesquisa Nacional por Amostra de Domicílios. PNAD Segurança Alimentar 2009.* Instituto Brasileiro de Geografia e Estatística, Rio de Janeiro, Brazil.

Kawani, Néri, M. and Son (2006) *Crescimento pro Pobre, o Paradoxo Brasileiro.* Fundação Getulio Vargas (FGV) Rio de Janeiro, Brazil.

Levy-Costa, R. (2005) Disponibilidade domiciliar de alimentos no Brazil: distribuição e evolução (1974–2003). *Revista de Saúde Pública* 39, 530–540.

Lima, A.L.L., Silva, A.C.F., Konno, S.C., Conde, W.L., Aquino, M.H.B. and Monteiro, C.A. (2010) Causas do declínio acelerado da desnutrição infantil no Nordeste do Brasil (1986–1996–2006). *Revista de Saúde Pública* 44, 17–27.

Ludwig, D.S., Peterson, K.E and Gortmaker, S.L. (2001) Relation between consumption of sugar-sweetened drinks and childhood obesity: a prospective, observational analysis. *The Lancet* 357, 505–508.

Maluf, R. (2007) *Segurança Alimentar e Nutricional.* Editora Vozes, Rio de Janeiro, Brazil.

Maluf, R. and Burlandy, L. (2007) *Poverty Inequality and Social Policies in Brazil.* Working Paper No. 1, Centro de Referência em Segurança Alimentar e Nutricional (CERESAN), CPDA/UFRRJ/UFF/IBASE, Rio de Janeiro, Brazil.

MDA (2003) *Lei 10696 de 2 de Julho de 2003. Institui o Programa de Aquisição de Alimentos. Diario Oficial da Uniao,* 2 Jul. Ministério do Desenvolvimento Agrário, Brasília.

MDA (2008) *Decreto 6447 de 7 de Maio de 2008. Regulamenta o Artigo 19 da Lei 10696 que Institui o Programa de Aquisição de Alimentos. Diário Oficial,* 07 Mai. Ministério do Desenvolvimento Agrário, Brasília.

MDS (2003) *Medida Provisória n° 132, de 20 de Outubro 2003. Cria o Programa Bolsa Família e dá Outras Providências. Diário Oficial da União,* 20 out. Ministério do Desenvolvimento Social e Combate à Fome, Brasília.

MDS (2010) *Balanço de Avaliação da Execução do Programa de Aquisição de Alimentos – PAA 2003 a 2010.* Ministério do Desenvolvimento Social e Combate à Fome, Brasília.

MEC (2006) *Fundo Nacional de Desenvolvimento da Educação. Resolução CD No 32, de 10 de Agosto de 2006. Estabelece as Normas para a Execução do Programa Nacional de Alimentação Escolar. Diário Oficial da União.* Ministério da Educacão, Brasília.

MEC (2009) *Lei n° 11.947, de 16 de Junho de 2009 Dispõe sobre o Atendimento da Alimentação Escolar e do Programa Dinheiro Direto na Escola aos Alunos da Educação Básica.* Ministério da Educacão, Brasília.

MEC/MS (2006) *Portaria Interministerial MS/MEC 1010 de 08/05/2006 que Regulamenta as Ações de Promoção da Alimentação Saudável nas Escolas. Diário Oficial,* 08 Mai. Ministério da Educacão e Ministério da Saúde, Brasília.

MS (2005a) *Sistema das Nações Unidas. 32ªSessão – Comitê Permanente de Nutrição. Estudo de Caso Brasileiro.* Ministério da Saúde, Brasília.

MS (2005b) *Série C. Projetos, Programas e Relatórios. Departamento de Atenção Básica. Coordenação geral da Política de Alimentação e Nutrição. Avaliação do Programa Bolsa-alimentação.* Segunda Fase. Secretaria de Atenção à Saúde, Ministério da Saúde, Brasília.

MS (2009) *Pesquisa Nacional de Demografia e Saúde da Criança e da Mulher – PNDS 2006: Dimensões do Processo Reprodutivo e da Saúde da Criança.* Ministério da Saúde, Brasilia.

Monteiro, C.A., Conde, W. and Konno, S. (2006) *Análise do Inquérito Chamada Nutricional 2005.* Faculdade de Saúde Pública, Universidade de São Paulo (FSP/USP), São Paulo, Brazil.

Morris, S.S., Olinto, P., Flores, R., Nilson, E.A.F. and Figueiredo, A.C. (2004) Conditional cash transfers are associated with a small reduction in the rate of weight gain of preschool children in northeast Brazil. *Journal of Nutrition* 34, 2336–2341.

Néri, M.C. (ed.) (2006) *Miséria, Desigualdade e Estabilidade: O Segundo Real.* Fundação Getulio Vargas (FGV), Rio de Janeiro, Brazil.

Nestle, M. (2003) *Food Politics: How the Food Industry Influences Nutrition and Health.* University of California Press, Berkeley and Los Angeles, California.

Presidency of the Federative Republic of Brazil (2006) *Lei 11.346, de 15 de Setembro de 2006, que Cria o Sistema Nacional de Segurança Alimentar e Nutricional.* Presidente da República Federativa do Brasil, Brasília.

Saboia, A.L. (2008) *Síntese de Indicadores Sociais: Uma Análise das Condições de Vida da População Brasileira (Apresentação).* Instituto Brasileiro de Geografia e Estatística Pesquisa Nacional por Amostra de Domicílios (IBGE-PNAD), Brasília.

Schmitt, C.J. and Guimarães, L.A. (2008) O mercado institucional como instrumento para o fortalecimento da agriculta familiar de base agroecológica. *Revista Agriculturas: Experiências em Agroecologia* 5(2), 7–13.

Schutter, O.D. (2009) *Report of the Special Rapporteur on the Right to Food*. United Nations Mission to Brazil, Geneva, Switzerland.

Segall-Corrêa, A.M. and Marin-León, L. (2008) *Cai a Insegurança Alimentar no Brasil – Dados da PNAD 2004 e PNDS 2006*. Universidade Estadual de Campinas (UNICAMP), Campinas, Brazil.

Segall-Correa, A.M., Marin-Leon, L., Helito, H., Perez-Escamilla, R., Santos, L.M.P. and Paes-Souza, R. (2008) Transferência de renda e segurança alimentar no Brasil: análise dos dados nacionais. *Revista de Nutrição (Campinas)* 21(Suplemento), 39–51.

Silva, M.C.M., Assis, A.M.O., Santana, S.M.C.P., Santos, N.S. and Brito, E. (2007) Programa Bolsa Família e segurança alimentar das famílias beneficiárias: resultados para o Brasil e regiões [Bolsa Família programme and food security of beneficiary families: Results in Brazil and regions]. In: Vaitsman, J. and Paes-Sousa, R. (eds) *Avaliação de Políticas de Programas do MDS – Resultados, Volume 2 – Bolsa Família e Assistência Social [Evaluation of MDS Policies and Programmes – Results, Volume 2 – Bolsa Família and Social Assistance]*. Secretaria de Avaliação e Gestão da Informação/Ministério do Desenvolvimento Social e Combate à Fome (SAGI/MDS), Brasilia, pp. 67–96.

Sparovek, G. (2007) *Estudo Comparado sobre a Efetividade das Diferentes Modalidades do Programa de Aquisição de Alimentos no Nordeste [Comparative study on the effectiveness of the different modes of the food acquisition program (PAA) in the Northeast]*. In: Vaitsman, J. and Paes-Sousa, R. (eds) *Avaliação de Políticas de Programas do MDS, Volume 1 – Segurança Alimentar e Nutricional [Evaluation of MDS Policies and Programmes, Volume 1 – Food and Nutrition Security]*. Secretaria de Avaliação e Gestão da Informação/Ministério do Desenvolvimento Social e Combate à Fome (SAGI/MDS), Brasília, pp. 15–48.

WHO/FAO (2003) *Diet, Nutrition and the Prevention of Chronic Diseases. Report of the Joint WHO/FAO Expert Consultation*. WHO Expert Consultation Technical Report Series No. 916, World Health Organization, Geneva, Switzerland with Food and Agriculture Organization of the United Nations, Rome.

WHO (2004) *Global Strategy on Diet, Physical Activity and Health*. World Health Organization, Geneva, Switzerland.

WHO (2006) *Child Growth Standards. Length/height-for-age, Weight-for-age/weight-for-length, Weight-for-height and Body Mass Index-for-age: Methods and Development*. World Health Organization, Geneva, Switzerland.

10 The Gender Informed Nutrition and Agriculture (GINA) Alliance and the Nutrition Collaborative Research Support Program (NCRSP)

Cheryl Jackson Lewis*

US Agency for International Development, Washington, DC, USA

Summary

The US Agency for International Development's (USAID) Gender Informed Nutrition and Agriculture (GINA) Alliance, piloted in Uganda, Mozambique and Nigeria, has proven effective in reducing hunger and poverty. The programme employed a gender-focused, community-based approach to improving household food and nutrition security in sub-Saharan African communities, with a particular emphasis on the nutritional status of children under 5 years. Overall, the GINA programmes in the three countries were able to reduce inadequate weight-for-age of 3000 children under 5 years during the period from the programme baseline to follow-up evaluation. Additionally, GINA resulted in increased availability of nutritious foods in participating households; increased awareness and understanding of the basic causes of malnutrition; increased food production, leading to greater consumption of nutritious foods and increases in income; a link between markets and GINA farmer groups; and the development of gender-diverse farmer groups complete with a well-functioning organizational structure. GINA's focus on gender roles led to an upgrading in the status of women and recognition of them as producers and processors of food. As a result, women's control over their assets, as well as the size of their assets, increased. As a result of the successful pilot, USAID is now scaling up the GINA model through a new US$15 million Nutrition Collaborative Research Support Program (Nutrition CRSP) and Nutrition Innovation Laboratory. This research is specifically designed to build the evidence base to demonstrate how agricultural interventions implemented and co-located with health activities may lead to improvements in the nutritional status of women and children at scale.

Description of the GINA Programme

The Gender Informed Nutrition and Agriculture Alliance (GINA) piloted in Uganda, Mozambique and Nigeria has proven effective in reducing hunger and poverty. GINA's success has largely been based on recognizing that women are central to improving household food and nutrition security in sub-Saharan African communities. Women in this region are the households' main caretakers in food production, preparation and consumption. It has been demonstrated that when women have access to and control of increased household resources, they utilize these resources to improve the well-being of their families,

---

*Contact: cheryl.lewis@fns.usda.gov

especially their children. GINA teams in Mozambique, Uganda and Nigeria partnered with women producer associations to improve food and nutrition security for the most vulnerable, particularly children under 5 years of age. GINA promoted improved agriculture and nutrition practices, increased agricultural productivity and addressed traditional gender inequities detrimental to maternal and child nutrition.

The GINA programme combined five important elements:

- The introduction of nutritious crops and animal food sources that provide protein, essential micronutrients and other nutrients to complement basic staples.
- Technical support to farmer groups to increase yields through better planting, harvesting, storage and processing technologies.
- Nutrition education to ensure that a better and more diversified food supply translated into adequate diets, especially for infants and young children.
- Women's empowerment with knowledge and skills to improve their capacity to care for their children while at the same time increasing their access to resources, incomes and decision-making roles in their households and communities.
- The promotion of the nutrition dimension in development, poverty and food security plans, policies and budgets through reporting on decision making at multiple levels.

While GINA's predecessor, The Agriculture and Nutrition Advantage (TANA) programme, developed capacity and advocacy for nutrition and food security initiatives at the national level, GINA focused on community-level interventions. Each country team identified the underlying causes of malnutrition in the GINA communities selected to clarify the relationship between the problem and the proposed interventions. In all three countries, the causes of malnutrition were a combination of agricultural, nutritional, gender, political and cultural factors. Consequently, GINA teams developed linked agriculture and nutrition interventions with

a focus on gender to combat the high levels of malnutrition. Each country team developed its own strategy, plan of action and partnerships, depending on the particular underlying causes of malnutrition.

The GINA conceptual framework also helped each country team to define its plan of action. The conceptual framework incorporated actions and structures at the household and institutional levels. The framework illustrated how nutritional outcomes are determined by household resources, how these resources are utilized, and how broader institutions, which typically operate with no or very little participation from households, have an impact on food security at the household level. The action plans developed by GINA country teams directly responded to gaps in the nutrition–agriculture pathway featured in the conceptual framework. Ultimately, each of the country teams, utilizing their respective action plans, was responsible for contributing to the project goal of reducing malnutrition.

The GINA programme was implemented in Uganda for 24 months and in Mozambique and Nigeria for 18 months with funding from the USAID/Washington (US Agency for International Development at Washington – USAID/W) Bureau for Economic Growth, Agriculture and Trade (EGAT) and the USAID Africa Bureau's Initiative to End Hunger in Africa (IEHA). USAID/W's resources were complemented by resources from USAID/Nigeria and World Vision in Mozambique.

Programme Objectives

Each country had specific objectives. The objectives for Mozambique included: (i) to improve the availability of nutrient-rich crops; and (ii) to implement community-based nutrition activities in targeted localities. Uganda had three objectives: (i) to incorporate and operationalize nutrition into the multi-sectoral poverty alleviation programmes, in particular the Plan for Modernization of Agriculture (PMA) and the Poverty Eradication Action Plan (PEAP); (ii) to enhance awareness, knowledge, skills and practices among service providers and farmer groups about the importance of nutrition in social/economic development at the district and sub-county level; and (iii) to promote integrated nutrition and agricultural practices at the community level that are informed by gender analysis. Nigeria's (three) objectives were: (i) to implement priority nutrition and agriculture activities using a ranking system developed with the community Project Implementation Committee (PIC/Community-based Monitoring and Evaluation Committee (CBMEC)); (ii) to develop appropriate linkages between GINA and existing donor, civil society and local government-supported activities in project operational areas; and (iii) to implement activities that best complement integrated community-based projects.

Programme Evaluation

At the conclusion of the GINA programme, an evaluation was conducted to:

- assess the extent to which project interventions under GINA had been responsible for reducing malnutrition and hunger, as measured by weight-for-age of children under 5 years;
- extract and consolidate lessons learned from GINA activities implemented in the three project countries; and
- provide recommendations for expanding the approaches and interventions that had been used beyond sub-Saharan Africa towards a global mechanism for reducing malnutrition.

The evaluation team conducted site visits to all GINA communities in Mozambique, Uganda and Nigeria, where they observed project agricultural, health and nutrition activities. The team also conducted key informant interviews with officials from the ministries of health, representatives from various NGOs (non-governmental organizations) and USAID mission and programme staff. Further, the team interviewed clinical personnel, programme promoters/coordinators and GINA participants (individually and via community and focus groups).

In addition, they reviewed various USAID documents, and recent research on food security and development in Africa.

The evaluation also relied on secondary data. All weight-for-age results cited by the evaluation report were based on data collected and reported by GINA teams in the three countries. The evaluation team was able to verify that the volunteers who weighed the children had been trained by nutrition experts, and were regularly supervised by technically qualified field coordinators who were themselves provided regular technical support. District technical and monitoring and evaluation personnel tabulated results from the individual growth monitoring sessions. The team observed weighing and charting techniques of a sample of GINA volunteer growth promoters in Mozambique and Uganda, and found them to be competent. The qualitative evaluation data were analysed using content analysis techniques, and univariate analyses were conducted on the quantitative data. The data and findings for each country were integrated into country-specific case studies.

Findings

The programme evaluation was composed of nine questions that broadly addressed GINA's effectiveness in reducing inadequate weight-for-age among children under 5 years old, empowering women, responding to the needs of HIV-affected households with children under 5 years, and supporting other USAID efforts to combat hunger and malnutrition.

How effective was GINA in reducing inadequate weight-for-age in children under 5 years?

The first question asked in the evaluation was to what extent had linked agriculture and nutrition interventions been effective in contributing to the achievement of GINA's primary objective: reducing inadequate weight-for-age of children under 5 years?

A comparison of data from national and regional demographic and health surveys in all three countries with GINA baseline data indicated that the proportion of underweight children in the GINA communities was much higher than that in the national and regional rates of underweight children in the host countries (Table 10.1). Overall, GINA programmes reduced the percentage of inadequate weight-for-age children under 5 years in all three countries between 2006 and 2007 (Table 10.2). However, in Nigeria, this reduction was only modest.

A number of conclusions related to agriculture, income and prevalence of malnutrition, as well as to nutritional knowledge and behaviour, were reached for each country. They included the following:

1. Rates of malnutrition were reduced.
2. The availability of nutritious foods increased in participating households. Based on the premise that having enough food is not sufficient to improve undernutrition, GINA helped participants learn that adequate health and good nutritional practices, as well as increased and diversified food supplies, are needed to combat malnutrition.

3. Participating farmers gained a better understanding of the basic causes of malnutrition. Participants were able to prepare more balanced and nutritious meals. In addition, they were able to plant a variety of crops in rotation to ensure food availability and the maintenance of soil nutrients.
4. Women's knowledge about infant and young child feeding (IYCF) increased. They became more aware of the need for exclusive breastfeeding for the first 6 months. Awareness was raised through several channels that included regular growth monitoring and promotion (GMP) at the community level, frequent production group education sessions, food demonstrations, mother-to-mother support and, in Uganda, weekly radio broadcasts.
5. Links were established among health services and the promotion of key child health interventions and education: hygiene, immunization, bed nets, etc. Sanitation and safety measures improved at the personal, household and community levels. This reduced the incidence of diarrhoea, malaria and associated morbidity.
6. Women's knowledge about nutritious foods and the causes of malnutrition

Table 10.1. Proportion of children under 5 years old who are underweight for their age[a] in GINA target countries.

Country	National average (DHS)[a]	Regional average (DHS)	GINA communities (baseline)
Mozambique	23.8% (2003)	26.8%	52%
Nigeria	28.7% (2003)	23.6%	24%
Uganda	15.9% (2006)	19.3%	21.2%

[a]Demographic and Health Survey (DHS) definitions: 'An underweight child has a weight-for-age Z-score that is < −2 sd based on the NCHS/CDC/WHO international reference population. This condition can result from either chronic or acute malnutrition or a combination of both' (NCHS, National Center for Health Statistics; CDC, US Centers for Disease Control and Prevention; WHO, World Health Organization).

Table 10.2. Underweight trends among GINA-registered children[a] in GINA target areas.

Mozambique		Nigeria		Uganda	
Baseline	Follow-up (06/2007)	Baseline (11–12/2006)	Follow-up (07–08 /2007)	Baseline (06–07/2006)	Follow-up (06/2007)
52.0%	9.0%	24.6%	22.9%	21.2%	10.2%

[a]Children <59 months old with a weight-for-age score below −2 sd based on the NCHS/CDC/WHO international reference population (NCHS, National Center for Health Statistics; CDC, US Centers for Disease Control and Prevention; WHO, World Health Organization).

increased. They learned skills for preventing or reversing malnutrition; they also strengthened their capacity to care for their children and access technical resources to improve food production and/or food processing. The status of women in their households and communities increased as they improved the nutritional status of their children.

7. Increases in income were controlled either by the women themselves or through joint decision making with their husbands.

8. GINA groups established links to markets. The groups established market links with local traders, sold produce to local hotels, supplied 'home-grown' school feeding programmes and made direct sales in local markets.

9. GINA community production groups became functioning entities with offices and bank accounts. These groups were ready and eager to serve as community platforms for disseminating additional agriculture and nutrition inputs and were eager to continuously enhance the health and nutrition knowledge of group members.

10. Both men and women farmers were included in GINA production groups. The reported benefits of the inclusion of both genders were: increased participation of women in household decision making, women enhancing their status by serving as group leaders and GMP volunteers, the greater involvement of women in community dialogue, and their better understanding (along with men) of the causes of malnutrition and how to prevent it.

The above results were dependent on several factors:

- The first was that men and women in food-insecure communities were willing and able to form production groups, and to devote time to meetings, training sessions and additional fieldwork to benefit their children and households.
- The second was that field staff were well trained and supervised and received consistent technical guidance from nutrition and agriculture experts. The support of well-trained health workers and social promoters was essential for effective

dialogue with mothers and caretakers, and for increased community engagement. As a result, health and social promoters were more easily able to promote better nutritional practices, reinforcing the proper utilization of food on a regular basis.

- The third was that dynamic volunteers from communities were trained to be catalysts for local agriculture and nutrition development activities, especially GMP.
- The fourth was that partner leaders were put in place who understood the GINA concept and guided project resources and activities to ensure nutrition outcomes.
- The last was that local government partners were involved. Through meetings and trainings, previously isolated government employees learned to assist communities and use their limited resources to achieve local food and nutrition security practices.

Did GINA's team meet the stated objectives in their action plans or proposals?

The evaluation team found that, except for some project areas in Nigeria, programme activities were implemented as planned. Training records were reviewed and trained staff and volunteers were interviewed, and, in all cases, the evaluation team concluded that the quality of training had been satisfactory or better than satisfactory. In all but a few instances, GINA country teams met or exceeded their life of project (LOP) targets (Table 10.3).

What role, if any, has attention to gender played in achieving GINA's results?

GINA's participants, implementers and the evaluation team all agree that gender considerations played a critical role in generating community interest and support for the project. This interest and support resulted in significant reductions in malnutrition, improvement in the general health status of children, increased production of nutritious crops and improved capacity of communities to implement community-based food security programmes.

Table 10.3. GINA performance indicators: target versus actual over life of project (LOP).

Indicator	Mozambique (target/actual)	Uganda (target/actual)	Nigeria (target/actual)
No. agriculture-related firms benefiting directly from training	2/3	40/21	9/9
No. partner organizations and institutional members of those organizations	4/4	50/15	42/42
No. producer organizations, water associations, trade, business and community organizations assisted	42/42	30/60	18/18
Female attendance in training	412/469	150/2471	57/50
Male attendance in training	412/453	150/353	81/73
No. public–private partnerships formed	2/2	15/15	10/4
No. technologies made available for transfer	12/12	4/6	11/11
No. women's associations assisted	42/42	50/60	9/9

To what extent do GINA's activities complement other USAID efforts to reduce childhood malnutrition in the three countries?

No one activity can sufficiently respond to the multiple complex dimensions of hunger and malnutrition. USAID has initiated several efforts to reduce malnutrition under the Presidential Initiative to End Hunger in Africa (IHEA). These efforts are designed to integrate vulnerable communities into sustainable development processes by increasing productive assets and breaking the cycle of poverty. Examples of USAID health activities aimed at reducing childhood malnutrition in Mozambique, Uganda and Nigeria include: (i) the Expanded Program of Immunization (EPI); (ii) micronutrient supplementation; (iii) nutrition; (iv) control of malaria; (v) control of diarrhoea; (vi) family planning; (vii) prevention of HIV/AIDS; and (viii) epidemic response to cholera and meningitis. The focus areas of these programmes were included in the GINA model for the three countries.

Based on the qualitative assessment of GINA, it appears that community-based interventions had a greater impact on the reduction of childhood malnutrition than institutional- or facility-based interventions. In particular, educational messages had a strong impact on the improvement of nutritional practices by GINA participants. Nutritional messages were targeted towards both men and women, making it possible for

households to reach consensus on the adoption of good nutritional practices. In addition, the focus on the development of the asset base of GINA participants (especially women) made it possible for the majority of programme participants to have the resources needed for better nutritional practices.

Further, analyses showed that community-based programming approaches were effective in a variety of settings, including rural, peri-urban and small settings as well as in moderately dense communities. This held true even with varying degrees of inadequate resources, limited manpower and cultural practices detrimental to child and maternal nutrition and well-being. Overall, the success of these interventions had a positive impact on the community and, as such, helped to address malnutrition.

Given the level of resources provided under GINA, what was the magnitude of impact?

In Mozambique, the programme benefited from World Vision's Development Assistance Programme and shared resources. It also benefited from World Vision's institutional capacity for managing similar projects. In Uganda, GINA profited immensely from Makerere University's Department of Food Science and Technology [now the Department of Food Technology and Human Nutrition] institutional memory and liaison with government ministries and departments. In Nigeria,

GINA benefited from the strong nutrition expertise at the implementing NGO and from collaboration with the COMPASS (Community Participation for Action in the Social Sector: a USAID/Nigerian government partnered project) and BASICS (Basic Support for Institutionalizing Child Survival): also a USAID partnered project) projects. These two projects, through a partnership with the implementing NGO, conducted some of the nutrition activities in Kano and Akwa Ibom.

Project costs for GINA consisted of direct costs for purchasing materials, salary payments and other direct expenses incurred while implementing programme activities, as well as indirect costs, or costs that the programme beneficiaries had to pay, mostly in terms of labour and time. Successful programmes were able to cover all of the indirect costs (while also attracting more participants), a substantial amount of the direct costs and some recurrent costs. Given the positive impact of the programme on reducing underweight among children under 5 years and the high level of commitment among programme participants, GINA had significant impact and should be scaled up in order to achieve a broader impact.

Overall, the GINA project demonstrated that relatively modest amounts of money supporting linked nutrition, health and agriculture interventions can have significant benefits for the poor. It also showed that the programme could relatively easily be scaled up, expanded and/or replicated in other localities within the project countries. At the community level, the model was implemented in ways that were locally appropriate and were shaped by the operational context. As a result, the time frames, inputs, outputs and impacts of the model varied across the three countries. Table 10.4 presents some aspects of this variation.

How effective was the project in supporting the objectives of IEHA in the IEHA countries?

GINA reduced malnutrition for children under 5 years, improved household health practices, increased the production, processing and marketing of nutrient-rich crops, and improved local capacity to manage community-based nutrition and agriculture interventions that combat malnutrition. In an effort to reduce malnutrition, GINA created a demand for nutritious foods, provided nutrition and health training, and enhanced the supply of nutritious crops in project communities. Gender relations were significantly improved, with increased cooperation between men and women within households. The division of labour according to gender became less rigid and community members, particularly women, improved their status and asset base. These achievements complemented and contributed to IEHA goals and objectives.

How effective was the project in informing CAADP of NEPAD on food and nutrition security options?

Member countries of NEPAD (New Partnership for Africa's Development) pursue the following objectives under CAADP (Comprehensive Africa Agriculture Development Programme): extending the area under sustainable land management and reliable water control; improving rural infrastructure and trade-related capacities for market access; increasing food supply; reducing hunger and improving responses to food emergency crises; and improving agricultural research and technology dissemination and adoption. Efforts to move the CAADP process beyond the political commitment and framework stage to implementation are at various stages in the member countries. These activities are primarily taking place at the national level and member countries must ensure that they translate into tangible benefits for all communities. The GINA project has played an essential role in demonstrating that relatively modest amounts of money that support combined nutrition, health and agriculture interventions can provide significant benefits to the poor. GINA is closely linked to Pillar III of CAADP, in that they both promote community-based approaches to food security.

The GINA project has provided many evidence-based success stories at the village level that may prove instructive to CAADP. GINA has been involved on both

Table 10.4. A comparison of GINA models in Mozambique, Uganda and Nigeria.

	Mozambique	Nigeria	Uganda
Time frame	Mar 2006–Aug 2007 (18 months)	Jan 2006–Jun 2007 (18 months)	Oct 2005–Sep 2007 (24 months)
Impact on weight/ age of children <5 (reduction in underweight among children admitted at baseline)	82%	7.5%	52%
Number of female farmers:			
Trained	469	50	2471
Adopted new technology	369	20	1725
Number of male farmers:			
Trained	453	73	353
Adopted new technology	453	100	1014
Number of field staff employed	District coordinator; agricultural extensionist (1) and auxiliaries (2); nurse/nutrition specialist (1); nutrition field assistants (2)	LGA[a] Project Officers (3); plus personnel provided by COMPASS[b] and BASICS[c]	District coordinators (3); agricultural extensionists (3); health assistants (3)
Volunteers	Growth monitors and Mothers' Group members	Growth monitors	Growth promoters
Major implementing organization	World Vision-Mozambique	Food Basket Foundation International	Department of Food Science and Technology, Makerere University[d]
Other partners	Institute of Agriculture Research Mozambique (AM), MOH,[e] District Government	BASICS, COMPASS, LGAs	District and Sub-county Government, MOH, NAADS[f]

[a]LGA Local Government Area; [b]COMPASS, Community Participation for Action in the Social Sector; [c]BASICS, Basic Support for Institutionalizing Child Survival; [d]now the Department of Food Technology and Human Nutrition; [e]MOH, Ministry of Health; [f]AADS National Agricultural Advisory Services.

the agriculture products supply side (growing nutrient-rich food crops) and demand side (consumption of the food). In addition, the project has conducted market access and linkage activities. GINA's country experiences and lessons learned are an invaluable resource to CAADP that can be utilized as CAADP moves forward. GINA informed national governments and CAADP through USAID project reporting structures and country management partners. Information was also relayed directly to national governments that are informing CAADP as it develops its Country Pacts.

How did the project contribute to the strategic direction for the implementation of the CAADP Pillar 3: 'Increasing food supply'?

GINA contributed to the implementation of CAADP Pillar 3 through improving food security (expansion of crop areas, improved crop output and crop marketing), nutrition and health interventions, enhancing capacity building and effectively disseminating targeted messages to vulnerable households.

Conclusions

Lessons learned

GINA had the explicit objective of addressing or preventing malnutrition. To achieve this objective, the programme focused on women because of their unique role as primary caregivers and producers, and processors of food at the household level. This gender focus distinguished GINA from many community-based development programmes or other poverty reduction efforts by ensuring that women took leadership roles. The programme also supported women by providing them with the resources they needed to effectively conduct their multifaceted role within the household. Male participation was also actively sought because of men's roles both in the allocation of household resources and the re-examination of cultural beliefs and customs detrimental to children's and mother's nutrition and health. The programme interventions were specifically targeted at the households of malnourished children under 5 years as measured by weight-for-age. Because past experience had shown that it was not enough to assume that nutrition improvement will arise from enhanced agricultural productivity and/or incomes, nutritional education messages with the goal of promoting better nutritional practices were a central part of the programme's activities. Concomitantly, a strong gender focus for interventions is a strong predictor for success. As such, in addition to specific nutrition interventions, women's roles in both household livelihoods and community organizations need to be considered in designing food security programmes. Hence, care should be taken to ensure that women continue to be involved participants and beneficiaries in programmes designed to enhance livelihoods and community capacities.

The GINA programme was based on a multi-sectoral programme design. It combined multiple interventions from a number of sectors (agriculture, marketing, nutrition education, hygiene and health care) to address undernutrition. GINA interventions were linked to ongoing activities in other sectors to ensure integration at both the national and district levels where planning and coordination with other partners, such as the Ministry of Health (MOH), was critical. These linkages maximized the limited programme financial and staffing resources. The GINA model also focused on promoting community involvement and ownership which, in turn, supported capacity development and sustainability efforts. GINA community groups can now act as a foundation for additional development efforts desired by the community, such as child spacing information and services and/or literacy and maths classes.

Lastly, the different project management systems in the three countries allowed for diversity in programmatic implementation. Similar diversity could be used for new projects that share GINA objectives, resources and target populations. In addition, the technical support provided to field staff from national managers and consultants was excellent. This reinforces the need to build institutional and individual management and implementation capacities appropriate to local context needs in ensuring the success of food security programmes.

Recommendations for future programme design changes

GMP by trained and supervised community volunteers is a valuable nutrition-enhancing tool and should be retained as an important element of the GINA model. The promotion of nutrition/feeding messages and/or referral for health services, as well as negotiation with mothers to take certain actions to benefit their children, are essential portions of the GINA model. The growth promoters that the evaluation team encountered were very dedicated and willing to spend entire days weighing, charting and counselling. However, in some cases, more technical expertise was required for reliable monitoring and evaluation of programme impact. The need for a more reliable monitoring and evaluation framework was deemed especially important if GINA is to be expanded to larger areas. Any such framework should include indicators (dietary, anthropometric, care, others) that are collected and tabulated by technically qualified professionals or trained para-professionals. A standardized baseline should be developed for all countries implementing GINA. This will allow for comparisons of the rate and nature of adoption of practices across countries. Individual countries could have the option to explore additional topics beyond the standardized core data set. In addition, a control group should ideally be selected early on as part of the design. Further, the evaluators recommended that the possibility of conducting a longitudinal, pre-post study on a subsample of child participants, as well as a study of the knowledge, attitudes, behaviour and practices of maternal knowledge and infant feeding practices, should be explored.

Nutrition status is an intergenerational phenomenon. Optimal nutritional status prior to pregnancy helps to ensure a healthy pregnancy and fetus. Similarly, malnutrition can start before birth and persist throughout life. Nutritional stress during adolescence and the reproductive years affects the health of women and, consequently, of the next generation. To break the cycle of the poor nutrition that passes from generation to generation, nutrition improvement programmes such as GINA must focus on women's nutritional needs. In addition, there is need to compile an inventory of the traditional beliefs and customs of various communities where GINA is operating. Qualitative research may be useful for better understanding of these beliefs and planning appropriate behaviour change strategies that can promote healthy customs and reduce harmful ones.

In all GINA programme countries, the health component was the weakest area of the programme. Positive results based on supplying nutritious food to children younger than 5 years can be reduced or reversed by poor hygiene and/or waterborne diseases. The poor quality of drinking water and lack of toilets in countries, together with poor and/or distant water sources, limited the success of the project. So measures should be taken to ensure that

the health component of future projects is adequately addressed to realize the full potential of increased consumption of nutritious food. In addition, water for agricultural purposes was a constraint in nearly every area the evaluation team visited. In Nigeria, for example, the community committees ranked water systems for dry season agriculture as an important component for achieving better food security. Although the project supported micro-irrigation technologies and increased the availability of water for households in response to community needs in Nigeria, this was not nearly enough. Based on these findings, support for the provision of water for irrigation and household use should be strengthened in future project designs.

Finally, GINA's experiences and materials should be communicated and shared. Radio programmes should be carefully assessed for impact. When positive outcomes are documented, certain generic messages and programmes should be developed centrally and shared for translation and adaptation with all GINA implementing partners for local broadcasting. There should be targeted dissemination of key findings to promote capacity strengthening. Each participating country should determine the target groups, with an aim of achieving the biggest impact in the shortest time possible. Communication messages should be conveyed in a form that is most effective to the specific target group (e.g. town hall meetings, press briefings, conferences, round table discussions, fact sheets, videos). A GINA web link should also be explored as a communication tool.

In conclusion, due to the successful pilot, USAID is now scaling up the GINA model through a new US$15 million Nutrition Collaborative Research Support Program (Nutrition CRSP, or NCRSP and Nutrition Innovation Laboratory). The Nutrition CRSP will work with missions, development partners and host countries through its Feed the Future Implementation Plan and Food Security Investment Plan to determine what kind of investments in agriculture-based strategies, health and nutrition, institutional and human capacity development and policies can be used to achieve large-scale and sustainable improvements in nutrition outcomes, numbers of households with improved dietary quality and diversity, infant and young child feeding practices, and national and community capacity to combat undernutrition. This research is specifically designed to build the evidence base to demonstrate how agricultural interventions implemented and co-located with health activities may lead to improvements in the nutritional status of women and children at scale.

Acknowledgements

This chapter is a synopsis of the GINA Evaluation Report.[1] The evaluators were M.D. Tanamly, G. Downer and D. Chikozorwe. The author would also like to acknowledge the Principal Investigators and Project Managers of GINA: Brian Hilton – World Vision, Mozambique; Isaac Akinyele – Food Basket Foundation International, Nigeria; and Joyce Kikafunda, Makerere University, Uganda.

Note

[1] Tanamly, M.D., Downer, G., and Chikodere, D. (2008) Evaluation of the Gender Informed Nutrition and Agriculture Project. University of Missouri, Columbia, Missouri.

11 Guyana's Hinterland Community-based School Feeding Program (SFP)

Suraiya J. Ismail,[1]* Edward A. Jarvis[2] and Christian Borja-Vega[3]

[1]Social Development Inc, Georgetown, Guyana; [2]Ministry of Education, Georgetown, Guyana; [3]The World Bank, Washington, DC, USA

Summary

Four of Guyana's ten administrative regions are inhabited largely by its indigenous peoples, the Amerindians, often in remote communities where poverty and food insecurity are common and access to basic services is limited. Food supplies come from subsistence agriculture, hunting, fishing and costly imports from coastal regions. The diet lacks diversity, chronic undernutrition levels are high and school attendance is poor. In 2006, the Ministry of Education established the Hinterland Community-based School Feeding Program (SFP), whose objectives include raising community participation in schools, increasing student attendance and academic performance, and improving the nutrition of primary schoolchildren. The impact evaluation of the SFP (2007–2009) covered 20 intervention schools and 44 control schools. Stunting rose by 3% in the control group but fell by 3% in the intervention group. The SFP increased attendance by 4.3%. Participation in learning activities improved in intervention schools but declined in control schools. Children in intervention schools performed better in national academic assessment tests. The SFP conferred the greatest benefit on children who had the poorest nutritional status at baseline. Parents participated fully in food production and meal delivery activities. Households benefited through increased employment and a more varied food supply. The SFP also contributed to preserving food security through a period of food price volatility, has a low cost per child relative to other programmes and has reduced dependence on imports. Outstanding challenges include increasing access to agricultural inputs and safe water, and reaching the most remote communities. Preliminary discussions indicate that communities are keen to continue the SFP, and can suggest ways to reduce the cost to the Ministry.

Introduction

School feeding activities have long been a part of many of the education policies of governments. More recently, the objectives of such programmes have focused on maximizing learning capacity through the relief of short-term hunger and improving attendance. Experiences from Chile, Peru, Jamaica and South Africa have shown that school feeding programmes can achieve improvements in attendance, dropout rates, academic achievement and nutritional status (Musgrove, 1991; Vial et al., 1991; McCoy, 1997; Grantham-McGregor et al., 1998; Jacoby et al., 1998; Simeon, 1998). Other benefits of such programmes include the relief of short-term hunger, improved classroom behaviour and better food consumption patterns. In addition to these possible benefits and objectives, school

*Contact: sjismail@yahoo.co.uk

feeding programmes are often seen as safety nets that achieve a transfer to households of the value of the meal or snack provided (Bundy *et al.*, 2009).

Guyana and its Hinterland Regions

Guyana is located on the north-eastern coast of South America, bordering the Atlantic Ocean, Brazil, Venezuela and Suriname. It covers an area of 215 000 km², and in 2008 its population was estimated as little over 761,000 (Bureau of Statistics, 2008); it is the only English-speaking country in South America. Although Guyana is part of mainland South America, it is culturally closer to the Caribbean, with an ethnically mixed population of approximately 43.5% East Indian, 30.2% Afro-Caribbean, 9.2% Amerindian (Guyana's indigenous peoples) and 17.5% mixed and other ethnicities. Guyana is rich in

natural resources, but it is the second poorest country in the Americas. For most of the 1980s, it was one of the world's most indebted countries, but by 1994, Guyana had successfully reduced significantly its debt burden and levels of poverty (World Bank, 2006).

The country is divided into ten administrative regions (Fig. 11.1), four of which are inhabited largely by the country's indigenous peoples, many of whom live in small, remote communities. These hinterland regions (Regions 1, 7, 8 and 9) encompass nearly 68% of the country's land area but less than 10% of its population (FAO, 2009). Access to many communities is difficult and expensive, and in the rainy seasons is virtually impossible. The provision of basic services, such as agriculture, health and education to these Amerindian communities thus presents a major challenge for the Government of Guyana.

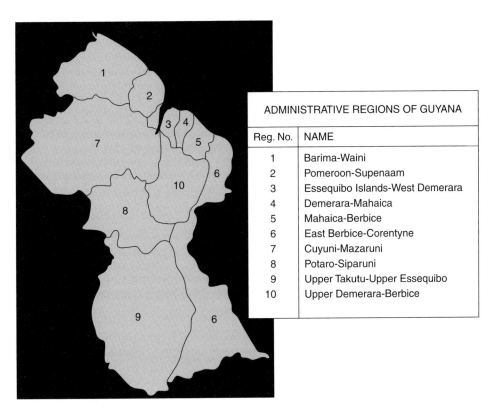

ADMINISTRATIVE REGIONS OF GUYANA	
Reg. No.	NAME
1	Barima-Waini
2	Pomeroon-Supenaam
3	Essequibo Islands-West Demerara
4	Demerara-Mahaica
5	Mahaica-Berbice
6	East Berbice-Corentyne
7	Cuyuni-Mazaruni
8	Potaro-Siparuni
9	Upper Takutu-Upper Essequibo
10	Upper Demerara-Berbice

Fig. 11.1. Map of Guyana by administrative regions. From Ministry of Health (2010).

The topography of the hinterland regions comprises tropical rainforest, savannah and mountainous and riverine areas. These regions are part of the Guiana Shield of South America, which also encompasses parts of Brazil, Suriname and Venezuela, an area of great importance for its biodiversity and its contribution to limiting climate change.

Economic activities include logging and mining for gold, diamonds and bauxite. Poverty, unemployment, underemployment, and food insecurity are common. Agriculture is constrained by the climate, pests and limited access to agricultural inputs. Food supplies come from subsistence agriculture (previously shifting, now more settled), hunting, fishing and, increasingly, from costly imports from the coastal regions and Brazil. The diet lacks diversity, especially in vegetables, fruits, legumes and dairy products. Primary nutritional problems include chronic undernutrition (stunting) and a high prevalence of anaemia, the latter related to a high prevalence of malaria. Table 11.1 highlights differences between coastal and hinterland regions in key health and nutrition indicators. The figures for stunting and wasting reflect the differences in ethnicity between coastal and hinterland populations: stunting is highest among the Amerindian children of the hinterland regions, while wasting is highest among the East Indian children of the coastal communities.

Guyana's Hinterland Community-based School Feeding Program

A previous study of school feeding programmes in Guyana provided evidence that the centralized provision of food was ineffective (Ismail and Hill, 2005). The food supply was inconsistent, delivery was sporadic and costly, and the outcomes did not bring the expected results. It is against this background that the Ministry of Education established the Hinterland Community-based School Feeding Program (SFP). An important finding of Jamaica's school feeding programme was that school feeding should be linked to improvements in the learning environment and the quality of education offered to the children (Grantham-McGregor, 1998; Simeon, 1998). In line with this finding, Guyana's Community-based SFP was developed as a component of the Education for All-Fast Track Initiative (EFA-FTI), which has the broad objective of improving access to and quality of primary education countrywide. The EFA-FTI is funded through a global catalytic trust fund and managed by the World Bank. Guyana's Community-based SFP began in 2006 and is still in progress. Its objectives include building better community participation in schools and their activities, and improving student attendance, student performance and the nutritional status of primary schoolchildren. Additionally, the SFP aims to improve community access to a more

Table 11.1. Guyana's health and nutrition indicators for the coastal and hinterland regions. From Bureau of Statistics and UNICEF (2006); Ismail and Roopnaraine (2009).

Indicator	Coastal regions	Hinterland regions
Prevalence of stunting (<5years; <−2 sd)	8.7%	22.7%
Prevalence of wasting (<5years; <−2 sd)	9.7%	3.7%
Prevalence of anaemia (<2years; haemoglobin <11g/dl)	63.5%	74.6%
Low birth weight (<2500 g)	18.6%	24.2%
Infant mortality/1000 live births	38	52
Mortality under 5 years/1000	47	68

varied diet and raise household incomes by stimulating increased and diversified local agriculture and creating employment within the programme.

The Ministry of Education, through funding from the EFA-FTI, provides one-time investment start-up funds equivalent to 2 months of the operating costs of the SFP for that school. Operating costs are calculated based on the school population at the rate of approximately US$0.875/child for each school day. Support, through the provision of advice from extension workers, is provided by the Ministry of Agriculture. Figure 11.2 shows the conceptual framework of the SFP.

All primary schools in Guyana's hinterland region (Regions 1, 7, 8 and 9) are eligible to participate in the programme. In order to participate, schools and their communities are required to submit project proposals for approval to the National School Feeding Committee, which is a multi-sectoral task force,[1] undergo a general orientation about the SFP and training in basic bookkeeping, food hygiene and the preparation of nutritious meals, using locally produced foods whenever possible. Communities must also ensure that school kitchens[2] meet the Ministry of Health guidelines for food safety and food hygiene, and trained cooks must undergo health tests and certification. Inevitably, this self-selecting

procedure means that some schools start in the programme earlier than others, and these are mostly the better organized schools and communities. Currently, 92 of the 138 primary schools in the eligible regions have started school feeding, and 14,625 children are fed each school day; those that remain are the smaller, more remote schools.

Impact Evaluation of the School Feeding Program

The impact evaluation of the SFP[3] began in 2007 with the collection of baseline data in 64 schools in Regions 1 and 7. Mid-term and final round surveys followed in 2008 and 2009. Twenty schools that began school feeding during the evaluation period formed the intervention group, and the remaining 44 schools constituted the control group. Students in Grades 2–4, 2–5 and 2–6 were included in the samples for years 2007, 2008 and 2009, respectively. This enabled the use of both longitudinal and cross-sectional samples. Where appropriate, sample selectivity was partially controlled for in the analysis.

Enumerators for the surveys were trained by staff of the Ministries of Education and Health, and of Social Development Inc. Questionnaires were administered to parents,

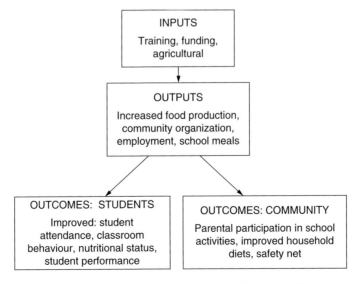

Fig. 11.2. Guyana's Hinterland School Feeding Program: a conceptual framework. From Ismail *et al.* (2010).

head teachers, class teachers and students. In addition to basic questions on the households and the schools, questionnaires also gathered information on parental participation in school activities related school feeding, and on absenteeism and reasons for absence. Children's weights and heights were measured and student attendance was obtained from class registers. Trained enumerators observed classes to record student behaviour, namely signs of active participation and of disconnect (distraction) with classroom activities. Parents responded to questions from a short food frequency questionnaire. Focus group discussions were held in each community, with parents, farmers and members of the community's school feeding committee. Academic performance was assessed by means of students' scores in national assessment tests. These are routinely administered by the Ministry of Education to all children in Grades 2, 4 and 6. Table 11.2 shows the sample sizes achieved for each survey round.

The impact evaluation addressed the following questions:

- Has the programme raised parental participation in school activities?
- Has the programme improved the diets of households?
- Has the programme provided a safety net against food price increases?
- Has the programme had a positive impact on students' school attendance and nutritional status?
- Has the programme led to improvements in students' classroom participation, behaviour and academic performance?

The answers to these questions are examined in the following two sections.

Impact of the School Feeding Program: the communities

Results from the parental questionnaires, the food frequency questionnaire and the focus group discussions highlighted a number of encouraging findings, and parents expressed overwhelming support for the programme, for a number of reasons:

- The programme provided or increased employment for some families (as cooks and as farmers) and had raised incomes.
- It improved the food supply in the community, in terms of both quality and quantity.
- The children's school attendance, academic performance and nutrition visibly improved.
- Children of the poorest families could now count on receiving at least one nutritionally balanced meal every school day.

In general, discussions revealed a high sense of ownership of the programme, and a willingness to contribute more resources if necessary. Farmers stated that even though the prices paid for their produce by the school were frequently below market prices, most continued to sell to the school because the programme benefited the community's children.

The period of the evaluation (2007 to 2009) coincided with a period of uncertainty and high volatility in the prices of food and agricultural commodities. An increase in food prices diminishes the spending capacity of households, and a daily meal to children in poor households represents a safety net mechanism from adverse price shocks.

Table 11.2. The sizes of the evaluation samples used in the impact evaluation of the Guyana School Feeding Program in 2007–2009. From Ismail *et al.* (2010).

	2007	2008	2009
Questionnaire or recording form	Grades 2–4	Grades 2–5	Grades 2–6
Class observations	105	172	170
Class teachers	112	140	162
Head teachers	64	61	58
Parents (incl. food frequency)	581	583	569
Students	2430	3006	3877

On average, before the food price shocks, a household in a control community spent US$2.40 less/month on food, compared to intervention households. During and after the food price shocks, control areas spent US$9.00 less/month on food. Thus, during and after the price increases, an estimated 510 more children in control areas were at risk of falling into poverty.

Figures 11.3 and 11.4 illustrate the impact of the SFP and of the food price shocks on the diversity of diets consumed by control and intervention households, and the frequency of consumption of key foods.[4] While improving the diets of schoolchildren was a primary aim of the SFP, it was hoped that the diets of other members of the household would also improve through greater access to a diverse food supply and through a better understanding of what constitutes a nutritionally balanced meal. At baseline, diets in the intervention communities were clearly superior in terms of diversity of commodities, reflecting

the selectivity bias of the sample of intervention schools. Owing to the rise in food prices, diet diversity and the frequency of consumption of key foods fell in both control and intervention communities. However, they fell significantly less in the intervention areas than in control areas, indicating the cushioning effect of the SFP.

Parents were also asked what kind of breakfast their child had received, if any.[5] The short-term hunger that occurs if a child receives an inadequate breakfast and/or has a long and arduous journey to school is a major contributor to poor classroom behaviour and academic achievement. Single parents were least likely to offer a full breakfast to their children. An important finding of the evaluation was that students attending intervention schools were significantly less likely to receive a full breakfast. So the question arises as to whether the parents of intervention schoolchildren are withholding a full breakfast because they know the child will receive

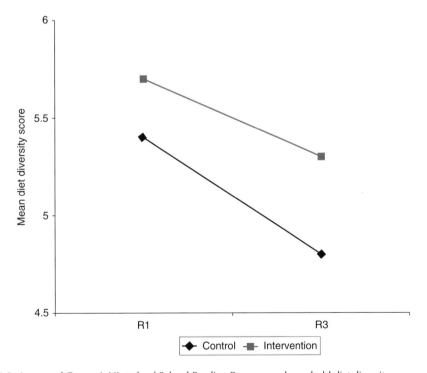

Fig. 11.3. Impact of Guyana's Hinterland School Feeding Program on household diet diversity scores (number of different foods consumed). R1, evaluation round 1 (2007, baseline); R3, evaluation round 3 (2009). From Ismail *et al.* (2010).

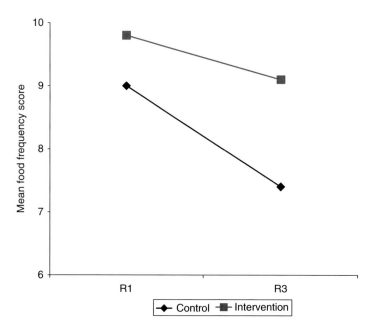

Fig. 11.4. Impact of Guyana's Hinterland School Feeding Program on household food frequency scores (weekly frequency of consumption of certain key foods). R1, evaluation round 1 (2007, baseline); R3, evaluation round 3 (2009). From Ismail et al. (2010).

a substantial lunch. If this is indeed the case, then the training offered by the SFP needs to stress the importance of an adequate breakfast, even when a full lunch is to be offered at noon.

Impact of the School Feeding Program: the students

Nutritional status, classroom behaviour, student attendance and academic performance all improved in intervention schools in comparison with control schools.

Students' classroom behaviour

Almost two thirds of head teachers and class teachers from intervention schools consistently noted that the behaviour of students changed with the SFP. These statements were corroborated by survey data. Students' participation in and disconnect from learning activities were assessed by means of direct observations at each survey round. Participation and disconnect (or distraction) scores were calculated, based on the percentage of children showing signs of active participation, such as volunteering responses, or of distraction, such as engaging in non-relevant or inappropriate activities. The results showed that participation fell sharply in control schools but improved in intervention schools over the period 2007 to 2009: mean participation scores rose from 21.1 to 22.3 in intervention schools and fell significantly from 22.5 to 19.0 in control schools. Conversely, distraction from classroom activities showed a significant reduction in intervention schools, from 6.8 to 2.1, and no significant change in control schools (from 5.3 to 4.7).

Nutritional status

It is well accepted that poor linear growth (stunting) can be the result of a number of factors, largely related to the environment, socioeconomic factors and education. Nutrition, infections and mother–infant interactions have been cited as environmental factors with the greatest influence on child growth (Waterlow, 1994). Other authors (Martorell *et al.*, 1988) have highlighted the link between stature and poverty. In the context of nutrition, poor stature is associated with diets of poor quality, i.e. diets deficient or marginal in micronutrients or protein rather than in energy. Specific micronutrients mentioned in various studies include zinc, calcium and vitamin A, but there may be others that have not yet been studied. While breastfeeding practices and mother–infant interactions are generally excellent in Amerindian communities in Guyana, diets are often monotonous and low in vegetables, dairy products, legumes and fruits[6] and infections are widespread. A study conducted in Regions 8 and 9 compared the stature of children of two tribes: the Wapishana in Region 9 and the Patamona in Region 8 (Dangour, 2001). The Wapishana villagers were substantially wealthier and had access to a more diverse diet than the Patamona villagers, who lived in relatively remote areas. The Wapishana children were on average more than 3 cm taller than their Patamona counterparts.

The results of the impact evaluation of the SFP confirm the findings of earlier studies in the region: that there were still high levels of stunting and a low prevalence of wasting (less than 3%). Even at baseline, the prevalence of stunting (height-for-age < −2 Z-scores) was higher in control schools (20%) than in intervention schools (16%). By the third round of the evaluation (2009), the prevalence of stunting had fallen by nearly three percentage points among intervention children, and risen by more than three percentage points among the children attending control schools. The differences in the prevalence of stunting between the two groups had thus risen from four percentage points in 2007 to ten in 2009.

Growth in children is divided into three phases: infancy, childhood and puberty. By the time a child reaches primary school, the first two phases are completed. Studies on immigrant and adopted children suggest that improving the child's environment can reverse at least some of the growth deficit experienced in early childhood. Results from Guyana's SFP would seem to support this.

A point to note is that the children in the intervention group would not only have benefited from a nutritionally balanced lunch at school, but would also have received a more diverse diet at home. This additional benefit highlights the importance of a programme that is community based and enables the entire community to improve its access to a better and more varied food supply.

Student attendance

Absenteeism in the 2 weeks before the survey day was obtained from class registers, and teachers and students were asked to give reasons for their absence. There was a net increase in attendance of 4.3% in the intervention group, after controlling for sample selectivity. After illness, the main reason for absence was labour at home or on the farm: 22.4% of students were kept at home to provide labour for the family in housework, farm work or childcare. Travel to the school can be arduous and prolonged for many children, often involving either long walks or long canoe trips or both, and sometimes in bad weather when roads and paths are flooded and rivers impassable. Over 7% of children were absent in the 2 weeks before the survey date because of bad weather or difficulties with transportation. In 2009 (the final survey round), 127 children (6.6%) were absent for economic reasons (no food, no money, no uniform, no stationery). All children except one who stated that they were absent because of lack of food were from the control schools where no lunch was provided.

Academic performance

An important finding of the impact evaluation was that the greatest improvements in academic performance (using National Assessment Test Scores) were seen among children who were stunted (height-for-age < −2 Z-scores) or at risk of stunting (height-for-age < −1 Z-score) at baseline. This subgroup of children represented 58.1% of the control group and 46.2% of the intervention group.

Between 2007 and 2009, National Assessment Test Scores for English rose significantly in the intervention group – from

38.1% to 49.6%. It also improved in the control group – from 40.2% to 43.4%, although this increase was not significant; this gave a net improvement of 8.3 percentage points for the intervention group (Fig. 11.5). For maths, scores rose significantly in the intervention group – from 42.2% to 47.6%, but fell in the control group – from 48.1% to 44.1%; this gave a net increase of 9.4 percentage points for the intervention group (Fig. 11.6).

Issues Arising from the School Feeding Program

Costs

The budget of the EFA-FTI provides funding for the operating costs of the SFP at the rate of nearly US$0.875/child each school day. In addition, a one-off start-up sum, equivalent to 2 months of a school's SFP operating cost is supplied. The operating budget covers the cost of food, cooks' stipends, cooking fuel, water and cleaning materials. The start-up sum is used to help equip a school with the supplies (goods) they will need to execute their community-based school feeding proposal.

The unit cost of Guyana's SFP of US$0.875 compares favourably with the equivalent unit cost of India's Midday Meal Program of US$1.14/child for each school day. However, the unit costs of Guyana's programme are likely to fall if it was to be expanded to cover other less remote schools, as food costs for items that need to be purchased are lower in these areas. The community-based approach

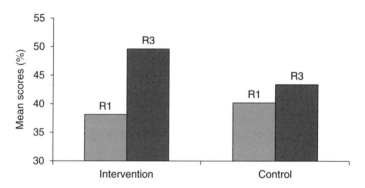

Fig. 11.5. English scores: impact of Guyana's Hinterland School Feeding Program on children stunted at the baseline. R1, evaluation round 1 (2007, baseline); R3, evaluation round 3 (2009). From Ismail *et al.* (2010).

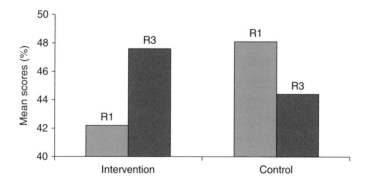

Fig. 11.6. Mathematics scores: impact of Guyana's Hinterland School Feeding Program on stunted children. R1, evaluation round 1 (2007, baseline); R3, evaluation round 3 (2009). From Ismail *et al.* (2010).

can not only bring benefits to a target population with reasonable programme costs, it can also serve as a means to achieve a financially sustainable programme that takes advantage of local agricultural markets to stimulate local economies. As such, the local purchasing of food for school feeding is seen as a force multiplier, benefiting both children and the local economy at the same time.

Addressing sustainability

External funding for the SFP will come to an end in October 2012, bringing into question its long-term sustainability, if the government of Guyana is unable to absorb the costs in their entirety. In July 2010, an in-depth consultation was held with a number of programme communities to determine in what ways and to what extent communities were willing to contribute more to the SFP so as to reduce the financial burden on the Ministry of Education. The draft results of the consultation clearly indicate the strong sense of community ownership of the SFP and recognition of its importance to schoolchildren and to the wider community, and this bodes well for its sustainability. Communities offered suggestions for activities and approaches that could assist with programme sustainability. These suggestions included:

- the creation of school gardens;
- using the school's kitchen facilities for income-generation activities, such as catering, preparation and sale of snacks;
- sale of surplus agricultural production at nearby markets, and where feasible, in the coastal regions and
- partnerships of various forms with the private sector, churches and other religious bodies and non-governmental organizations (NGOs) working in the area (private sector partnerships were considered to be especially likely in areas where mining and logging companies operated, especially those that were foreign owned).

An issue that was raised by many communities was the almost total absence of access to credit in these regions. Consultations with banks operating in Guyana may prove fruitful in helping to establish lines of credit for households and communities who would otherwise be unable to qualify for loans.

Conclusions and Outstanding Challenges

Primary challenges facing the Ministry of Education in its efforts to improve academic achievement in the hinterland regions of Guyana include:

- poor student attendance;[7]
- high levels of stunting, associated with a poor, nutritionally imbalanced diet; and
- poverty and limited access to essential resources, services and the foods needed to provide a nutritionally balanced diet.

The design of Guyana's Hinterland Community-based School Feeding Program (SFP) was such as to create a sustainable programme with a strong community base that also addresses aspects of the communities' developmental challenges, in addition to the need for improving education in Amerindian communities. As a side effect, the programme has provided employment opportunities by increasing local agricultural production and by providing jobs for a limited number of community women as cooks.

The main significant findings of the impact evaluation are as follows:

- The SFP increased average attendance by 4.3% between 2007 (the baseline) and 2009 (the round 3 evaluation) in intervention schools.
- Control schools showed consistently higher levels of stunted children in all survey rounds, perhaps partly because of their poorer economic status (selectivity). The prevalence of stunting fell significantly– by 3% – in intervention schools, but rose by the same amount in control schools.
- Children's classroom behaviour improved with the introduction of a nutritionally balanced school meal. By the round 3 evaluation (in 2009), students in intervention schools had higher

levels of class participation than those in control schools. Conversely, students' disconnect and distraction from classroom activities fell in intervention schools.

- Among children who were stunted at baseline, significant improvements were found among children attending intervention schools in National Assessment Test scores for both maths and English. Better attendance, improved student participation in classroom activities and better nutritional status, when combined with the EFA-FTI's efforts to improve schools' human and physical resources, must ultimately promote the Ministry's aim of improving academic achievement in the hinterland regions even further.
- Community participation in school feeding-related activities has been achieved: parents actively participate in cooking and serving meals, and in growing and providing food commodities.
- The programme's implementation coincided with a period of uncertainty and high volatility in the prices of food and agricultural commodities. It improved diet diversity and the frequency of food consumption in communities where school feeding was in progress, as compared with control communities, despite higher food prices. During the food price shocks the gap in food consumption frequency and diet diversity between control and intervention groups increased substantially. The programme has thus successfully provided a safety net against food price increases. Expansion could also bring a safety net mechanism to regions and communities facing economic hardship.

The evaluation findings and the experiences of the SFP raise a number of important issues and challenges that need the attention of the Ministry of Education:

- Although attendance was indeed better in intervention schools, absenteeism remains a serious concern. More than 59% of all children included in the evaluation were absent for at least 1 day in the 2 weeks before the survey day. Of these children, more than 22% gave labour of some kind as a reason for their absence – this included the care of younger siblings and work on the farm or in the home.
- A further 6.6% of truant children in the 2 weeks preceding the survey were absent because of the household's economic condition: there was no food, nor uniform, cash or stationery. Interestingly, of those who gave lack of food as the reason for absence, all children except one attended control schools where no lunch was offered.
- The short-term hunger that occurs if a child receives an inadequate breakfast and/or has a long and arduous journey to school is a major contributor to poor classroom behaviour and academic achievement. A third of all children stated that they had received an inadequate breakfast or no breakfast at all. This raises the issue of providing a snack at the start of a school day. It also highlights the need for basic education of parents on the importance of breakfast (even when the child can expect a nutritious lunch), as well as on nutrition in general.
- On the whole, Guyana's SFP is a remarkably comprehensive programme, encompassing aspects of community development, increasing employment and improving food security. One outstanding omission is nutrition education for students. An activity that brings together nutrition education with the establishment of school gardens would contribute substantially to ensuring that benefits endure beyond the years of schooling.
- Programme monitoring, as well as discussions with communities, revealed that some communities at least would benefit from greater support from the Ministry of Agriculture's extension workers and from a better supply of agricultural inputs, such as pesticides, fertilizer and seeds.
- The issue of bringing on board schools that are currently not participating in the SFP is a difficult one. These schools

are located in the least well-endowed communities – those that are remote and hard to access, but are also most in need of the programme.

- Finally, the Ministry of Education may wish to consider opening discussions with the Ministry of Finance and the banking and other private sector institutions on the provision of access to credit to farmers in hinterland communities.

In summary, Guyana's SFP for hinterland primary schools has achieved a great deal in regions of the country that present enormous challenges to development efforts. These achievements need now to be sustained and strengthened.

Acknowledgements

This chapter presents the findings of a 3 year impact evaluation that was financed by the World Bank and the Education for All-Fast Track Initiative in Guyana. The impact evaluation was developed, field work carried out, and analysis, writing and editing of the chapter was completed in partnership with the World Bank team, Social Development Inc. and the Government of Guyana team. Overall guidance and editing were provided by Angela Demas, Senior Education Specialist at the World Bank, and valuable inputs were provided by Evelyn Hamilton, Chief Planning Officer of the Guyana Ministry of Education. We are grateful for the contributions of the enumerators, to the partnering agencies, including staff at the Ministries of Education, Health, Agriculture, Amerindian Affairs and in local government. We are also grateful for the support provided by staff of the EFA-FTI and the regional education offices. Lastly, we would like to thank the hinterland school communities for their willingness and enthusiasm to participate in the impact evaluation of their Community-based School Feeding Program.

Notes

[1]The National School Feeding Committee task force includes representatives of the Ministries of Education, Agriculture, Health, Amerindian Affairs and Local Government, as well as Social Development Inc. (a consultancy firm that specializes in programme design, research, monitoring and impact evaluations in areas including public health nutrition).

[2]In general, the programme insists that the community provides a school kitchen, but outsourcing the provision of meals is an option allowed in certain cases.

[3]The evaluation was designed and implemented by the Ministry of Education, the World Bank and Social Development Inc.

[4]The diet diversity score was calculated by simply summing the number of different foods consumed. The food frequency score was calculated by summing the frequency of consumption, during 2 weeks, of a limited number of key foods.

[5]This information was corroborated by similar questions asked of the students.

[6]The level of consumption of these foods varies substantially with location.

[7]It should be noted that this issue is not unique to the hinterland regions.

References

Bundy, D., Burbano, C., Grosh, M., Gello, A., Jukes, M. and Drake, L. (2009) *Rethinking School Feeding: Social Safety Nets, Child Development, and the Education Sector*. World Food Programme/World Bank, Washington, DC.

Bureau of Statistics (2008) *Census 2008*. Bureau of Statistics, Georgetown, Guyana.

Bureau of Statistics and UNICEF (2006) *Guyana: Monitoring the Situation of Children and Women. Multiple Indicator Cluster Survey*. Bureau of Statistics/United Nations Children's Fund, Georgetown, Guyana.

Dangour, A.D. (2001) Growth of upper- and lower-body segments in Patamona and Wapishana Amerindian children (cross-sectional data). *Annals of Human Biology* 28, 649–663.

FAO (2009) *Country Profile: Food Security Indicators – Guyana*. Food and Agriculture Organization of the United Nations, Rome.

Grantham-McGregor, S.M., Chang, S. and Walker, S.P. (1998) Evaluation of school feeding programs: some Jamaican examples. *The American Journal of Clinical Nutrition* 67, 785S–789S.

Ismail, S. and Hill, H. (2005) *Report of a Study on School Feeding in Guyana*. Social Development Inc., for the Ministry of Education, Georgetown, Guyana.

Ismail, S. and Roopnaraine, T. (2009) *The Impact Evaluation of Guyana's Basic Nutrition Program – Integrated Report*. Social Development Inc., for the Ministry of Education, Georgetown, Guyana.

Ismail, S., Borja, C. and Jarvis, E. (2010) *Guyana's Hinterland Community-based School Feeding Programme: Impact Assessment, 2007–2009*. Report, Latin America and the Caribbean Regional Office, The World Bank, Washington, DC.

Jacoby, E.R., Cueto, S. and Pollitt, E. (1998) When science and politics listen to each other: good prospects from a new school breakfast program in Peru. *The American Journal of Clinical Nutrition* 67, 795S–797S.

Martorell, R., Mendoza, F. and Castillo, R. (1988) Poverty and stature in children. In: Waterlow, J.C. (ed.) *Linear Growth Retardation in Less Developed Countries*. Nestlé Nutrition Workshop Series, Vol. 14. Vevey/Raven Press, New York, pp. 57–73.

McCoy, D. (1997) *An Evaluation of South Africa's Primary School Nutrition Programme*. Child Health Unit, Health Systems Trust, Durban, South Africa.

Ministry of Health (2010) *National Nutrition Strategy 2010–2015*. Ministry of Health, Georgetown, Guyana.

Musgrove, P. (1991) *Feeding Latin-America's Children: An Analytical Survey of Food Programs*. Report No. 9526-LAC, Latin America and the Caribbean Regional Office, Human Resources Division, Technical Department, Washington, DC.

Simeon, D.T. (1998) School feeding in Jamaica: a review of it evaluation. *The American Journal of Clinical Nutrition* 67, 790S–794S.

Vial, I., Muchnik, E. and Kain, J. (1991) The evolution of Chile's main nutrition intervention programmes. *Food and Nutrition Bulletin* 13, 170–178 (2).

Waterlow, J.C. (1994) Summary of causes and mechanisms of linear growth retardation. In: Waterlow, J.C. and Schürch, B. (eds) *Causes and Mechanisms of Linear Growth Retardation Proceedings of an I/D/E/C/G/ Workshop held in London January 15–18, 1993. European Journal of Clinical Nutrition* 48(Suppl.1), S210–S211.

World Bank (2006) *Guyana Poverty Assessment*. Washington, DC.

12 The Impact of School Food Standards on Children's Eating Habits in England

Michael Nelson,[1]* Jo Nicholas,[2] Dalia Haroun,[3] Clare Harper,[4]
Lesley Wood,[2] Claire Storey[5] and Jo Pearce[6]
[1]*Public Health Nutrition Research, London, UK (former Director of Research
and Nutrition, Children's Food Trust)*; [2]*Children's Food Trust (formerly the School
Food Trust), Sheffield, UK*; [3]*Zayed University, Dubai, United Arab Emirates*;
[4]*ISS Education, Northolt, UK*; [5]*formerly of the School Food Trust, Sheffield, UK*;
[6]*University of Nottingham, UK*

Summary

School food has been provided to pupils in England for many decades. From the mid-1970s, however, both the number of meals provided and the quality of the food declined. Legislation was introduced in 2001 to ensure that school catering services provided healthy options, but surveys of consumption in 1997 and 2004–2005 showed that the improved availability of healthy options in school had little or no impact on children's eating habits. In February 2005, Jamie Oliver presented a series of television programmes highlighting the poor quality of school food. The UK government responded by setting up the School Meals Review Panel to make recommendations on how to improve school food, and the School Food Trust (now the Children's Food Trust), a Non-Departmental Public Body to promote the education and health of children and young people by improving the quality of food supplied and consumed in schools. Legislation was introduced in 2006–2008 that set out what caterers could and could not provide for children in schools. At the same time, the Trust worked with caterers, schools, pupils, parents, manufacturers, food distributors, institutions providing further education for catering staff, and others, in a coordinated programme of change. This chapter reports clear evidence of the improvements in provision, choice and consumption of food in schools that have followed the introduction of legislation and of a national programme of work to change catering practices and the attitudes of pupils, parents and others towards healthier food provision in schools. It also provides objective evidence of the impact of healthier food on children's learning behaviour in the classroom, and of the overall costs and benefits of healthier school meals.[1]

Introduction

Teachers know that a hungry child cannot learn. From the mid-19th century, parish schools in England began to provide food to pupils to ensure that they could concentrate on their studies. This provision was voluntary, however – and recognition by the government that a more structured programme of support for food and nutrition was necessary did not emerge until well into the 20th century.

Following the introduction of the welfare state in 1948, nutritional standards for school food were introduced to promote the provision

---

*Contact: michael.nelson@phnresearch.org.uk

of healthier food. The parameters of what was meant by 'healthier' changed over time, of course, as nutritional knowledge improved, and the guidance on school food provision changed accordingly. A legal requirement was placed on local authorities to provide food at lunchtime for pupils from low-income families.

School meals in the 1960s and 1970s were not highly regarded. About two thirds of pupils had a main meal at midday. Meals were provided by school catering services organized by the local education authority, but there were few training courses for school cooks, nor a requirement for specific qualifications, and the quality of food on offer was sometimes poor. By 1980, it was clear that the take-up of school lunches was on the decline, as the service lagged behind pupils' and parents' expectations. Food culture was also changing, and there was an expectation of greater choice and growing competition from what was on offer in the high street.

In 1980, the government deregulated the school meals service, and nutritional standards were no longer applied to the provision of meals. The requirement remained for local authorities to provide food for pupils from low-income households in receipt of selected benefits but, in 1986, the rules changed again and 400,000 pupils from low-income families whose parents were working lost their entitlement to free school meals (FSM). The introduction of Compulsory Competitive Tendering (CCT) in 1988 meant that local authorities were required by law to tender for school catering services (they could no longer simply opt to provide their own services) and, by law, they were required to take the lowest bid. This resulted in a further deterioration in the nutritional quality of the food on offer. By 1990, school food take-up had fallen to just over 40%, and the food provided and consumed was typically high in fat, salt and sugar, all of which were at levels above government guidelines on healthy eating.

By 2000, the government recognized that the number of children who were becoming overweight and obese was increasing dramatically, and that the diets of many children were either low in foods from specific food groups (such as fruits and vegetables), or deficient in nutrients (such as iron, zinc,

folate, vitamin A, dietary fibre, etc.). In an attempt to harmonize public health messages about healthy eating with what was on offer in schools, the government introduced legislation in 2001 (The Education Regulations, 2001) to regulate school food. This ensured that catering services in schools provided healthy options for children, but did not restrict the sales of foods high in fat, salt and sugar, nor actively promote the healthier options in a meaningful way. A comparison of food consumption in schools in 2004–2005 (Nelson *et al.*, 2004, 2006) with that in 1997 (Food Standards Agency, 2000, 2006) showed that the availability of healthy options per se had had little or no impact on children's eating habits in school (Nelson *et al.*, 2007).

The Start of Change

In February and March of 2005, the celebrity chef Jamie Oliver presented a series of television programmes on school food. These showed graphically to the British public that much of what was on offer to pupils in schools was of poor quality, made from the cheapest ingredients, and often high in fat, salt and sugar. There was a marked inconsistency between what children were being taught about healthy eating in the classroom and what was being offered in the dining room. Packed lunch quality was no better (Evans *et al.*, 2010).

In response to public outcry and Oliver's *Feed me better* campaign, the government (Department for Education and Skills (DfES)) set up the School Meals Review Panel. This body, which had representatives from school food catering (both local authority and private catering providers), food manufacturers, pressure groups promoting healthier food provision and consumption, academics and government, met between April and August 2005, and in September 2005 made recommendations to the government about how to improve school food catering services (School Meals Review Panel, 2005). At the heart of this recommendation was the introduction of legislation to control what could and could not be served in schools.

At the same time (in 2005), the government established the School Food Trust (now the Children's Food Trust). The Trust was given the unique remit of transforming school food and food skills. It was set up as a Non-Departmental Public Body (NDPB) with £15 million of funding from the-then DfES (which was replaced by the Department for Children, Schools and Families (DCSF) and, subsequently, by the current Department for Education (DfE)) to promote the education and health of children and young people by improving the quality of food supplied and consumed in schools. The Trust's remit was to:

- ensure that all schools meet the food-based and nutrient-based standards for lunch and non-lunch food;
- increase the take-up of school meals;
- reduce diet-related inequalities in childhood through food education and school based initiatives; and
- improve food skills through food education, and school and community initiatives.

The first task of the Trust was to work closely with the government to draft and implement the legislation necessary to govern catering provision at school. This was introduced in a phased way over 3 years, starting with interim food-based standards introduced in 2006 (The Education Regulations, 2006) to final food-based and nutrient-based standards for all schools in place by September 2009 (The Education Regulations, 2007, 2008, 2011).To inform this work, the Trust undertook a review comparing school food standards in ten countries (Harper and Wells, 2007) and school meal provision in 18 countries (Harper et al., 2008).

At the same time, the Trust began a structured nationwide programme of engagement with the many stakeholders involved in the provision of school food: cooks, catering managers, catering companies (both local authority and private) and associations (such as the Local Authority Caterers Association, LACA), pupils, parents, head teachers, school governors and others. This aimed to determine the attitudes of the various stakeholders to school food, their views on what needed to change and on how the changes might be implemented. From these initial consultations emerged a programme of work that has occupied the Trust for the last 7 years. This has been an integrated programme, based soundly on the principles of behavioural economics, and delivered within the context of legislation. Between 2006 and 2012, the Trust developed a wide range of guidance, products and support services and training, mostly available free of charge, that were designed to underpin the efforts of all those involved in transforming the school food service and improving pupils' eating habits at school. It also engaged directly with central government to lobby in favour of the elements of infrastructure necessary to deliver healthy meals (adequate kitchens and dining rooms when planning new schools and refurbishing old ones, training programmes for catering staff, the inclusion of cooking in the curriculum, etc.).

The Trust was established with five divisions: Communications, Delivery, Partnerships and Programmes, Research and Nutrition, and Corporate Services.[2] Each of these divisions had a clear set of roles and responsibilities, and they evolved together to deliver the Trust's remit. The work of the Trust (under its new name) is described in full on its web site (Children's Food Trust, 2013a).

Developing a Theoretical Framework

The first stage of work for the Trust had three main aims: to identify who was involved in either providing or purchasing school food, and to understand their issues, needs and the barriers to change; to work closely with every stakeholder group to learn (and provide evidence for) which approaches to change were likely to be effective; and, finally, to publicize and help to embed this learning.

A systems map of the people and factors (nodes of influence) involved in promoting healthier eating of food in schools was developed iteratively over a period of several months. The first draft was widely circulated among the stakeholders and Trust staff were also asked to identify at which point(s) they felt their own particular area of work was having an impact. The result is shown in Fig. 12.1.

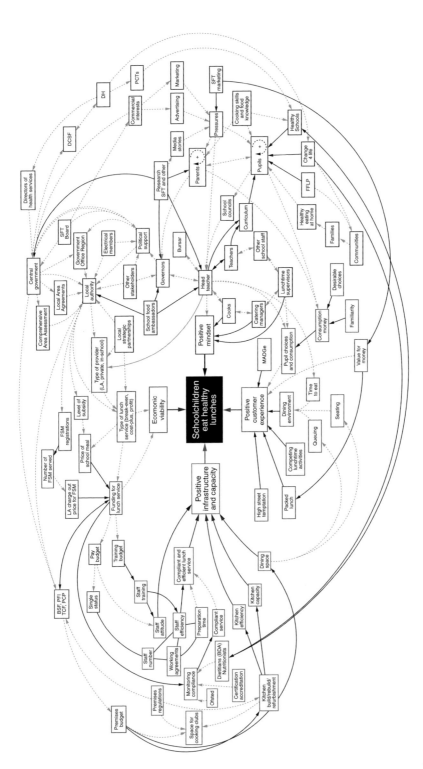

Fig. 12.1. Systems map showing main spheres of influence and key nodes relating to changes in school food provision and consumption by pupils of healthier food in schools. BDA, British Dietetic Association; BSF, Building Schools for the Future; DCSF, Department for Children, Schools and Families; DH, Department of Health; FFLP, Food for Life Partnership; FSM, free school meals; LA, Local Authority; MADGe, Marketing and Design Generator; Ofsted, (UK) Office for Standards in Education, Children's Services and Skills; PCP, Primary Capital Programme; PCTs, Primary Care Trusts; PFI, Private Finance Initiative; SFT, School Food Trust; TCP, Targeted Capital Fund (see http://www.education.gov.uk/vocabularies/educationtermsandtags/5820).

The map suggested that there were four key areas of influence:

- Positive customer experience.
- Positive mindset.
- Economic viability of service.
- Positive infrastructure and capacity.

Ignoring any one of these elements was likely to result in stalemate or stagnation at a local level. For example, pupils needed to have a positive experience in the dining room. So not only was it important to work closely with school councils (representative student bodies) in each school to make sure that they understood and communicated to their peers the need for change, but also to ensure that the caterers were agreeable to changing established habits and had the training to do so, that there were adequate kitchen and dining facilities in the school, that head teachers and parents were on board with the changes and that ultimately, the service would be financially viable. Ignoring any one of these spheres of influence was likely to result in failure or a reduction in the amount of change likely to occur.

Making the changes that were required, therefore, involved undertaking a large number of parallel or carefully sequenced activities to engage all of the stakeholders likely to have an influence at each stage of change and to understand the motivations for each stakeholder group. This drew upon a second set of theoretical understandings; these related to the ways in which change can be introduced, and in which stakeholders could be engaged, helped to see how their own role would contribute to change, and thereby become willing to take responsibility for their own stage in the process. Insights from psychology, marketing, customer insight and economics allowed the Trust to understand better what motivates decision making, and provided a range of possible new policy design themes that could operate in each setting. These included:

- *Choice design:* the way in which choices are presented to individuals can affect the choices they make.

- *Framing:* the way that losses, gains and risks are presented to people can affect their behaviour.
- *Social norms and expectations:* the thoughts and actions of others can (for better or worse) influence and guide individual behaviour.
- *Defaults:* people's inertia means they tend to accept readily the default option presented to them.
- *Aligning long- and short-term preferences:* so as to prevent individuals' short-term desires overriding and damaging their longer term preferences, short-term incentives or self-commitment devices can be used effectively.

The application of these principles to the design of interventions is illustrated throughout the work of the Trust. A good example can be seen in relation to the needs that pupils have at lunchtime and how those needs can be satisfied. Figure 12.2 shows the results from research with focus groups of pupils and their parents.

The hierarchy of needs to satisfy grows increasingly complex as children get older, involving more and more psychological elements (Ashfield-Watt, P.A.L., Dow, B., Abbot, R., Anderton, A. and Nelson, M. (2013) *Improving Adolescent Nutrition: Engaging Secondary School-Children with School Food.* Children's Food Trust, Sheffield, UK. In preparation). At the same time, there is a range of other factors that may be mediating against the adoption of healthier eating habits at lunchtime.

First, factors that relate to price:

- School meals are seen as 'expensive'.
- Packed lunches are seen as cheaper and more likely to satisfy 'consumption confidence' (the feeling on the part of both child and parent that the lunch provided will be eaten).
- Price affects low-income families not eligible for FSM.
- Free school meals (FSM) are not always a straightforward choice because of:
  - the stigma attached to them;
  - parents being intimidated by the FSM registration process; and
  - parents being unaware of FSM eligibility.

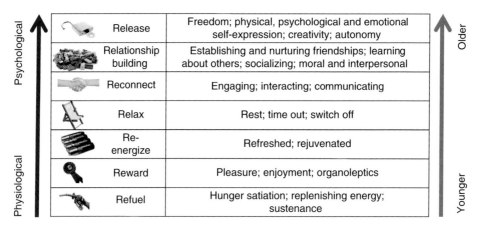

Fig. 12.2. Needs that pupils aim to satisfy at lunchtime.

Secondly, a mixture of other factors:

- Barriers to choice:
  - peer, parent and teacher approval or disapproval;
  - kudos attached to foods other than those served at lunchtime;
  - need for choice, variety and portability; and
  - healthy food feels 'imposed' or a restriction.
- The dining room:
  - atmosphere, decor, noise, queues, time to eat;
  - layout and seating;
  - method of payment;
  - school lunch staff attitudes and training; and
  - menus and information.
- Competition:
  - high street; and
  - lunchtime activities.

Each Division in the Trust had a specific role to play in analysing these factors. Ignoring any of them was likely to undermine even the best thought-through programme of pupil engagement. Unless each of these elements was addressed in ways which related to theoretical constructions that underpin people's behaviour and their willingness to change, effective and timely change was unlikely to occur.

A more recent paradigm for action priorities, the Nuffield Ladder of Intervention (Nuffield Council on Bioethics, 2007) has recently been promoted by the government in England, but it is clear that action at every level is needed to bring about comprehensive change.

Demonstrating the Impact of the Work of the Trust

The main focus of this chapter is to provide evidence that shows clearly how, over the last 7 years, the activities of the Trust have resulted in substantial change in the provision, choice and consumption of food in schools in England. The main responsibility for monitoring changes in provision, consumption, compliance with standards, and assessing the impact of changes on nutritional status, pupil behaviour and educational attainment through surveys and intervention studies, lies with the Trust's Division of Research and Nutrition. The research outputs of the Trust are summarized on the Trust's web site (Children's Food Trust, 2013b).

The evidence that has been collected demonstrates clearly how promoting better feeding practices in schools has made a difference to meal take-up, dietary intakes and learning behaviours in school. This provides a powerful message to head teachers: schoolchildren who eat healthier food in a nicer dining environment at lunchtime are likely to pay more attention in their classes after lunch and have higher levels of well-being. This, in turn, may lead to better achievement and attainment, although the evidence for this is modest (Stevens *et al.*, 2008; Belot and James, 2009). Recent findings from a study carried out by Newcastle University on the impact of changes in school food provision and consumption on wider eating habits in schoolchildren age 4–7 years and 11–14 years suggest that the benefits of healthier eating at school have an impact on total diet (Adamson *et al.*, 2011). There is also preliminary evidence of the impact of healthier eating on healthy growth and the avoidance of overweight and obesity in primary schoolchildren (Nelson, 2012).

Annual survey of school lunch take-up

Since 2006, the Trust has conducted an annual survey of school food catering services at local authority (LA) level. The survey is emailed to all LAs in England in March of each year. Each LA is asked to report take-up of paid-for and free school meals in primary, secondary and special schools for their own catering services and to collect take-up data for those provided by private or in school caterers. In addition, the survey asks about services offered to schools by LAs, meal prices and costs, catering facilities, factors associated with changes in take-up, financial issues, policy and strategy, staffing and pay, and progress towards meeting school food standards.

Since 2008–2009, the survey has used a standardized methodology to determine school lunch take-up (the percentage of pupils on roll taking a school lunch), and this has been adopted nationally. The data collection is supported by the use of questionnaires in MS Excel (with notes and prompts to encourage the clarity of data entries) and relevant data templates for LAs and schools, together with example calculations. The DfE or the Trust sends a letter to Directors of Children's Services and head teachers, and the Trust writes to private caterers nationally to encourage their participation.

A particular emphasis is placed on the accurate reporting of take-up data because the Trust and the DfE believe this is a good

measure not only of the increase in the proportion of schoolchildren who are likely to be eating more healthily at lunchtime, but also a general indicator of engagement with the child well-being agenda. A school with high take-up is focused on:

- balanced nutritional meals – better for short-term and long-term health;
- time and space to eat – promotes calm, recuperation from daily stresses, social interactions, communication skills – supports mental well-being;
- friendly environment – feels good to be there;
- respect for pupils as customers – encourages self-esteem;
- better understanding of food– nutrition, cooking, balanced diet, shopping, eating out – lifelong economic and social skills; and
- improved behaviour/concentration and hence learning.

Findings from the 2011–2012 annual survey

The most recent survey (2011–2012; Nelson *et al.*, 2012) shows that the long decline in the percentage of pupils taking a school lunch (Fig. 12.3) was reversed in 2008–2009, and that take-up has continued to increase since then (Fig. 12.4). In England as a whole, over 270,000 more pupils are now taking lunch at school compared with 2008–2009. There is also evidence that schools are providing meals that are compliant with the standards (Nelson *et al.*, 2012). Over two thirds of schools are reported to be compliant with the three components of the standards: food-based, nutrient-based and food other than lunch.

Further analysis of the data from 2010 has looked at the key associations between take-up and compliance and a range of factors that characterize catering service provision and policy (Nelson *et al.*, 2011). In the primary sector,[3] the key associations were: having full-production kitchens, support from head teachers, training for catering staff, keeping prices low, using software and professional support for menu planning and nutrient analysis, and writing to

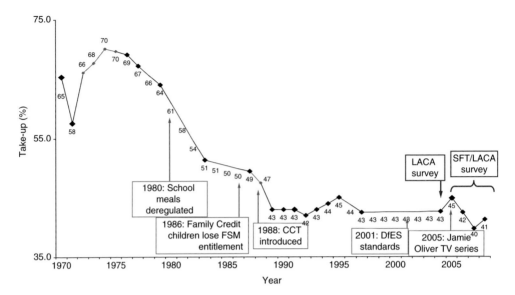

Fig. 12.3. Changes in school meal take-up for primary and secondary schools (combined) in England, and related historical events, 1970–2008. CCT, Compulsory Competitive Tendering; DfES, Department for Education and Skills; FSM, free school meals; LACA, Local Authority Caterers Association; SFT, School Food Trust.

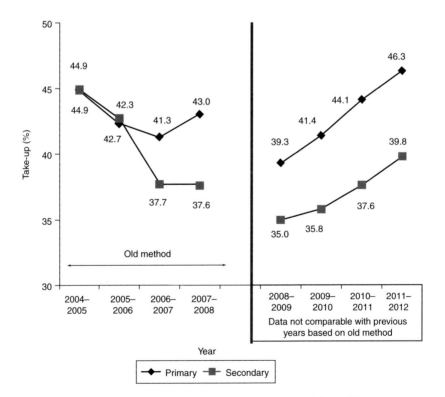

Fig. 12.4. Percentage take-up of school lunches in schools in England, paid for and free, in primary (including special) and secondary schools, 2004–2012. Left: data based on old survey method. Right: data based on new standardized survey methodology.

head teachers (by the LA) and to parents (by the head teacher) to encourage free school meal registration and take-up. In the secondary sector, the key associations were: use of cashless systems for payment in the dining room, reported levels of support from head teachers and governors, staff training, use of software for menu planning and nutrient analysis, paying for professional support, having a stay-on-site policy and (a negative association) having hot food transported from elsewhere.

These findings relate to associations, based on Pearson correlation coefficients and stepwise multiple regression. They cannot be said to be causal in nature, but they do suggest a range of factors that logically might be expected to support higher levels of take-up and compliance. The virtue of the analyses is that they provide a sense of priority relating to which influences are commonly observed nationally. There may, of course, be other activities undertaken at a local level which are not undertaken as consistently throughout England and so do not appear as significant in the analyses but which, nevertheless, are associated with higher levels of take-up (both paid-for and free) and compliance with the school food standards.

Primary school food study

In 2009, the Trust undertook a national survey of provision, choice and consumption in 139 primary schools in England. Data were recorded on catering practices and the provision of food and drink at lunchtime, and were used to assess compliance with the school food standards. In addition, 6690 pupils having a school lunch and 3481 pupils having packed lunches provided information on the food and drink choices of pupils and on the consumption and wastage of food and drink. Fieldwork was carried out in February, March and April 2009; each school was visited over 5 consecutive days during lunchtime. The methodology followed that used in a similar survey carried out in 2005 (Nelson et al., 2006). As the school food standards were introduced in 2006, the survey provided the opportunity to assess the overall impact of the Trust's work and that of the catering providers in the 2 years following the introduction of the standards. Full reports on the survey's implementation and findings have been published (Haroun et al., 2010a,b).

Figure 12.5 shows the changes in the percentages of foods offered by caterers between 2005 and 2009. There were statistically

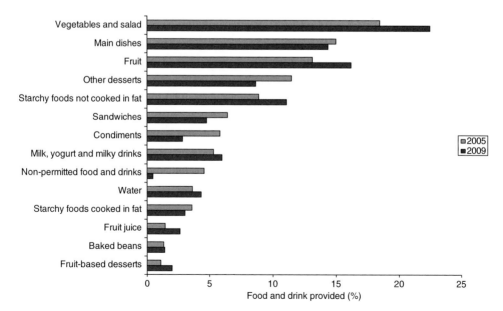

Fig. 12.5. Percentages of different food and drink groups provided, as a percentage of all food and drinks, in nationally representative samples of primary schools in England, 2005 and 2009.

significant increases in the provision of vegetables and salad, fruit, starchy foods not cooked in fat or oil, milk, yogurt and milk-based drinks, water, fruit juice and fruit-based desserts. There were declines in 'other' desserts (not fruit-based), sandwiches, condiments, 'non-permitted' food and drink (sweet and savoury snacks, soft drinks, confectionery, etc.; see the guidance on food- and nutrient-based standards from the School Food Trust, 2007), and starchy foods cooked in fat (e.g. chips – French fries).

The consequence of this change in provision is shown in Fig. 12.6. The number of pupils taking water increased by over 20%, vegetables and salad by almost 15%, fruit juice by 9% and fruit-based desserts by 8%; other positive changes were seen in relation to starchy foods not cooked in fat, and fruit. As a consequence, the consumption of fruit and vegetables was seen to have increased by 60%, from an average of 1.0 portion in 2005 to 1.6 portions in 2009. Foods regarded as less healthy, such as non-fruit-based desserts, condiments, starchy foods cooked in fat, and non-permitted food and drinks, were all taken less often.

When this is translated into changes in the average nutrient consumption from school lunches, levels of vitamin A, zinc, folate and dietary fibre increased (Fig. 12.7). At the other end of the spectrum, the consumption of non-milk extrinsic sugar (NMES), fat, saturated fatty acids (SFA) and sodium all fell substantially – sodium by almost a third. Energy intake also fell, which may contribute to healthier weight gain, but the evidence on growth is not yet available. Iron intake also fell, in spite of efforts by caterers to increase the iron density of many school recipes (Boaden *et al.*, 2008).

Changes of this magnitude on a national scale are remarkable in such a short period of time. The findings do not represent individual interventions in a handful of schools, but average changes in 17,000 primary schools across England. We do not know of any other intervention on this scale that shows such dramatic, consistent and robust evidence of healthier eating in children over such a short time period.

There is also strong evidence of the impact of standards in individual schools (Haroun *et al.*, 2011). Not all schools met all of the standards, but where standards were met there was a direct influence on the food taken by children. When a school met a given

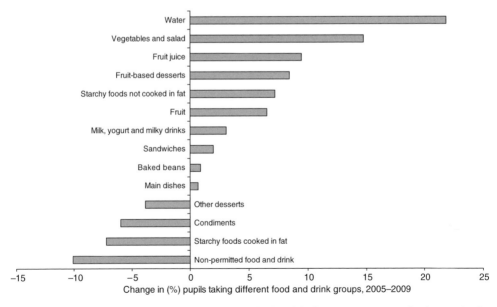

Fig. 12.6. Change in percentage of pupils taking different food and drink groups in primary schools in England, 2005–2009.

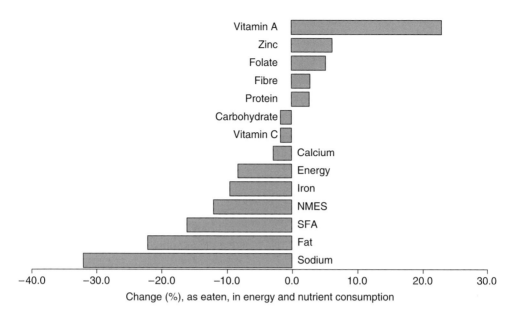

Fig. 12.7. Changes in the level of energy and nutrients eaten at lunchtime in primary schools in England in 2009 compared with 2005. NMES, non-milk extrinsic sugars; SFA, saturated fatty acids.

standard, it was more likely that pupils in that school would take and eat meals that were healthier. For example, in schools that met the standard for NMES, 74% of pupils took a meal that also met the standard, and 80% of meals as eaten met the standard. In schools that did not meet the standard, the values were 52% and 62%, respectively. There is, therefore, a direct relationship between the school meeting the standard and the proportion of pupils taking and eating healthier meals.

Secondary school food study

A study comparable to that in the primary sector was conducted in a nationally representative sample of 80 secondary schools in England in 2011 (Nicholas *et al.*, 2012). As in the primary sector, it was possible to compare the results from the current survey with findings collected in 2004 (Nelson *et al.*, 2004) in order to assess the impact of the new school food legislation and changes in catering provision and practice in the secondary sector. Again, the key findings suggest that the introduction of compulsory school food standards

has resulted in substantial improvements in food choices and nutrient intakes. The consumption of fruits, vegetables and starchy food not cooked in fat increased (Fig. 12.8), while energy intake, and consumption of fat, saturated fat, sugar and salt all decreased dramatically (Fig. 12.9). This contrasts markedly with the lack of improvement between 1997 and 2004 following the introduction of the 2001 guidelines, which required only that schools provide healthy options but placed no restrictions on the sales of high fat, sugar or salt foods, or constraints on the balance of provision.

School lunch and learning behaviours

There is anecdotal evidence from teachers and parents that children's behaviour and academic performance improve when they eat healthier food. However, there is a lack of robust evidence (Ells *et al.*, 2006) that this is the case. Most previous studies have focused on single foods or nutrients or meals, and been carried out in populations or settings in which the findings cannot be generalized to schools and pupils, and observations of

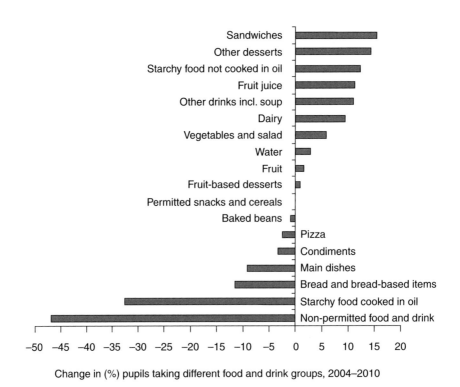

Change in (%) pupils taking different food and drink groups, 2004–2010

Fig. 12.8. Secondary schools: change in percentage of pupils taking specified foods, 2004–2010.

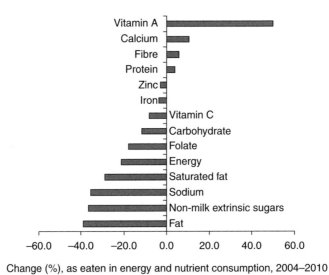

Change (%), as eaten in energy and nutrient consumption, 2004–2010

Fig. 12.9. Secondary schools: average percentage change, nutrients as eaten, 2004–2010.

behaviour have been largely subjective. One cannot conclude, therefore, that improved food results in improved behaviour.

In order to address this question, the Trust carried out two randomized controlled intervention studies, one in primary schools and the other in secondary schools. The hypothesis was that providing and promoting healthier school food at lunchtime, and improving the dining room environment, would have a positive impact on pupils' learning-related behaviours in the classroom after lunch.

In the primary school study (Golley *et al.*, 2010), four intervention schools had a 12 week intervention and two control schools were wait listed (i.e. the intervention was provided at the end of the study after the final behavioural measurements were made). At baseline, a systematic assessment of the dining environment was carried out in each school, and the food consumption at lunchtime of 131 pupils was measured on 5 consecutive days. Systematic observations of the pupils' learning-related behaviours were carried out in the classroom in the 60–90 min immediately after lunch by observers trained in a standardized technique. Pupils' learning behaviours were classified as 'on-task' or 'off-task' and the 'social mode' was noted: whether the pupil was working alone, with others or with a teacher. All of these observations were carried out at baseline and immediately after the 12 week intervention period. Results are expressed as the odds ratio (OR, the likelihood of observing the behaviour in children in the intervention schools compared with the control schools).

Table 12.1 shows the results in the primary school study. On-task and off-task behaviours were observed and used as proxy measures for concentration and disengagement (disruption), respectively. Teacher–pupil on-task engagement was 3.4 times more likely in the intervention schools than in the control schools (OR = 3.40; 95% CI: 1.56, 7.36; $P = 0.009$[4]). Teacher–pupil interaction represents about 80% of the time spent in primary school classrooms. However, on-task pupil–pupil behaviour was less likely in the intervention group (adjusted model OR = 0.45; 95% CI: 0.28, 0.70; $P < 0.001$). Similarly, off-task pupil–pupil behaviour was more likely in the intervention group than in the control group (adjusted model OR = 2.28; 95% CI: 1.25, 4.17; $P = 0.007$). Pupil–pupil interaction represents about 11% of the time spent in the classroom in primary schools. The study offers some support for the hypothesis that a school food and dining room intervention can have a positive impact on pupils' alertness. However, if raised alertness is not appropriately channelled and supervised, it may result in increased off-task behaviour when pupils are working together without adequate learning objectives or supervision.

Table 12.1. Occurrence of on-task and off-task behaviour overall and for each social mode separately in intervention schools (healthier school food promoted at lunchtime, and dining room environment improved) combined relative to wait listed (non-intervention) control schools.

	Group (intervention:control)		
	Odds ratio (OR)[a]	95% CI	*P*
On-task behaviour (concentration)			
All settings	1.14	0.87, 1.49	0.86
By setting:			
Individual on-task	1.34	0.74, 1.83	0.27
Pupil–pupil on-task	0.45	0.28, 0.70	<0.001
Teacher–pupil on-task	3.40	1.56, 7.36	0.009
Off-task behaviour (disengagement)			
All settings	0.83	0.74, 1.19	0.31
By setting:			
Individual off-task	0.71	0.37, 1.35	0.29
Pupil–pupil off-task	2.28	1.25, 4.17	0.007
Teacher–pupil off-task	1.09	0.35, 3.45	0.89

[a]Statistical analysis adjusted for class size (<22 versus ≥22), presence of additional adults in the classroom, English as an additional language (EAL), sex, free school meal (FSM) eligibility, special educational need (SEN) status, ethnicity and lunch type (school meal or packed lunch).

A similar study (Storey *et al.*, 2011) was carried out in seven intervention and four control secondary schools over 15 weeks and observed 136 pupils. Again, the control schools were wait listed. The intervention consisted of a range of approaches to improve the quality and presentation of the food on offer, to engage with pupils and to improve the dining environment (decorations, changed layout, reduced queuing, etc.) All the schools were offered a £2000 incentive to improve their dining environments.

Table 12.2 shows the results for the secondary school study. At follow-up, intervention group pupils were 18% more likely to be on-task (OR 1.18, 95% CI 1.05 to 1.33) and 14% less likely to be off-task (OR 0.86, 95% CI 0.75 to 0.98) compared with control group pupils, again controlling for potential confounders. The main contribution to the on-task behaviours came from pupils working well on their own (representing about 50% of the time spent in the classroom). The study suggests that modifying food provision and dining environment can improve learning-related behaviours of secondary school pupils in the post-lunch period. As in the primary study, the findings support ongoing investment and interventions by local

authorities across the UK to improve school food and lunchtime dining facilities.

The Trust has recently conducted research into the relationship between improved lunchtime provision and environment, the broader elements of need satisfied at lunchtime (see Fig. 12.2) and behaviour in the classroom after lunch (Kaklamanou, 2012).

Cost and impact

Over a period of 6 years, from 2005 to 2011, the DfE (in its various incarnations) provided programme grants of £15.4 million (2005–2008) + £22.6 million (2008–2011), a total of £38 million to set up and run the School Food Trust (SFT). During this same period, approximately 270,000 more pupils began taking school meals. Although there was an initial decline in take-up following the TV broadcasts in 2005 by Jamie Oliver about the poor quality of some school food, national take-up has increased since 2008–2009 (to 2010–2011) by about 5% in primary schools and about 2.5% in secondary schools. This represents an increase by 2010–2011 of approximately 270,000 more pupils taking a school lunch than in 2007–2008; it includes both paid-for

Table 12.2. Likelihood (OR) of on-task and off-task learning behaviours in intervention schools (improved quality and presentation food on offer, improved dining environment) compared with control schools, by social mode, taking potential confounders[a] into account.

	Group (intervention:control)			
	Odds ratio[a]	Lower CI	Upper CI	*P*
On-task behaviour (concentration)				
All settings	1.18	1.05	1.33	0.005
By setting:				
Individual on-task	1.24	0.97	1.58	0.088
Pupil–pupil on-task	1.04	0.86	1.25	0.716
Teacher–pupil on-task	0.82	0.64	1.04	0.103
Off-task behaviour (disengagement)				
All settings	0.86	0.75	0.98	0.021
By setting:				
Individual on-task	0.88	0.68	1.14	0.321
Pupil–pupil on-task	0.87	0.71	1.06	0.171
Teacher–pupil on-task	1.03	0.78	1.36	0.820

[a]Statistical analysis adjusted for class size (<22 versus ≥22), presence of additional adults in the classroom, English as an additional language (EAL), sex, free school meal (FSM) eligibility, special educational need (SEN) status, ethnicity and lunch type (school meal or packed lunch).

and free school meals. In relation to the direct funding for the SFT, therefore, it has cost approximately £38 million/270,000 = £141 for each pupil new to taking a school lunch. While the long-term impact of taking a school lunch is not fully known, from a public health perspective, £141 represents a small cost in relation to a change in eating habits in keeping with government guidelines – and with the potential to affect lifetime eating habits (and concomitant improvements in health) that may accrue from an introduction to healthier eating in school. If it is assumed that healthier eating habits at school are likely to have wider impacts on pupils' eating habits outside school and into adulthood, and that better school food is associated with better learning and achievement, then this represents a reasonable investment in the future of each child, and is likely to be more than offset in adulthood by health benefits and employment opportunities (London Economics, 2008).

In 2010–2011, there were approximately 3 million school meals served each day in England. This has varied slightly over time according to take-up and the numbers of pupils on roll. Evidence from the national studies of school food provision, choice and consumption in primary (Haroun et al., 2010a) and secondary (Nicholas et al., 2012) schools in England suggests that the balance of consumption has become healthier. There is also persistent evidence over many years that school lunches are more nutritionally sound than packed lunches (Evans et al., 2010; Pearce et al., 2011; Stevens et al., 2012). Hence, for the purposes of the present analysis, it can reasonably be argued that the average school lunch consumed in both the primary and secondary sectors is more nutritionally healthy than it was prior to the introduction of school food standards in England. The annual cost/child to have access to and consume a healthier school lunch (in relation to the costs of setting up and running the SFT over 6 years) would therefore be £38 million divided by 3 million meals/day divided by 6 years = £38 million/(3 million × 6 years) = £2.11. This approach takes into account the actual number of school meals served, as not every child has a school meal every day,

so £2.11 represents the cost/child-equivalent across the entire year.

The Trust's spend can be expressed in terms of the number of meals served over the period in which it has been running. If the annual spend/child-equivalent is approximately £2.11, and there are roughly 190 trading days/school year, then the Trust's spend/school lunch = £2.11/190 days = 1.1 p/lunch. A penny per meal signifies how tiny has been the level of investment needed to finance a change management organization that has had a demonstrable impact on the pace and extent of change in school food services over a 6 year period, and on children's eating habits nationally. The recent evaluation of the impact of the new standards on total diet (Adamson et al., 2011), which suggests that the healthier eating gains evident within school carry over to the total diet, means that the improved profile of eating in school is not compensated for by worse dietary habits outside school.

Finally, it is important to note that over this same period (2005–2011), the DfE provided a ring-fenced school lunch grant. From 2005 to 2008, this was £240 million specifically to subsidize ingredients, which equates to £240 million/(3 million × 3 years × 190 days) = 14 p/meal. Over the 2008–2011 period, the DfE provided a further £240 million. This money was again ring-fenced, and covered both food and other items (such as small pieces of kitchen equipment, software for menu and nutrient analysis, professional support from a nutritionist or dietician to implement the standards), which equated to about 11 p/meal (Nelson, 2013).

These subsidies were intended to be transitional to help schools and caterers meet the costs of transition. It cannot be said to what degree this additional funding was responsible for the change in school food provision, but it clearly helped to support the economic viability of the service. The subsidy will continue as part of the general grant provided to schools by central government, but will no longer be ring-fenced. In addition, the DfE in England decreed in September 2010 that schools which adopt Academy status (i.e. become independent of local authority control) are no longer required by law to follow the standards for school food. It will be important to evaluate the impact of the loss of ring-fencing of this subsidy to catering services and the loss of compulsory standards on provision and consumption over the coming years.

Conclusions

This chapter presents robust evidence of the impact of the combination of school food regulations and the approaches taken by the School Food Trust (and now the Children's Food Trust) in generating significant, persistent and beneficial changes in children's eating habits over a relatively short period of time. There is also evidence of the positive impact of healthier food and improved dining spaces at lunchtime on learning behaviour in the classroom after lunch.

The Trust believes that the introduction of compulsory school food standards in England has been effective in improving children's eating habits only because it was underpinned nationally and locally by four elements: ensuring that catering services were economically viable; making sure that parents, pupils, teachers and governors understood that healthier eating was desirable; engaging with pupils to ensure that they had a positive experience in the dining room; and working to develop a positive infrastructure (relating to food procurement, caterer training, etc.) to support the delivery of healthier food. This included support for audits and inspection of the service to determine compliance with the standards.

This approach provides a robust and generalizable model for intervention that can be applied at local, regional and national levels. It also provides a platform for transforming children's eating habits, using school as the hub for both learning and practice relating to healthy lifestyles, and engaging pupils and parents in the development of cooking skills that support healthier eating. These strategies will not only improve the nutrition provided to children in school, but are expected to have an impact on their choice of diet, health and attainment both

outside school and as adults. Evidence relating to this wider impact is being generated.

Looking forward

From October 2011, the School Food Trust was no longer a Non-Departmental Public Body (NDPB), but operates as a charity under the new name (as from 2012) of the Children's Food Trust. The aim is to provide products and services to schools, local authority and central Government. The Trust continues to advise governments in England and elsewhere on a range of activities. It is also sharing the lessons it has learned with non-governmental organizations (NGOs) and governments both inside and outside the UK through conferences, workshops and other means of networking, marketing and dissemination. The Trust has developed consultancy and research services (with appropriate links) to support these activities.

Evidence of the impact of school food legislation on diet both inside and outside school, and on obesity, is currently being collected through the National Diet and Nutrition Survey, a national, rolling survey of a representative cross-section of the UK population (National Diet and Nutrition Survey Rolling Programme, 2011). In the future, there will be the need to link more strongly nutrition education in schools with practice. The components are: classroom – dining room – cooking – garden – consumption at home (Fig. 12.10). The process is iterative at every stage, that is, the loops are all overlapping and reinforcing.

To that end, the Trust's Research and Nutrition team works closely with the Let's Get Cooking (LGC) programme on the evaluation of the impact of the programme in 5000 schools in England (Children's Food Trust, 2012). This project engages both pupils and parents in facilitated cookery sessions that focus on the preparation of healthy food (the LGC team works closely with the nutrition team in the Trust on the recipes and portion sizes that are appropriate by age). It carries the messages from school to home and

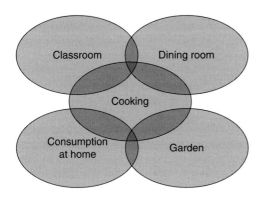

Fig. 12.10. Overlapping relationships between spheres of influence on children's eating habits and development of understanding of food.

embeds them firmly in the family, and engages not just the women but other family and community members. The Trust sees this as a powerful, evidence-based model for changing people's knowledge, skills, norms and expectations. In developing countries, similar approaches have been used to facilitate the development of better nutrition-related health and social support, as well as to promote the extension of the school day (Bundy *et al.*, 2009).

A new focus of the Children's Food Trust is on early years. Better provision of healthy food in the early years provides a powerful model for engagement with mothers and families around good nutrition. In 2010, the Trust provided secretariat support to the

DfE-appointed Advisory Panel on Food and Nutrition in Early Years. The remit of the Advisory Panel was to consider the need for the development of food and drink guidelines for practitioners working in early years' settings, and to make recommendations to the DfE on the implementation of these guidelines. The Panel's report and background papers prepared for consideration are available on the Trust's web site (Advisory Panel on Food and Nutrition in Early Years, 2011). The recommendations of the Advisory Panel addressed not only issues relating to healthy food but also wider issues of obesity and dietary balance – a quarter of pupils currently arrive at the reception class in primary school already either overweight or obese. The Panel's recommendation of food-based guidelines, underpinned by a nutrient framework, was accepted, and the Trust has developed and published guidance to help early years' providers and practitioners to meet the Early Years Foundation Stage (EYFS) welfare requirement for the provision of healthy, balanced and nutritious food and drink (School Food Trust, 2012). Again, there will be a need to evaluate the impact of the introduction of guidance and for relevant support on practice. To that end, the Trust is currently carrying out a survey in early years' settings (children aged 12 months to 4 years) to identify the characteristics of food provision and consumption in these settings, and to compare these with the guidelines.

Notes

[1]This chapter is based on a paper delivered in Rome in December 2010. The text has been updated (to 2012) to reflect subsequent changes in the status of the School Food Trust (now the Children's Food Trust) and to reflect recent findings and research. The references were last updated in 2013.

[2]From 1 October 2011, after the UK government discontinued the status of Non-Departmental Public Body (NDPB), the School Food Trust is no longer an NDPB, but operates as a charity. Starting in 2012, the 'Children's Food Trust' became the new name for the School Food Trust. The divisional structure described reflected the needs of the new organization and has since changed, but research and the development of a robust evidence base to inform policy and understand policy impact remain a priority.

[3]Special schools were excluded from this analysis because their characteristics are different from the majority of primary schools.

[4]Adjusted for class size, presence of additional adults in the classroom (yes/no), English as an additional language (EAL), free school meal eligibility (FSM), sex, special educational need (SEN) status, ethnicity (White British or 'other') and lunch type (school lunch or packed lunch).

References

Adamson, A., White, M. and Stead, M. (2011) *The Process and Impact of Change in the School Food Policy on Food and Nutrient Intake of Children Aged 4–7 and 11–12 Years Both In and Out of School; A Mixed Methods Approach*. Report of work undertaken by Newcastle University and the University of Stirling as part of the Public Health Research Consortium (funded by the UK Department of Health Policy Research Programme). Available at: http://phrc.lshtm.ac.uk/papers/PHRC_B5-07_Final_Report.pdf (accessed 11 June 2013).

Advisory Panel on Food and Nutrition in Early Years (2011) School Food Trust [now Children's Food Trust], Sheffield, UK. Available at: http://www.childrensfoodtrust.org.uk/advice/eat-better-start-better/advisory-panel (accessed 11 June 2013).

Belot, M. and James, J. (2009) *Healthy School Meals and Educational Outcomes*. Working Paper No. 2009-1, Institute for Social and Economic Research, University of Essex, Colchester, UK. Available at: https://www.iser.essex.ac.uk/publications/working-papers/iser/2009-01 (accessed 11 June 2013).

Boaden, D., French, C. and Bacon, P. (2008) *Report on the Development of Secondary School Lunch Recipes with Increased Iron Content*. School Food Trust [now Children's Food Trust], Sheffield, UK. Available at: http://webarchive.nationalarchives.gov.uk/20100210190918/http://schoolfoodtrust.org.uk/UploadDocs/Library/Documents/iron_enriched_recipes.pdf (accessed 11 June 2013).

Bundy, D., Burbano, C., Grosh, M., Gelli, A., Jukes, M. and Drake, L. (2009) Rethinking School Feeding: Social Safety Nets, Child Development, and the Education Sector. World Food Programme/The World Bank, Washington, DC. Available at: http://siteresources.worldbank.org/EDUCATION/Resources/278200-1099079877269/547664-1099080042112/DID_School_Feeding.pdf (accessed 11 June 2013).

Children's Food Trust (2012) *Evaluation of the Let's Get Cooking [Big Lottery Funded] Programme. Final Report*. School Food Trust [now Children's Food Trust], Sheffield, UK. Available at: http://www.childrensfoodtrust.org.uk/assets/research-reports/LGC%20%20Big%20Lottery%20evaluation%20FINAL_Technical_report_31_Jan_12.pdf (accessed 11 June 2013).

Children's Food Trust (2013a) About the Trust. Children's Food Trust, Sheffield, UK. Available at: http://www.childrensfoodtrust.org.uk/our-mission/about-the-trust (accessed 11 June 2013).

Children's Food Trust (2013b) Research. Children's Food Trust, Sheffield, UK. Available at: http://www.childrensfoodtrust.org.uk/research (accessed 11 June 2013).

Ells, L.J., Hillier, F.C. and Summerbell, C.D. (2006) *A Systematic Review of the Effect of Nutrition, Diet and Dietary Change on Learning, Education and Performance of Children of Relevance to UK Schools*. Food Standards Agency, London. Available at: http://www.food.gov.uk/multimedia/pdfs/systemreview.pdf (accessed 11 June 2013).

Evans, C.E., Cleghorn, C.L., Greenwood, D.C. and Cade, J.E. (2010) A comparison of British school meals and packed lunches from 1990 to 2007: meta-analysis by lunch type. *British Journal of Nutrition* 104, 474–487.

Food Standards Agency (2000) *National Diet and Nutrition Survey: Young People Aged 4 to 18 Years. Volume 1: Report of the Diet and Nutrition Survey*. Prepared for the UK Food Standards Agency by Gregory, J.R., Lowe, S., Bates, C.J., Prentice, A., Jackson, L.V., Smithers, G., Wenlock, R. and Farron, H. The Stationery Office, London.

Food Standards Agency (2006) *National Diet and Nutrition Survey. Young People Aged 4 to 18 Years: Revised Consumption Data for Some Food Groups*. Prepared for the UK Food Standards Agency. The Stationery Office, London. Available at: http://www.food.gov.uk/science/dietarysurveys/ndnsdocuments/ndnsprevioussurveyreports/ndnssurvey4to18 (accessed 11 June 2013).

Golley, R., Baines, E., Bassett, P., Wood, L., Pearce, J. and Nelson, M. (2010) School lunch and learning behaviour in primary schools: an intervention study *European Journal of Clinical Nutrition* 64, 1280–1288. Available at: http://www.nature.com/ejcn/journal/vaop/ncurrent/full/ejcn2010150a.html (accessed 11 June 2013).

Haroun, D., Harper, C., Pearce, J., Wood, L., Sharp, L., Poulter, J., Hall, L., Smyth, S., Huckle, C. and Nelson, M. (2010a) *Primary School Food Survey 2009 – Full Technical Report, rev. 2012*. School Food Trust [now Children's Food Trust], Sheffield, UK. Available at: http://www.childrensfoodtrust.org.uk/assets/research-reports/primary_school_food_survey_2009_full_technical_report_revised2012.pdf (accessed 11 June 2013).

Haroun, D., Harper, C., Wood, L. and Nelson, M. (2010b) The impact of the food-based and nutrient-based standards on lunchtime food and drink provision and consumption in primary schools in England.

Public Health Nutrition 14, 209–218. Available at: http://journals.cambridge.org/action/displayAbstract?aid=7871394 (accessed 11 June 2013).

Haroun, D., Harper C., Wood, L. and Nelson, M. (2011) Nutrient-based standards for school lunch complement food-based standards and improve pupils' nutrient intake profile. *British Journal of Nutrition* 104, 472–474. Available at: http://journals.cambridge.org/action/displayAbstract?fromPage=online&aid=8346540 (accessed 11 June 2013).

Harper, C. and Wells, L. (2007) School Meal Provision in England and Other Western Countries: A Review. Sheffield, School Food Trust [now Children's Food Trust], Sheffield, UK. Available at: http://www.childrensfoodtrust.org.uk/assets/research-reports/school_meals_review_may07.pdf (accessed 11 June 2013).

Harper, C., Wood, L. and Mitchell, C. (2008) *The Provision of School Food in 18 Countries*. School Food Trust [now Children's Food Trust], Sheffield, UK. Available at: http://www.childrensfoodtrust.org.uk/assets/research-reports/school_food_in18countries.pdf (accessed 11 June 2013).

Kaklamanou, D. (2012) *School Lunch, Perception and Behaviour Study: Focus Group Analysis*. Report prepared for the School Food Trust by Daphne Kaklamanou. School Food Trust [now Children's Food Trust], Sheffield, UK. Available at: http://www.childrensfoodtrust.org.uk/assets/research-reports/sft_slab3_focus_groups_findings.pdf (accessed 11 June 2013).

London Economics (2008) *Estimating the Economic Impact of Healthy Eating. Final Report for the School Food Trust. Prepared by London Economics*. School Food Trust [now Children's Food Trust], Sheffield, UK. Available at: http://www.childrensfoodtrust.org.uk/assets/research-reports/estimating_economic_impact_of_healthy_eating.pdf (accessed 11 June 2013).

National Diet and Nutrition Survey Rolling Programme (2011) Department of Health, London. Available at: http://webarchive.nationalarchives.gov.uk/20130107105354/http://www.dh.gov.uk/en/Publicationsandstatistics/PublishedSurvey/ListOfSurveySince1990/Surveylistlifestyle/DH_128165 (accessed 11 June 2013).

Nelson, M. (2012) School Lunch Take Up and Obesity. Research Note prepared by Michael Nelson on behalf of the School Food Trust [now Children's Food Trust], Sheffield, UK. Available at: http://www.childrensfoodtrust.org.uk/assets/research-reports/research_note_take_up_and_obesity.pdf (accessed 11 June 2013).

Nelson, M. (2013) School food cost–benefits: England. *Public Health Nutrition* 16, 1006–1011.

Nelson, M., Bradbury, J., Poulter, J., McGee, A., Msebele, S. and Jarvis, L. (2004) *School Meals in Secondary Schools in England*. Research Report No. RR557, prepared for the UK Food Standards Agency, Department for Education and Skills, London. Available at: http://webarchive.nationalarchives.gov.uk/20130401151715/https://www.education.gov.uk/publications/RSG/publicationDetail/Page1/RR557 (accessed 11 June 2013).

Nelson, M., Nicholas, J., Suleiman, S., Davies, O., Prior, G., Hall, L., Wreford, S. and Poulter, J. (2006) *School Meals in Primary Schools in England*. Research Report No. RR753, prepared for the UK Food Standards Agency, Department for Education and Skills, London Available at: http://webarchive.nationalarchives.gov.uk/20130401151715/https://www.education.gov.uk/publications/RSG/publicationDetail/Page1/RR753 (accessed 11 June 2013).

Nelson, M., Lowes, K., Hwang, V. and Members of Nutrition Group, School Meals Review Panel, Department for Education and Skills (2007) The contribution of school meals to food consumption and nutrient intakes of young people aged 4–18 years in England. *Public Health Nutrition* 10, 652–662.

Nelson, M., Nicholas, J. and Wood, L. (2011) *Fifth Annual Survey of Take Up of School Lunches in England 2009–2010: Key Findings from Further Analysis*. School Food Trust [now Children's Food Trust], Sheffield, UK. Available at: http://www.childrensfoodtrust.org.uk/assets/research-reports/fifth_annual_survey2009-2010further_analysis.pdf (accessed 11 June 2013).

Nelson, M., Nicholas, J., Riley, K., and Wood, L. (2012) *Seventh Annual Survey of Take Up of School Lunches in England [2011–2012]*. School Food Trust/[now] Children's Food Trust, Sheffield, UK. Available at: http://www.childrensfoodtrust.org.uk/assets/research-reports/seventh_annual_survey2011-2012_full_report.pdf (accessed 11 June 2013).

Nicholas, J., Wood, L. and Nelson M. (2012) *Secondary School Food Survey 2011: 1. School Lunch: Provision, Selection and Consumption*. Research Report prepared for the School Food Trust/[now] Children's Food Trust, Sheffield, UK. Available at: http://www.childrensfoodtrust.org.uk/assets/research-reports/secondary_school_food_provision_selection_consumption.pdf (accessed 11 June 2013).

Nuffield Council on Bioethics (2007) The intervention ladder. From Chapter 3: Policy process and practice. In: *Public Health Ethical Issues*. Nuffield Council on Bioethics, London, pp. 29–47 ['The intervention ladder' is covered on pp. 41–42.]. Available at: http://www.nuffieldbioethics.org/public-health/public-health-policy-process-and-practice (accessed 11 June 2013).

Pearce, J., Harper, C., Haroun, D., Wood, L. and Nelson, M. (2011) Short communication: key differences between school lunches and packed lunches in primary schools in England in 2009. *Public Health Nutrition* 14, 1507–1510.

School Food Trust (2007) *A Guide to Introducing the Government's Food-based and Nutrient-based Standards for School Food*. School Food Trust/[now] Children's Food Trust, Sheffield, UK. Available at: http://www.childrensfoodtrust.org.uk/assets/sft_nutrition_guide.pdf (accessed 11 June 2013).

School Food Trust (2012) *Voluntary Food and Drink Guidelines for Early Years Settings in England – A Practical Guide*. School Food Trust [now Children's Food Trust], Sheffield, UK. Available at: http://www.childrensfoodtrust.org.uk/assets/eat-better-start-better/CFT%20Early%20Years%20Guide_Interactive_Sept%2012.pdf (accessed 11 June 2013).

School Meals Review Panel (2005) *Turning the Tables – Transforming School Food. Appendices: Development and Implementation of Nutritional Standards for School Lunches*. Department for Education and Skills, London. Available at http://www.childrensfoodtrust.org.uk/assets/research-reports/turning_the_tables_appendices.pdf (accessed 11 June 2013).

Stevens, L., Oldfield, N., Wood, L. and Nelson, M. (2008) *The Impact of Primary School Breakfast Clubs in Deprived Areas of London: Findings*. School Food Trust [now Children's Food Trust], Sheffield, UK. Available at: http://www.childrensfoodtrust.org.uk/assets/research-reports/sft_breakfast_club_findings_dec08.pdf (accessed 11 June 2013).

Stevens, L., Nicholas, J., Wood, L. and Nelson, M. (2012) *Secondary School Food Survey 2011: 2. School Lunches versus Packed Lunches*. School Food Trust [now Children's Food Trust], Sheffield, UK. Available at: http://www.childrensfoodtrust.org.uk/assets/research-reports/secondary_school_lunches_v_packed_lunches.pdf (accessed 11 June 2013).

Storey, C., Pearce, J., Ashfield-Watt, P., Wood, L. and Nelson, M. (2011) A randomized controlled trial of the effect of school food and dining room modifications on classroom behaviour in secondary school children. *European Journal of Clinical Nutrition* 65, 32–38. Available at: http://www.nature.com/ejcn/journal/v65/n1/full/ejcn2010227a.html (accessed 11 June 2013).

The Education Regulations (2001) *Statutory Instrument 2000 No. 1777. Education (Nutritional Standards for School Lunches) (England) Regulations 2000*. The Stationery Office, London. Available at: http://www.legislation.gov.uk/uksi/2000/1777/contents/made (accessed 11 June 2013).

The Education Regulations (2006) *The Education (Nutritional Standards for School Lunches) (England) Regulations 2006. Statutory Instrument No. 2381*. The Stationery Office, London. Available at: http://www.legislation.gov.uk/uksi/2006/2381/contents/made (accessed 11 June 2013).

The Education Regulations (2007) *The Education (Nutritional Standards and Requirements for School Food) (England) Regulations 2007. Statutory Instrument No. 2359*. The Stationery Office, London. Available at: http://www.legislation.gov.uk/uksi/2007/2359/contents/made (accessed 11 June 2013).

The Education Regulations (2008) *The Education (Nutritional Standards and Requirements for School Food) (England) (Amendment) Regulations 2008. Statutory Instrument No. 1800*. The Stationery Office, London. Available at: http://www.legislation.gov.uk/uksi/2008/1800/contents/made (accessed 11 June 2013).

The Education Regulations (2011) *The Education (Nutritional Standards and Requirements for School Food) (England) (Amendment) Regulations 2011. Statutory Instrument No. 1190*. The Stationery Office, London. Available at: http://www.legislation.gov.uk/uksi/2011/1190/contents/made (accessed 11 June 2013).

13 Animal Source Foods as a Food-based Approach to Improve Diet and Nutrition Outcomes

Charlotte G. Neumann,[1]* Nimrod O. Bwibo,[2] Constance A. Gewa[3] and Natalie Drorbaugh[4]

[1]*University of California, Los Angeles (UCLA), California, USA;* [2]*University of Nairobi, Nairobi, Kenya;* [3]*George Mason University, Fairfax, Virginia, USA;* [4]*Public Health Nutrition Consultant, Los Angeles, California, USA*

Summary

Animal source foods (ASFs), particularly meat of a wide variety, fish, fowl meat, milk, eggs, snails, worms and other small animals supply not only high-quality and readily digested protein and energy, but also readily absorbable and bioavailable micronutrients. The inclusion of ASFs in the diet promotes growth, cognitive function, physical activity and health, and is particularly important for children and pregnant women. The importance of ASF consumption for health and nutritional outcomes has been documented in observational settings and, more recently, in intervention studies. A recent Kenyan study provides causal evidence that adding even a modest amount of meat to the diet of schoolchildren improves cognitive function and school performance, physical activity, growth (increased lean body mass), micronutrient status and morbidity. Outcomes from several nutrition interventions promoting ASF production and consumption have also demonstrated improvements in nutritional outcomes. Non-governmental organizations (NGOs) have played a key role in promoting ASFs in the diets of populations in low-income countries and in addressing issues that constrain household production and utilization of ASFs, and the chapter provides examples of the activities of several NGOs operating in Africa. In addition to current strategies, small freshwater fish and rabbits are two ASF sources with great potential for addressing nutritional deficiencies that have not received sufficient attention. Even modest amounts of meat and other ASFs in the diet from a variety of sources can greatly improve the overall nutrition and micronutrient status, health and function of rural populations.

Introduction

The inclusion of animal source foods (ASFs) in the diet is an important food-based strategy for improving nutrition outcomes globally. Fish, fowl, milk, eggs and insects or other protein sources, such as worms, snails, molluscs and other small animals, supply not only high-quality and readily digested protein and energy, but also readily absorbable and bioavailable micronutrients (Neumann *et al.*, 2002). ASFs are inherently richer sources of specific micronutrients, particularly iron, zinc, riboflavin, vitamin A, vitamin B_{12} and

---

*Contact: cneumann@ucla.edu

calcium than are plant foods (Murphy and Allen, 2003). Meat and milk are not nutritionally equivalent, and milk cannot be a substitute for meat as it does not provide the same nutrient mix as meat; therefore, meat and milk are not interchangeable (Table 13.1). Overall, red meat (beef, lamb, pork) has a somewhat higher zinc and iron content than other meats, such as poultry and fish. Milk, eggs and fish are important sources of preformed vitamin A, and fish and milk provide calcium and phosphorus (Hansen et al., 1998). Vitamin B_{12} is provided nearly exclusively by meat and milk (Watanabe, 2007).

The inclusion of ASFs in the diet has been shown to promote growth, cognitive function, physical activity and health. The relatively high fat content of ASFs increases energy density, which is particularly useful in young children, given their relatively small gastric volume. Milk and other dairy products and meat provide high-quality, readily digestible and complete protein containing all the essential amino acids (Williamson et al., 2005). The need for ASFs is particularly important during pregnancy when iron, zinc, calcium,

vitamin B_{12}, folic acid and high-quality protein are necessary to support maternal nutritional needs, fetal growth and development, and preparation for lactation (Allen, 2005). ASFs are important complementary foods in preschool and school-aged children for supporting optimal growth and development (Brown et al., 1995). Schoolchildren also need ASFs for adequate nutrition to sustain and improve cognitive development, physical activity and behaviours conducive to learning (Grantham-McGregor and Ani, 1999; Neumann et al., 2002; Black, 2003). Children in developing countries frequently suffer infections that lead to a decrease in total food intake, impaired absorption and increased nutrient losses, which can result in impaired linear growth.

Additionally, typical weaning diets contain little or no ASFs, except for varying, but usually small, amounts of non-human milk with very low available iron, zinc and vitamin A. The diets are also very low in energy density, and in order to obtain an adequate intake the child would have to greatly exceed its gastric volumetric capacity. Even modest amounts of

Table 13.1. Major micronutrients (per 100 g) contained in selected animal source foods (ASFs).[a] From Leung et al. (1972); West et al. (1987); DeFoliart (1992); Nettleton and Exler (1992); American Academy of Pediatrics (1997); Pennington (1998); Grantham-McGregor and Ani (1999); Shils et al. (1999); Neumann et al. (2002); Murphy and Allen (2003); Roos et al. (2003b); USDA (2006).

Animal source food (ASF)	Iron (mg)	Zinc (mg)	Vitamin B_{12} (µg)	Vitamin A[b] (µg RAE[c])	Calcium (mg)
Meat					
Beef, medium fat, cooked	0.32 (available)	2.05 (available)	1.87	15	8
Goat meat (moderately fat)	2.3	4.0	1.13	0	11
Liver, beef	10	4.9	52.7	1500	8
Mutton	2	2.9	2.2	10	10
Pork	1.8	4.4	5.5	2	11
Poultry	1.1	4.0	0.10	85	10
Milk					
Whole, unfortified	0.01	0.18	0.39	55	119
Fish					
Freshwater fish, raw	1.8	0.09	2.2	43 IU[d]	175
Small fish (<25 cm)	5.7	0.33	2.1	100	776
Other ASFs					
Caterpillars	2.3	At least 10	Not available	Not available	185
Hen's eggs, cooked	3.2	0.9 (raw)	2.0 (raw)	500	61
Rabbit	2.4	2.4	6.5	0	20
Termites (fresh)	1.0	Not available	Not available	0?	12

[a]Nutrient content values are approximate and based on multiple sources; [b]Vitamin A content varies with cooking method; [c]RAE, retinol activity equivalents; [d]IU, international unit.

ASFs (2 oz/day, ~59 ml/day) incorporated into weaning diets can increase the diet energy density, through their fat content, and can supply vitamin B_{12}, preformed vitamin A, available iron and zinc from haem iron, and protein of high biological value (Neumann et al., 2003, 2007). Additionally, ASFs can contribute to alleviation of protein-energy malnutrition (PEM) and various micronutrient deficiencies. Hence, their inclusion in the diet of these population groups (pregnant women, preschool and school-aged children) is an essential strategy for improving intake of essential nutrients and nutritional status.

Food-based approaches offer more protection and sustainability than the use of non-food supplements. The addition of modest amounts of meat, fish, poultry and other ASFs to the diet can greatly improve the health, micronutrient and overall nutrient status and function of rural populations, particularly of women and children (Marquis et al., 1997; Neumann et al., 2002; Allen, 2005). The importance of ASF consumption for improving health, nutritional status and cognitive function has been documented in observational settings and, more recently, in intervention studies (Neumann et al., 2003).

Evidence on the Impact of the Consumption of Animal Source Foods (ASFs)

Early observational evidence

The beneficial role of ASFs in the diets of pregnant women and young children was highlighted by findings from the Human Nutrition Collaborative Research Support Program (NCRSP). This longitudinal observational study, which was conducted from 1983 to 1987 in rural Kenya, rural Mexico and a semi-rural area of Egypt, reported significant statistical associations between the intake of ASFs and increased rates of growth and cognitive development, high levels of physical activity, positive pregnancy outcomes and decreased morbidity in three parallel longitudinal observational studies (Allen et al., 1992; Kirksey et al., 1992;

Neumann et al., 1992). In the NCRSP studies, it emerged that those children who consumed little or no animal products, particularly meat, performed least well on cognitive tests measuring verbal comprehension, and abstract and performance perceptual abilities, as evaluated by the Raven's Progressive Matrices (RPM) (Raven, 1960). In addition, those children consuming the fewest animal products were the least attentive in the classroom, less physically active and showed the least amount of leadership behaviour in the playground during free play (Sigman et al., 1989; Espinosa et al., 1992). Additionally, the greatest deficits in linear growth were found in those with little or no ASF in their diets (Neumann and Harrison, 1994). The evidence from these longitudinal observational studies (after statistically controlling for an array of covariates) strongly suggested a positive link between the intake of ASF and improved cognitive, behavioural and physical development (Sigman et al., 1989; Allen et al., 1992; Kirksey et al., 1992; Neumann et al., 1992; Neumann and Harrison, 1994).

Additional observational evidence on the positive association of intake of ASF and linear growth was obtained in a study of 12–15 month-old Peruvian toddlers (Marquis et al., 1997). Complementary foods – consisting of ASFs and breast milk – were all found to promote the linear growth of toddlers. Growth was also positively associated with intake of ASFs in children with low intakes of complementary foods. Intake of animal protein (meat, fish) showed a positive and statistically significant relationship with height in studies in New Guinea (Smith et al., 1993) and in South and Central America (Allen et al., 1992; Black, 1998).

In addition to human milk, both cow's and goat's milk consumption have been linked to improvement in the physical growth of children. Non-governmental organizations (NGOs) working with dairy cattle and goats (Heifer Project International, Farm Africa and an International Livestock Research Institute study in Ethiopia) have presented data that show increased milk consumption and child growth in households raising livestock (Shapiro et al., 1998). Increased income generation may also be a factor in improved growth, mediated through improved health care and the purchase of animal products, although this was not documented. A number of studies with varying designs in various disparate locations all show that cow's milk consumption by infants and young children promotes physical growth, particularly in length or height (Takahashi, 1984; Walker *et al.*, 1990; Guldan *et al.*, 1993).

Experimental evidence of the positive impact of ASF consumption

The positive associations observed between meat intake and physical growth, cognitive function and school performance and physical activity in the NCRSP studies (described above) stimulated a further study in Kenya from 1998 to 2001, which used a randomized, controlled feeding intervention study design. Results from this 2 year Child Nutrition Project (CNP) provided causal evidence for the important benefits of meat on growth, cognition, behaviours and activity in rural Kenyan school-aged children.

The CNP study was designed as a randomized, controlled isocaloric feeding intervention study with three different additions to the local traditional plant-based dish *githeri* (made of maize, beans and greens): ground beef (meat group), whole milk (milk group), or vegetable fat to render the plain *githeri* group isocaloric. A control group received no intervention school feeding but was compensated by the gift of milk goats at the end of the study, at one per family – a gift of the parent's choice. Children received mid-morning 'snacks' every day they attended school. The control group participated in all measurements but did not receive this intervention feeding. The snacks for all three intervention groups were based on *githeri*, as described above. For the meat group, finely minced beef (Farmer's Choice, Nairobi, Kenya), with 10–12% fat, was added to the *githeri*. Members of the milk group were given a glass (250 ml) of ultra-heat treated (UHT) whole cow's milk in addition to the basic *githeri*. The plain *githeri* group received *githeri* with extra oil (Kimbo, Unilever, East African Industries, Nairobi,

Kenya), which was added to equalize the energy content of the three snacks. The oil was used in all three types of *githeri*, but the greatest amount was added to the plain *githeri*. Midway through the study, the oil was found to be fortified with retinol (37 μg/g), although it had not initially been labelled as such. Ingredients were increased by ~25% after a year as the children increased in size and drought conditions continued. Feedings were designed to offer ~20% of the required daily energy intake. Snacks furnished ~250 kcal (~1060 kJ)/day (Table 13.2). This design allowed an examination of cause and effect relationships between meat intake and functional outcomes and also allowed controlling for intervening confounding variables.

Twelve schools in Embu District of Kenya were randomized to one of the three types of feeding or to the control group, with three schools assigned to each condition. Feeding occurred on every day that children attended school. Data were collected at baseline and longitudinally over seven 3-month school terms (2.25 years). There were two cohorts, with ~500 children and ~375 children, respectively, enrolled exactly a year apart. The second cohort was enrolled because of a 6 week teachers' strike early in the study and a prolonged drought throughout the first year. The usual daily intake was assessed by semi-quantitative 24 h recall from the mother and from the child, if present. Measurements of head and upper arm circumference, height, weight, and of triceps and subscapular skin folds, were obtained longitudinally. Mid-upper arm circumference and fat folds were used to derive indices such as arm fat area, arm muscle area and body mass index (BMI). Behavioural and activity assessments, and cognitive tests, were carried out. Cognitive testing included the Verbal Meaning Test designed in East Africa, Digit Span – a measure of short-term memory for children aged 7 years and over (Weschler, 1974), and Raven's Progressive Matrices (RPM) – a nonverbal test of performance, abstract reasoning, perception and problem solving (fluid intelligence) (Raven, 1960). End-of-term examination scores were obtained from the head teacher's office. Physical activity and behaviours were measured by observation techniques

Table 13.2. Nutrient content of school snacks containing the local plant-based dish of *githeri* in Kenya.

	Githeri + meat	*Githeri* + milk	Plain *githeri* + extra oil
Year 1			
Serving size	185 g (includes 60 g meat)	100 g + 200 ml milk	185 g + 3 g oil
Energy, kcal	239	241	240
Energy, kJ	1028	1063	1032
Protein, g	19.2	12.7	7.9
Iron, mg (total)	2.42	1.52	3.16[a]
Zinc, mg (total)	2.38	1.46	1.35
Vitamin B_{12}, µg	0.75	0.96	0.0
Years 2 and 3: Jan 1999–Mar 2001			
Serving size	225 g (includes 85 g meat)	100 g + 250 ml milk	230 g + 3.8 g oil
Energy, kcal	313	313	313
Energy, kJ	1346	1346	1346
Protein, g	21.7	15.2	8.4
Iron, mg (total)	2.94	1.57	3.93[a]
Zinc, mg (total)	2.89	1.66	1.68
Vitamin B_{12}, µg	0.91	1.16	0.0

[a]Total iron presented. The actual percentage absorbed would be ~5 owing to the high phytate and fibre content of the plant-based *githeri*.

using time sampling to obtain estimates of child physical activity, behaviours and social interaction during unstructured play in the schoolyard, and activity and attentiveness in the classroom. Venous blood samples were obtained at baseline and at the end of years 1 and 2. Biochemical analyses of micronutrients were carried out only for cohort I. Morbidity data were collected every 1–2 months, with 15 home visits per child over the 2.25 years. Fifteen morbidity outcome variables were assessed; these consisted of signs and symptoms found in commonly prevalent conditions.

At baseline, total protein intake was normal, but little or no animal source protein was consumed. Stunting and underweight were present in ~30% of children. Biochemical and food intake analyses confirmed anaemia and multiple micronutrient deficiencies (of iron, zinc, vitamin B_{12}, vitamin A, riboflavin and calcium) at baseline (Siekmann et al., 2003). The mean age of children at baseline was 7.4 years (range 6–14 years).

Cognitive function and school performance

The results of the intervention showed that compared with all other groups, the meat group exhibited the greatest statistically significant rate of increase in scores over time in the RPM test, which measures abstract reasoning, problem solving, reasoning by analogy and perceptual awareness of sequences (Fig. 13.1) (Neumann et al., 2007). No significant differences were seen in scores on tests of verbal meaning and in Digit Span tests. The plain *githeri* and meat groups performed significantly better over time in tests of arithmetic ability than did the milk and control groups (Whaley et al., 2003). Improvements in zone-wide end-of-term school examinations showed that the meat group obtained statistically significantly greater gains in total test scores and scores in arithmetic tests compared with all other groups (Fig. 13.2).

Playground activity

The greatest increase in the amount of time students spent in high levels of physical activity during free play and the greatest decrease in time spent in low levels of physical activity were seen in the meat group (Sigman et al., 2005). Moreover, the meat group showed the greatest increase in initiative and in leadership behaviours among peers during recess free play (Sigman et al., 2005). All increases were statistically significant. Children in the plain *githeri* group were also more active and displayed more initiative and leadership behaviours than those in

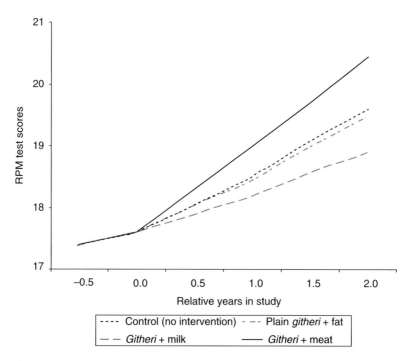

Fig. 13.1. Changes in Raven's Progressive Matrices (RPM) test scores of Kenyan schoolchildren given different intervention diets, or with no intervention (control) by relative years in study, over a 2 year period from 1998 to 2001. From Neumann *et al.* (2007). *Githeri* is a local plant-based dish.

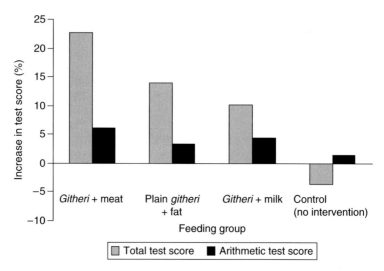

Fig. 13.2. Increases in end-of-term examination scores (total test scores and arithmetic test scores) of Kenyan schoolchildren (Cohort II, see text) given different intervention diets, or with no intervention (control), from 1998 to 2001. From Neumann *et al.* (2007).

the milk and control groups, although not nearly as much so as in the meat group. The milk group performed the most poorly of the three intervention groups.

Growth

The meat group and, to a lesser extent, the milk group, showed the steepest and most highly statistically significant gain in arm muscle area (indicative of lean body mass) compared with all other groups (Grillenberger et al., 2003, 2006) (Fig. 13.3). Compared with the control group, increases in weight were observed in all children supplemented with any type of intervention feeding. Although no overall significant differences in height were seen in any one of the groups, in the 6–7 year old children and the stunted children, the milk group showed improved linear growth rates. Milk was also found to improve both weight gain and growth in the stunted and the younger children in the study. None of the other groups showed any significant rate of gain in height.

Micronutrient status

After the first year of the intervention feeding, plasma concentrations of vitamin B_{12}, haemoglobin, serum iron and retinol increased significantly in all groups (all $P < 0.01$) (Siekmann et al., 2003). The greatest improvement was seen in vitamin B_{12} status and was observed mainly in the meat and milk groups (Siekmann et al., 2003; McLean et al., 2007). In the meat group, median plasma vitamin B_{12} concentrations increased from 131 pmol/l to 189 pmol/l, and in the milk group, concentrations increased from 164 pmol/l to 236 pmol/l ($P < 0.01$ for both groups) (Siekmann et al., 2003). The increases in plasma vitamin B_{12} concentration were not significantly different between the milk and meat groups; in both of these groups, the prevalence of severe vitamin B_{12} deficiency decreased – from 46.8% to 21.4% in the meat group and from 30.6% to 9.7% in the milk group (Siekmann et al., 2003).

Morbidity

The control group showed the highest prevalence of occurrences of morbidity and the least decline in morbidity over time of all groups. The meat group had a significant decline in diarrhoeal diseases ($P = 0.037$) and typhoid ($P = 0.050$) compared with all other groups, and in jaundice compared with the plain *githeri* group. The milk group showed a significant decrease in upper respiratory infections compared with other groups ($P < 0.05$). For malaria and total illness, the significantly

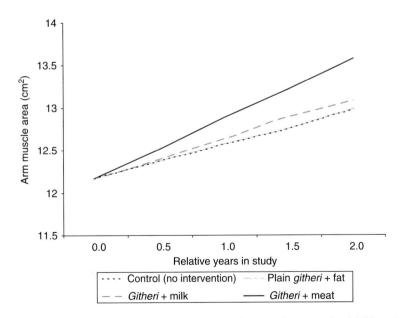

Fig. 13.3. Increases in lean body mass (measured as arm muscle area) of Kenyan schoolchildren given different intervention diets, or with no intervention (control), from 1998 to 2001. Note that the plain *githeri* + fat and the control groups have nearly identical slopes. Adapted from Neumann et al. (2010). *Githeri* is a local plant-based dish.

greatest declines were seen in the plain *githeri* and the meat groups. The slightly greater decline in total illness observed in the plain *githeri* group compared with the meat group was not statistically significant and may possibly have been due to the substantial vitamin A fortification of the fat that was added to the plain *githeri* supplement to equalize its energy content with that of the milk and meat snacks. The brand of cooking fat used (Kimbo) had been fortified with vitamin A by the manufacturer, but had not been labelled as such until later on in the study.

This was the first randomized, controlled intervention study to show positive causal effects of meat intake on cognitive and school performance, physical activity levels, behaviours, lean body mass, nutritional status and selected morbidity measures. These findings demonstrate that the inclusion of meat in the diet has multiple positive functional impacts. Schoolchildren need diets containing adequate quantity and quality for optimal learning.

Other evidence for positive impacts of ASF on health and development

Recent studies have also documented the benefits of food-based approaches that integrate meat or other ASFs. A recently completed study in Guatemalan children reports improvements in vitamin B_{12} status and development following supplementation with beef or vitamin B_{12} (Allen *et al.*, 2007).

A quasi-experimental community-based dietary intervention in Malawi, involving dietary diversification with an increase in fish utilization, found significant improvement in the lean body mass of stunted children and a lower incidence of anaemia after 12 months. Further, common infections, reported by mothers in their children, were lower in the intervention group (Yeudall *et al.*, 2002).

In Asia, results from the Homestead Food Production (HFP) Program, which combines instruction for women of poor households in home gardening, small livestock production for the consumption of eggs, meat and liver, and nutrition education, show that this approach has led to increased intake of micronutrient-rich foods in Bangladesh (Iannotti *et al.*,, 2009). Additionally, improvement in vitamin A intake and anaemia prevalence in mothers and children participating in the HFP intervention group (compared with the control group) has been reported (Stallkamp *et al.*, 2007). In Nepal, a decline in anaemia prevalence in women in the HFP intervention group (compared with the control group) has been reported (Talukder *et al.*, 2007). In children in Nepal and Cambodia under the HFP programme, only non-significant declines in anaemia prevalence were reported in the Nepalese children, and no change was seen in the Cambodian children (Talukder *et al.*, 2007).

In Vietnam, reductions in the incidence of diarrhoeal infections, respiratory infections, pneumonia/severe pneumonia and stunting were observed in children in intervention group households, following an intervention that included nutrition education and household food production (English *et al.*, 1997; Schroeder *et al.*, 2002; Sripaipan *et al.*, 2002).

New and Ongoing Randomized Feeding Trials

The Kenya CNP randomized controlled feeding study has stimulated various other studies on the amelioration of nutrient deficiencies in both infants and children using a variety of types of meat. In China, an intervention is in progress that is providing pureed pork as a complementary food to toddlers from age 6 to 18 months; this is being compared with the provision of a complementary food based on a plant recipe. Local doctors supervise the distribution and the feeding of the meat (lean pork) meal or the plant meal daily in the homes of the participant families 7 days a week. Longitudinal measures, including growth, infections and cognitive development are being assessed (M. Hambidge, personal communication, 2008).

Another study is just beginning in rural Vietnam to assess the effect of ASF supplements (alternating days of seafood, fish, meat and fowl) before and during pregnancy on a number of outcomes, including birth weight, prematurity rate, infant growth and infections (J. King, personal communication, 2010).

A further study is currently under way in Eldoret, Kenya, as part of the Academic Model Providing Access to Healthcare (AMPATH) at Moi University (Eldoret, Kenya) in collaboration with Indiana University. This study is assessing the impact of meat biscuits versus soy biscuits versus control wheat biscuits in a randomized, controlled study of HIV-positive drug-naive women and their affected and infected children. The main outcomes being assessed are body composition (particularly lean body mass), muscle strength, nutritional status, immune function, morbidity, child growth and development, physical activity measured by time allocation observations, and biochemical nutrient status (Ernst *et al.*, 2008).

Discussion

Challenges in increasing ASF consumption in low-income populations

The role of non-governmental organizations (NGOs)

In Africa, NGOs play an important role in the promotion of ASF production and consumption. Small animal husbandry for household consumption, and secondarily for income-generation, is being promoted by a number of NGOs as a strategy for improving nutritional outcomes in populations with little access to ASFs. At the household level, small animals can provide a variety of products, including meat, milk, butter, yogurt and fat, to meet nutritional needs. Two projects are under way in Malawi, through World Vision. In the Orphaned and Vulnerable Children Enablement Project, households are provided with chicken, goats or rabbits for breeding, and offspring are given to other households. The Integrated Fish Farming Project supplies local farmers with the training and resources to raise pond fish (such as tilapia) to improve local diets.

The Farm Africa Kenya Dairy Goat and Capacity Building Project provides Toggenburg goats to communities in Ethiopia and other East African countries, along with training on how to cross-breed with local goats to produce high-milk-yielding goats. Another NGO – Heifer Project International – provides livestock and animal care training to improve the nutrition of families and generate income. This organization provides animal donations to families as 'living loans', and in exchange for their livestock and training, the families agree to give one of their animal's offspring to another family in need; this is called Passing on the Gift. The animals provided to families are specific to the conditions of the area. In Kenya, Heifer provides goats, which mainly supply milk for consumption by the family. Extra milk is sold for income generation or to make other products. Manure from the goats can also be used to fertilize gardens.

Freedom from Hunger provides credit and micro-loans to poor women. Frequent loan repayment meetings include intense nutrition education. This type of microcredit can help to promote nutrition improvement in combination with maternal education and income generation by providing small loans to start small businesses. Small animal husbandry is being tested in multiple sites in Ghana though the GLCRSP (Global Livestock Collaborative Research Support Program) and Freedom From Hunger project called 'Enhancing Child Nutrition through Animal Source Food Management' (ENAM) (Global Livestock CRSP, 2005). This project has documented an increased diversity of ASFs in the diet when mothers had ASF-based income generation (Global Livestock CRSP, 2007; Sakyi-Dawson *et al.*, 2009). Just as important as the income generation is the mother's increase in knowledge of nutrition and the importance of ASFs.

Issues with raising livestock in Africa

A number of issues pose challenges in raising livestock and other small animals, particularly in Africa, but elsewhere as well. Insufficient grazing land and forage impose certain limitations on livestock raising in Africa, as access to or ownership of land is often necessary for this. Poultry that are not free range require feed, which is often costly, and also need immunizations. Veterinary care, including immunizations and disease care, is scant and expensive, with poor households having limited access to such services. There is also a shortage of agricultural extension education and services by women for women. These services are badly needed, because women and children provide the bulk of care for small household animals (Ayele and Peacock, 2003; Smitasiri and Chotiboriboon, 2003). Some innovative programmes that have begun to address these issues include the training and utilization of community-based women animal health workers in various districts of Kenya. In the Paravet programmes, Kenyan women veterinarians train local women to take care of animals, provide simple treatments for minor conditions and carry out immunizations (Jones *et al.*, 1998; Mugunieri *et al.*, 2004, 2005). This has been a great success, albeit not a very widespread programme.

Another problem with rearing animals, including fish, for consumption, is the need for preservation of the meat to prevent spoilage in the absence of refrigeration. Household and community initiatives for food preservation are needed to prevent wastage and to ensure a steady supply of ASF, especially for poor areas and households where purchasing meat in the cash economy is not affordable. Various preservation techniques and methods of incorporating ASF into diets have been successful. Creative solutions have included blood biscuits and cereals fortified with dried blood, which are utilized in Latin America and in parts of Africa, and have resulted in improved iron status (Calvo *et al.*, 1989; Olivares *et al.*, 1990; Walter *et al.*, 1993; Kikafunda and Sserumaga, 2005).

Smoking and solar drying are common options for producing safe, shelf-stable products under controlled conditions. Although canned meat products are widely consumed in the Pacific Islands, they are not generally affordable, available, or culturally acceptable as food for children in rural sub-Saharan Africa. In the Kenyan NutriBusiness project, community women's groups produce weaning foods by solar drying excess legumes and vegetables. Rabbit and chicken meat have been dried to produce finger foods such as chips that can also be powdered for inclusion in weaning porridge (Muroki *et al.*, 1997;

Maretzki and Mills, 2003; Maretzki, 2007; Mills *et al.*, 2007). Also in the NutriBusiness project, weaning mixes are sold for income generation, as are products that do not contain meat. This successful approach is now being carried out in several African countries.

Neglected available sources of high-quality ASF

Small freshwater fish

Small freshwater fish provide an important source of protein, iron, zinc, calcium and preformed vitamin A, and they are an excellent source of calcium when consumed whole (Roos *et al.*, 2003a,b, 2007). Studies in Bangladesh have documented how *mola* fish can potentially ameliorate vitamin A, calcium and other micronutrient deficiencies (Roos *et al.*, 2003a,b). In Africa, the *omena* (*Rastrineobola argentea*) fish has great potential as an ASF food source to address multiple nutritional issues.

The *omena* is a small freshwater fish about 2 inches (~5 cm) long and is found in Lake Victoria and other large lakes in East Africa. It is known by multiple names, including *omena* in Kenya, *mukene* in Uganda and *fulu* in Tanzania. On the Kenyan side, it comprises about 44% of the total catch of fish from Lake Victoria, and at one time *omena* comprised 70% of the fish catches in Lake Victoria (Abila, 2003). It is considered a 'poor man's fish' and a 'low-value' product due to its relatively low commercial value (Kabahenda and Husken, 2009). Yet, because of their low price, these fish are accessible to poor rural and urban populations in large areas of Africa. *Omena* has a relatively long shelf life and can be sold fresh. However, the fish is more often salted and dried and this product is available for purchase in many markets in East Africa. The dried form is relatively affordable and has a long shelf life. When eaten whole, it provides a source of complete protein, in addition to oil, iron, zinc, calcium, magnesium and other micronutrients, and can make a major contribution to food security and diet quality improvement (Table 13.3). *Omena* has been used occasionally in hospitals and clinics to supplement the diet of patients, and in

Table 13.3. Nutrient content (per 100 g) of *omena* fish (*Rastrineobola argentea*) and rabbit. From Pennington (1998); Kabahenda and Husken (2009).

	Carbohydrates	Protein	Fat	Iron (mg)	Zinc (mg)	Calcium (g)	Vitamin B$_{12}$ (µg)
Omena fish	66.1 (%)	29.2 (%)	0.78 (%)	8.2	10.1	159.2	Data not available
Rabbit	0.0 (g)	30.4 (g)	8.4 (g)	2.4	2.4	0.02	6.5

combination with maize–soy blend products provided by international organizations, with reports of improved nutritional outcomes. While few evaluations of the use of *omena* have been published, there has been one recent study presented that used *omena* fish to prevent and control iron deficiency anaemia in adolescent girls (Masabe, 2010).

Ironically, *omena* is being greatly diverted from human consumption and now comprises a large proportion (50–65%) of the fishmeal used for livestock and feed for larger fish species (such as the Nile perch) (Abila, 2003). There has been an increase in demand for *omena* by neighbouring African countries, as well as by Saudi Arabia, Europe and Japan. This poses a major threat to food security for poor local populations. There are continuing reports of increasing malnutrition occurring in populations that live in major fish-exporting areas of East Africa. Trade control measures are needed to ensure that the availability of *omena* for local human consumption and food security is in balance with exports of this product.

Rabbits

Small-scale rabbit husbandry is a practical solution to supply meat at the household level in many parts of the world. Rabbit meat is a rich source of energy, protein and micronutrients, especially iron, zinc and calcium (Table 13.3). It also provides more protein, less fat and energy per gram than beef, pork, lamb or chicken. Currently, the bulk of rabbits are raised for consumption in Europe and the USA (Lebas *et al.*, 1997), but high-scale urban restaurants in Africa and elsewhere are now serving rabbit meat as a luxury dish. While rabbit meat production has increased in parts of Africa and Asia, in many countries livestock is still the generally preferred meat source (Lebas *et al.*, 1997).

Rabbits offer multiple advantages as a source of ASF. In captivity, they are relatively disease free, consume a wide variety of fibrous vegetation and breed rapidly (Cheeke, 1984). In ideal conditions, some species produce as many as eight to nine litters a year, with four to eight offspring per litter (Cheeke, 1984). This means that one male and four females could produce approximately 3000 offspring (or 1450 kg of meat) in a year. Rabbits are also able to tolerate moderate amounts of heat and other harsh conditions. Cages for protection from rain and predators can be made from simple materials such as used wooden crates or wire mesh. Rabbit raising is now being incorporated into scattered school programmes, such as in boarding schools or rural day schools, in Africa. Rabbits enjoyed sporadic and short-lived attention from FAO (Food and Agriculture Organization of the United Nations) and certain NGOs in the 1990s; however, this neglected ASF source now deserves reconsideration as it has potential to address nutrient deficiencies at the household level at very low cost – because the food and housing needs of these animals are minimal.

Concluding Remarks

The addition of modest amounts of meat and other ASFs to the diet from a variety of sources can greatly improve the overall energy, protein and micronutrient status, health and function of rural populations (Neumann *et al.*, 2002, 2003; Allen, 2005). Investing in diet improvement for children and women of reproductive age would maximize the chances of improving growth, cognitive development and school performance of children, and pregnancy outcomes (Neumann *et al.*, 2002). ASF would also improve adult work performance and productivity by improving iron and overall nutrition status (Diaz *et al.*, 1991).

Nutrition improvement is vital and should be an integral part of health, education and development efforts. Food-based approaches using ASFs in rural areas with many subsistence families are more likely to be sustainable in improving diet quality and energy density than 'pill-based' approaches. While food-based solutions are more complex and interdisciplinary in nature, and require long-term commitments, they are more likely to address malnutrition at its source, leading to long-term sustainable improvements. Additional intervention studies are needed to document the impact and complexities of using ASFs as a food-based approach to the improvement of nutrition and health. Interventions that are currently under way that promote ASF consumption need to include more rigorous evaluation to document strategies, problems and outcomes.

Putting 'meat on the table' requires a supply of small animals within the production capabilities of smallholder farmers and their families. Extension workers, preferably women, need to provide technical support and nutrition education to women to assist in household animal production and in the preparation, preservation and feeding of such ASFs, principally meat, to children and young women of reproductive age. The inclusion of ASFs is a potentially sustainable approach to improve nutrition at the household level, particularly through strategies that involve small animal husbandry and fish raising at the household level, mainly for household consumption but with some degree of income generation. Improved nutritional status is important in building human capital and is a first and fundamental step to reducing poverty and promoting social and economic development.

Acknowledgements

The Child Nutrition Project (CNP) study 'Role of Animal Source Foods to Improve Diet Quality and Growth and Development in Kenyan SchoolChildren' was supported by the Global Livestock Collaborative Research Support Program (GL-CRSP) directed by Montague W. Demment, whose broad vision encompassed the inclusion of human nutrition as part of livestock development; it was also supported by USAID (Subgrant No. DAN-1328-G-00-0046-00), by the James A. Coleman African Study Center (UCLA), and was funded in part by the National Cattlemen's Beef Association (PCE-G-98-00036-00). Dr Marian Sigman, a child development expert, directed the cognitive, activity and behavioural aspects with the assistance of Dr Shannon Whaley. Dr Robert Weiss directed statistical analyses. Dr Lindsay H. Allen directed biochemical assessment. Dr Suzanne Murphy directed the food intake analysis and developed the nutrient database for Embu. Monika Grillenberger, Erin Reid and Jonathan Siekmann also conducted fieldwork and analysis of data. Pía Chaparro contributed to the development of this chapter. The authors thank the families and schools of Embu who participated in the study and the Ministry of Health.

References

Abila, R.O. (2003) *Fish Trade and Food Security: Are They Reconcilable in Lake Victoria?* FAO Fisheries Report No. 708, Food and Agriculture Organization of the United Nations, Rome.

Allen, L.H. (2005) Multiple micronutrients in pregnancy and lactation: an overview. *The American Journal of Clinical Nutrition* 81, 1206S–1212S.

Allen, L.H., Backstrand, J.R., Chávez, A. and Pelto, G.H. (1992) *People Cannot Live by Tortillas Alone: The Results of the Mexico Nutrition CRSP. Final Report of Mexico Project.* Human Nutrition Collaborative Research Program, US Agency for International Development, Washington, DC/ Department of Nutritional Sciences, University of Connecticut, Storrs, Connecticut/Instituto Nacional de Ciencias Médicas y Nutrición Salvador Zubirán, Mexico City, Mexico.

Allen, L.H., Ramirez-Zea, M., Zuleta, C., Mejia, R.M., Jones, K.M., Demment, M.W, and Black, M. (2007) Vitamin B-12 status and development of young Guatemalan children: effects of beef and B-12 supplements. In: *Experimental Biology 2007 Meeting, April 28–May 5, 2007, Washington, DC.* ASPET (The American Society for Pharmacology and Experimental Therapeutics, Bethesda, Maryland. *The FASEB Journal* 21(Meeting Abstracts Suppl.) A681:674.3. Available at: http://www.fasebj.org/cgi/content/meeting_abstract/21/5/A681 (accessed 13 June 2013).

American Academy of Pediatrics (1997) *Pediatric Nutrition Handbook.* American Academy of Pediatrics, Evenston, Illinois.

Ayele, Z. and Peacock, C. (2003) Improving access to and consumption of animal source foods in rural households: the experiences of a women-focused goat development program in the highlands of Ethiopia. *Journal of Nutrition* 133(11, Suppl. 2), 3981S–3986S.

Black, M.M. (1998) Zinc deficiency and child development. *The American Journal of Clinical Nutrition* 68 (2, Suppl.), 464S–469S.

Black, M.M. (2003) Micronutrient deficiencies and cognitive functioning. *Journal of Nutrition* 133(11, Suppl. 2), 3927S–3931S.

Brown, K.H., Creed-Kanashiro, H. and Dewey, K.G. (1995) Optimal complementary feeding practices to prevent childhood malnutrition in developing countries. *Food and Nutrition Bulletin* 16, 320–339.

Calvo, E., Hertrampf, E., de Pablo, S., Amar, M. and Stekel, A. (1989) Haemoglobin-fortified cereal: an alternative weaning food with high iron bioavailability. *European Journal of Clinical Nutrition* 43, 237–243.

Cheeke, P.R. (1984) Potential of rabbit production in tropical and subtropical agricultural systems. *Journal of Animal Science* 63, 1581–1586.

DeFoliart, G.R. (1992) Insects as human food. *Crop Protection* 11, 395–399.

Diaz, E., Goldberg, G.R., Taylor, M., Savage, J.M., Sellen, D., Coward, W.A. and Prentice, A.M. (1991) Effects of dietary supplementation on work performance in Gambian laborers. *The American Journal of Clinical Nutrition* 53, 803–811.

English, R.M., Badcock, J.C., Giay, T., Ngu, T., Waters, A.M. and Bennett, S.A. (1997) Effect of nutrition improvement project on morbidity from infectious diseases in preschool children in Viet Nam: comparison with control commune. *British Medical Journal* 315, 1122–1125.

Ernst, J., Ettyang, G., Neumann, C.G., Nyandiko, W.M., Siika, A. and Yiannoutsos, C.T. (2008) *Introduction to the HIV Nutrition Project (HNP): Increasing Animal Source Foods (ASF) in Diets of HIV-infected Kenyan Women and Their Children.* Research Brief 08-01-HNP, Global Livestock Collaborative Research Support Program (CRSP), Davis, California. Available at: http://crsps.net/wp-content/downloads/Global%20Livestock/Inventoried%207.16/2-2008-2-175.pdf (accessed 12 June 2013).

Espinosa, M.P., Sigman, M., Neumann, C.G., Bwibo, N.O. and McDonald, M.A. (1992) Playground behaviors of school-age children in relation to nutrition, schooling, and family characteristics. *Developmental Psychology* 28, 1188–1195.

Global Livestock CRSP (2005) *Global Livestock CRSP: Annual Report 2005.* Collaborative Research Support Program, University of California, Davis, California.

Global Livestock CRSP (2007) *Global Livestock CRSP: Annual Report 2007.* Collaborative Research Support Program, University of California, Davis, California.

Grantham-McGregor, S.M. and Ani, C.C. (1999) The role of micronutrients in psychomotor and cognitive development. *British Medical Bulletin* 55, 511–527.

Grillenberger, M., Neumann, C.G., Murphy, S.P., Bwibo, N.O., van't Veer, P., Hautvast, J.G. and West, C.E. (2003) Food supplements have a positive impact on weight gain and the addition of animal source foods increases lean body mass of Kenyan schoolchildren. *Journal of Nutrition* 133(11, Suppl. 2), 3957S–3964S.

Grillenberger, M., Neumann, C.G., Murphy, S.P., Bwibo, N.O., Weiss, R.E., Jiang, L., Hautvast, J.G. and West, C.E. (2006) Intake of micronutrients high in animal-source foods is associated with better growth in rural Kenyan school children. *British Journal of Nutrition* 95, 379–390.

Guldan, G.S., Zhang, M.Y., Zhang, Y.P., Hong, J.R., Zhang, H.X., Fu, S.Y. and Fu, N.S. (1993) Weaning practices and growth in rural Sichuan infants: a positive deviance study. *Journal of Tropical Pediatrics* 39, 168–175.

Hansen, M., Thilsted, S.H., Sandstrom, B., Kongsbak, K., Larsen, T., Jensen, M. and Sorensen, S.S. (1998) Calcium absorption from small soft-boned fish. Journal of Trace Elements in Medicine and Biology 12, 148–154.

Iannotti, L., Cunningham, K. and Ruel, M. (2009) *Improving Diet Quality and Micronutrient Nutrition: Homestead Food Production in Bangladesh.* IFPRI Discussion Paper 00928, International Food Policy

Research Institute, Washington, DC (accessed 22 November 2010). Available at: http://www.ifpri.org/sites/default/files/publications/ifpridp00928.pdf (accessed 4 June 2013).

Jones, B.A., Deemer, B., Leyland, T.J., Mogga, W. and Stem, E. (1998) Community-based animal health services in Southern Sudan: the experience so far. In: *Proceedings of the 9th International Conference of Association of Institutes of Tropical Veterinary Medicine (AITVM), Harare, 4th–18th September, 1998*, pp. 107–133. Available at: http://www.eldis.org/fulltext/comsud.pdf (accessed 12 June 2013).

Kabahenda, M.K. and Husken, S.M.C. (2009) A review of low-value fish products marketed in the Lake Victoria region. Project Report 1974. WorldFish, Penang, Malaysia.

Kikafunda, J.K. and Sserumaga, P. (2005) Production and use of a shelf-stable bovine blood powder for food fortification as a food-based strategy to combat iron deficiency anaemia in subsaharan Africa. *AJFAND (African Journal of Food Agriculture and Nutritional Development)* 5:1. Available at: https://tspace.library.utoronto.ca/bitstream/1807/7695/1/nd05007.pdf (accessed 12 June 2013).

Kirksey, A., Harrison, G.G., Galal, O.M., McCabe, G.A., Wachs, T.D. and Rahmanifar, A. (1992) The Human Cost of Moderate Malnutrition in an Egyptian Village, Final Report Phase II. Nutrition CRSP (Collaborative Research Support Program), Purdue University, Lafayette, Indiana.

Lebas, F., Coudert, P., de Rochambeau, H. and Thébault, R.G. (1997) *The Rabbit – Husbandry, Health and Production*. FAO Animal Production and Health Series No. 21, Food and Agriculture Organization of the United Nations, Rome.

Leung, W.-T.W., Butrum, R.R., Chang, F.H., Rao, M.N. and Polacchi, W. (1972) *Food Composition Table for Use in East Asia*. Food and Agriculture Organization of the United Nations, Rome and US Department of Health, Education, and Welfare, Washington, DC.

Maretzki, A.N. (2007) Women's nutribusiness cooperatives in Kenya: an integrated strategy for sustaining rural livelihoods. *Journal of Nutrition Education and Behavior* 39, 327–334.

Maretzki, A.N. and Mills, E.W. (2003) Applying a nutribusiness approach to increase animal source food consumption in local communities. *Journal of Nutrition* 133(11, Suppl. 2), 4031S–4035S.

Marquis, G.S., Habicht, J.P., Lanata, C.F., Black, R.E. and Rasmussen, K.M. (1997) Breast milk or animal-product foods improve linear growth of Peruvian toddlers consuming marginal diets. *The American Journal of Clinical Nutrition* 66, 1102–1109.

Masabe, P. (2010) Poster presentation. In: *4th Africa Nutritional Epidemiology conference (ANEC IV), Nairobi, Kenya, 4–8 October 2010*.

McLean, E.D., Allen, L.H., Neumann, C.G., Peerson, J.M., Siekmann, J.H., Murphy, S.P., Bwibo, N.O. and Demment, M.W. (2007) Low plasma vitamin B-12 in Kenyan school children is highly prevalent and improved by supplemental animal source foods. *Journal of Nutrition* 137, 676–682.

Mills, E.W., Seetharaman, K. and Maretzki, A.N. (2007) A nutribusiness strategy for processing and marketing of animal-source foods for children. *Journal of Nutrition* 137, 1115–1118.

Mugunieri, G.L., Irungu, P. and Omiti, J.M. (2004) Performance of community-based animal health workers in the delivery of livestock health services. *Tropical Animal Health and Production* 36, 523–535.

Mugunieri, L.G., Omiti, J.M. and Irungu, P. (2005) Animal health service delivery systems in Kenya's marginal districts. In: Omamo, S.W., Babu, S. and Temu, A. (eds) *The Future of Smallholder Agriculture in Eastern Africa: The roles of States, Markets, and Civil Society*, pp. 401–453. IFPRI (International Food Policy Research Institute) Eastern Africa Food Policy Network, Kampala, Uganda.

Muroki, N.M., Maritim, G.K., Karuri, E.G., Tolong, H.K., Imungi, J.K., Kogi-Makau, W., Maman, S., Carter, E. and Maretzki, A.N. (1997) Involving rural Kenyan women in the development of nutritionally improved weaning foods: nutribusiness strategy. *Journal of Nutrition Education* 29, 335–342.

Murphy, S.P. and Allen, L.H. (2003) Nutritional importance of animal source foods. *Journal of Nutrition* 133(11, Suppl. 2), 3932S–3935S.

Nettleton, J.A. and Exler, J. (1992) Nutrients in wild and farmed fish and shellfish. *Journal of Food Science* 57, 257–260.

Neumann, C.G. and Harrison, G.G. (1994) Onset and evolution of stunting in infants and children. Examples from the Human Nutrition Collaborative Research Support Program. Kenya and Egypt studies. *European Journal of Clinical Nutrition* 48(Suppl. 1), S90–S102.

Neumann, C.G., Bwibo, N.O. and Sigman, M. (1992) Final Report Phase II: Functional Implications of Malnutrition, Kenya Project. Human Nutrition Collaborative Research Support Program (CRSP), University of California, Los Angeles, California.

Neumann, C.G., Harris, D.M. and Rogers, L.M. (2002) Contribution of animal source foods in improving diet quality and function in children in the developing world. *Nutrition Research* 22, 193–220.

Neumann, C.G., Bwibo, N.O., Murphy, S.P., Sigman, M., Whaley, S., Allen, L.H., Guthrie, D., Weiss, R.E. and Demment, M.W. (2003) Animal source foods improve dietary quality, micronutrient status, growth and cognitive function in Kenyan school children: background, study design and baseline findings. *Journal of Nutrition* 133(11, Suppl. 2), 3941S–3949S.

Neumann, C.G., Murphy, S.P., Gewa, C., Grillenberger, M. and Bwibo, N.O. (2007) Meat supplementation improves growth, cognitive, and behavioral outcomes in Kenyan children. *Journal of Nutrition* 137, 1119–1123.

Neumann, C.G., Demment, M.W., Maretzki, A.N., Drorbaugh, N. and Galvin, K.A. (2010) The livestock revolution and animal source food consumption: benefits, risks, and challenges in urban and rural settings of developing countries. In: Steinfeld, H., Mooney, H.A., Schneider, F. and Neville, L.E. (eds) *Livestock in a Changing Landscape: Drivers, Consequences, and Responses.* Island Press, Washington, DC, pp. 221–248.

Olivares, M., Hertrampf, E., Pizarro, F., Walter, T., Cayazzo, M., Llaguno, S., Chadud, P., Cartagena, N., Vega, V., Amar, M. and Stekel, A. (1990) Hemoglobin-fortified biscuits: bioavailability and its effect on iron nutriture in school children. *Archivos Latinoamericanos de Nutrición* 40, 209–220.

Pennington, J.A.T. (1998) *Bowe's and Church's Food Values of Portions Commonly Used.* Lippincot-Raven Publishers, Philadelphia, Pennsylvania.

Raven, T.C. (1960) *Raven's Progressive Matrices: Guide to Standard Progressive Matrices.* Psychological Corporation, New York.

Roos, N., Islam, M. and Thilsted, S.H. (2003a) Small fish is an important dietary source of vitamin A and calcium in rural Bangladesh. *International Journal of Food Sciences and Nutrition* 54, 329–339.

Roos, N., Islam, M. and Thilsted, S.H. (2003b) Small indigenous fish species in Bangladesh: contribution to vitamin A, calcium and iron intakes. *Journal of Nutrition* 133(11, Suppl. 2), 4021S–4026S.

Roos, N., Wahab, M.A., Chamnan, C. and Thilsted, S.H. (2007) The role of fish in food-based strategies to combat vitamin A and mineral deficiencies in developing countries. *Journal of Nutrition* 137, 1106–1109.

Sakyi-Dawson, O., Marquis, G.S., Lartley, A., Colecraft, E.K., Ahunu, B.K., Butler, L.M., Reddy, M.B., Jensen, H., Lonergan, E. and Quarmime, W. (2009) *Impact of Interventions on Caregiver's Nutrition Knowledge and Animal Source Food Intake in Young Children in Ghana.* Global Livestock Collaborative Research Support Program (GLCRSP), Davis, California.

Schroeder, D.G., Pachon, H., Dearden, K.A., Kwon, C.B., Ha, T.T., Lang, T.T. and Marsh, D.R. (2002) An integrated child nutrition intervention improved growth of younger, more malnourished children in northern Viet Nam. *Food and Nutrition Bulletin* 23(4, Suppl.), 53–61.

Shapiro, B.I., Haider, J.G., Wold, A. and Misgina, A. (1998) The intra-household economic and nutritional impacts of market-oriented dairy production: evidence from the Ethiopian highlands. In: Jabbar, M.A., Peden, D.G., Mohamed Saleem, M.A. and Li Pun, H. (eds) *Agro-ecosystems, Natural Resources Management and Human Health Related Research in East Africa.* International Livestock Research Institute (ILRI), Addis Ababa, pp. 109–123.

Shils, M.E., Olson, J.A., Shike, M. and Ross A.C. (eds) (1999) *Modern Nutrition in Health and Disease.* Williams and Wilkins, Baltimore, Maryland.

Siekmann, J.H., Allen, L.H., Bwibo, N.O., Demment, M.W., Murphy, S.P. and Neumann, C.G. (2003) Kenyan school children have multiple micronutrient deficiencies, but increased plasma vitamin B-12 is the only detectable micronutrient response to meat or milk supplementation. *Journal of Nutrition* 133(11, Suppl. 2), 3972S-3980S.

Sigman, M., Neumann, C.G., Jansen, A. and Bwibo, N.O. (1989) Cognitive abilities of Kenyan children in relation to nutrition, family characteristics and education. *Child Development* 60, 1463–1474.

Sigman, M., Whaley, S.E., Neumann, C.G., Bwibo, N., Guthrie, D., Weiss, R.E., Liang, L.J. and Murphy, S.P. (2005) Diet quality affects the playground activities of Kenyan children. *Food and Nutrition Bulletin* 26(2, Suppl. 2), S202–S212.

Smitasiri, S. and Chotiboriboon, S. (2003) Experience with programs to increase animal source food intake in Thailand. *Journal of Nutrition* 13 (11, Suppl. 2), 4000S–4005S.

Smith, T., Earland, J., Bhatia, K., Heywood, P. and Singleton, N. (1993) Linear growth of children in Papua New Guinea in relation to dietary, environmental and genetic factors. *Ecology of Food and Nutrition* 31, 1–25.

Sripaipan, T., Schroeder, D.G., Marsh, D.R., Pachon, H., Dearden, K.A., Ha, T.T. and Lang, T.T. (2002) Effect of an integrated nutrition program on child morbidity due to respiratory infection and diarrhea in northern Viet Nam. *Food and Nutrition Bulletin* 23(4, Suppl.), 70–77.

Stallkamp, G., Akhter, N., Karim, R., Jinnatunnesa, R., Habib, A., Baten, A., Uddin, A., Talukder, A. and de Pee, S. (2007) Homestead food production improves micronutrient status in mothers and young children in Bangladesh. In: *Micronutrient Forum, 2007, Istanbul, Turkey*, Abstract W15, p. 102. Available at: http://www.micronutrientforum.org/meeting2007/MN%20Forum%20Program%20Part%20II_ Abstracts.pdf (accessed 12 June 2013).

Takahashi, E. (1984) Secular trend in milk consumption and growth in Japan. *Human Biology* 56, 427–437.

Talukder, A., Stallkamp, G., Karim, R., Sapkota, G., Kroeun, H., Witten, C., Haselow, N. and de Pee, S. (2007) Homestead food production and its impact on the prevalence of anemia among non-pregnant women and children in Asia (Bangladesh, Nepal and Cambodia). In: *Abstracts, Micronutrient Forum, 2007, Istanbul, Turkey*, Abstract W18, p. 102. Available at: http://www.micronutrientforum.org/meeting2007/ MN%20Forum%20Program%20Part%20II_Abstracts.pdf (accessed 12 June 2013).

USDA (2006) National Nutrient Database for Standard Reference, Release 19. US Department of Agriculture, Washington, DC.

Walker, S.P., Powell, C.A. and Grantham-McGregor, S.M. (1990) Dietary intakes and activity levels of stunted and non-stunted children in Kingston, Jamaica. Part 1. Dietary intakes. *European Journal of Clinical Nutrition* 44, 527–534.

Walter, T., Hertrampf, E., Pizarro, F., Olivares, M., Llaguno, S., Letelier, A., Vega, V. and Stekel, A. (1993) Effect of bovine-hemoglobin-fortified cookies on iron status of schoolchildren: a nationwide program in Chile. *The American Journal of Clinical Nutrition* 57, 190–194.

Watanabe, F. (2007) Vitamin B12 sources and bioavailability. *Experimental Biology and Medicine* 232, 1266–1274.

Weschler, D. (1974) *Weschler Intelligence Scale for Children*, rev. edn. Psychological Corporation, New York.

West, C.E., Pepping, F., Scholte, I., Jansen, W. and Albers, H.F. (1987) ECSA and CTA (1987) Food composition table for energy and eight important nutrients in foods commonly eaten in East Africa. Technical Centre for Agricultural and Rural Cooperation, Wageningen, Netherlands (CTA) and East, Central and Southern African Health Community (ECSA), Arusha, Tanzania.

Whaley, S.E., Sigman, M., Neumann, C., Bwibo, N., Guthrie, D., Weiss, R.E., Alber, S. and Murphy, S.P. (2003) The impact of dietary intervention on the cognitive development of Kenyan school children. *Journal of Nutrition* 133(11, Suppl. 2), 3965S–3971S.

Williamson, C.S., Foster, R.K., Stanner, S.A. and Buttriss, J.L. (2005) Red meat in the diet. *Nutrition Bulletin* 30, 323–355.

Yeudall, F., Gibson, R.S., Kayira, C. and Umar, E. (2002) Efficacy of a multi-micronutrient dietary intervention based on haemoglobin, hair zinc concentrations, and selected functional outcomes in rural Malawian children. *European Journal of Clinical Nutrition* 56, 1176–1185.

14 Adapting Food-based Strategies to Improve the Nutrition of the Landless: A Review of HKI's Homestead Food Production Program in Bangladesh

Emily P. Hillenbrand[1]* and Jillian L. Waid[2]

[1]*Helen Keller International (HKI), Asia-Pacific Regional Office, Phnom Penh, Cambodia;* [2]*HKI, Bangladesh Country Office, Dhaka, Bangladesh*

Summary

Helen Keller International's (HKI) homestead food production (HFP) model is a food-based strategy to increase the micronutrient intake of individuals, improve household food security and advance women's empowerment. The standard HFP intervention includes gardening, poultry production, group marketing, and nutrition behaviour change communication (BCC). The model has historically been implemented with smallholder households that have a minimal amount of land. However, individuals in ultra-poor households with minimal land access are among the most food-insecure and malnourished in Bangladesh, and they require food-based interventions targeted to their unique capabilities. Recognizing the urgent nutritional needs of the growing number of landless households in Bangladesh, HKI has been adapting its HFP model to reach this marginalized population. Targeting HFP to the landless, ultra-poor households in Bangladesh requires modification of the HFP package of support to focus on technologies that maximize yields and promote nutritionally rich varieties that can be produced on microplots. Given their limited production capacity and immediate income needs, interventions for the ultra-poor should also include skill-building and income-earning opportunities that are linked to agricultural production. Along with improving incomes or agricultural skills to improve access to food, the provision of nutrition education and counselling is essential for improving nutrition outcomes. Using the available literature and data sets from HKI's 20 year history of HFP in Bangladesh, this chapter briefly reviews the evidence of HFP's nutritional impact on the land constrained, summarizes programmatic challenges in working with this group, and proposes modifications to ensure that the most marginalized can derive equitable nutrition benefits from this food-based intervention.

Introduction

In Bangladesh, 56 million individuals (over 40% of the population) do not consume the minimum number of calories required to sustain a healthy life (BBS, 2007). In addition, because of a lack of dietary diversity, an even greater share of the population suffers from the hidden hunger of micronutrient malnutrition, which is related to cultural food preferences as well as to

---

*Contact: ehillenbrand@care.org

problems of income poverty (FPMU, 2009). Most households subsist on a diet consisting mainly of rice, which provides an estimated 69% of food energy but is low in fat, essential amino acids and micronutrients (Darnton-Hill *et al.*, 1988; FPMU, 2009). Animal source foods, which provide high-quality protein and bio-available iron and vitamin A, make up less than 3% of household total energy intake (FAO, 2010). For poor and ultra-poor households, consumption patterns are even more limited and rice based, as poverty is a barrier to purchasing the variety of foods that are needed for dietary quality (BBS, 2007). Nationally, rice production has kept pace with population growth; however, cultural food preferences for a heavily rice-based diet and lack of knowledge about the need for a diversified diet create limited demand for more diversified agriculture production systems.

Food-based approaches that focus on dietary diversification are effective strategies for reducing micronutrient and macronutrient deficiencies in malnourished populations (Tontisirin *et al.*, 2002; Bhattacharjee *et al.*, 2007; Allen, 2008). HKI's model has been recognized as one of the most successful food-based nutrition interventions in the world (Iannotti *et al.*, 2009; Bread for the World Institute, 2010). In Bangladesh, Helen Keller International (HKI) was one of the pioneer organizations to introduce and scale up dietary diversification strategies that combined homestead food production (HFP) and nutrition behaviour change communication (BCC). Many local and international non-governmental organizations (NGOs), as well as the Government of Bangladesh, have adopted similar food-based strategies throughout the country. In addition, the government's National Food Policy names investing in homestead gardening as one key strategy for reducing malnutrition among vulnerable groups (FPMU, 2009).

One of the general caveats related to food-based approaches to nutrition is that, by definition, they may fail to serve one of the most needy and food-insecure populations – the rural landless (Kennedy, 1994). In recent decades, average land-size holdings in Bangladesh have declined significantly. The proportion of landless households in rural areas is increasing, posing long-term threats to national food and nutrition security (BBS, 2008; FAO and WFP, 2008). Land and livelihood security are closely linked in Bangladesh (FAO and WFP, 2008); a greater proportion of the landless are ultra-poor than of those with some land (BBS, 2007), and landlessness is also associated with higher rates of malnutrition (BBS and UNICEF, 2007). In sum, the landless ultra-poor have insufficient or irregular income to access nutrient-rich foods, and they have less horticultural production capacity to produce sufficient food for their own consumption.

Given the steady erosion of land access and the increased policy attention to the plight of the ultra-poor in Bangladesh, it is critical and timely to consider how a food-based approach such as HKI's HFP model can be adapted to tackle malnutrition within this vulnerable group. The first section of this chapter will look more closely at the problem of landlessness in Bangladesh, and specifically at how landlessness is correlated with extreme poverty and nutrition insecurity. It will then present the design and evolution of the HFP model in Bangladesh and demonstrate the outcomes that can be attributed to this model. Finally, the chapter will discuss the specific challenges to and proposed approaches to/tools for developing a successful food-based HFP model for the landless.

The chapter draws on published and unpublished quantitative and qualitative data from a number of HFP projects that have been undertaken by HKI Bangladesh. Table 14.1 below lists the years of operation, geographic reach, and number of beneficiaries for each of the cited projects. Particular projects will be referred to throughout the chapter using the short form of the project's name, which is given in the last column of Table 14.1. When figures that have not previously been published are cited, the description of the data set used for secondary analysis will be given in the footnote.

Food Insecurity and Malnutrition Among the Landless in Bangladesh

Despite steady economic growth and near self-sufficiency in rice production, rates of

Table 14.1. List of Homestead Food Production (HFP) Program projects of Helen Keller International (HKI) Bangladesh to date, briefly summarizing projects implemented from 1988 to 2010.

Years	Project name	Area	HFP beneficiary households	In text reference
1988–1990	The vitamin A home gardening and promotion of consumption for prevention of nutritional blindness pilot	Kaliaganj Union	150	Pilot Project
1990–1993	The vitamin A home gardening and promotion of consumption for prevention of nutritional blindness project	Panchagaor District	1000	Vit-A home gardening
1993–2003	National Gardening and Nutrition Surveillance Project	178 Sub-districts, throughout Bangladesh	888,087	NGNESP
2003–2005	Improving nutrition and food security through homestead food production in the riverine islands and flood plains of Bangladesh	Northern Char	10,250	Char 1
2004–2009	Jibon-o-Jibika (Life and Livelihood)	Southern Coastal Belt	26,840	JOJ
2005–2007	Improving nutrition and food security through homestead food production in the riverine islands and flood plains of Bangladesh (Phase 2)	Northern Char	10,250	Char 2
2005–2007	Chittagong Hill Tracts Homestead Food Production Project	Chittagong Hill Tracts	10,250	CHT-HFP
2008–2011	Development Initiatives for Sustainable Household Activities in Riverine Islands	Northern Char	10,425	DISHARI
2008–2010	Reconstruction, Economic Development and Livelihoods Project	Southern Coastal Belt	20,252	REAL
2009–2012	Making markets work for women	Chittagong Hill Tracts	450	M²W²

poverty and malnutrition remain high in Bangladesh. In this agrarian economy, there is a distinct correlation between landlessness and poverty. Due to a growing population and the expansion of urban areas and industry, agricultural land has diminished from 65% of Bangladesh's total land area in 1990 to 55% today (Ministry of Agriculture, 2007). Average land holdings have declined, and the proportion of landless rural households is increasing (BBS, 2008). The Agriculture Census of 2008 shows that the percentage of absolute landless rural farming households (those that do not have any access to cultivable land) had increased by more than 26% in the previous 12 years, from 10.2% to 12.8% (BBS, 2008).[1] With the predicted rise in sea level related to climate change, it is likely that the amount of land available for cultivation will further diminish in the future (Hossain, 2010).

Fractured and dwindling land holdings constitute a significant structural impediment to diversified food production and food security in Bangladesh (Rahman and Manprasert, 2006; BBS, 2007). Extreme land scarcity limits individual household capacity to produce adequate food to meet year-round nutritional and/or income needs. Loss of land is linked to diminished capacity to accumulate other assets, and is often accompanied by a shift to agricultural day labour or by migration to other areas of Bangladesh for employment (Rahman and Manprasert, 2006; Chowdhury, 2009). In addition, the rural economy is poorly diversified, offering limited non-farm opportunities. Of the vast majority of the rural ultrapoor, 72% are engaged as agricultural day labourers, a seasonal occupation that can leave households without income for several months of the year (Matin et al., 2008; Van Haeften and Moses, 2009). In turn, malnutrition related to seasonal hunger compromises the most critical livelihood capital of the landless – their physical labour capacities. Illness associated with poor health and undernutrition translates into lost working days and decreased income, thus exacerbating the cycle of poverty and malnutrition among the landless (Jha *et al.*, 2009).

Rates of ultra-poverty are also highest among the landless. While 28% of the total rural population lives below the lower expenditure poverty line, 50% of the absolutely landless (defined in this chapter as owning less than 0.05 acres of land) live in ultra-poverty (Ahmed *et al.*, 2007; BBS, 2007). Among ultra-poor households in Bangladesh, nutritional status and micronutrient adequacy are severely compromised. About 75% of the daily calories in this wealth group come from rice alone – 5% more than the already high proportion consumed by the population overall (BBS, 2007). A greater proportion of children from landless households are malnourished, compared with children from households with greater land access (BBS and UNICEF, 2007). In the wake of the 2008 price hikes, the nutrition security of the poor and ultra-poor was further compromised; poor households spent up to 86% of household expenditures on food in the wake of recent price spikes, which was a 16% point rise from the same season before the price rise (FAO and WFP, 2008). This spending shift corresponds with a sharp reduction in the consumption of non-rice and nutritious foods, with negative nutrition implications that compromise the labour capacity and human capital of this group (WFP *et al.*, 2009).

The landless ultra-poor are not only poorer than others but also have distinct livelihood strategies and vulnerabilities. In Bangladesh, ultra-poor households are more likely than others to be headed by a family member with no education and to have fewer income-earning members per household (BBS, 2007; FAO and WFP, 2008). Without land or other livelihood assets, the ultra-poor are excluded from many microfinance organizations and the social capital that such groups can provide (HKI, 2009, 2010a; Tango International, 2009). They face various forms of social exclusion and

marginalization, which may preclude them from accessing existing safety nets.

In spite of this, ultra-poor women generally have greater mobility than women of higher wealth groups, who are restricted to the homestead (HKI, 2009). Their acute need for income compels ultra-poor women to transgress cultural constraints to seek day labour opportunities, although this transgression simultaneously deepens their social exclusion (HKI, 2009). Their livelihood strategies entail time-consuming investments in making themselves visible to patrons, for example by providing unpaid and degrading labour to wealthy residents in the village in the hopes of being supported by that patron later (Matin *et al.*, 2008; Van Haeften and Moses, 2009). The opportunity cost of attending group meetings or nutrition trainings is steeper for the ultra-poor, who may end up missing vital opportunities for day labour.

While a number of programmes and organizations in Bangladesh are currently targeting the ultra-poor, most of these interventions adopt an income-based approach and do not address nutritional deficits (particularly micronutrient deficiencies). Typical ultra-poor interventions include social safety nets, such as the Government of Bangladesh's Vulnerable Group Development programme, temporary cash-for-work or food-for-work programmes and asset transfer packages. Few of these approaches are nutrition-sensitive or nutrition centred. For example, food-for-work programmes or government food distribution programmes are generally rice based, and provide calories but not sufficient micronutrients for optimal health. There is abundant evidence that poverty-reduction schemes alone – while expanding the access of households to food – do not automatically result in improved dietary practices or reductions in stunting and micronutrient-deficiency disorders (Kennedy, 1994; Mascie-Taylor *et al.*, 2010).

Ensuring balanced and nutritious food for the ultra-poor is a key performance indicator in the Government of Bangladesh's National Food Policy (FPMU, 2009). Given that 80% of the rural poor in the country depend on agriculture for their livelihoods, investing in a food-based, nutrition-centred approach such as homestead gardening continues to be an important strategy for addressing malnutrition and food security for a plurality of rural groups (FPMU, 2009). However, the landless ultra-poor are the group simultaneously most in need of and historically least able to take advantage of existing agriculture-based dietary diversification approaches. Before discussion of possible modifications to the HFP programme in order to better assist the landless ultra-poor, the chapter will first review how HKI's model has worked in the past and how it has nutritionally benefited the land-constrained.

HKI's Homestead Food Production Program in Bangladesh

HKI's Homestead Food Production (HFP) Program is a food-based agriculture strategy designed specifically to reduce food insecurity and micronutrient deficiencies. Begun as a pilot project in 1988, HFP initially presented a sustainable, food-based solution to the widespread problem of vitamin A deficiency (HKI, 2006a). The basic HFP programme components focus on providing beneficiaries with the technical agricultural skills to grow year-round, diverse plant varieties rich in vitamin A. Beneficiaries are organized into groups for ease of training and mutual support. To ensure the sustainability of the agriculture component, HFP establishes a demonstration plot and nursery at community level, later referred to as the Village Model Farm (VMF). The owner of the VMF receives support to demonstrate improved gardening techniques and to produce a supply of seeds and saplings of micronutrient-rich plant varieties for the benefit of the community. More information about the scale up of the HFP programme in Bangladesh can be found in Talukder *et al.* (2000).

As vitamin A deficiency was a generalized health problem at the start of the HFP programme,[2] beneficiary selection was not based on strict poverty or nutrition criteria but primarily on the beneficiaries having sufficient land and interest to participate. Even the earliest projects (Vitamin A home gardening, 1990–1993) set a land ownership ceiling

of 0.35 acres for project beneficiaries. From the start, the HFP programme historically reached a population of marginal farmers, a group that government agricultural extension services often fail to support. HFP always provided valuable agriculture and nutrition support to the poor – if not the ultra-poor or the landless.

In the 20 years since the programme began, HFP has been shown to be a flexible, nutrition-sensitive intervention that can be adapted to meet different target populations and to support various goals, including poverty reduction, maternal and child health, and women's empowerment. HFP has enabled project beneficiaries to increase egg and lentil consumption, nearly triple garden production and double the varieties of vegetables produced (Iannotti *et al.*, 2009). In addition, certain projects that had a more comprehensive evaluation structure show that HFP can drastically reduce rates of anaemia. Figure 14.1 illustrates the impact of the programme on anaemia rates for mothers and children under 5 years of age from two HFP projects that were undertaken in the mid-2000s. The reduction of anaemia rates for the beneficiaries is in sharp contrast to the slight rise in anaemia rates among the comparison population.

Over the years, the HFP programme evolved into a more comprehensive approach to food security, developing greater income-earning opportunities for beneficiaries in addition to the original nutrition aims of the programme. From its outset, HFP included a nutrition component to educate beneficiaries on the importance of consuming vitamin A-rich foods and a more diverse diet. As the programme evolved, it expanded to address more broad-based nutrition issues, such as infant and young child feeding practices and the importance of increased consumption of food and micronutrients during pregnancy. The nutrition education programme includes growth monitoring and promotion activities in the community, home visits for one-on-one nutrition counselling and interactive group courtyard sessions (HKI, 2010b,c). Activities for addressing gender inequality, a root cause of malnutrition, were also integrated into the project core.

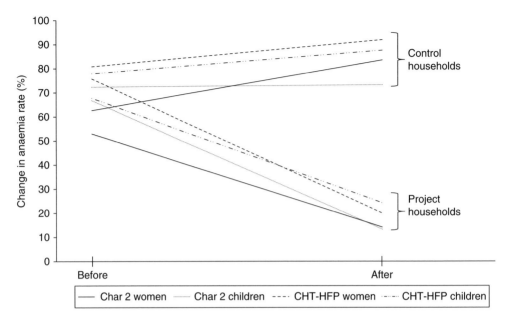

Fig. 14.1. Reduction in anaemia rates in women and children from two homestead food production (HFP) projects (with a poultry component) implemented by Helen Keller International (HKI) in Bangladesh from 2005 to 2007. Char 2, a Phase 2 project in Northern Char on improving nutrition and food security through HFP in riverine islands and flood plains; CHT-HFP, an HFP project in the Chittagong Hill Tracts.

In 2002, during the last year of NGNESP (National Gardening and Nutrition Surveillance Project), HKI added a poultry-rearing component, based on evidence that the vitamin A from animal source foods is more easily absorbed than that from plant sources (Nielsen *et al.*, 2003; Leroy and Frongillo, 2007). The poultry programme has had multiple positive impacts, including poverty alleviation. In 2009, InterAction (an international NGO) recognized HKI Bangladesh's Improved Poultry Program (IPP) as a best practice in agriculture, for its multiple benefits, including nutrition outcomes, contributions to women's empowerment, women's income, poverty reduction and agricultural productivity (InterAction, 2010). Since 2005, a goat-rearing component has been added as an asset transfer for the poorest women.

The main measures of HFP success were increases in dietary diversification, a proxy indicator for food security and reduced micronutrient malnutrition. Anthropometric measurements were also made from the earliest projects, but a sizeable effect on this indicator

has never been shown, perhaps due to short evaluation cycles. Other key outcomes are changes in agricultural production techniques that emphasize greater plant varieties and year-round production. Evaluations of HFP programmes have also documented noticeable gains in women's control over household decisions and income generated from the sale of surplus HFP products.

Inclusion of the Landless in HKI's Homestead Food Production Program

In concert with the evolutions in programme design, HKI has increasingly turned its attention to those in greatest need of homestead food production. As stated earlier, the most food-insecure and nutritionally vulnerable populations in Bangladesh tend to be the land constrained and those living in environmentally insecure areas, such as riverbanks and riverine islands, where land tenure is insecure and soil is constantly eroding. A review of the history of HFP programmes reflects a downward shift in the average amount of land operated by project beneficiaries at the time of beneficiary selection. As the HKI programme strove to reach more vulnerable populations in more remote and environmentally insecure locations, the mean land size that was available also dropped. In the recent DISHARI project (see Table 14.1), initiated in 2008 and targeting a subgroup of landless beneficiaries, the average land holding is the lowest to date, only 0.17 acres. Figure 14.2 below shows the drop in mean size of land owned by beneficiaries of HFP programmes over a period of time.[3]

HKI Bangladesh first explicitly targeted a beneficiary group defined as 'ultra-poor' within the context of a 5 year Food for Peace programme funded by USAID (United States Agency for International Development). In this project, HKI was responsible for delivering its HFP package to beneficiaries enrolled in a maternal/child health nutrition (MCHN) intervention led by Save the Children USA. As target households were households with a child under 2 years of age, they were not necessarily the neediest in the locality. After a mid-term review, however, a group of highly food-insecure households that initially were not enrolled in the MCHN component because they did not have a child under 2 years old were included. In order to include these households, HKI reached out to the poorest of the poor (landless women and female heads of household) and modified the HFP intervention to meet the needs of this group. The ultra-poor received an asset-transfer package of small livestock (goats) and livestock management training. Since that pilot intervention, HKI has included landless ultra-poor beneficiaries in several HFP projects, together with its traditional demographic of marginal smallholders. Subsequent HKI HFP programmes (including DISHARI, REAL and M^2W^2; see Table 14.1) have provided a more comprehensive package to the ultra-poor, including asset transfer, gardening support and poultry support, and nutrition BCC.

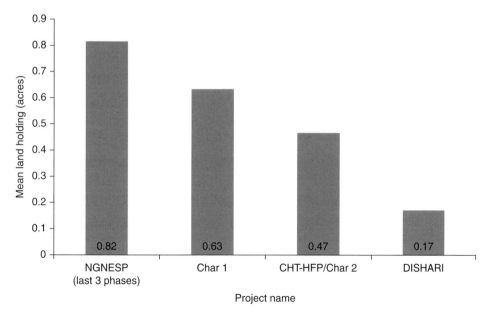

Fig. 14.2. Changes in the mean size of land owned by beneficiaries of Helen Keller International (HKI) homestead food production (HFP) projects from 1999 to 2008. NGNESP, National Gardening and Nutrition Surveillance Project throughout Bangladesh (1993–2003); Char 1, a Phase 1 project in Northern Char on improving nutrition and food security through HFP in riverine islands and flood plains (2003–2005); CHT-HFP, an HFP project in the Chittagong Hill Tracts (2005–2007); Char 2, Phase 2 of the Northern Char project (2005–2007); DISHARI, Development Initiatives for Sustainable Household Activities in Riverine Islands in Northern Char (2008–2011).[3]

Table 14.2. Sampled households in Homestead Food Production (HPF) Program data sets from three projects that operated in Bangladesh in the last decade (Char 1, Char 2 and CHT-HFP; see Table 14.1) categorized by land holding size, with numbers and percentages of households by size of land owned.

Size of land operated in decimals (≈1/100 acre, or 40.46 m^2	No. households in data set	%
<5	1528	31
5–50	2151	44
>50	1192	24

For three HFP projects that took place in the last decade (Char 1, Char 2 and CHT-HFP; see Table 14.1), information on nutrition impact is available and can be disaggregated by beneficiaries' access to land.[4] Table 14.2 gives the numbers and percentages of households in the data set for each land ownership category; the majority of households owned between 0.50 and 0.05 acres of land.

The impact that can be attributed to HKI's food-based nutrition programmes is a marked increase in women's weighted food frequency scores (FFS, calculated using a food consumption score, FCS, for the mother of the small child in each household),[5] and a sizeable decrease in women's and children's anaemia scores. Overall, women's FFS increased 22 points among project beneficiaries (from 22.2 at baseline to 44.0 at end line), while it rose only 4 points in the control group (from 19.5 to 23.2). Among all sampled beneficiary women, the prevalence of anaemia dropped from 57.5% at baseline to 28.8% at end line, while it rose among sampled non-beneficiary women over the same time period (63.8% to 75.8%). Among beneficiary households, the anaemia rate among children aged 6–59 months fell from 69.4% to 28.3%, but in children from control households, anaemia rates went from 73.0% to 68.5%, a comparatively smaller improvement.

These results are broken down by land ownership category in Table 14.3. The first part of the table displays changes in the FFS of sampled mothers. Households in all land ownership categories benefited from the intervention in comparison with those in the control group,

though the benefits attributable to the programme were greater for women in households with larger land holdings. At baseline, the difference in FFS between beneficiary mothers in landless households (owning <0.05 acres of land) and those in landed households (owning >0.5 acres of land) was significant (adjusted Wald test, $P < 0.000$), while the difference between the landless and the middle group (those land holdings of 0.05–0.50 acres) was not significant (adjusted Wald test, $P < 0.105$). At end line, however, the maternal FFS of the landless group was significantly lower than those of both the middle and upper land ownership groups (adjusted Wald test, $P < 0.000$).[6] Although landless households appear to have lower anaemia rates at end line (see the last two parts of Table 14.3), this difference was not statistically significant – but this finding does merit further exploration.

This brief analysis reveals that dietary diversity strategies such as HKI's HFP model can improve the dietary quality and micronutrient status of individuals in highly land-constrained households. All groups, regardless of their land holdings, saw noticeable improvements in their dietary diversity and anaemia rates over the course of the programme. At the same time, the data show that landless households have had limited opportunities in the past to reap the full potential nutritional benefits that HFP can deliver. This suggests that supplemental or revised interventions may be required to yield equitable results with this relatively more marginalized population. The next section outlines some challenges and promising approaches for maximizing nutritional gains with the landless group.

Programmatic Challenges of Addressing Nutrition of the Landless

As HKI expanded its work with landless subgroups, the organization also conducted qualitative and participatory research to gain insights into their characteristics and livelihood strategies. This research, coupled with national studies of ultra-poverty and field experience from local staff, gave the recommendations for working with the ultra-poor.

Table 14.3. Comparison of baseline and end-line results for food frequency consumption (as estimated by the food frequency score, FFS) and maternal and child anaemia levels in three homestead food production (HFP) projects implemented by Helen Keller International (HKI) Bangladesh in 2003–2008.[4–6] Asterisks indicate level of significance.

Maternal food frequency score

Land holding		Baseline	End line	Mean difference	Increase attributable to programme
Landless (<0.05 ha)	Control	18.8 (17.7–20.0)	23.7 (22.3–25.1)	4.8**	12.3
	Beneficiary	20.3 (18.8–21.8)	37.5 (34.2–40.7)	17.1**	
Functionally landless (0.05–0.50 ha)	Control	19.0 (17.8–20.2)	22.6 (21.5–23.6)	3.6**	18.4
	Beneficiary	21.5 (20.5–22.6)	43.5 (42.5–44.6)	22.0**	
Landed (>0.5 ha)	Control	22.4 (20.4–24.3)	24.5 (22.7–26.2)	2.1	19.6
	Beneficiary	24.7 (23.3–26.2)	46.5 (45.1–47.8)	21.7**	

Maternal anaemia levels

Land holding		Baseline	End line	Mean difference	Reduction attributable to programme
Landless (<0.05 ha)	Control	61.2% (0.568–0.656)	68.9% (0.637–0.741)	7.7%*	−45.0%
	Beneficiary	58.6% (0.524–0.649)	21.3% (0.129–0.298)	−37.3%**	
Functionally landless (0.05–0.50 ha)	Control	63.9% (0.596–0.683)	77.5% (0.743–0.808)	13.6%**	−40.5%
	Beneficiary	57.0% (0.529–0.612)	30.1% (0.267–0.336)	−26.9%**	
Landed (>0.5 ha)	Control	69.9% (0.635–0.763)	80.3% (0.75–0.856)	10.4%*	−39.7%
	Beneficiary	57.4% (0.521–0.627)	28.1% (0.235–0.327)	−29.3%**	

Childhood anaemia levels

Land holding		Baseline	End line	Mean difference	Reduction attributable to programme
Landless (<0.05 ha)	Control	73.1% (0.696–0.766)	63.3% (0.588–0.678)	−9.8%*	−31.2%
	Beneficiary	72.5% (0.681–0.769)	31.5% (0.228–0.402)	−40.9%**	
Functionally landless (0.05–0.50 ha)	Control	74.1% (0.677–0.804)	72.1% (0.682–0.76)	−2.0%	−43.0%
	Beneficiary	72.8% (0.676–0.779)	27.8% (0.238–0.318)	−44.9%**	
Landed (>0.5 ha)	Control	68.1% (0.637–0.725)	71.2% (0.645–0.779)	3.0%	−43.3%
	Beneficiary	67.9% (0.626–0.733)	27.7% (0.222–0.331)	−40.2%**	

In particular, this chapter draws on three qualitative research reports that form HKI's understanding of the ultra-poor: (i) a participatory livelihoods analysis to design a pilot project adapting HFP for vulnerable, extreme-poor farming and fishing communities in the environmentally insecure and extremely remote area of Char Fasson, conducted within the JOJ (Jibon-o-Jibika – Life and Livelihood; see Table 14.1) project;[7] (ii) a gender analysis that studied the distinct social contexts and livelihood strategies between extreme-poor and poor women in the REAL project (Reconstruction, Economic Development and Livelihoods Project, an economic growth-focused intervention; see Table 14.1);[8] and (iii) a social analysis conducted among the landless ultra-poor of the ethnically marginalized groups of the Chittagong Hill Tracts that formed the basis of the M^2W^2 (Making markets work for women) project (see Table 14.1) (HKI, 2010). The section below illustrates some of the suggested HFP modifications for working successfully with the landless ultra-poor.

Technologies for nutrition-oriented production on microplots

Agriculture technologies promoted in the HFP model are geared towards creating a 'developed garden', which is defined as producing a diversity of micronutrient-rich crops in multiple growing seasons on fixed, rather than scattered, plots. The production technologies demonstrated by the VMFs included creating a drainage system through raised beds, establishing a compost pit and using live fencing (Talukder et al., 2000).[9]

While these technologies greatly improve crop quality and productivity on mid-sized plots, households with minimal land need to utilize different technologies and vegetable varieties. Typically, field staff encouraged the ultra-poor to produce 'pit crops' – gourd-type varieties that require minimal land and labour and often generate good income. While some pit crop varieties (such as orange fleshed pumpkin) are rich in vitamin A, the majority of traditional gourds grown in Bangladesh are not. The land-constrained

ultra-poor are less able to produce – and therefore less likely to consume – the leafy vegetables that can be grown elsewhere, as these generally require more land and labour to produce; they are also generally richer in micronutrients (Weinger, 2010). Maximizing the micronutrient benefits from homestead production on microplots requires attention to new growing technologies and the promotion of seed varieties that are dense in micronutrients but require minimal space to grow.

The ultra-poor generally have access only to poor quality and insecure land, such as seasonal flood plains or riverine areas. During the flood period, the gardens of some VMFs and many beneficiaries become fully submerged, leading some programme participants to cease gardening until the floodwaters have receded (HKI, 2010, personal communication, DISHARI Project Staff Meeting, Helen Keller International Bangladesh). This makes year-round, diversified food production a challenge when targeting the extremely vulnerable.

The HFP model has been implemented in diverse agro-ecological zones of Bangladesh, including the flood-prone chars (flood sediment islets) of northern Bangladesh and the cyclone-prone areas of the Coastal Belt, and it has integrated disaster risk reduction guidance into the standard model. In these environmentally insecure areas, all beneficiaries are taught some disaster-preparedness techniques; for example, to store seeds safely and to produce 'flood-resistant' and quickly germinating varieties for consumption or for income-generation during lean periods.

However, because of their greater environmental vulnerability, the landless HFP participants may require greater support and technologies for food storage for the lean season. In addition, ensuring year-round food security for this group may require the integration of non-food-based support during critical times of the year. An example of this mixed agriculture and non-agriculture HFP intervention was applied in Char Fasson. During the participatory livelihoods analysis in Char Fasson, ultra-poor respondents stated that their most critical needs were for access to work during the lean season, as this would reduce the cyclical distress caused by seasonal joblessness and hunger (Tango International,

2009). While most participants were greatly interested in homestead production activities, they also requested support for off-farm livelihood skills to diversify their skills portfolios and enable them to weather seasonal food crises (Tango International, 2009).

In response, HKI developed a mixed intervention, including cash-for-work and cash-for training components, asset transfer and training on 13 on- and off-farm livelihood skills. The interventions were tailored to meet the needs of different target groups within the population – such as adolescent boys and girls, day labourers, and destitute and labour-constrained female-headed households. The focus on homestead food production, together with marketing, food processing, income generation and livelihood skills training, provided a mix of short-term and longer term support to meet food security and nutrition needs.

Input packages required for immediate and long-term nutrition gains

One of the advantages of homestead food production is its minimal implementation cost, which favours scalability and sustainability. The basic delivery package to beneficiaries consists of seeds, financial and technical support for gardening and poultry rearing, and technical training. The standard delivery package was based on the assumption that beneficiaries would have some land holding and minimal income. Historically in Bangladesh, HFP inputs were allocated based on land size and production capacity;[10] which resulted in uneven outcomes among the beneficiaries.

At the start of the REAL project, for example, both poor and ultra-poor participants were included in the same HFP training groups. All participants were given equal support on poultry and seeds. The gender analysis of the REAL project revealed that the less poor beneficiaries (those with larger land holdings) were able to invest their own savings, their spouse's earnings, or their own vegetable income in expanding their poultry rearing activities. This enabled them to generate substantial income and egg production within a short time. However, the ultra-poor households were unable to supplement the support

from the project and so did not immediately realize the nutritional and income benefits that were gained by the other economic groups (HKI, 2009). Despite their greater need for food and nutrition security, the ultra-poor beneficiaries, because of their lower starting points and household assets, had greater difficulty than the poor in translating the support from the project into rapid income or food production gains.

In sum, the landless have the least capacity to produce horticultural goods and yet they have the most urgent need for nutritious food and income. Therefore, when targeted at a more vulnerable population, the minimal 'package' of inputs needs to be modified to ensure substantial improvements to the nutrition and livelihood security of the ultra-poor. The design and evaluation of an appropriate mix of inputs for landless beneficiaries– so to ensure production gains and nutritional outcomes – needs to be taken into consideration at the start of the project. When beneficiary groups include women from different wealth strata (poor and ultra-poor), stratifying appropriate benefit packages within a single project may be a challenge, but it is one that needs to be considered during project design.

For the ultra-poor – who are often trapped in a vicious cycle of debt, food insecurity and ill health – an appropriate package of support may entail a mixture of food- and non-food-based benefits, which can both meet their immediate needs and secure their intermediate-term livelihood security. One form of intermediate-term support that is commonly used in strategies targeting the ultra-poor is asset transfer of livestock, such as goats. In other parts of South Asia, where milk and cheese products are more widely consumed, goat or sheep rearing is inherently part of a food-based nutrition strategy. In Bangladesh, where fresh milk products are not in demand and the commonly bred goats are poor milk producers, goat rearing is primarily an asset-transfer strategy and safety net. Small livestock are essentially a savings account that can be liquidated in times of crisis or sold routinely for extra income (Matin et al., 2008; HKI, 2009). This enables extreme-poor beneficiaries to invest in other livelihood assets or enterprises, to maintain food security during lean seasons and to meet unexpected expenses without spiralling into debt. Goats can be ideal assets for the land and labour constrained because they require minimal care or costs for upkeep and can graze on open land.[11]

Since 2008, HKI has distributed goats to landless, ultra-poor beneficiaries to supplement their package of gardening and poultry support. This ultra-poor livestock intervention has been enthusiastically received by the beneficiaries and has translated into substantial income gains once the goats begin producing kids. The average goat in the REAL project has sold for about US$23.[12] Because the Black Bengal goat variety breeds twice a year and often produces twins, this asset-transfer approach can help to secure long-term food security for the nutritionally vulnerable. Moreover, project data show that a number of ultra-poor beneficiaries are using income from goats to lease land and invest in diversified homestead food production activities (REAL Annual Review Meeting Minutes, Patuakhali, Bangladesh, May 2010, personal communication). In Bangladesh then, while the rearing of goats does not have direct nutritional benefits for their owners, it can be an essential supplementary component to a food-based dietary diversification strategy.

Understanding the social aspects of ultra-poverty in Bangladesh

Understanding the specific needs and capacities of different beneficiary groups within a project is critical to ensuring equitable benefits for all when designing food-based intervention programmes. Modifying a food-based approach to meet the nutritional security of the landless ultra-poor also demands recognition of the social forces and livelihood strategies that characterize their food security, their nutritional needs and their income-generating constraints and opportunities. As discussed earlier, the ultra-poor have extremely weak social capital, are excluded from most microfinance networks and are not on the participant lists for many NGO benefit programmes (Matin *et al.*, 2008). Adapting the HFP model to view the beneficiary group itself as a vital social resource may help the poor and

ultra-poor alike to translate project support into social capital resources.

Social capital is known to be a critical resource for women's asset accumulation, and microfinance programmes are based on the principle that women – without any other collateral – can use the social capital of the lending groups to obtain loans and assets (Kumar and Quisumbing, 2010). Strengthening the group cohesion and social capital generated through HFP programmes may facilitate asset accumulation and greater decision making within their households, which could translate into better nutritional and health-related actions.

The current HFP programmes cluster beneficiaries into several groups of 20 women around a single VMF, primarily for the purposes of facilitating group training and input distribution. The programme, which does not require a loan or repayment, is potentially more inclusive than those such as microfinance groups, which exclude those with the least capacity to repay. However, a gender analysis conducted by HKI in the REAL project showed that members in a given beneficiary group displayed limited social solidarity across wealth groups, and there was minimal interaction or social support among members outside specific training events. Recently, the social resource of the group participants was leveraged through group marketing activities, in which a cluster of women producers market their produce in bulk at a designated collection point (often the VMF). The ultra-poor generally have less surplus produce to sell, owing to their limited productive capacity on marginal land, but the group marketing approach, including training on market information and business planning skills, is equally important to them and can enhance their livelihood strategies.

HKI's group-based nutrition activities offer another mechanism for strengthening social solidarity within the beneficiary groups and for building the social capital of landless members within their communities. These activities include growth promotion and the use of participatory maps to monitor the nutrition challenges and achievements of group members. Both of these tools are effective in working with the ultra-poor and make good use of the social resource of the group to motivate sustainable behaviour change. Illiterate group leaders and group members are capable of understanding child growth charts and they respond with great enthusiasm to growth monitoring sessions, which also provide opportunities for close follow-up and counselling (HKI, 2010, personal communication, DISHARI Project Staff Meeting, Helen Keller International Bangladesh). Some ultra-poor beneficiaries, who are likely to have minimal opportunities for education, have noted that the education on and knowledge of nutrition and gardening that they gain from the project raises their profile in the eyes of their family members and others in the community.

When working with a group-based approach that includes the ultra-poor though, certain considerations must be taken into account. The opportunity cost of lost day-labour wages can prohibit the ultra-poor from participating in project-related training courses and, in some cases, the timing of training sessions may need to be adjusted to accommodate their livelihood strategies. In other cases, HKI has offered a daily training wage for ultra-poor participants, with the compensation equivalent to the current day-labour rate; this enables them to invest their time in training activities and education opportunities that strengthen their long-term food security capacity. In addition, extreme-poor women in Bangladesh are able to take advantage of livelihood opportunities – such as participation in mixed-gender skills training, cash-for-work jobs or training sessions conducted by male trainers – that are socially disallowed for women in a less-poor category. This has enabled HKI to provide the ultra-poor with livelihood occupations, such as mobile poultry vaccinators.

These different social contexts and needs again highlight the imperative to tailor different packages of food- and income-based interventions to different wealth groups. Yet the reality is that distributing stratified benefits within a heterogeneous training group may cause intra-group conflict, counteracting the potential social capital gains. In modifying the HFP model to include the landless ultra-poor, it may be beneficial to work with smaller, more economically homogenous groups, as well as to build in specific training segments related to group cohesion and the benefits of cooperative action.

Focusing nutrition interventions on the context of the ultra-poor

Food security and nutrition programmes often measure success in changes in the anthropometric outcomes of children. As nutrition is the central focus of HKI's HFP programmes, HFP nutrition interventions are geared towards stopping the intergenerational cycle of malnutrition and almost exclusively target women of reproductive age, especially pregnant women and mothers of children less than 2 years of age. The approach is counselling intensive and focuses on breastfeeding and infant and young child feeding practices. Many of the ultra-poor, however, tend to be older or widowed and may be beyond reproductive age; therefore, donor programmes that are focused on nutrition outcomes in children less than 2 years old may inadvertently exclude many of the most nutritionally needy, ultra-poor from participating in a given intervention. Standard nutrition behaviour change communication approaches that focus on child health outcomes may not be applicable to this group.

Whether of reproductive age or not, the ultra-poor have chronically energy-deficient diets and suffer a constellation of health problems and struggles to access health care. Adapting the model to include the landless ultra-poor requires a deeper understanding of the root causes of their nutritional deficiencies and health needs. The nutrition education package for the landless ultra-poor, for example, may emphasize macronutrient and fat consumption or the connection between physical labour and nutrition requirements, rather than have an exclusive focus on maternal nutrition and infant–young child feeding practices. Training materials and messages for this group of people may also need to be designed to reflect their health-seeking behaviours and capacities, and communication outreach strategies may need to be modified to reach them in places where they work and reside.

Promising Nutrition Approaches to Working with the Ultra-poor

While there is yet limited HKI data that is disaggregated by land-size group and intervention basket, the programme experiences outlined above offer some preliminary lessons that can be developed and refined into a comprehensive strategy for meeting the needs of land-constrained groups. While further research is needed, a set of basic observations follows below.

Expansion of technologies to intensify nutrition-sensitive microplot production

The standard technical training provided to HFP beneficiaries emphasizes techniques that can improve the productivity of medium-scale plots, through raised bed drainage systems, the use of live fencing and the creation of compost pits. However, ultra-poor women may lack the family support for the traditionally male aspects of gardening labour, such as raising beds, building a fence or taking their surplus produce to market (HKI, 2009). Field reports suggest that the landless cannot follow this technical approach; the standard advice that they are given is to plant pit crops, which are hardy, fast growing, require minimal space and tend to generate a quick and sizeable income. Effective technologies to maximize poor-quality and flooded land do exist (such as rooftop gardening or floating gardens), and can be applied in targeted geographical zones of Bangladesh. Promising techniques, such as the hydroponic technologies being tested by other NGOs, could be considered in an HFP programme targeting the ultra-poor living in flood-prone regions or with minimal land holdings (Saha, 2010).

Intensifying the year-round productivity of microplots not only calls for new mechanical technologies and/or hardier, micronutrient-rich varieties, but also for the consistent use of training approaches and planning tools that capitalize on beneficiaries' understanding of seasonality and their particular land characteristics. HKI uses participatory land mapping and garden-planning exercises with beneficiaries, which develop their capacity to plan year round and to modify their production strategies at different times of the year. This process, facilitated by field staff, encourages the beneficiaries to consider the nutritional as well as the income goals for their garden, and to design a growing strategy based on the particular capacities and limitations of their land plot. Ultimately, this enables the ultra-poor to make the greatest use of limited resources and builds the planning skills that represent an important livelihood capital for the extreme poor.

Equity-centred approach based on livelihoods and nutritional analysis

An equity-centred approach is based on a clear understanding of who is malnourished within a beneficiary population and why, and what different capabilities the subgroups have (Kennedy, 1994). Landless poor beneficiaries are involved in irregular day-labour activities, face greater time constraints than less poor beneficiaries and have urgent income and nutrition needs. For these beneficiaries, HFP agriculture-related interventions (seed support and gardening training) need to be complemented with more immediate, short-terms benefits. HKI has successfully introduced cash-for-work and cash-for-training components into its HFP programme, and these enable the landless ultra-poor to meet their needs while building human and financial capital for agro-based microenterprises. Other complementary strategies might include direct asset transfer, conditional cash transfers and group-based access to savings accounts, agriculture credits or leased land.

An equity-centred approach to HFP requires a revision of input distribution according to the differentiated needs of the beneficiaries. Working with smaller, more homogeneous, groups for training, income-generating and group savings activities may be more costly to implement, but it may ultimately be more effective in helping the ultra-poor to leverage social, labour and financial support from the programme. A participatory livelihoods or social analysis during the programme design stage would identify the livelihood capitals (beyond land) that different groups within a population can access or need to acquire to improve their immediate and long-term nutrition security.

Emphasis on subsidized poultry rearing for nutrition and income

HKI's Improved Poultry Program (IPP) is particularly appropriate for the landless ultra-poor, as it requires minimal land to produce a sustainable source of animal source foods. The emphasis of the poultry programme is on intensive production of eggs, through supplemental feeding and better chick rearing practices (creep feeding). Poultry rearing maximizes the productivity of microplots and generates immediate income and animal source foods for consumption. Data from HKI show that poultry, as opposed to livestock or other agricultural assets, are more likely to remain under women's control (HKI, 2006b). Furthermore, the poultry programme has resulted in significant impacts on anaemia rates in women and children (Interaction, 2010).

A further benefit of the poultry programme is that it creates livelihood opportunities for ultra-poor women, who tend to have greater mobility than less poor women. Within the HFP programme, HKI has trained a number of ultra-poor women as mobile community vaccinators, who are then linked to the government for supplies and charge a fee for providing both individual and mass vaccinations. In one USAID-funded HFP project, 244 ultra-poor, landless women were trained as community-based vaccinators. These women were dependent on government safety nets, such as the Vulnerable Group Development programme, which provides the equivalent of roughly US$8/month. In the course of this project, high-performing vaccinators were earning as much as Taka 4000–5000/month (US$57–71), while those at the lower end of the scale were earning around Taka 500–1500/month (US$7–21).[13] This improves the income status of the individual vaccinator, and meets a critical need of smallholder producers throughout the community by filling the demand that government extension services are not able to meet (InterAction, 2010).

Development of agro-enterprises with emphasis on nutritional outcomes

Building on the success of the community-based vaccinator programme described above, modifications of the HFP model could consider additional agro-based occupations for which HFP generates demand. Skill training

in these occupations should be specifically targeted to the landless HFP participants, who are less able to benefit from the homestead gardening component. One opportunity built into the HFP programme is an emphasis on distributing local (rather than hybrid) poultry breeds, which are less disease prone. Given the steady demand for quality, local-variety poultry birds in HFP programme areas, building up ultra-poor women into certified local poultry breeders would be a sustainable solution that would generate benefits to the ultra-poor, as well as to the broader smallholder community.

Other agro-based occupations might include mobile seed selling (to reach smallholders located far from the VMF), sapling production, large livestock vaccination, mobile promotion of farm technologies (such as micro-irrigation equipment) or tree grafting. In HKI projects, the poultry programme has also been shown to create local employment for carpenters, who produce the sheds that are required. Female ultra-poor beneficiaries could also be trained in this skill, which would not only create income but would transform social norms about gendered occupations.

Incorporation of market research and value-addition processes

In the original HFP programme design, income generation from sales of vegetables and poultry was a positive side effect, rather than the primary purpose of the programme. Data from HKI projects show that almost all HFP families with land generate and sell some surplus produce and that this income-generating aspect of the programme is significant for the associated gains in women's autonomy and decision making. HKI has gradually increased focus on the marketing component of its programmes, developing approaches such as group marketing that enable women to generate profit with minimal inconvenience or time loss.

Incorporating a market-oriented approach into HFP that strengthens linkages with the private sector may create alternative livelihood opportunities for the ultra-poor. It can also have benefits for the broader community by facilitating access to quality inputs, and creating a cheaper, more diverse and nutritious food supply in the local markets and for households. Apart from being a demonstration farmer, the owner of the VMF could also be trained in business plan development and supported to establish linkages with private-sector market actors.

Nutrition-sensitive sub-sector and value-chain analyses conducted at the outset of the HFP programme can identify niche crops where value addition can provide employment for the ultra-poor and greater profits for all producers in the group. In addition to basic postharvest grading and handling processes, primary and secondary processing can add significant value to products and enable sales during the off season. In HFP catchment areas where primary postharvest processing can be done at the beneficiary level, the functionally landless producers can be trained and equipped to participate in value-addition processes, including packaging or home-based processing. Technologies that can be introduced at the beneficiary level include solar driers, rice-husking machines and canning processes. Processing and storing food can also serve the overall purpose of providing access to nutritious food year round. However, maximizing the nutritional gains of food storage techniques will depend on selecting appropriate technologies for preserving the micronutrient content of the selected product (Bhattacharjee *et al.*, 2007).

Nutrition behaviour change communication for different populations

The risk of incorporating market-oriented approaches into the HFP programme is that the emphasis on income will displace nutrition goals. In some cases, sudden or rapid access to income for cash-poor households allows them to access foods that are perceived as 'higher status', although these may not be nutritionally valuable. Much malnutrition relates to intra-household allocation problems or to inappropriate adolescent, maternal and young-child feeding practices. Research shows that intensive nutrition education

alone – without micronutrient supplements – can improve the status of moderately malnourished children (Roy *et al.*, 2005). From the outset, the HFP programme united nutrition communication with agricultural training. The combination of homestead food production with nutrition education has brought about significant reductions in anaemia rates and improvements in dietary diversity in diverse project areas. Within a single year of a pilot Essential Nutrition Actions (ENA) project in 2008, the ENA training in essential nutrition actions (ENA) – integrated into an existing food security and nutrition intervention (the JOJ project; see Table 14.1) – was found to have a statistically significant supplemental impact on child underweight in the project area (HKI, 2010b).

For most of the landless ultra-poor, a focus on income generation is critical to enable them to purchase the nutritious foods that they are not able to produce on their homesteads. There is clear evidence of the critical role that nutrition education plays here, and this would need to be included as a core component along with the other livelihood strategies outlined in this chapter. Moreover, specific nutritional research and training materials may need to be designed to ensure that nutrition messages and programmes address the specific vulnerabilities of ultra-poor groups, including the elderly and those of non-reproductive age.

Discussion

The conditions and approaches detailed above are highly specific to the context of Bangladesh, where land scarcity is extreme and constitutes a defining characteristic of food insecurity and malnutrition. Nevertheless, the challenge of evolving tried-and-true food-based, nutrition-sensitive approaches to reach more marginalized populations will be a global imperative in the decades to come, as climate change, urbanization and population pressures limit the resources (including water) that are available for diversified agriculture production. HKI's research and field experience has shown that landless beneficiaries are very enthusiastic about being included in HFP interventions, which are seen as providing a stable source of food, potential income and social capital. However, to ensure that the landless ultra-poor are able to gain equitably from HFP, certain modifications to critical areas of the 'standard' HFP model are required.

HKI's homestead food production programme, which places a central focus on nutrition, has been shown to be a flexible production model that can have positive nutrition benefits for the landless. Adapting the model for the landless calls for an equity-centred approach, based on a clear understanding of how and why different populations are malnourished, and what different capabilities the subgroups have to produce or access nutritious foods. This equity-centred approach also entails stratifying support packages for different subgroups.

Food-based interventions are unique in that they specifically promote nutrition outcomes, which have long been neglected in poverty reduction and agriculture extension programmes. The landless ultra-poor are the most nutritionally compromised and malnourished, and have limited access to health services. The livelihood strategies of the most vulnerable tend to be more diverse and varied, and they have to employ nutritionally risky coping mechanisms. For this reason, the capacity to produce even a small quantity of home-based, nutritious food, with minimal labour or time inputs, can be an especially valuable intervention for the ultra-poor. Having better nutrition and fewer nutrition-related health complications can translate into sustainable livelihood gains for the ultra-poor, for whom physical labour capacity is often their most important livelihood resource.

HKI's experience to date indicates that to maximize their capacity to benefit from the HFP strategy, the ultra-poor require both food-based and income-oriented supports, which enable them to meet immediate needs while building up longer term food security and stability. This

may include a combination of agro-based microenterprises, emphasis on food storage techniques and combinations of asset transfer and livelihood skill building. Developing nutrition-sensitive agro-enterprises in a community-based model can also yield nutrition benefits for the broader community, as it can expand the availability of and demand for a diversified horticultural food basket.

Training in nutrition and nutrition-sensitive agricultural planning is an indispensable component of any food-based intervention, particularly one that targets the ultra-poor, although communication approaches to improve the nutritional practices of the ultra-poor are not identical to those promoting child growth outcomes. To have lasting impact on the nutrition status of the ultra-poor, a behavioural change communication strategy must be designed for them that is based on an understanding of the underlying determinants of their malnutrition and their nutrition strategies.

These essential programme modifications have implications for intervention costs as well as for further research and evaluation needs. More extension research is also required into growing technologies and seed varieties, including flood-sensitive varieties, that can maximize the year-round productivity of poor-quality and small plots of land. As food-based nutrition interventions are modified to address the ultra-poor, disaggregation of nutrition outcomes by wealth quintile and rigorous monitoring of intervention types will be critical to determining the most cost-effective and efficacious strategies.

Acknowledgements

Our acknowledgements go to Diane Lindsey, Country Director, Bangladesh, HKI and to Akoto Osei, Regional Nutrition Advisor, APRO, HKI.

Notes

[1] As this proportion is only calculated from rural households, the figure may understate the growth in landlessness by not counting families who have migrated to urban areas as a result of loss of land.

[2] In 1990, vitamin A deficiency was defined as a public problem by the World Health Organization (WHO) based on a prevalence of childhood night blindness that was higher than the cut-off of 1% among children 12–59 months of age.

[3]The data used to create this graph were drawn from the eight baseline data sets of five HKI programmes: Fifth round NGNESP (719 observations); Sixth round NGNESP (719 observations); Seventh round NGNESP (860 observations); Char 1 (420 observations); Char 2 (400 observations); CHT-HFP (400 observations); and DISHARI (499 observations). In the graph, land holding is defined by land-ownership. See Table 14.1 for further project details.

[4]This analysis was completed using six data sets, three baseline surveys and three end-line surveys from each of the Char 1, Char 2 and CHT-HFP projects (see Table 14.1 for further details). Each data set included a sample of ~400 beneficiary households and ~400 control households from nearby villages who were not included in the programme. The sample was drawn from the subset of households in each community that contained a child under the age of 5 years. In each household, one child under 5 years of age and his/her mother were surveyed and measured and had their blood haemoglobin level tested using a Hemocue machine. All three programmes were of the same length, began and ended in the same season, and baseline and end-line surveys were conducted in the same season. Sampling structures for all three surveys were the same and the questionnaire was nearly identical. Analysis was done using Stata 11.0 software and utilizing the svyset commands to account for the clustered survey design.

[5]The analysis of food frequency (to produce a food frequency score – FFS) was done by calculating a food consumption score (FCS) for the mother of the small child in each household. This score is a measure of food security, dietary diversity and food frequency designed and promoted by the United Nations World Food Programme (WFP). Though this indicator is usually constructed for the whole household as a food security measure, constructing the indicator on an individual captures the nutritional status of that individual. The methodology for the construction this indicator can be found in WFP (2008).

[6]The estimated gain in maternal food frequency score (FFS) from the project was constructed by measuring the difference in food consumption score (FCS; see Endnote 5) between baseline and end line for all groups and then subtracting the difference between the treatment and the control group for that category of land holding.

[7]Char Fasson is an area in Bhola District, Barisal Division. It is surrounded by the Bay of Bengal on three sides and is vulnerable to land erosion and severe cyclones. The research discussed here was undertaken as part of the Jibon-o-Jibika Food for Peace Title II Project, carried out from 2004 to 2009.

[8]The REAL project was an income-oriented project to rehabilitate households that lost livelihoods in the wake of Cyclone Sidr.

[9]For these reasons VMF (Village Model Farm) owners were required to have a demonstration plot of a minimum of 0.15 acres (600 m^2), although the average VMF plot size in 2006 was closer to 0.25 acres (HKI, 2006a). The direct beneficiaries of the HFP programme typically had access to only the homestead land around the house.

[10]A household with more land would have received a greater amount of inputs such as seeds.

[11]Case studies from across South Asia point to some of the challenges of small ruminant management, which relate to low productivity, poor-quality extension services or susceptibility to diseases (SAPPLPP, 2010). In its work with small livestock, however, HKI has developed a set of best practices to keep mortality to a minimum, of an average of 5%. The most critical of these practices is to purchase livestock from extremely local markets, rather than purchasing them in bulk or from large-scale markets. This purchase practice significantly reduces rates of disease and mortality, although it also extends the amount of time (and therefore costs) of distribution to beneficiaries. In addition to local purchase of livestock, training in vaccination and linkages to the government services is essential to the success of the programme (REAL Annual Review Meeting Minutes, Patuakhali, Bangladesh, May 2010, personal communication).

[12]If this were considered to be the monthly income, it would be equivalent to twice the per capita upper poverty line.

[13]This income estimate is based on a conversion rate of 70 Bangladesh Taka (BDT) to US$1.

References

Ahmed, A.U., Vargas Hill, R., Smith, L.C. and Frankenberger, T. (2007) *Characteristics and Causes of Severe Poverty and Hunger*. 2020 Focus Brief on the World's Poor and Hungry People, International Food Policy Research Institute (IFPRI), Washington, DC. Available at: http://conferences.ifpri. org/2020Chinaconference/pdf/beijingbrief_ahmed2.pdf (accessed 14 June 2013).

Allen, L.H. (2008) To what extent can food-based approaches improve micronutrient status? *Asia Pacific Journal of Clinical Nutrition* 17(S1), 103–105.

BBS (2007) *Household Income and Expenditure Survey*. Bangladesh Bureau of Statistics, Planning Division, Ministry of Planning, Government of the People's Republic of Bangladesh, Dhaka.

BBS (2008) *Preliminary Report of Agriculture Census*. Planning Division, Ministry of Planning, Government of the People's Republic of Bangladesh, Dhaka.

BBS and UNICEF (2007) *Child and Mother Nutrition Survey of Bangladesh 2005*. Bangladesh Bureau of Statistics, Planning Division, Ministry of Planning, Government of the People's Republic of Bangladesh and United Nations Children's Fund, Dhaka.

Bhattacharjee, L., Kumar Saha, S. and Nandi, B.K. (2007) *Food-based Nutrition Strategies in Bangladesh: Experience of Integrated Horticulture and Nutrition Development*. RAP Publication 2007/05, Department of Agriculture Extension, Government of Bangladesh, Dhaka and Regional Office for Asia and the Pacific, Food and Agriculture Organization of the United Nations, Bangkok.

Bread for the World Institute (2010) *Our Common Interest: Ending Hunger and Malnutrition, 2011 Hunger Report. Twenty-first Annual Report on State of World Hunger*. Bread for the World Institute, Washington, DC.

Chowdhury, M.I. (2009) *Impact of Increasing Landlessness on Access to Food: Experience of Small and Marginal Farmers in Rural Bangladesh*. Unnayan Onneshan – The Innovators, Dhaka. Available at: http://www.bdresearch.org.bd/home/attachments/article/221/Impact_of_Increasing_Landlessness.pdf (accessed 14 June 2013).

Darnton-Hill, I., Hussein, N., Kann, R. and Duthic, M.R. (1988) *Tables of Nutrient Composition of Bangladeshi Foods: English version with Particular Emphasis on Vitamin A Contents*. Helen Keller International Bangladesh, Dhaka.

FAO (2010) Consumption, Table D2 – Share of dietary components in total energy consumption (2005–2007). In: *FAO Statistical Yearbook 2010*. Food and Agriculture Organization of the United Nations, Rome. Available at: http://www.fao.org/economic/ess/ess-publications/ess-yearbook/ess-yearbook2010/yearbook2010-consumption/en/ (accessed 9 July 2013).

FAO and WFP (2008) *Special Report: FAO/WFP Crop and Food Supply Assessment Mission to Bangladesh, 28 August 2008*. Food and Agriculture Organization of the United Nations and World Food Programme, Rome. Available at: ftp://ftp.fao.org/docrep/fao/011/ai472e/ai472e00.pdf (accessed 14 June 2013).

FPMU (2009) *National Food Policy Plan of Action (2008–2015)*. Monitoring Report, Food Planning and Monitoring Unit, Ministry of Food and Disaster Management, Government of the People's Republic of Bangladesh, Dhaka.

HKI (2006a) *Economic and Social Impact Evaluation*. Internal unpublished report available on request. Helen Keller International Bangladesh, Dhaka.

HKI (2006b) *Female Decision-making Power and Nutritional Status within Bangladesh's Socio-economic Context*. Nutritional Surveillance Project Bulletin No. 20, Helen Keller International Bangladesh, Dhaka. Available at: http://www.hki.org/research/NSP%20Bulletin%2020.pdf (accessed 13 June 2013).

HKI (2009) *A Gender Analysis of Sidr Reconstruction Efforts in the REAL Project*. Bulletin No. 5, Helen Keller International Bangladesh, Dhaka. Available at: http://www.hki.org/research/HKI%20Bulletin%20Bangladesh%20May%2010%20Gender%20Analysis_REAL%20Project.pdf (accessed 13 June 2013). This is a summary of the full report, which is available on request from HKI Bangladesh.

HKI (2010a) *A Social analysis in Laxmichari Upazila Making Markets Work for Women Project (M²W²)*. Bulletin No. 10, Helen Keller International Bangladesh, Dhaka. Available at: http://www.hki.org/research/HKI%20Bulletin%20Bangladesh%20Oct%2010%20Social%20Analysis%20in%20Laxmichari.pdf (accessed 13 June 2013).

HKI (2010b) *Training Communities on Essential Nutrition Actions*. Bulletin No. 4, Helen Keller International Bangladesh, Dhaka. Available at: http://www.hki.org/research/HKI%20Bulletin%20Bangladesh%20April%2010%20Training%20Communities%20on%20ENA.pdf (accessed 13 June 2013).

Hossain, M.A. (2010) Global warming induced sea level rise on soil, land and crop production loss in Bangladesh. In: *19th World Congress of Soil Science, Soil Solutions for a Changing World: Global Challenges and Soil Salination, Brisbane, Australia, 1–6 August. Working Group 3.4: Challenges and Soil Salination*, pp. 77–80. Available at: http://www.iuss.org/19th%20WCSS/Symposium/pdf/WG3.4.pdf (accessed 14 June 2013).

Iannotti, L., Cunningham, K. and Ruel, M. (2009) Diversifying into healthy diets: homestead food production in Bangladesh. In: Spielman, D.J. and Pandya-Lorch, R. (eds) (2009) *Millions Fed: Proven Successes in Agricultural Development*. International Food Policy Research Institute (IFPRI), Washington, DC, pp. 145–151.

InterAction (2010) *Best Practices and Innovations (BPI) Initiative: Agriculture and Rural Livelihoods. Improved Poultry Program, Helen Keller International, Best Practice Award for Livestock Production. Best Practices and*

Innovations [in Agriculture] Initiative Round 1 Awards. Available at: http://www.interaction.org/sites/default/files/BPI%20Round%201%20-%20HKI%20-%20FINAL.pdf (accessed 14 June 2013).

Jha, R., Gaiha, R. and Sharma, A. (2009) Calorie and micronutrient deprivation and poverty nutrition traps in rural India. *World Development* 37, 982–991.

Kennedy, E.T. (1994) Approaches to linking agriculture and nutrition. *Health Policy and Planning* 9, 295–305.

Kumar, N. and Quisumbing, A.R. (2010) *Does Social Capital Build Women's Assets? Disseminating Agricultural Technologies to Individuals versus Groups in Bangladesh*. Evaluating the Long-Term Impact of Anti-poverty Interventions in Rural Bangladesh, Project Note – August 2010, International Food Policy Research Institute (IFPRI), Washington, DC and Chronic Poverty Research Centre, Manchester, UK. Available at: http://www.ifpri.org/sites/default/files/publications/ifpricprcnote_kumarquisumbing1.pdf (accessed 14 June 2013).

Leroy, J.L. and Frongillo, E.A. (2007) Can interventions to promote animal production ameliorate undernutrition? *Journal of Nutrition* 137, 2311–2316.

Mascie-Taylor, C.G.N., Marks, M.K., Goto, R. and Islam, R. (2010) Impact of a cash-for-work programme on food consumption and nutrition among women and children facing food insecurity in rural Bangladesh. *Bulletin of the World Health Organization* 88, 854–860.

Matin, I., Sulaiman, M. and Rabbani, M. (2008) *Crafting a Graduation Pathway for the Ultra-poor: Lessons and Evidence from a BRAC programme*. CRPC Working Paper No. 109, Chronic Poverty Research Centre, Manchester, UK. Available at: http://www.chronicpoverty.org/publications/details/crafting-a-graduation-pathway-for-the-ultra-poor-lessons-and-evidence-from-a-brac-programme/ss (accessed 14 June 2013) [archived site].

Ministry of Agriculture (2007) Table 5.01 Cropping Intensity 1980-81 to 2004-05. In: *Handbook of Agricultural Statistics, December 2007*. Ministry of Agriculture, Government of the People's Republic of Bangladesh, Dhaka. Available at http://www.moa.gov.bd/statistics/Table5.01CI.htm (accessed 25 November 2010).

Nielsen, H., Roos, N. and Thilsted, S.H. (2003) The impact of semi-scavenging poultry production on the consumption of animal source foods by women and girls in Bangladesh. *Journal of Nutrition* 133 (11, Suppl.), 4027S–4030S.

Rahman, M.H. and Manprasert, S. (2006) Landlessness and its impact on economic development: a case study in Bangladesh. *Journal of Social Sciences* 2, 54–60.

Roy, S.K., Fuchs, G.J., Mahmud, Z., Ara, G., Islam, S., Shafique, S., Akter, S.S. and Chakraborty, B. (2005) Intensive nutrition education with or without supplementary feeding improves the nutritional status of moderately malnourished children in Bangladesh. *Journal of Health, Population, and Nutrition* 23, 320–330.

Saha, S.K. (2010) Soilless cultivation for landless people: an alternative livelihood practice through indigenous hydroponic agriculture in flood-prone Bangladesh. *Ritsumeikan Journal of Asia Pacific Studies* 27, 139–152. Available at: http://www.apu.ac.jp/rcaps/uploads/fckeditor/publications/journal/RJAPS_V27_Saha.pdf (accessed 14 June 2013).

SAPPLPP (2010) Small Ruminants. South Asia Pro-Poor Livestock Policy Programme, New Delhi. Available at: http://sapplpp.org/thematicfocus/small-ruminants (accessed 28 November 2010).

Talukder, A., Kiess, L., Huq, N., de Pee, S., Darnton-Hill, I. and Bloem, M.W. (2000) Increasing the production and consumption of vitamin A-rich fruits and vegetables: lessons learned in taking the Bangladesh homestead gardening programme to a national scale. *Food and Nutrition Bulletin* 21, 165–172.

Tango International (2009) *Char Fasson Assessment Design Document*. Prepared for Save the Children Bangladesh, Dhaka, Tango International, Tucson, Arizona.

Tontisirin, K., Nantel, G. and Bhattacharjee, L. (2002) Food-based strategies to meet the challenges of micronutrient malnutrition in the developing world. *The Proceedings of the Nutrition Society* 61, 243–250.

Van Haeften, R. and Moses, P. (2009) *USAID Office of Food for Peace Bangladesh Food Security Country Framework FY 2010–2014*. Food and Nutrition Technical Assistance Project (FANTA-2), Academy for Educational Development (AED), Washington, DC. Available at: http://pdf.usaid.gov/pdf_docs/PDACU310.pdf (accessed 14 June 2013).

Weinger, S. (2010) *A Sustainability Review of Helen Keller International's NGO Gardening and Nutrition Education Surveillance Project*. Draft document, Helen Keller International Bangladesh, Dhaka.

WFP (2008) *Food Consumption Analysis. Calculation and Use of the Food Consumption Score in Food Security Analysis*. Technical Guidance Sheet, Vulnerability Analysis and Mapping Branch, World Food

Programme, Rome. Available at: http://documents.wfp.org/stellent/groups/public/documents/manual_guide_proced/wfp197216.pdf (accessed 14 June 2013).

WFP, UNICEF and IPHN (2009) *Household Food Security and Nutrition Assessment in Bangladesh, November 2008–January 2009.* World Food Programme, Rome, United Nations Childrens' Fund (UNICEF Bangladesh), Institute of Public Health Nutrition (IPHN) for Ministry of Health and Family Welfare, Government of Bangladesh, Dhaka. Available at: http://www.unglobalpulse.org/sites/default/files/reports/Attachment_0.pdf (accessed 14 June 2013).

15 The Growing Connection Project – With a Mexico Case Study

Bob Patterson[1]* and Margarita Álvarez Oyarzábal[2]

[1]*Former Liaison Office for North America, Food and Agriculture Organization of the United Nations, Washington, DC, USA;* [2]*Former Coordinator in Mexico for The Growing Connection, Guadalajara, Mexico*

This chapter does not fall into the mainstream of detailed research or knowledge-shifting papers that have been presented at this symposium. We would particularly like to thank Brian Thompson and his colleagues in the Nutrition Division of FAO for inviting our low-key, low-budget and 'unofficial' initiative – 'The Growing Connection' to participate in this symposium.

The Growing Connection

The Growing Connection (TGC) operates in 12 countries in Latin America, the Caribbean, Africa, the USA and Canada. There are about 130 garden/production and demonstration sites worldwide, some very small, some very large. The project itself is funded through a registered, tax-exempt non-profit organization (NGO) that we operate out of FAO's Liaison Office for North America, in Washington, DC. FAO's supportive participation in TGC is through in-kind coordination and support: portions of salary, office space for me and one FAO colleague, plus partial funding of travel and communication costs incurred to operate the project. FAO has

agreed to absorb these costs as they are seen to be entirely consistent with the 'liaison' function of the Washington office – engaging people directly into FAO's mandate of fighting hunger through sustainable agriculture.

TGC is operated in the field by NGOs. All growing sites are self-financed – meaning directly by the growers/participants themselves (e.g. schools, women's associations, etc.), or by benefactors – donors, foundations, philanthropic institutions and corporate social activities. The Growing Connection has no employees, no staff. In one sense, that makes coordination more difficult; on the other hand, it means that the participants are involved because they like what they do – and because they like the results.

We have learned much from the people who comprise The Growing Connection, and we have learned that people, everywhere, respond well to opportunities to directly participate in their own nutritional (and taste) improvement. Wherever we introduce ourselves and our activities, we ask a couple of questions of our participants and audiences: Did you grow up on a farm? Did your parents or grandparents? Was there a vegetable garden? Are you now a gardener? Do you grow vegetables? The responses to these questions

*Contact: robertpatterson57@gmail.com

tell us that the vast majority of people are not that far removed from the food production/growing process. Usually they have a direct history of growing/gardening, or it is one or two generations removed.

We have also seen that there is a 'growing' trend, almost everywhere, in which people, families, communities and institutions are seeking ways and means to become directly involved in production, even if this only means growing some fresh herbs and heirloom tomatoes. As we ask these questions very frequently, we see that more hands than ever are going up on that last question.

There is a 300% increase in the purchase of vegetable seeds in the USA over that of 2 years ago. Some analysts will no doubt say that this results from rising food costs and a weak economy. Whichever is the case, we find it really encouraging, and feel that it points to 'fertile ground' for our project – TGC.

Over the course of this symposium, we have become exposed to multiple, most interesting research and developments in human nutrition, particularly as regards 'at-risk' populations. This has been an education for us and we have learned a considerable amount about food-based nutrition programmes and research, and why food-based approaches result in better nutrition. Research, development and deeply considered analysis, however, are not what we do in TGC. Rather, we work with gardeners, teachers, growers, communities and families. Much of what this symposium addresses deals with the 'why'; we are going to talk a little bit about the 'how'.

The TGC approach focuses on *how* to get people gardening, growing, producing fresh food, *how* to increase people's access to fresh fruits and vegetables by direct, personal activities with appropriate, affordable tools and information. On the nutrition side, this presentation reinforces and repeats the advice that we all received from our mothers and grandmothers: 'Eat your vegetables'.

TGC combines two seemingly diverse innovations: (i) innovations in growth – meaning agricultural/horticultural growth, and innovations in growing food – essentially to grow the vegetables as close to the household as you can; and (ii) innovations in communications technology – access to information to enhance and share the ability to grow food.

Most simply, TGC is about access to useful tools – how to acquire them affordably and how to use them effectively and, we hope, how to share that knowledge about how to use them. We also hope that TGC participants will document their experiences and will share these locally and globally with others. While, quite obviously, we want good gardeners to become curious about our project, more importantly, we use IT/communications technology, computers, phones, etc. to broadcast our message on the Web, which we hope will engage participants and interested parties in a worldwide network of practitioners sharing best practices, advice and innovations.

I want now to focus on some simple and practical tools and innovations in horticulture. These methods and tools complement very well what we have learned at this symposium, particularly from our colleagues who are working in Bangladesh. In TGC, we have tried to find a 'tool kit' that will allow people to easily become gardeners, to easily grow food and to do that virtually anywhere. We work in rural and urban areas, with people who are rich and poor; the only qualification to join TGC is a positive reply to the question, 'Do you want to grow vegetables?'. To the extent possible, TGC enables actions that follow this positive reply.

We try to make the tools and practices we promote in TGC as accessible and as simple as possible. We promote easy methods, such as household or institution-level water collectors. I recently (2 weeks ago) saw schoolchildren in Toronto mounting half-pipe ducting on the chain-linked fences around their school playground (Fig. 15.1). They collect water for their garden, just down below. It works on gravity alone, and is really clever: the children have designed it to look like an eagle.

In addition to water collection, traditional composting and worm composting can be done almost anywhere. Nothing special is needed. Vermiculture is the most productive and environmentally friendly way to fertilize plants.

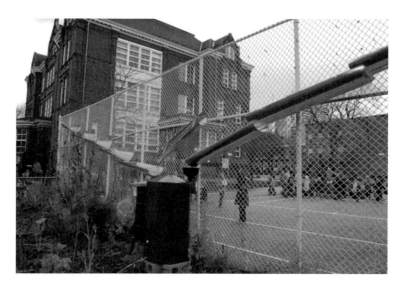

Fig. 15.1. Water collectors in Toronto, Ontario, Canada. Photo courtesy of Syd Patterson.

At many of our sites – particularly those where, for example, a women's group is engaged in 'market production', hoop houses (informal greenhouses) (Fig. 15.2) in various forms have proven to be excellent investments. One can significantly extend the growing season with a bit of plastic, some wood, wire, bags and tyres: these are not necessarily very elegant, but they certainly work.

Finally, in TGC we use many different types of containers – containerized production enables production to be carried out on the doorstep. It also effectively 'creates' fertile land, often where none existed before. Let's look at our particular favourite, the earth box.

The earth box is the type of innovation that typifies how anyone who is interested in taking a direct role in enhancing their own nutrition can immediately become directly involved and successfully engaged in vegetable production. We use this tool in all of our sites for several key reasons:

- It needs 80% less water than an in-ground drip system.
- It takes 50% less fertilizer, and even if you decide to use conventional, chemical-based fertilizers, they are entirely contained within the system and there is no contamination of soils or water tables.

- It requires about 90% less labour. Once you have planted, you just water and deal with above ground pests; there is no weeding, no continual cultivation, and no fertilization.

In TGC we have proven that this tool can be used virtually anywhere: mountaintops, rooftops or balconies, or in peripheral areas or on a large scale, such as the row of 500 planted at an orphanage in South Africa. Using this and similar containers is, essentially, a recreation of one third of a square metre of fertile land, and this land will be recreated anywhere you want it.

The earth box is a commercial product (known as EarthBox), but we use it because it works. Indeed, virtually everywhere we go with this box, people copy it, innovate or come up with artisanal versions, and we entirely welcome that. One can take a few planks of wood, put them together, line the resulting box with plastic and it will work. The key to this system is the reservoir of water on the bottom – 12 l – and a 'wicking' substratum (always local). This is a coco peat from Mozambique, which is local if you are in South Africa, where this box comes from. Put water in the tube, capillary action begins and the vegetable plants get the nutrients they need. It's really simple (Fig. 15.3).

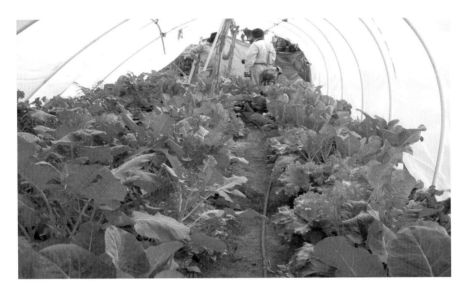

Fig. 15.2. Hoop houses. Photo courtesy of Margarita Álvarez.

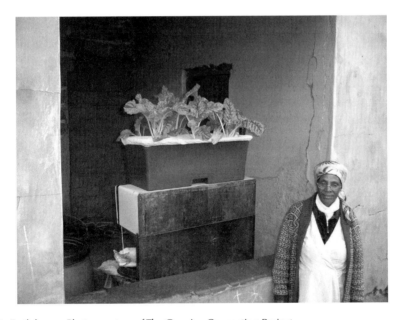

Fig. 15.3. Earth boxes. Photo courtesy of The Growing Connection Project.

These tools for composting, vermiculture, water management and microclimates, particularly when combined with the containers, demonstrate to people that it is easy to grow food. The tools themselves act as facilitators and catalysts, drawing people into the process of growing food, demonstrating success and inspiring further curiosity and action (Fig. 15.4).

At every TGC site, we work with local agriculturists – often universities but also NGOs — to make sure we're adopting these

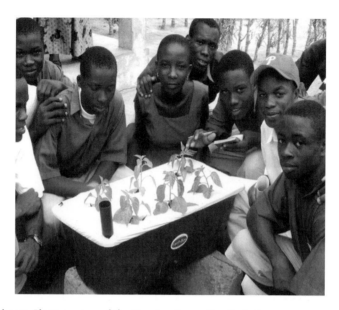

Fig. 15.4. Earth boxes. Photo courtesy of The Growing Connection Project.

tools as locally and practically as possible. We work extensively with local agronomists to develop appropriate and affordable local substrata with the proper crop nutrients for earth boxes (Fig. 15.5).

While, in TGC, I have always been sure we can make our techniques work with success, we're also always careful to make the 'tool kits' as affordable as possible. We have one essential ground rule regarding our tools, i.e. there are no motors and the mantra is 'no cost or low cost'. The decision for not having motors is based on my 30 years of fieldwork with FAO. If you have a motor, someone steals it, or it will break, so there are no motors. That also makes our tools easier to use, easier to maintain, accessible (especially to women), durable and have a higher rate of success.

In Ghana, where we started this project, we had the good luck to work with the University of Cape Coast team who were training many of the agricultural extension officers there. This team has been very eager to develop school farms and gardens using improved, innovative techniques. However, as we toured and visited schools, we learned that many of the children who were working in the gardens were doing so on detention,

effectively being put to farm and work on gardens as a punishment, which is not really a good way to convince children to like it!

When one considers the difficulty of their work, breaking up hard ground in the Ghanaian dry season, hauling water, etc., you quickly realize that this is exceptionally hard work; it is punishing. But several months after we introduced these earth boxes, together with some simple water collection and artisanal composters, the cool kids started to migrate towards the gardens. It was clear that incentive rather than punishment worked in the gardens. The children liked what was happening: they saw that it had results. The innovative tools acted as a magnet, drew them in and made them curious and interested. That same school, 2 years later, won the President's Prize for best school farm! Those same children have gone on to improved cassava production, organic pest management and diversified vegetable production. As they became engaged in growing, and as they achieved success, they also saw the returns.

The right tools will always act as a magnet and will act as a catalyst, because as soon as you start working with something like this, you start asking yourself questions about

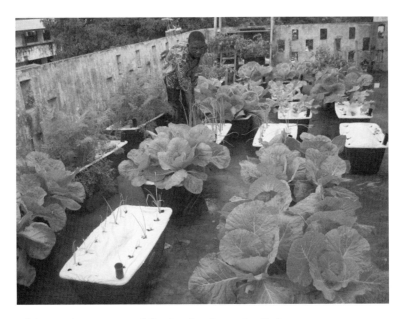

Fig. 15.5. Earth boxes. Photo courtesy of The Growing Connection Project.

water management, about composting. How does soil compost in this? What about pest management? Crop rotation? These are fundamental questions of horticulture and agriculture, the basic things one needs to know in order to have something fresh and tasty in one's mouth every day. When this happens, you help people to scale up and afterwards you can make yourself available to answer any questions, so that your students are able to carry on independently afterwards.

We've spoken about our simple basic tool kit. There is another reason why we keep it uniform and simple: it facilitates communications. When we are able to use IT to connect, for example, the schoolchildren in Ghana with those in Washington, DC, they have something directly in common: the same tools and the same experiences. They talk to each other about their growing experiences, certainly, then they talk about clothes and TV shows, and they share how they have learned to produce things together – they exchange recipes.

TGC in Mexico

TGC in Mexico started in 2004 in partnership with the Science and Agronomy Campus of the University of Guadalajara. At the beginning, TGC worked directly with one of the poorest and most isolated communities in Jalisco, Mexico, the Huicholes, thanks to the University's rural extension programme. Activities in Mexico have since expanded to rural schools, to groups of women in indigenous communities, and also to government projects and health centres throughout the country, particularly in Oaxaca and Chiapas. Later, we included urban sites (schools, clinics and women's associations) in low-income areas (Fig. 15.6).

As you have seen, one can always plant a garden on a rooftop or in an alley. TGC also has sites at a handicapped community and employment centre, and recently we started to collaborate with the private sector in nutrition programmes for employees and their families. In this latter example, TGC has built rooftop vegetable gardens to diversify the workers' daily diets by adding fresh green vegetables and herbs; the hope is to build continuing and sustained interest in urban food production at household level (Fig. 15.7).

Based on more than 5 years of research and experiments at the University of Guadalajara, we have adapted the earth box to local conditions and to inputs that are

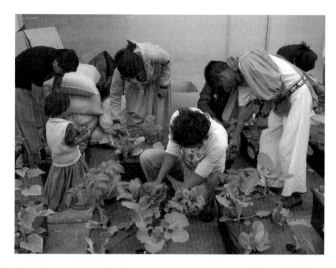

Fig. 15.6. The Growing Connection Project in Mexico. Photo courtesy of Margarita Álvarez Oyarzábal.

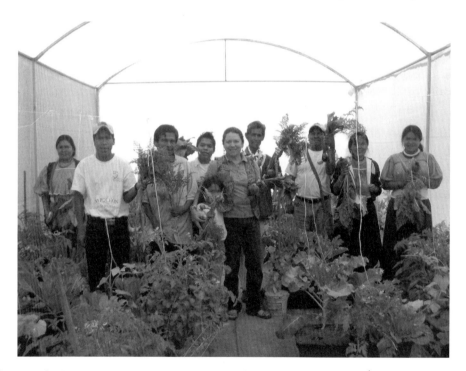

Fig. 15.7. The Growing Connection Project in Mexico. Photo courtesy of Margarita Álvarez Oyarzábal.

locally available in Mexico at low cost. This includes the use of locally available worm castings (vermiculture) and *estopa de coco* – dried and milled coconut fibre. When building sites at the high-altitude areas we use hoop houses and tunnels to extend cropping seasons, and we take advantage of the boxes for very efficient use of water. This has allowed TGC to demonstrate and convince people to grow vegetables in areas where previously it was not possible. We have initiated organic production among communities and schools. An additional advantage is that these activities have increased people's interest in organic farming.

Even though many of our teaching/demonstration/production sites are located in schools in Mexico, we have engaged diverse groups of participants in TGC; in almost every case, including schools, we think that the direct and driving participation/support of women is a key to success. It is the women who prepare and share the meals with the whole family, and it is the women who collect and pass on their knowledge to their children and across the rest of the community. We have learned over the past 6 years that the project can be taken up by almost anyone because it is easily understood, it is very simple, and it is for all ages and all conditions. That is good, of course. However, where there is women's participation in decision making and setting priorities, the chances of success increase greatly.

Personally, the best part of TGC has been to see project participants gain satisfaction and pride from growing their own vegetables. They have discovered new foods and learned new recipes. Many of the women in indigenous communities had not previously heard of spinach or broccoli. They would ask: what is this for? At the outset, at our very first cropping cycles, they would give spinach or broccoli to their chickens and rabbits because they had no idea of how to prepare them or of their nutritional value. Following careful extension work in the preparation of soups and simple recipes using these products, they are now regularly part of the diets of participating villages, and the results have been fewer eye and skin infections among the children. The fresh produce

has improved their nutrition as well as their creativity and dignity (Fig. 15.8).

It is clear that in TGC communities we have seen changes in nutrition and health among people that we work with, particularly in young children: their skin and eyes show it. We have also seen the engagement of a diverse group of people that has started growing or want to grow their vegetables.

To conclude, I would like to express my gratitude for all your excellent presentations of research findings and of the diverse projects that you have shared with us and which can build a platform to move ahead and take action.

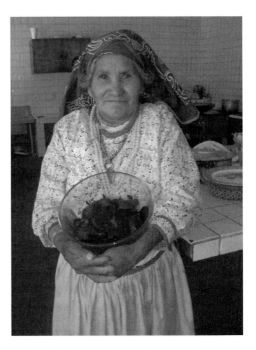

Fig. 15.8. The Growing Connection Project in Mexico. Photo courtesy of Margarita Álvarez Oyarzábal.

16 Biofortification: A New Tool to Reduce Micronutrient Malnutrition*

Howarth E. Bouis,[1†] Christine Hotz,[2] Bonnie McClafferty,[3] J. V. Meenakshi[4]
and Wolfgang H. Pfeiffer[5]
[1]International Food Policy Research Institute (IFPRI), Washington, DC, USA;
[2]Nutridemics, Toronto, Ontario, Canada; [3]Global Alliance for Improved Nutrition
(GAIN), Washington, DC, USA; [4]Delhi School of Economics, Delhi, India;
[5]International Center for Tropical Agriculture (CIAT), Cali, Colombia

Summary

The density of minerals and vitamins in food staples eaten widely by the poor may be increased either through conventional plant breeding or through the use of transgenic techniques, a process known as biofortification. HarvestPlus seeks to develop and distribute varieties of food staples (rice, wheat, maize, cassava, pearl millet, beans and sweet potato) that are high in iron, zinc and provitamin A through an interdisciplinary, global alliance of scientific institutions and implementing agencies in developing and developed countries. In broad terms, three things must happen for biofortification to be successful. First, the breeding must be successful – high nutrient density must be combined with high yields and high profitability. Secondly, efficacy must be demonstrated – the micronutrient status of human subjects must be shown to improve when they are consuming the biofortified varieties as compared with what is normally eaten. Thus, sufficient nutrients must be retained in processing and cooking and these nutrients must be sufficiently bioavailable. Finally, the biofortified crops must be adopted by farmers and consumed by those suffering from micronutrient malnutrition in significant numbers. Biofortified crops offer a rural-based intervention that, by design, initially reaches those more remote populations that comprise a majority of the undernourished in many countries, and then penetrates to urban populations as production surpluses are marketed. In this way, biofortification complements fortification and supplementation programmes, which work best in centralized urban areas and then reach into rural areas with good infrastructure. Initial investments in agricultural research at a central location can generate high recurrent benefits at low cost as adapted, biofortified varieties become available in country after country across time at low recurrent costs.

Rationale for Biofortification

Modern agriculture has been largely successful in meeting the energy needs of poor populations in developing countries. In the past 40 years, agricultural research in developing countries has met Malthus's challenge by placing increased cereal production at its centre. However, agriculture must now focus on a new paradigm that will not only produce more food, but deliver better-quality food as well.[1]

---

*Reprinted (with minor modifications) with permission from the *Food and Nutrition Bulletin*.
†Contact: h.bouis@cgiar.org

Through plant breeding, biofortification can improve the nutritional content of the staple foods poor people already eat, providing a comparatively inexpensive, cost-effective, sustainable, long-term means of delivering more micronutrients to the poor. This approach not only will lower the number of severely malnourished people who require treatment by complementary interventions, but also will help them maintain improved nutritional status. Moreover, biofortification provides a feasible means of reaching malnourished rural populations who may have limited access to commercially marketed fortified foods and supplements.

Unlike the continual financial outlays required for traditional supplementation and fortification programmes, a one-time investment in plant breeding can yield micronutrient-rich plants for farmers to grow around the world for years to come. It is this multiplier aspect of biofortification across time and distance that makes it so cost-effective.

Comparative Advantages of Biofortification

Reaching the malnourished in rural areas

Poor farmers grow modern varieties of crops developed by agricultural research centres supported by CGIAR (formerly known as the Consultative Group on International Agricultural Research) and by national agricultural research and extension systems (NARES), and disseminated by non-governmental organizations (NGOs) and government extension agencies. The biofortification strategy seeks to put the micronutrient-dense trait in the most profitable, highest yielding varieties targeted to farmers and to place these traits in as many released varieties as is feasible. Moreover, marketed surpluses of these crops make their way into retail outlets, reaching consumers in both rural and urban areas. The direction of the flow, as it were, is from rural to urban in contrast to complementary interventions that begin in urban centres.

Cost-effectiveness and low cost

Biofortified staple foods cannot deliver as high a level of minerals and vitamins per day as supplements or industrially fortified foods, but they can help to bring millions over the threshold from malnourishment to micronutrient sufficiency. Figure 16.1 shows this potential schematically for when a high percentage of the iron-deficient population is relatively mildly deficient. For those who are severely deficient, supplements (the highest cost intervention) are required.

In an analysis of commercial fortification, Horton and Ross (2003) estimated that the present value of each annual case of iron deficiency averted in South Asia was approximately US$20.[2]

Consider the value of 1 billion cases of iron deficiency averted in years 16 to 25 after the biofortification research and development project was initiated (100 million cases averted a year in South Asia). The nominal value of US$20 billion (1 billion cases times a value of US$20/case) must be discounted because of the lags involved between the time that investments are made in biofortification and the time benefits are realized. At a 3% discount rate, the present value would be approximately US$10 billion, and at a 12% discount rate, the present value would be approximately US$2 billion. This benefit is far higher than the cost of breeding, testing and disseminating high-iron and high-zinc varieties of rice and wheat for South Asia (<US$100 million in nominal costs).

Sustainability of biofortification

Once in place, the system described in the previous section is highly sustainable. The major fixed costs of developing the varieties and convincing the nutrition and plant science communities of their importance and effectiveness are being covered by programmes such as HarvestPlus (http://www.harvestplus.org), a Challenge Program of the CGIAR. However, the nutritionally improved varieties will continue to be grown and consumed year after year. Recurrent expenditures are required for monitoring and maintaining these traits in crops, but these recurrent costs are low

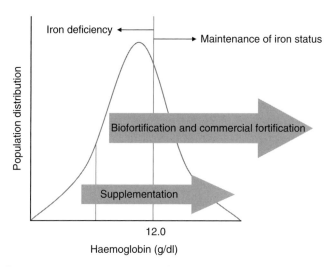

Fig. 16.1. Biofortification improves nutrient status (in this case of iron) for those less deficient and maintains status for all at low cost.

compared with that of the initial development of the nutritionally improved crops and the establishment, institutionally speaking, of nutrient content as a legitimate breeding objective.

Limitations of Biofortification

Varying impact throughout the life cycle

Biofortified staple foods can contribute to body stores of micronutrients such as iron, zinc and vitamin A (the three target nutrients under HarvestPlus) throughout the life cycle, including those of children, adolescents, adult women, men and the elderly. The potential benefits of biofortification are, though, not equivalent across all of these groups and depend on the amount of staple food consumed, the prevalence of existing micronutrient deficiencies and the micronutrient requirement as affected by daily losses of micronutrients from the body and special needs for processes such as growth, pregnancy and lactation (Hotz and McClafferty, 2007).

Time dimension to deliver biofortified crops and to build up and maintain body stores

It will take a decade before a first wave of biofortified crops is widely adopted in several developing countries. It is only when this happens and the attributable impact is confirmed, as measured by significant reductions in the prevalence of iron, zinc and vitamin A deficiencies, that biofortification will take its place beside supplementation, fortification and nutrition education as an effective strategy for reducing micronutrient malnutrition.

Implementing Biofortification

For biofortification to be successful, three broad questions must be addressed:

- Can breeding increase the micronutrient density in food staples to reach target levels that will have a measurable and significant impact on nutritional status? (Pfeiffer and McClafferty, 2007).
- When consumed under controlled conditions, will the extra nutrients bred into the food staples be bioavailable and absorbed at sufficient levels to improve micronutrient status? (Hotz and McClafferty, 2007).
- Will farmers grow the biofortified varieties and will consumers buy and eat them in sufficient quantities?

Much of the evidence available to address these questions has been generated under the

HarvestPlus Challenge Program. HarvestPlus is an interdisciplinary alliance of research institutions and implementing agencies that is developing biofortified varieties of rice, wheat, maize, cassava, pearl millet, beans and sweet potato, as shown in Table 16.1. HarvestPlus activities are presented along a pathway of impact and are classified into three phases of discovery, development and dissemination (Fig. 16.2). Research developments at any one stage may necessitate revisiting the previous stages to refine and ensure high quality of the biofortified products.

Discovery and development research includes standardizing analytical methodologies, protocols and proof of concept research in relation to crop improvement, testing and nutritional efficacy (Grusak and Cakmak, 2005). Dissemination activities are highly dependent on the success of the discovery and development phases, as well as on establishing partnerships between HarvestPlus and country agencies that will lead to the delivery of biofortified seeds to farmers and the introduction of biofortified crops to consumers.

Stage 1: Identifying target populations and staple food consumption profiles

The overlap of cropping patterns, consumption trends and incidence of micronutrient malnutrition determines target populations. This, in turn, determines the selection and geographic targeting of focus crops.

For each of the seven staple food crops listed in Table 16.1, the following activities have been undertaken:

• Identification of countries with high per capita consumption of the food staple (based on Food and Agriculture Organization (FAO) databases).

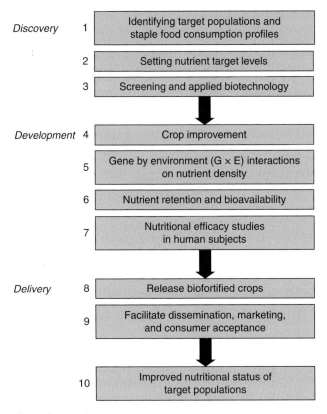

Fig. 16.2. HarvestPlus pathway to impact.

Table 16.1. Schedule of product release of biofortified crops (by year).

Crop	Nutrient	Countries of first release	Agronomic trait	Release year[a]
Sweet potato	Provitamin A	Uganda, Mozambique	Disease resistance, drought tolerance, acid soil tolerance	2007
Cassava	Provitamin A	Nigeria, Democratic Republic of Congo	Disease resistance	2011
Bean	Iron, zinc	Rwanda, Democratic Republic of Congo	Virus resistance, heat and drought tolerance	2012
Maize	Provitamin A	Zambia	Disease resistance, drought tolerance	2012
Pearl millet	Iron, zinc	India	Mildew resistance, drought tolerance	2012
Maize	Provitamin A	Zambia	Disease resistance, drought tolerance	2012
Rice	Zinc, iron	Bangladesh, India	Disease and pest resistance, cold and submergence tolerance	2013
Wheat	Zinc, iron	India, Pakistan	Disease and lodging resistance	2013

[a]Year approved for release by national governments after intensive multi-location testing for agronomic and micronutrient performance.

- Establishment of estimates of the prevalence of iron, zinc and vitamin A deficiencies for these countries.
- Gathering of information on existing and planned expansion and effectiveness of alternative micronutrient interventions in these countries.
- Identification of countries in which biofortification would have the highest potential impact using the information mentioned above.
- Preliminary evaluation of the feasibility of developing and delivering biofortified crops in the high-potential-impact countries, including an assessment of:
  - the scientific capability and institutional strength of the NARES;
  - the present levels of adoption of improved, modern varieties by poor farmers, the level of development of seed distribution systems and the feasibility of realizing significant adoption of high-yielding/high-profit biofortified varieties combined with superior agronomic characteristics of newly introduced varieties; and
  - the political stability and strength of supporting governmental and non-governmental enabling institutions.

Formal *ex ante* impact and benefit–cost analyses were conducted to help refine the targeting exercise. This involved developing a methodology for undertaking *ex ante* benefit–cost analysis (Stein *et al.*, 2005). Other publications (Meenakshi *et al.*, 2007; Qaim *et al.*, 2007; Stein *et al.*, 2007, 2008) are based on this methodology.

Stage 2: Setting nutrient target levels

Nutritionists work with breeders to establish nutritional breeding targets based on the food intake of target populations, nutrient losses during storage and processing, and the bioavailability of nutrients related to the presence or absence of complementary compounds. One of the first questions asked by breeders and nutritionists in the development of the HarvestPlus Program strategy was 'By how much do we need to increase the micronutrient content of our crops to improve the micronutrient status of their consumers?'.

The additional micronutrient intake resulting from biofortification, as a food-based strategy, would ideally be enough to fill the gap between current intakes and the amount that would result in the majority of the population having intakes above the theoretical mean dietary requirement level (the estimated average requirement, or EAR) for the respective micronutrient. Universal food fortification programmes recommend this approach in their design (Allen *et al.*, 2006). However, quantitative information on micronutrient intakes for most potential target populations does not exist or exists only in very limited form. There are also differences in staple food processing, storage and cooking practices and the inclusion of other foods that can result in large differences in the micronutrient content and bioavailability in the staple food across different populations.

HarvestPlus set preliminary 'minimum' target levels for micronutrient content using gross assumptions about: staple food intake (g/day); bioavailability (% nutrient absorbed) or, in the case of vitamin A, the retinol equivalency of provitamin A carotenoids; losses of the target nutrient with milling, processing, storage and cooking; and the proportion of the daily nutrient requirement that should be achieved from the additional amount of micronutrient in the staple food. Table 16.2 presents examples of the types of data used to estimate target levels for micronutrient contents of biofortified crops. As information of this type becomes available for specific populations, target levels for micronutrient contents in different staple food crops can be refined and adjusted. If preliminary target levels are determined to be inadequate for a specific population, the breeding process will continue until breeders reach or surpass the necessary micronutrient content.

As with universal fortification of staple foods, biofortification will lead to some degree of increased micronutrient intakes among individuals in all life stages. A possible exception is exclusively breastfed children but, even in this case, increased intakes of provitamin A by lactating women may result in increased content in the breast milk and hence transfer to the breastfed infant. Young children and women of reproductive age typically suffer the greatest consequences of micronutrient deficiencies because of their increased requirements for growth and for pregnancy and lactation, and so may be considered the primary targets for this strategy. Biofortification as the sole micronutrient

strategy may not be sufficient to cover the deficit in micronutrient intakes by very young children (i.e. under 2 years of age), who have particularly high micronutrient needs and relatively low staple food intakes. Therefore, HarvestPlus estimated appropriate target levels for the micronutrient contents of biofortified foods, taking into account the potential impact in children approximately 4–6 years of age and in non-pregnant, non-lactating, premenopausal women (Table 16.2). It is estimated that with the lower staple food intakes by younger children (i.e. 1–3 years of age), who may still be breastfed, the same target levels for biofortified foods may cover approximately one quarter to one third of their micronutrient requirements. The potential biological intake of a lower increment in micronutrient impact would need to be determined.

Researchers will compile empirical data on staple food intakes for different age groups in a variety of populations in order to refine these estimates. How these levels of increased micronutrient intake translate into changes in nutrition and health status remains to be determined. As breeding for biofortification progresses, the achievable micronutrient content may exceed the current minimum target level and thus make a greater contribution to the micronutrient needs among those groups with elevated requirements.

Stage 3: Screening and applied biotechnology

The global germplasm banks of the CGIAR institutes and the germplasm banks held in trust by national partners provide a reservoir of germplasm of staple crops for screening by HarvestPlus. Genetic transformation provides an alternative strategy to incorporate specific genes that express nutritional density.

The first step in conventional breeding is to determine whether sufficient genetic variation exists to breed for a particular trait of interest – in the specific case of HarvestPlus, whether breeding parents can be found with target levels (or higher) of iron, zinc and provitamin A. Researchers have analysed approximately 300,000 samples for trace minerals or

Table 16.2. Information and assumptions used to set target levels for micronutrient content of biofortified staple food crops.

		Rice (polished)	Wheat (whole)	Pearl millet (whole)	Beans (whole)	Maize (whole)	Cassava (FW)[a]	Sweet potato (FW)
Per capita consumption	Adult women (g/day)	400	400	300	200	400	400	200
	Children 4–6 years (g/day)	200	200	150	100	200	200	100
Iron	EAR[b] (%) to achieve				~30			
	EAR, non-pregnant, non-lactating women (µg/day)				1460			
	EAR, children 4–6 years (µg/day)				500			
	Micronutrient retention after processing (%)	90	90	90	85	90	90	90
	Bioavailability (%)	10	5	5	5	5	10	10
	Baseline micronutrient content (µg/g)	2	30	47	50	30	4	6
	Additional content required (µg/g)	11	22	30	44	22	11	22
	Final target content (µg/g)	13	52	77	94	52	15	28
	Final target content as dry weight (µg/g)	15	59	88	107	60	45	85
Zinc	EAR (%) to achieve				~40			
	EAR, non-pregnant, non-lactating women (µg/day)				1860			
	EAR, children 4–6 years (µg/day)				830			
	Micronutrient retention after processing (%)	90	90	90	90	90	90	90
	Bioavailability (%)	25	25	25	25	25	25	25
	Baseline micronutrient content (µg/g)	16	25	47	32	25	4	6
	Additional content required (µg/g)	8	8	11	17	8	8	17
	Final target content (µg/g)	24	33	58	49	33	12	23
	Final target content as dry weight (µg/g)	28	38	66	56	38	34	70
Provitamin A	EAR (%) to achieve				~50			
	EAR, non-pregnant, non-lactating women (µg/day)				500			
	EAR, children 4–6 years (µg/day)				275			
	Micronutrient retention after processing (%)	50	50	50	50	50	50	50
	Bioavailability ratio (µg to RAE)[c]	12:1	12:1	12:1	12:1	12:1	12:1	12:1
	Baseline micronutrient content (µg/g)	0	0	0	0	0	1	2
	Additional content required (µg/g)	15	15	20	30	15	15	30
	Final target content (µg/g)	15	15	20	30	15	16	32
	Final target content as dry weight (µg/g)	17	17	23	34	17	48	91

[a]FW, fresh weight; [b]EAR, estimated average requirement; [c]RAE, retinol activity equivalent.

for provitamin A carotenoids during screening (Menkir *et al.*, 2008). The second step is to determine from the screening results whether sufficient genetic variation exists to breed for high-zinc rice and wheat, high-iron beans and pearl millet, and high-provitamin A cassava, maize and sweet potato.

Stage 4: Crop improvement

Crop improvement and nutritional bioavailability and efficacy (Stage 7 below) make up the two largest stages of all research activities. Crop improvement includes all breeding activities falling within a product concept that produce varieties containing those traits that (in target populations, in target areas) improve nutrient content, while also giving high agronomic performance and preferred consumer quality (Stangoulis *et al.*, 2007; Harjes *et al.*, 2008).

Biofortification crop improvement is divided into three phases:

- Early-stage product development and parent building (Phase 1).
- Intermediate product development (Phase 2).
- Final product development (Phase 3).

Phases 1 and 2 are undertaken at CGIAR centres. Final product development (Phase 3) for a particular growing 'mega-environment' may take place at the relevant CGIAR centre or NARES. Once promising high-yielding, high-nutrient lines emerge from final product development, they are tested by the NARES in multi-location trials throughout the target country (sometimes referred to as 'genotype by environment – G × E – testing').

A subset of these promising lines that do well on average across these several in-country sites is then submitted formally to Varietal Release Committees (VRCs) for testing for official release. VRCs perform independent, multi-location trials before officially approving varieties for release. During these multi-location trials, in anticipation of a favourable decision by the

VRCs and to save time, NARES often begin to multiply seed prior to prelaunch.

This entire process may take up to 6–8 years to complete. Table 16.3 characterizes current progress throughout the five-phase breeding pipeline for seven crops. Progress is measured by the nutrient levels (expressed as percentages of the absolute target levels given) in breeding lines in a specific phase of development. High-yielding, high-nutrient biofortified varieties currently emerging from the end of this breeding 'pipeline' may have lower levels of nutrients and/or lower yields than prototype lines currently entering the front of the pipeline – owing to new discoveries, such as the identification of higher nutrient germplasm (breeding parents) – made while the lines about to be released have been making their way through the breeding pipeline.

For example, all orange sweet potato varieties – whether currently being tested for official release (Stage 5) or currently just under initial development (Phase 1) – have at least 100% of the target levels of 30 µg/g of provitamin A carotenoids. By contrast, for cassava, much recent and rapid progress has been made in developing lines that meet the target of 15 µg/g of provitamin A carotenoids. Thus, only varieties currently in Phase 1 of the breeding process have 100% of the target level of provitamin A carotenoids. High-yielding yellow cassava varieties with 30–50% of the target level are currently being tested for release (Stage 5), reflecting a relative lack of progress in attaining high provitamin A levels just 2.3 years ago. Even though varieties currently in Stage 5 have provitamin A levels well below target levels, they are high yielding and so can be approved for release.

Finally, the fast-track options shown in Table 16.3 refer to lines that, due to their high yields and favourable agronomic characteristics, are in the regular breeding programme but have been discovered (serendipitously during germplasm screening) to be relatively high in iron, zinc or provitamin A. Breeding for high nutrient levels is then not necessary. These are coursed directly through multi-location testing and then (assuming favourable results) to the VRCs.

Table 16.3. Breeding progress as of August 2007/8, showing iron, zinc and provitamin A expressed as a percentage of the breeding target levels in lines in the programmes/countries shown and at the stage of breeding indicated.

Crop/ programme	Screening — Screening gene/ trait identification validation	Early development parent building	Crop improvement — Intermediate product development	Final product development	G × E testing — Performance G × E testing in target countries	Launch — Release prelaunch seed multiplication
Programme			NARS[a] Uganda	Programme	Introductions	NARS Uganda
Sweet potato						
Breeding	Provitamins A	100% target	100%	100%	100%	100%
Fast track	Uganda, Mozambique				100%	100%
Maize						
Breeding	Provitamins A	100% target	60%	50%	n.a.[b]	
Cassava						
Breeding	Provitamins A	100% target	>75%	>75%	50%	≥30%
Fast track	DR Congo[c]					n.a.
Beans						
Breeding	Iron	100% target	60%	40–50%	40–50%	
Fast track	Rwanda					40–50%
Rice, polished						
Breeding	Zinc	100% target	100%	75–100%	75–100%	≥30%
Wheat						
Breeding	Zinc	100% target	100%	≥30%	≥30%	
Pearl millet						
Breeding	Iron	100% target	100%	75–100%	50–75%	

[a]NARS, National Agricultural Research System (of Uganda); [b]n.a., not available; [c]DR Congo, Democratic Republic of Congo.

Stage 5: G × E interactions on nutrient density

Germplasm is tested in target countries for its suitability for release. G × E interactions can greatly influence genotypic performance across different crop-growing scenarios. HarvestPlus researchers are looking for high and stable expression of high micronutrient content across environments, as well as alternative farming practices that enhance the uptake of nutrients in the edible portion of the crop.

By 2008, all crops were entering or were about to enter G × E trials. Table 16.3 presents the progress of the first and successive generations of biofortified crops as of 2007/8. G × E analysis of sweet potato, for example, shows that varieties were demonstrating 100% of the target levels of provitamin A. G × E analyses of cassava currently finishing all stages of breeding had accomplished 50% of the target level

of provitamins A, but those improved varieties that were just entering the cassava breeding process and had built on the successes of previous generations were demonstrating their ability to reach 100% of the target.

Stage 6: Nutrient retention and bioavailability

HarvestPlus nutrition teams are measuring the effects of the usual processing, storage and cooking methods on micronutrient retention for biofortified crops and evaluating practices that could be used by target populations to improve retention.

Recent research results are suggestive that retention of micronutrients may also be genetically determined, which then adds retention heritability to the plant breeding portfolio. Nutritionists use various methods to study the degree to which the nutrients bred into crops are absorbed by using *in vitro* and animal models and, with the most promising varieties, by direct study in humans in controlled experiments. These studies guide plant breeders in refining their breeding objectives (Pedersen and Eggum, 1983; Villareal *et al.*, 1991; Iglesias *et al.*, 1997; K'osambo *et al.*, 1998; Hagenimana *et al.*, 1999; Sungpuang *et al.*, 1999; Bechoff *et al.*, 2003; Grewal and Hira, 2003; Chavez *et al.*, 2004, 2007; Howe and Tanumihardjo, 2006; Sison *et al.*, 2006; Van Jaarsveld *et al.*, 2006; Kidmose *et al.*, 2007; Li *et al.*, 2007; Bengtsson *et al.*, 2008; Wu *et al.*, 2008; Bechoff *et al.*, 2009; Tako *et al.*, 2009; Thakkar *et al.*, 2009).

Stage 7: Nutritional efficacy studies in human subjects

Although nutrient absorption by the body is a prerequisite to preventing micronutrient deficiencies, ultimately the change in prevalence of micronutrient deficiencies with long-term intake of biofortified staple foods needs to be measured directly. Hence, randomized, controlled efficacy trials demonstrating the impact of biofortified crops on micronutrient status will be required to provide evidence to support the release of biofortified crops at the level of nutrient density so far achieved (i.e. the minimum target level).

As outlined under Stage 2 above, nutrient targets have been set for breeders based on assumptions about the retention of micronutrients in the staple food crop following the usual processing and cooking methods, and how bioavailable these nutrients will be when consumed by micronutrient-deficient populations. These assumptions need to be studied and tested empirically. Eventually, efficacy needs to be evaluated as well (Haas *et al.*, 2005; Van Jaarsveld *et al.*, 2005).

In general, the findings show that retention and bioavailability are higher than assumed. If these promising results are validated with further research to be undertaken under HarvestPlus II, this could eventually allow for a lowering of the minimum target levels for breeders. If, however, breeders can attain the targets already set, the thus-far-promising results suggest that impacts could be higher than expected.

Stage 8: Release biofortified crops

Varietal release regulations differ by country and often by states within countries. Proof that the variety is new and distinguishable and adds value must be established in order to register new varieties of crops. HarvestPlus works with NARES to gather the relevant information for registration and formal release of biofortified crops in target regions.

Stage 9: Facilitate dissemination, marketing and consumer acceptance

Market chain analysis, seed development and production capacity, consumer acceptance studies and the cultivation of an enabling policy environment for the uptake and production of biofortified crops in a country are essential cornerstones for the development of a sustainable, independent, demand-driven, national biofortification research and implementation programme.

The dissemination strategy for nutrients that are invisible (iron and zinc) is to benefit from the superior agronomic characteristics of the newly introduced varieties that will drive their adoption and larger share of the total supply and thereby consumption in a given country. For example, high-iron beans that are drought and heat tolerant are undergoing national release trials in Africa. High-zinc wheat varieties to be released in India and Pakistan will be resistant to newly evolved yellow rust viruses, to which current popular varieties are not resistant.

For nutrients that are visible – e.g. high-provitamin A sweet potato, maize and cassava are orange or yellow – nutritional messages must be delivered simultaneously with the release of high-yielding, high-profit biofortified varieties to effect a switch from the production and consumption of white varieties (which is currently the norm) to the production and consumption of orange or yellow varieties.

The experience of HarvestPlus in the dissemination of biofortified crops is limited to orange sweet potato, which is very high in provitamin A. A published pilot study in Mozambique showed that behaviour can be changed among farmers who switched from production of white to orange varieties and whose families then consumed the orange varieties. As a result, vitamin A deficiency among preschoolchildren in treatment villages declined from 60% to 38%, while vitamin A deficiency remained constant in control villages (Low *et al.*, 2007). HarvestPlus is now concentrating on identifying activities and messages that will effect this same behaviour change at the lowest cost possible.

In 2006, HarvestPlus embarked upon its first dissemination activity of high-provitamin A carotenoid (pVAC) sweet potato in Uganda and Mozambique. Researchers and implementation specialists are gathering lessons learned in strengthening seed systems, developing markets and generating consumer demand through behaviour change for this nutrient-dense orange variety of sweet potato. Best practices will be applied to the expansion of sweet potato to other regions of the world and to instruct dissemination strategies for other pVAC-dense (orange) biofortified staple crops.

Stage 10: Improved nutritional status of target populations

Ultimately, biofortified crops are expected to improve the nutritional status of populations. Baselines and post-dissemination impact and effectiveness surveys are conducted in target regions with and without the intervention to determine whether biofortified crops can improve human health in the absence of experimental conditions. Some work has been conducted relating to the dissemination of orange sweet potato in Uganda and Mozambique (see above), and final results were reported in 2011.

Conclusions

The biofortification strategy seeks to take advantage of the consistent daily consumption of large amounts of food staples by all family members, including women and children, who are most at risk of micronutrient malnutrition. As a consequence of the predominance of food staples in the diets of the poor, this strategy implicitly targets low-income households.

After a one-time investment in developing seeds that fortify themselves, recurrent costs are low and germplasm can be shared internationally. It is this multiplier aspect of plant breeding across time and distance that makes it so cost-effective. Further, once in place, the production and consumption of nutritionally improved varieties are highly sustainable, even if government attention and international funding for micronutrient issues fade.

Biofortification provides a feasible means of reaching malnourished populations in relatively remote rural areas, and delivers naturally fortified foods to people with limited access to commercially marketed fortified foods, which are more readily available in urban areas. Biofortification and commercial fortification, therefore, are highly complementary.

Ultimately, good nutrition depends on adequate intakes of a range of nutrients and other compounds, in combinations and at levels that are not yet completely understood. Thus, the best and final solution to eliminating undernutrition as a public health problem in developing countries is to provide increased consumption of a range of non-staple foods. However, this will require several decades and informed government policies to be realized, and a relatively large investment in agricultural research and other public and on-farm infrastructure (Graham *et al.*, 2007).

In conceptualizing solutions for a range of nutritional deficiencies, interdisciplinary communication between plant scientists and human nutrition scientists holds great potential. Human nutritionists need to be informed, for example, about the extent to which the vitamin and mineral density of specific foods, as well as compounds (e.g. prebiotics) that promote and inhibit their bioavailability, can be modified through plant breeding. Plant breeders need to be aware of both the major influence that agricultural research may have had on nutrient utilization in the past (e.g. the bioavailability of trace minerals in modern varieties versus their bioavailability in traditional varieties) and the potential of plant breeding for future improvements in nutrition and health.

Notes

[1] An important part of the overall solution is to improve the productivity of a long list of non-staple food crops. Due to the large number of foods involved, achieving this goal requires a very large investment, the dimensions of which are not addressed here.

[2] A World Bank study in 1994 assigned a present value benefit of US$45 to each annual case of iron deficiency averted through fortification (a mix of age-sex groups). The same study gives a present value of US$96 for each annual case of vitamin A deficiency averted for preschoolers.

References

Allen, L., de Benoist, B., Dary, O. and Hurrell, R. (eds) (2006) *Guidelines on Food Fortification with Micronutrients*. World Health Organization, Geneva, Switzerland and Food and Agriculture Organization of the United Nations, Rome (available at: http://whqlibdoc.who.int/publications/2006/9241594012_eng.pdf) (accessed 17 June 2013).

Bechoff, A., Westby, A., Dufour, D., Dhuique-Mayer, C., Marouze, C., Owori, C., Menya, G. and Tomlins, K.I. (2003) Effect of drying and storage on the content of provitamin A of orange fleshed sweet potato (*Ipomoea batatas*): Direct sun radiations do not have significant impact. Poster presentation to: *Proceedings of the Thirteenth Triennial Symposium of the International Society for Tropical Root Crops (ISTRC): Tropical Root and Tuber Crops: Opportunities for Poverty Alleviation and Sustainable Livelihoods in Developing Countries, Arusha, Tanzania, 10–14 November 2003*.

Bechoff, A., Dufour, D., Dhuique-Mayer, C., Marouzé, C., Reynes, M. and Westby, A. (2009) Effect of hot air, solar and sun drying treatments on provitamin A retention in orange-fleshed sweet potato. *Journal of Food Engineering* 92, 164–71.

Bengtsson, A., Namutebi, A., Alminger, M.L. and Svanberg, U. (2008) Effects of various traditional processing methods on the all-trans-β-carotene content of orange-fleshed sweet potato. *Journal of Food Composition and Analysis* 21, 134–43.

Chavez, A.L., Sanchez, T., Tohme, J., Ishitani, M. and Ceballos, H. (2004) Effect of processing on beta-carotene content of cassava roots. Poster presentation to: *Sixth International Scientific Meeting of the Cassava Biotechnology Network, 8–14 March 2004*. Centro Internacional de Agricultura Tropical, Cali, Colombia. Available at: http://isa.ciat.cgiar.org/catalogo/listado_tools.jsp?pager.offset=25&tema=CASSAVA (accessed 17 June 2013).

Chavez, A.L., Sanchez, T., Ceballos, H., Rodriguez-Amaya, D.B., Nestel, P., Tohme, J. and Ishitani, M. (2007) Retention of carotenoids in cassava roots submitted to different processing methods. *Journal of the Science of Food and Agriculture* 87, 388–393.

Graham, R.D., Welch, R.M., Saunders, D.A., Ortiz-Monasterio, J.I., Bouis, H.E., Bonierbale, M., de Haan, S., Burgos, G., Thiele, G., Dominguez, M.R.L., Meisner, C.A., Beebe, S.E., Potts, M.J., Kadian, M., Hobbs, P.R., Gupta, R.K. and Twomlow, S. (2007) Nutritious subsistence food systems. *Advances in Agronomy* 92, 1–74.

Grewal, H.K. and Hira, C.K. (2003) Effect of processing and cooking on zinc availability from wheat (*Triticum aestivum*). *Plant Foods for Human Nutrition* 58, 1–8.

Grusak, M.A. and Cakmak, I. (2005) Methods to improve the crop-delivery of minerals to humans and livestock. In: Broadley, M.R. and White, P.J. (eds) *Plant Nutritional Genomics*. Blackwell Publishing, Oxford, UK, pp. 265–286.

Haas, J.D., Beard, J.L., Murray-Kolb, L.E., del Mundo, A.M., Felix, A. and Gregorio, G.B. (2005) Iron-biofortified rice improves the iron stores of non-anemic Filipino women. *Journal of Nutrition* 135, 2823–2830.

Hagenimana, V., Carey, E.E., Gichuki, S.T., Oyunga, M.A. and Imungi, J.K. (1999) Carotenoid contents in fresh, dried and processed sweetpotato products. *Ecology of Food and Nutrition* 37, 455–473.

Harjes, C.E., Rocheford, T., Bai, L., Brutnell, T.P., Kandianis, C.B., Sowinksi, S.G., Stapleton, A.E., Vallabhaneni, R., Williams, M., Wurtzel, E.T., Yan, J. and Buckler, E.S. (2008) Natural genetic variation in lycopene epsilon cyclase tapped for maize biofortification. *Science* 319, 330–333.

Horton, S. and Ross, J. (2003) The economics of iron deficiency. *Food Policy* 28, 51–75.

Hotz, C.C. and McClafferty, B. (2007) From harvest to health: challenges for developing biofortified staple foods and determining their impact on micronutrient status. *Food and Nutrition Bulletin* 28, S271–S279.

Howe, J.A. and Tanumihardjo, S.A. (2006) Carotenoid-biofortified maize maintains adequate vitamin A status in Mongolian gerbils. *Journal of Nutrition* 136, 2562–2567.

Iglesias, C., Mayer, J., Chavez, A.J. and Calle, F. (1997) Genetic potential and stability of carotene content in cassava roots. *Euphytica* 94, 367–373.

Kidmose, U., Christensen, L.P., Agili, S.M. and Thilsted, S.H. (2007) Effect of home preparation practices on the content of provitamin A carotenoids in coloured sweet potato varieties (*Ipomoea batatas* Lam.) from Kenya. *Innovative Food Science* and *Emerging Technologies* 8, 399–406.

K'osambo, L.M., Carey, E.E., Misra, A.K., Wilkes, J. and Hageni-mana, V. (1998) Influence of age, farming site, and boiling on pro-vitamin A content in sweet potato (*Ipomoea batatas* (L.) Lam.) storage roots. *Journal of Food Composition and Analysis* 11, 305–321.

Li, S., Tayie, F.A.K., Young, M.F., Rocheford, T. and White, W.S. (2007) Retention of provitamin A carotenoids in high β-carotene maize (*Zea mays*) during traditional African household processing. *Journal of Agricultural and Food Chemistry* 55, 10744–10750.

Low, J.W., Arimond, M., Osman, N., Cunguara, B., Zano, F. and Tschirley, D. (2007) A food-based approach introducing orange-fleshed sweet potatoes increased vitamin A intake and serum retinol concentrations in young children in rural Mozambique. *Journal of Nutrition* 137, 1320–1327.

Meenakshi, J.V., Nancy, J., Manyong, V., De Groote, H., Javelosa, J., Yanggen, D., Naher, F., Garcia, J., Gonzales, C. and Meng, E. (2007) How cost-effective is biofortification in combating micronutrient malnutrition? An *ex ante* assessment. HarvestPlus Working Paper 2, International Food Policy Research Institute (IFPRI), Washington, DC.

Menkir, A., Liu, W., White, W.S., Maziya-Dixon, B. and Rocheford, T. (2008) Carotenoid diversity in tropical-adapted yellow maize inbred lines. *Food Chemistry* 109, 521–529.

Pedersen, B. and Eggum, B.O. (1983) The influence of milling on the nutritive value of flour from cereal grains. *Plant Foods for Human Nutrition* 33, 267–278.

Pfeiffer, W.H. and McClafferty, B. (2007) Biofortification: breeding micronutrient-dense crops. In: Kang, M.S. and Priyadarshan, P.M. (eds) *Breeding Major Food Staples for the 21st Century*. Blackwell Publishing, Oxford, UK, pp. 61–91.

Qaim, M., Stein, A.J. and Meenakshi, J.V. (2007) Economics of biofortification. *Agricultural Economics* 37, 119–133.

Sison, M.E.G.Q., Gregorio, G.B. and Mendioro, M.S. (2006) The effect of different milling times on grain iron content and grain physical parameters associated with milling of eight genotypes of rice (*Oryza sativa* L.). *Philippine Journal of Science* 135, 9–17.

Stangoulis, J.C.R., Huynh, B.L., Welch, R.M., Choi, E.Y. and Graham, R.D. (2007) Quantitative trait loci for phytate in rice grain and their relationship with grain micronutrient content. *Euphytica* 154, 289–294.

Stein, A.J., Meenakshi, J.V., Qaim, M., Nestel, P., Sachdev, H.P.S. and Bhutta, Z.A. (2005) *Analyzing the Health Benefits of Biofortified Staple Crops by Means of the Disability-adjusted Life Years Approach: A Handbook Focusing on Iron, Zinc and Vitamin A.* HarvestPlus Technical Monograph Series 4, International Food Policy Research Institute (IFPRI), Washington, DC.

Stein, A.J., Nestel, P., Meenakshi, J.V., Qaim, M., Sachdev, H.P.S. and Bhutta, Z.A. (2007) Plant breeding to control zinc deficiency in India: how cost effective is biofortification? *Public Health Nutrition* 10, 492–501.

Stein, A.J., Meenakshi, J.V., Qaim, M., Nestel, P., Sachdev, H.P.S. and Bhutta, Z.A. (2008) Potential impacts of iron biofortification in India. *Social Science and Medicine* 66, 1797–1808.

Sungpuag, P., Tangchitpianvit, S., Chittchang, U. and Wasantwisut, E. (1999) Retinol and beta carotene content of indigenous raw and home-prepared foods in Northeast Thailand. *Food Chemistry* 64, 163–167.

Tako, E., Laparra J.M., Glahn, R.P., Welch, R.M., Lei, X.G., Beebe, S. and Miller, D.D. (2009) Biofortified black beans in a maize and bean diet provide more bioavailable iron to piglets than standard black beans. *Journal of Nutrition* 139, 305–309.

Thakkar, S.K., Huo, T., Maziya-Dixon, B. and Failla, M.L. (2009) Impact of style of processing on retention and bioaccessibility of β-carotene in cassava (*Manihot esculenta*, Crantz). *Journal of Agricultural and Food Chemistry* 57, 1344–1348.

van Jaarsveld, P.J., Faber, M., Tanumihardjo, S.A., Nestel, P., Lombard, C.J. and Benade Spinnler, A.J. (2005) β-Carotene-rich orange-fleshed sweet potato improves the vitamin A status of primary school children assessed with the modified-relative-dose-response test. *The American Journal of Clinical Nutrition* 81, 1080–1087.

van Jaarsveld, P.J., Marais, D.W., Harmse, E., Nestel, P. and Rodriguez-Amaya, D.B. (2006) Retention of β-carotene in boiled, mashed orange-fleshed sweet potato. *Journal of Food Composition and Analysis* 19, 321–329.

Villareal, C.P., Maranville, J.W. and Juliano, B.O. (1991) Nutrient content and retention during milling of brown rices from the international rice research institute. *Cereal Chemistry* 68, 437–439.

Wu, X., Sun, C., Yang, L., Zeng, G., Liu, Z. and Li, Y. (2008) β-Carotene content in sweet potato varieties from China and the effect of preparation on β-carotene retention in the Yanshu No. 5. *Innovative Food Science* and *Emerging Technologies* 9, 581–586.

17 Medium-scale Fortification: A Sustainable Food-based Approach to Improve Diets and Raise Nutrition Levels

Miriam E. Yiannakis,[1]* Aimee Webb Girard[2] and A. Carolyn MacDonald[1]
World Vision International, based at World Vision Canada, Mississauga, Ontario, Canada; [2]Emory University, Atlanta, Georgia, USA

Summary

This chapter examines the success and sustainability potential of medium-scale fortification (MSF) and small-scale fortification (SSF) to increase rural access to and usage of fortified flours within the Canadian International Development Agency (CIDA)-funded Micronutrient and Health (MICAH) Programme in Malawi. World Vision implemented the MICAH programme (1996–2005) to address anaemia and micronutrient malnutrition of women and children in Malawi. MICAH consisted of a package of community-based multi-sectoral interventions implemented with multiple partners. SSF and MSF of maize flour consumed by the general population, and a specially formulated local complementary food (*likuni phala*), were part of an anaemia control package that also included small animal production and consumption, backyard gardens, community-based iron supplementation, deworming of children and malaria control. Project evaluations provided strong evidence of impact over the 9 years of implementation. For example: anaemia in children under 5 years decreased from 86% (1996) to 60% (2004); anaemia in non-pregnant women decreased from 51% (2000) to 39% (2004). The Domasi Fortification Unit, the MSF operation initiated by MICAH, has continued (to date, 2010) as a self-sustaining, fully commercialized producer of fortified foods, supplying other fortification units and feeding programmes throughout Malawi. Linking SSF sites with MSF operations is a promising approach to successful scale up and sustainability of community-based fortification.

Background

Project overview

The Domasi Fortification Unit (DFU) in Zomba, Malawi is an example of a successful medium-scale fortification (MSF) initiative. The DFU was initiated as one of multiple approaches within a large multi-sectoral Micronutrient and Health (MICAH) Programme in Malawi that was aimed at improving the iron and iodine status of women and children, as these were major public health concerns (see Supplemental Table 17.2 at the end of the chapter for interventions included as part of the MICAH programme). The DFU was linked with small-scale fortification (SSF) mills and integrated with other interventions, including iron and iodine supplementation, diet diversity and modification, promotion of centrally iodized salt,

---

*Contact: miriam_yiannakis@worldvision.ca

disease control (particularly preventing and treating malaria, hookworm, schistosomiasis), improving water and sanitation, and HIV/AIDS prevention. World Vision initiated and managed the MICAH programme, which ran from 1996 to 2005, funded by the Canadian International Development Agency (CIDA) and World Vision Canada.

The DFU is part of the Domasi Community Nutrition Project in Zomba (the southern region of Malawi), one of World Vision Malawi's nine implementing partners (i.e. the different offices that World Vision Malawi worked with) for MICAH.[1] The DFU fortifies both the national staple of maize flour, targeted to improve iron status among women, and a specially formulated local complementary food called *likuni phala*, targeted to children under 5 years. A post-project assessment in 2008 that examined the scale and sustainability of MICAH's anaemia control package rated the DFU as functioning independently, thus contributing to ongoing sources of iron, whereas some other key interventions (e.g. weekly iron supplementation) were not sustained (Siekmans *et al.*, 2009). The DFU had become, and continues to be (2010), a self-sustaining, fully commercialized producer of micronutrient-fortified foods and pre-blend. It supplies surrounding communities with fortified products, feeding initiatives throughout Malawi with fortified *likuni phala* and SSF units with fortified pre-blend.

In addition to the DFU medium-scale operation, MICAH initiated small-scale fortification (SSF) through 19 privately owned village mills in project sites across the country. If scaled up, SSF has potential to reach a large proportion of the rural population with essential micronutrients, but there are significant barriers to achieving this, particularly related to quality control and affordability. The DFU experience demonstrates that an MSF unit can overcome these challenges more readily, and that the most promising option for expanding SSF may be through forming partnerships between an MSF unit and its neighbouring SSF mills. Some of the SSF efforts initiated by MICAH Malawi outside Domasi have also been sustained since the programme ended, but they continue to rely on direct support from World Vision.

Project evaluations provide strong evidence of impact over the 9 years of MICAH implementation. For example, anaemia in children under 5 years decreased from 86% (1996) to 60% (2004) and anaemia in non-pregnant women decreased from 51% (2000) to 39% (2004) (Berti *et al.*, 2010). While these overall improvements cannot be attributed to fortification alone, it is likely that the consumption of fortified foods contributed to the decrease in anaemia, as 12% of households in the MICAH interventions areas (versus 2% in non-MICAH areas) were consuming fortified maize flour at the end of the programme in 2004 (MacDonald *et al.*, 2010).

MICAH Fortification Activities

Rationale for including small- and medium-scale fortification

Malnutrition is a major public health problem in Malawi and little progress in combating it has been made over the past several decades (NSO and ORC Macro, 2001). In addition to general undernutrition, micronutrient deficiencies are common in adults and children. In 1996, MICAH's baseline survey in the project areas showed that 56% of Malawian children under 5 years were stunted (length/height-for-age Z-score (HAZ) < −2SD), and anaemia affected 84% of children under 5 years (Hb (haemoglobin) < 1.0 g/dl) and 59% of pregnant women (Hb < 11.0 g/dl). Similarly, the *Report of the National Micronutrient Survey 2001* (Ministry of Health and Population, Lilongwe, Malawi; unpublished document, 2003) reported approximately 60% of children under 5 years as vitamin A deficient, 80% anaemic and 1% suffering from cretinism. An estimated 60% of child anaemia was attributable to iron deficiency. Among women of child-bearing age, 57% were vitamin A deficient and 44% were anaemic; 47% of pregnant women were anaemic. Among men, 38% and 17% were vitamin A deficient and anaemic, respectively.

Maize is the principal food crop and dietary staple in Malawi. Malawians consume approximately 180 kg/year per capita, typically in the form of maize meal. However, maize is a poor source of micronutrients, largely because it contains a high concentration of phytates, which inhibit the absorption of critical micronutrients. To further exacerbate this problem, poverty limits the ability of households to diversify their diets to include foods that enhance absorption or are naturally rich sources of bioavailable micronutrients, particularly animal source foods such as meat, dairy products and eggs.

At the time that MICAH initiated its fortification activities, at least 80% of the general population, including even the poorest rural households,[2] used service hammer mills to process domestically consumed maize meal (Motts, 2003). Moreover, 86% of the national population resided in rural areas, according to Malawi's Central Statistics Office. Commercially packaged maize meal products were seldom distributed beyond the immediate urban zones of the nation's three major cities, because of insufficient demand that is largely related to affordability and preference for a specific grade of meal (Motts, 2003). Thus, central maize fortification was not a viable delivery mechanism for providing additional micronutrients to the majority of Malawians. In contrast, fortification through small mills had the potential to reach a large majority of the population.

Technical aspects of small- and medium-scale fortification

Small-scale mills typically produce less than 5 t of milled grain/day or less than 1 t/h (MI, 2004). In many cases, there may be only one or two employees milling grain either continuously or in batches. Customers manually clean the grain before milling and there may or may not be screens available for sifting. Medium-scale mills have a capacity of 1–3 t/h and can produce from 5 to 50 t/day of milled product. They are slightly larger operations, often privately owned and with 3–10 employees; they have more than one hammer mill, and produce more than one milled product at a time (MI, 2004). SSF and MSF involve adding micronutrients to milled products in small- and medium-sized milling units using a diluted micronutrient pre-blend with or without special dosing or blending equipment. The pre-blend may be added either during the milling process or after. This is achieved by using:

- a calibrated scoop/spoon to measure an amount proportional to the weight of grain;
- a sachet, containing an amount appropriate for a set weight of grain; or
- a small dosifier that dispenses an amount proportional to the weight of grain flow.

Markets for SSF mills are local, and are often situated in market places or other locations where people shop or live. There is little to no on-site quality assurance or quality control conducted by employees or owners. MSF mills tend to serve regional markets, and may have some capacity for quality assurance and quality control, though this may be inconsistent. While small-scale mills are more effective than large-scale mills at reaching rural populations with fortification – because they are accessed by such a large proportion of the rural and poor population (i.e. those that would most benefit from additional micronutrients), multiple barriers exist to fortifying at the small-scale level compared with centrally fortifying products. MSF units are a more feasible option and partnering MSF with small-scale mills holds promise as a model for scaling up community-based fortification for the greatest impact.

Overview and results of the MICAH fortification pilot

Recognizing the potential benefits of SSF for Malawi's rural poor, MICAH Malawi initiated a pilot project in 1998. The first activity involved partnering with the Domasi Likuni Phala Project, a component of the Domasi Mission Community Nutrition Project (DMCNP). The primary role of the DMCNP was the production of *likuni phala*, a maize/soya blend used for rehabilitative feeding of malnourished children and complementary feeding of infants. Although *likuni phala* contains adequate energy and protein for young children, the phytic acid content is high, iron and zinc content low, and the resulting bioavailable iron and zinc extremely low (Gibson *et al.*, 1998). MICAH worked with the Domasi Likuni Phala Project to improve the micronutrient density of *likuni phala* through fortification. Further strengthening of this partnership enabled the mill to expand its line of products and increase production overall. Eventually, the mill became an MSF unit known as the DFU.

The DFU also provided a grain milling service for the surrounding communities that included fortification using the Direct Addition methodology developed by MICAH. The positive outcome of this unique partnership between medium-scale production and small-scale service milling is that of cost sharing. Profit from higher margin products (fortified *likuni phala* primarily sold to larger organizations) enabled the business to provide fortification to the community at minimal cost.

In June 2001, MICAH Malawi expanded its pilot fortification project to support maize fortification in eight communities, each with one small-scale hammer mill. Households brought dehulled whole maize to the community mill, where a fortificant was added by the Direct Addition method (see Box 17.1) immediately before milling. By MICAH's final year (2005), SSF had reached at least 22,600 households via 19 community mills spread throughout Malawi's three regions (North, Central and South). However, this achievement has not been sustained following the close of the MICAH programme – except in a limited number of mills where

World Vision has continued to provide funding and support for SSF activities.

In 2005, the DFU became a commercially active and profitable medium-scale operation producing and fortifying whole maize flour, cream of maize, soya flour and *likuni phala*, as well as micronutrient pre-blend. The DFU's primary customer base included local grocery stores, the Blantyre Synod, and non-governmental organizations (NGO) and intergovernmental organizations. Most commercial customers were located within a 150 km radius (Baldwin Radford, 2005).

Community maize milling and SSF were regarded by the DFU as a necessary community service and therefore were offered to neighbouring communities despite minimal profitability (0.52% of product sales in 2004). In 2005, the DFU milling service had approximately 1000 visits/month and was supporting one other mill in a nearby village to provide fortification in its community milling service. These two small-scale outlets enabled access to fortified food for individuals milling their own grain; in addition the DFU also worked with 31 village committees to sell fortified flour products, including *likuni phala* (Baldwin Radford, 2005).

Following the end of MICAH funding, DFU continued to develop as a commercially viable business. In 2007, 2 years after MICAH, the DFU produced 408 t of *likuni phala*, 75 t of pre-blend and 870 t of fortified maize flour (Siekmans, 2007). Six additional mills in Senzani implementing SSF through other World Vision funding sourced their pre-blend

---

Box 17.1. Direct Addition method.

In Africa, small-scale fortification (SSF) is performed using hammer mills. Hammer mills use swivelled metal blades to grind the grain and blast it against a metal screen. The very high speeds of the rotating blades force the fine meal through the screen.

In Malawi, maize brought by community members to the mill for milling is weighed volumetrically in a calibrated bucket and a pre-blend containing the fortificant is added at the rate of one 150 g scoop/5 kg maize. The micronutrient pre-blend initially contained one part fortificant (Roche IS 254) and 199 parts milled maize (the carrier, 1:200 dilution ratio). The pre-blend is added to the maize before milling and briefly mixed by hand. The mixture is then sent through the mill. If a number of customers are lined up for milling, the mill is set to run continuously and each batch is added in succession. A hand-manipulated steel plate immediately below the in-feed hopper is opened or closed to admit the maize to the mill and thus keep each batch separate. This allows the pre-blend to be added to the next batch while the last of the earlier batch is still exiting the mill.

from the DFU (Baldwin Radford, 2005). As of 2009, the DFU had further expanded its product range to include chicken feed (produced using by-products of *likuni phala* production) and sachets of fortificant for household-level fortification of maize meal. In 2010, the business expanded its market further by working with a network of individuals who promote and sell DFU products in Blantyre in the Southern Region and in Lilongwe and Ntchisi in the Central Region.

Discussion

Two key areas are discussed below based on the case study results. First, the finding that the DFU is currently a self-sustaining business 5 years post programme, and providing fortified products to consumers in 31 surrounding communities, suggests the merit of increasing MSF units. Based on findings of the DFU pilot, MSF has strong potential for positively increasing nutrient availability among the general population, and is worth replicating.

Secondly, SSF presents many more challenges than MSF and so it should be a secondary focus. Nevertheless, by linking small mills to MSF units and by addressing additional key challenges, it may be operationally possible and affordable to implement national-scale hammer mill fortification.

Medium-scale fortification (MSF): the Domasi Fortification Unit

From 2005 to 2010, the DFU has produced and sold fortified foods to a range of customers, from local community members to national organizations operating large feeding programmes, through: (i) direct service milling with Direct Addition fortifying; (ii) bulk purchasing, milling, fortifying and packaging of maize for retail distribution and sale; and (iii) bulk production of fortified *likuni phala* for sale locally and to government and NGOs. Two main contributors to the success of the MSF pilot are: (i) technical expertise; and (ii) the evolution of the DFU into a sustainable and commercial MSF unit.

Technical contributions to DFU's success included: (i) the development of a successful methodology for delivering vitamins and minerals to milled maize; (ii) the development of a quality control and assurance plan; and (iii) an effective information, education and communication campaign that improved consumer acceptance and uptake of fortified foods. Key enabling factors that transitioned the DFU into a profitable and sustainable medium-scale commercial mill were: (i) technical support from external consultants, and the development of sustainable business plans and initial investments in human resources; (ii) the establishment of effective partnerships; and (iii) ongoing national-level advocacy work by World Vision and partners.

Technical contributors to programme success

IDENTIFYING A FORTIFICATION METHOD FOR HAMMER MILLS. The first key programme issue for MICAH Malawi was identifying a simple, low-cost, effective and contextually appropriate fortification method for hammer mills. The Direct Addition method that was identified by MICAH as meeting these criteria consists of simply measuring the micronutrient pre-blend in a calibrated scoop and manually adding an amount of pre-blend that corresponds to the weight of the maize being milled. Sampling and testing of fortified products demonstrated that this particular method of addition resulted in uniform mixing of fortificants (iron and zinc) into the maize or *likuni phala* product. The micronutrient concentrations of iron and zinc in the fortified products were tested in country by the Malawi Bureau of Standards and externally in Canada by Maxxam Analytical Laboratories, Mississauga, Ontario.

The Direct Addition method can be applied to the larger amounts of maize used in MSF production as well as at the scale of village mills, where Malawian women bring relatively small, varying quantities of maize to be milled at any one time. After harvest, quantities of 20–30 kg are brought weekly for milling, while in the lean season only about 1–5 kg are brought, often on a daily basis. The miller processes each customer's varying quantities of maize or other staple, one at a time. The customer is charged based on the quantity of maize processed measured with a calibrated tin bucket, usually holding up to approximately 18 kg of maize.

DEVELOPING QUALITY ASSURANCE AND QUALITY CONTROL. A second technical challenge in the MICAH programme was the absence of a formalized quality assurance and quality control mechanism for fortification for either medium- or small-scale mills in Malawi. In addition, regulations and legislation on fortification were not in place at the national level when the programme began. Even if legislation had existed, it would have been problematic to expect systematic enforcement of regulations given the plethora of medium- and small-scale mill sites in Malawi (more than 10,000). To address quality assurance, MICAH worked on two levels: (i) at the local level, building capacity at the DFU with resources from World Vision and partners; and (ii) at the national level, building partnerships to advocate for national standards, policies, legislation and financial support.

Locally, training on all aspects of fortification was provided to DFU staff by technical experts from MICAH, including a nutritionist, public health specialist, external milling specialist and local business person. Small-scale millers also participated in these training sessions.

Every 3 months the World Vision Fortification Coordinator and MICAH Coordinator visited all the mills and sampled the fortified products, as per standard industry milling sampling techniques recommended and taught by the external fortification/milling consultant. MICAH covered the cost of having samples analysed by the Malawi Bureau of Standards (MBS) and Maxxam Analytical Laboratories.

Initially, World Vision employed 'fortification monitors' at the DFU and at participating small-scale mills. The role of these monitors was to assist with both quality control and social marketing. Monitors controlled the pre-blend inventory, tracked the pilot process and encouraged customers to fortify their maize and *likuni phala*. Monitors also addressed customer concerns about fortification, recorded

whether customers did or did not fortify and played a crucial educational role.

The initial testing of the Direct Addition methodology highlighted ways to monitor the process through simple mathematical calculations, such as balance sheets and service milling records to show that the correct amount of premix had been used for that total quantity of maize. This system works when the quality assurance and quality control are implemented as required by supervisory staff at the medium-scale level. Technical expertise also provided examples of easy-to-use, end-product tests that can be carried out by site monitors.

Nationally, as a result of advocacy efforts by MICAH and partners, the MBS developed national food fortification standards for maize in 2002, and set up quality assurance and quality control processes. The DFU now carries MBS certification, indicating that it complies with all food standards, including quality assurance and quality control measures. Furthermore, the presence of international grocery store chains in Malawi has significantly increased the number and volume of fortified foods on the market, as well as the diversity of food products. This market development has continued the impetus to ensure that locally produced foods are of sufficient quality to compete with international brands.

CREATING AN EFFECTIVE SOCIAL MARKETING STRATEGY. Initially, fortification activities were generally resisted by community members, as people held many erroneous ideas about fortified foods. One pervasive myth was that the pre-blend contained poison or contraceptives. Thus the third technical challenge was to generate demand for fortified products and services. Time, combined with appropriate information, education and communication dispelled many misconceptions, and consumer acceptance of fortified foods reached 100% according to follow-up evaluations.

This was accomplished through a number of social marketing activities taken on by the DFU in partnership with MICAH and others. MICAH contracted the Center for Social Research to conduct a survey on attitudes towards and acceptance of fortified foods; data collected from this survey provided valuable inputs for national level discussions on fortification, social marketing campaigns and the individualized education of mill customers by Mill Monitors. Posters designed by local artists described the fortification process. These were displayed at the DFU and the community mills and used by the Monitors to educate customers. Social marketing campaigns were conducted through drama and entertainment groups as well as through sponsoring a local soccer team, the Domasi Fortifiers. In addition, local radio stations broadcast weekly nutrition information briefs that included messages about fortification as well as basic nutrition and health messages.

Transition of the DFU to a sustainable and profitable MSF unit

The second factor critical to the overall success of MICAH fortification activities was the transition of the DFU into a sustainable commercial MSF unit. Importantly, the MICAH programme built on an existing successful project (the Domasi Likuni Phala Project) to improve the micronutrient density of *likuni phala* through fortification. With additional technical, financial and managerial support to strengthen the capacity of the mill, MICAH enabled the DFU to eventually operate as a successful MSF business.

START-UP TECHNICAL AND FINANCIAL INPUTS TO THE DFU. To build the initial capacity and future sustainability of the DFU, MICAH provided training in several topics: business management, data analysis, financial planning and management, fortification quality assurance and quality control, and fortification sustainability, as well as training in nutrition, community participation and other MICAH interventions. MICAH also funded and provided technical support for two part-time DFU positions in operations and financial management. These positions were considered key to ensuring both accountability and strategic planning.

While the DFU initially received start-up funding from MICAH for fortification, this grant did not supersede the need for the early development of business plans for the mill's transition to sustainability and independence. The start-up financial support for DFU included initial equipment purchases, stock purchases and limited staffing and training. Financial support decreased gradually. By 2003, the DFU covered 100% of staffing costs, was purchasing raw materials to increase production and had opened a bank account. Funding from World Vision ended in 2005 and the DFU has not only continued as a viable business, but has expanded its product range and increased profits.

ESTABLISHING PARTNERSHIPS. MICAH brought together MSF and SSF producers with mill owners and operators to develop plans to improve and expand the production and quality of fortified foods. This included liaising between producers and the MBS to ensure quality through means feasible for this level of producer and to discuss micronutrient premix concentrate importation.

Partnerships with international and local NGOs provided technical inputs, assistance and support. SUSTAIN (Sharing US Technology to Aid in the Improvement of Nutrition) provided input on packaging, labelling and market identification. KIT (Royal Tropical Institute, Netherlands) provided technical assistance on equipment. Fortification and milling experts provided annual reviews, support and ongoing technical inputs invaluable for ensuring overall quality, for troubleshooting and for accountability. Nutrition technical experts from World Vision also provided ongoing technical review and assistance for determining fortification levels, strategies to overcome barriers to fortification acceptance and measuring effectiveness on nutritional outcomes of the beneficiary population. Research proposals were developed with an academic partner in order to rigorously study both the efficacy and effectiveness of community-based fortification, but funding for this work was not forthcoming.

NATIONAL-LEVEL ADVOCACY. At the national level, MICAH provided leadership and funding to establish the National Fortification Alliance (NFA). The NFA comprised various government departments, including the ministries of finance, customs, tax and excise, health and agriculture, as well as consumer associations, private sector representatives (both large- and medium-scale producers), United Nations agencies and World Vision. The NFA advocated changes to Malawi's food standards to include fortification, conducted events to promote fortification and advocated the removal of import tariffs on fortificants and fortification equipment. International technical experts were consulted and provided convincing arguments based on fortification experience in other countries. The Ministry of Health then acted as advocate with regulators and policy makers for the importance of fortification to improve the micronutrient intake of the population. The Consumer's Association of Malawi was also crucial in advocating the right of Malawian consumers to purchase safe fortified food products. Some results from these advocacy efforts include food standards being implemented for the fortification of sugar and maize flour, and the removal of import taxes on IS 254 (the Roche premix).

While much national level advocacy focused on large-scale fortification, it also created an environment more conducive to addressing general monitoring systems, food standards and importation issues. Further, there were national level discussions about the potential of harmonizing fortificant formulas in order to lower costs by facilitating larger quantity shipments.

Small-scale fortification (SSF): partnering with medium-scale units for a cost-effective, sustainable service

SSF has the potential to make a significant contribution to the improved intake of essential micronutrients by the rural subsistence-farming population of Malawi, although there are significant barriers to the sustained effective implementation of this approach. The two major barriers relate to quality assurance processes for accountability to standards of delivery, and affordability. Partnering one MSF unit with a manageable network of SSF units offers an opportunity to mitigate these challenges, as the Domasi example demonstrates.

Quality assurance for small-scale fortification

The NFA successfully advocated the putting in place of maize flour fortification standards for Malawi. However, even with these in place, it would not be feasible to support and regulate thousands of SSF mills across the country to apply these standards. MICAH recognized the need for a quality assurance process suited to the hammer mill level and brought together key stakeholders to develop plans for this. The DFU provided a hub for testing quality assurance approaches and training SSF millers to implement them.

Before starting fortification activities at small mills, MICAH brought millers to the Domasi site for training on the prevalence and impact of micronutrient deficiencies, the role of food fortification, pre-blend ingredients, how to properly add fortificant, fortification levels for maize versus *likuni phala*, business planning and marketing. This training, as well as ongoing technical assistance, was provided by technical experts from MICAH, who also supervised the actual fortification activities. As at the DFU, samples of fortified products from the small-scale mills were initially collected and analysed every 3 months, and MICAH-funded Fortification Monitors were initially employed at all participating SSF sites for the combined role of quality control and social marketing.

Low-cost fortificant source and dilution method

The key requirements for ensuring the affordability of SSF are identifying low-cost and locally sourced fortificants or premix, a low-cost dilution method and the cost-effective distribution of pre-blend to the SSF sites. In the Malawi case study, these challenges were solved, in part, through linking multiple SSF units with the medium-scale DFU.[3]

The DFU purchased premix and diluted it with maize flour to make the pre-blend. The pre-blend was packaged in bulk (50 kg sacks) and distributed by MICAH to rural hammer mills implementing SSF. All inputs were sourced locally, with the exception of the premix, which was imported from South Africa. The DFU ensured that the supply of pre-blend was available for all SSF sites, and thus became a critical player in sustaining SSF by providing locally produced and relatively affordable pre-blend.

An important challenge of the programme related to the pre-blend was identifying an appropriate and sustainable dilution ratio. Higher dilution ratios require more maize carrier and are more costly owing to the need for purchasing greater quantities of carrier and transporting larger volumes. Initially, the DFU used a 1:200 dilution ratio, but an external evaluation in 2003 deemed this unsustainable due to high costs. In fact, the review found that 'minimizing the dilution ratio is the greatest single factor affecting household level affordability of fortification' (Motts, 2003). Therefore, in 2005, after testing for uniformity of blending, the 1:200 ratio was decreased to 1:50 ratio (see Table 17.1). World Vision initially tested samples of the (new ratio) fortified maize meal from each mill every 3 months for blend uniformity, discontinuing this when tests indicated satisfactory blending. However, it should be noted that World Vision has not shown conclusively that the Direct Addition blending method is reliable within 20% variability, due to budgetary constraints and laboratory testing quality control issues.

The 2003 study of World Vision's medium- and small-scale fortification pilot commissioned by the Micronutrient Initiative (MI) found that national maize fortification through medium- and small-scale mills should be operationally possible and affordable provided that: (i) a pre-blend dilution ratio in the range of 1:100 or lower is workable; (ii) mill owners (or local community institutions) are willing to take responsibility for obtaining supplies of pre-blend from a decentralized unit (e.g. MSF unit); and (iii) fortification costs are partially subsidized on a declining basis for up to 8 years, to underwrite the costs necessary to enable widespread and high levels of consumer acceptance of and willingness to pay for maize fortification (Motts, 2003).

During the implementation of the MICAH programme in Malawi (1998–2005), where MSF and SSF ultimately covered a population of 120,000, the total fortification costs (direct and indirect) were US$1.87/year per capita (Siekmans, 2007). In 2007, when SSF was expanded to cover a larger population, the annual cost per capita decreased to US$1.37 (ibid.). The direct costs (i.e. excluding overheads for quality assurance monitoring, administering subsidies or information and education (IEC) costs) of providing the recommended daily allowance of iron through fortified

Table 17.1. Fortified maize product from two different premix formulations using 1:200 and 1:50 dilution ratios. From Baldwin Radford (2005).

Nutrients	Nutrients/100 g serving fortified maize product	
	Using premix with 1:200 dilution ratio[a]	Using premix with 1:50 dilution ratio[b]
Calcium		8.000 mg
Folic acid	0.11 mg	0.091 mg
Iron (reduced >95% through 325 mesh)	2.86 mg	3.500 mg
Nicotinamide	5.85 mg	2.500 mg
Pyridoxine HCl	0.77 mg	0.313mg
Riboflavin	0.52 mg	0.170 mg
Thiamine mononitrate	0.78 mg	0.221mg
Vitamin A (palmitate)	1415 IU[c]	695.304 IU
Zinc oxide (Zn)	3.74 mg	1.506 mg

[a]Premix used from 1998 to 2005 (IS 254) as supplied by Roche Products, South Africa: 1:200 ratio of premix to maize (0.15 kg premix added to 30 kg maize) to create pre-blend; 150 g pre-blend fortifies 5 kg maize.
[b]Revised premix distributed from June 2005 (IS 353) as supplied by DSM (formerly Roche), South Africa: 1:50 ratio of premix to maize (0.15 kg premix added to 7.5 kg maize) to create premix; 37.5 g premix fortifies 5 kg maize.
[c]IU, international unit.

maize at a 1:100 premix dilution rate have been estimated at approximately US$0.87/ year per capita (Motts, 2003).

Concluding Remarks

Lessons learned

The case of the DFU offers many lessons that can be applied to programmes aiming to improve the nutritional status of a population. MICAH's integrated approach demonstrates how this can be done with cooperation and collaboration. MSF is an innovative and practical community-based way of enabling essential nutrients to reach populations who are without access to centrally fortified foods.

Several components are essential for the success and sustainability of MSF initiatives. Those include:

- early development of a sound and realistic business plan that can guide the fortification initiative toward self-reliance;
- adequate human resources, and ensuring in the business plan that appropriate competencies exist, or are developed, in key staff;
- a well-defined advocacy strategy that addresses legislative as well as practical issues at national level through to household level;
- a plan for products to reach the poorest populations, including creative thinking to determine a costing mechanism that will ensure low-income households can benefit from fortification services;
- technical expertise assistance for milling, nutrition and business, which has benefits for advocacy as well as troubleshooting problems;
- ongoing quality assurance and quality control; and
- evaluation of the impact on nutritional status and health.

The continued success of the DFU has had significant – though unanticipated – positive consequences for the surrounding community in the form of employment. The Domasi area is rural and comparable

employment is unavailable. DFU employees enjoy a work environment that is safe and non-discriminatory and they earn a fair wage. This is no small achievement, given that many of the factory staff are living with HIV and would otherwise have little opportunity for gainful employment.[4] Furthermore, employee salaries improve not just an individual's life circumstance, but in typical African tradition, support entire families.

Recommendations for application

The following recommendations are proposed as priority steps for programmers and policy makers to implement in order to build on the Domasi experience, and scale up MSF with SSF partnerships for improved nutrition of the rural poor in Malawi.

Evaluate effectiveness of MSF to improve nutritional status

The actual nutritional impact of maize fortification at service hammer mills must be convincingly demonstrated through an adequately funded effectiveness trial that evaluates biological and functional indicators. This is a precondition for a next step in scaling up and adopting this fortification method as a key health intervention.

Validate the Direct Addition fortification method

While the most economic 1:50 dilution ratio was tested and adopted by the DFU, further assessment is needed of the uniformity and reliability of the blending method in the fortified maize at the lower dilution ratio that is corroborated by an external laboratory.

Develop an MSF business model, based on the DFU experience

The success and sustainability of the DFU merits further investigation into the financial viability of and considerations for using MSF in other locations with poor nutrition that results from heavy reliance on staples and limited access to centrally fortified foods.

In order to replicate and scale up the DFU experience, it is necessary to conduct a detailed business review of the DFU and to document the process, marketing, costs and relative proportion of the income from the various products and customers.

Determine optimal cost structure and systems for SSF

Currently, SSF activities are not being expanded because of the level of financial and technical support that is required.[5] Exploration into future SSF and MSF potential must include investigation into the optimal cost structure for scale up in the Malawi context. It is unlikely that the poorest households will be able to cover the complete costs of fortification. However, a cost-sharing arrangement between the consumer, the private sector and the government should be considered. Within this planning process, a reliable, independently functioning system for distribution of the fortification preblend from the MSF to SSF units needs to be developed.

Even though medium- and small-scale fortification may be more expensive per person than large-scale fortification, both the costs and benefits should be compared with those of other interventions aimed at improving micronutrient intake, such as supplementation programmes or dietary diversification. In the light of these more relevant comparisons, medium- and small-scale fortification costs compare well.

Strengthen quality assurance processes for SSF

The NFA and the MBS are the two organizations that currently oversee monitoring and legislation for fortification in Malawi. The MBS provides certification to companies producing fortified food in accordance with Malawi's national food standards.[6] Although it would be difficult to provide quality assurance and quality control for the estimated 10,000 small-scale hammer mills operating throughout Malawi, MBS would be likely to be able to adequately monitor additional MSF units if they were to begin fortification.

For SSF, it will be necessary to determine creatively how consumers or community groups can be empowered to monitor and ensure the accountability to standards at the local level.

Case study summary

Food insecurity and malnutrition are very prevalent in Malawi, and most Malawians still reside in rural areas and utilize small-scale hammer mills to process maize. While legislative developments have improved food safety and standards at the national level, most people in Malawi cannot access that food system. Thus, medium- and small-scale fortification have great potential to reach rural populations. As demonstrated by the MICAH Malawi case, ultimately, a collaborative approach between MSF and SSF units is likely to achieve the greatest reach and impact.

The DFU example demonstrates the possibility of achieving sustainable MSF. Programmers and policy makers should now prioritize the evaluation of effectiveness and then the scaling up of MSF units as cost-effective and sustainable means to improve the nutrient intakes of poor, rural populations.

A secondary priority is to scale up SSF units linked to MSF units in geographically defined areas of high nutritional need, and in locations where governments or other organizations can provide technical support and subsidies, especially for quality control and quality assurance monitoring.

Including medium- and small-scale fortification in food security and nutrition programmes can improve the potential impact of the overall programme and, more importantly, maximize the sustainability of positive micronutrient impact.

Acknowledgements

The authors express their appreciation to the Domasi Fortification Unit and the Church of Central Africa Presbyterian (CCAP) Blantyre Synod. We are grateful to Quentin Johnson

Supplemental Table 17.2. MICAH (Micronutrient and Health) Malawi programme activities by purpose.

Strategy	Specific activities	Delivery platform
Purpose 1: To improve micronutrient status through increased intake and bioavailability of micronutrients		
1A. Micronutrient supplementation	1A1. Provide weekly iron and folic acid supplements for women of child-bearing age (WCBA)	Community based: traditional birth attendants (TBAs), village health volunteers and community health workers
	1A2. Provide daily iron and folic acid supplements for pregnant women	
	1A3. Provide weekly iron and folic acid supplements for children	
	1A4. Distribute iodine capsule annually to women and children in iodine-deficient areas without access to iodized salt	
1B. Diet diversification and modification	1B1. Promote and support women-led micro-livestock production to increase consumption of animal source foods	
	1B2. Promote and support household and community production and consumption of iron-enhancing and/or vitamin A-rich fruits and vegetables, including indigenous varieties, through home and school gardens	
	1B3. Introduce, support and promote solar drying of fruits and vegetables to provide year-round access to micronutrient rich foods	
1C. Food fortification	1C1. Support community hammer mills for small-scale community fortification with iron and other micronutrients	Small-scale and medium-scale fortification
	1C2. Support larger mills for production of fortified maize–soya blends for use as complementary foods and rehabilitation (*likuni phala*)	
	1C3. Support one mill to expand capacity to produce fortified *likuni phala*, fortified maize flour for commercial use and production of premix for sale to community mills	
1D. Salt iodization	1D1. Advocate for importation of only iodized salt into the country	
	1D2. Provide equipment and support for salt testing	
1E. Promote optimal infant and young child feeding practices	1E1. Promote and support of Baby Friendly Hospital Initiatives (BFHI)	Facility-based BFHI practices; community-based IEC with village health volunteers and TBAs
	1E2. Provide information and education (IEC) on exclusive breastfeeding and appropriate complementary feeding, including food demonstrations	
Purpose 2: To reduce prevalence of diseases affecting micronutrient status		
2A. Water and sanitation	2A1. Support construction of safe water supplies for household and school use	
	2A2. Organize communities to establish water committees and designate pump maintenance workers	

Continued

Supplemental Table 17.2. Continued.

Strategy	Specific activities	Delivery platform
	2A3. Promote construction and use of latrines, garbage waste disposal and utensil drying racks	
2B. Control and treat common endemic diseases	2B1. Support immunization, growth monitoring and promotion, diarrhoeal control activities, deworming and health and nutrition education	
	2B2. Provide malaria prophylaxis (mainly to pregnant women)	
	2B3. Initiate Drug Revolving Fund (DRF) schemes in selected villages and trained committees to operate and manage these DRFs	
	2B4. Implement mass deworming campaigns for children in schistosomiasis-endemic areas and clear bushes where snails reproduce	
2C. Immunization	2C1. Provide logistical support to the Ministry of Health (MOH) immunization programme	
	2C2. Include importance of immunization as part of health and nutrition education to project communities	
Purpose 3: To build capacity to implement micronutrient programmes		
3A. Capacity building	3A1. Create and fund position of 'Micronutrient Coordinator' within the MOH with responsibility for coordinating all micronutrient programming in the country	
	3A2. Include two-line ministries (health and agriculture) as implementing partners and foster collaboration and complementarity between these two units	
	3A3. Strengthen national laboratory facilities, especially in analysis of urinary iodine, and provide training and equipment for regional- and community-level health facilities and laboratories, to increase capacity to monitor micronutrient status	

for his technical assistance and support. We acknowledge the MICAH Malawi programme manager, Rose Namarika, who led the implementation of the programme, and the whole MICAH Malawi and World Vision Malawi team who contributed to the programme implementation in Malawi from 1996 to 2006. MICAH Malawi was funded by the Canadian International Development Agency and World Vision Canada.

Notes

[1]Other partners included: the Agriculture Development Division of the Ministry of Agriculture (MoA), Community Health Sciences Unit of the Ministry of Health (MoH), Ekwendeni Mission Hospital, St Gabriel's Mission Hospital, the International Eye Foundation, Emmanuel International (EI) and four World Vision Malawi Area Development Programmes.

[2]Defined as households producing maize sufficient for a 3–4 month supply annually.

[3]The DFU (Domasi Fortification Unit) linked with 17 SSF (small-scale fortification) units around Malawi.

[4]Personal communication from the factory manager indicated that another benefit for those affected by HIV/AIDS is that factory staff contribute a portion of their salary to purchase nutritious food every 2 weeks for those whose disease progression is causing them to lose weight. Further, this staff fund assists in the payment of school fees for children of those infected. In a context such as rural Malawi, this benefit is unprecedented.

[5]World Vision has, however, undertaken small-scale fortification in one project location with financial support from the USA.

[6]These encompass not only food standards but also quality assurance and quality control measures. The MBS (Malawi Bureau of Standards) sets the standard for all food processing in the country and carries out the required periodic tests. An MBS Standard logo is provided for companies that adhere to the MBS food standards.

References

Baldwin Radford, K. (2005) *Small Scale Fortification at a Rural Hammermill*. World Vision Malawi Micronutrient and Health (MICAH) Programme, Lilongwe, Malawi.

Berti, P., Mildon, A., Siekmans, K., Main, B. and MacDonald, C. (2010) An adequacy evaluation of a 10-year, four-country nutrition and health programme. *International Journal of Epidemiology* 39, 613–629.

Gibson, R.S., Ferguson, E.L. and Lehrfeld, J. (1998) Complementary foods used in developing countries for infant feeding: their nutrient adequacy and improvement. *European Journal of Clinical Nutrition* 52, 764–70.

MacDonald, A.C., Main, B.J., Namarika, R.H., Yiannakis, M.E. and Mildon, A.M. (2011) Small-animal revolving funds: an innovative programming model to increase access to and consumption of animal-source foods by rural households in Malawi. In: Thompson, B. and Amoroso, L. (eds) *Combating Micronutrient Deficiencies: Food-based Approaches*. Food and Agriculture Organization of the United Nations, Rome and CAB International, Wallingford, UK, pp. 137–149.

MI (2004) *Fortification Handbook: Vitamin and Mineral Fortification of Wheat Flour and Maize Meal*. Micronutrient Initiative, Ottawa, Canada.

Motts, N. (2003) *Small Scale Fortification Study in Malawi: Case Study of the Workability of Fortification via Service Hammermills*. Micronutrient Initiative, Ottawa, Canada.

NSO and ORC Macro (2001) *Malawi Demographic and Health Survey 2000*. Zomba, Malawi and Calverton, Maryland.

Siekmans, K. (2007) *Analysis of Cost for Core Nutrition Interventions*. World Vision International Nutrition Taskforce, Toronto, Canada.

Siekmans, K., Colecraft, E.K. and Nkhoma, O.W.W. (2009) *Assessing the Scale and Sustainability of Anaemia Packages Implemented in Ghana and Malawi*. World Vision, Toronto, Canada.

18 Optimized Feeding Recommendations and In-home Fortification to Improve Iron Status in Infants and Young Children in the Republic of Tajikistan: A Pilot Project

Marina Adrianopoli,[1]* Paola D'Acapito,[1] Marika Ferrari,[1] Lorenza Mistura,[1] Elisabetta Toti,[1] Giuseppe Maiani,[1] Ursula Truebswasser,[2] Khadichamo Boymatova[3] and Santino Severoni[4]

[1]*National Research Institute on Food and Nutrition (INRAN), Rome, Italy; [2]World Health Organization (WHO), Harare, Zimbabwe; [3]WHO, Dushanbe, Republic of Tajikistan; [4]WHO, Copenhagen, Denmark*

Summary

Anaemia is a widespread public health problem that affects particularly infants and young children aged from 6 to 24 months. Nutrition has an important role in addressing this condition, and integrated food-based strategies can be adopted to improve complementary feeding (CF) patterns. The objective of this chapter is to evaluate the efficacy of age-specific Food-Based Complementary Feeding Recommendations (FBCFRs) and the long-term effectiveness and feasibility of an in-home fortification – using micronutrient powders (Sprinkles®) – in order to optimize CF and reduce anaemia in infants and young children in two regions of Tajikistan (Khatlon and GBAO). The study was designed as a 12 month pilot trial. Tajik infants ($n = 209$) aged 6–12 months with blood haemoglobin (Hb) concentrations >7 g/dl and <11g/dl at baseline, were assigned to Group A, which was fed according to the FBCFRs for that age, or to Group B, which was fed according to the FBCFRs but plus Sprinkles. Nutrition education for caretakers was undertaken regularly. Anthropometry, haematological indices, morbidity and dietary recall were assessed at 0, 3, 6 and 12 months. The prevalence of anaemic subjects decreased by 30.0% in Group A and by 47.2% in Group B. Improvements of Hb levels were observed at 3 months (10.16 ± 0.98 g/dl in Group A and 11.32 ± 1.53 g/dl in Group B), and at 12 months (10.8 ± 1.3 g/dl in Group A and 11.0 ± 1.4 g/dl in Group B). In both groups, compliance was generally higher among 12–23 month-old breastfed children. Integrated food-based approaches, supported by behaviour change communication and by strengthening community nutrition knowledge, represent a long-term strategy to improve CF patterns and to address specific micronutrient deficiencies in early life.

Introduction

Anaemia, defined by the World Health Organization (WHO) as blood haemoglobin (Hb) concentration below the established cut-off levels (11.0 g/dl in children under 5 years of age) (WHO, 2001) represents one of the world's most serious health risk factors

---

*Contact: marina.adrianopoli@gmail.com

(WHO, 2001; WHO/UNICEF, 2004). Iron deficiency is one of the main contributing factors to anaemia, with major consequences for human health, including premature death, impaired mental and physical growth, and impaired social and economic development due to reduced work and cognitive performance and productivity (de Benoist *et al.*, 2008). Iron deficiency anaemia (IDA) constitutes one of the most prevalent nutritional deficiencies in the world and is identified among the ten most serious risks in countries with high infant mortality (WHO, 2000); it affects women and children in particular, as they are vulnerable to IDA due to their higher requirements for iron. Iron deficiency commonly develops after 6 months of age if complementary foods do not provide sufficient absorbable iron, even for exclusively breastfed infants (WHO, 2001); therefore, it needs to be prevented in early life and throughout the life cycle.

Iron deficiency and anaemia can be prevented and treated through food-based strategies to improve dietary diversity, together with food fortification and supplementation programmes to increase both iron intake and iron bioavailability. WHO recommends supplementation for all infants and children from 6 to 23 months of age in areas where the prevalence of anaemia exceeds 20–30% (WHO, 2001, 2003).

In-home fortification represents a practical way to add micronutrient premix to foods at the domestic level. This relatively new approach is mainly adopted for preventing and improving micronutrient deficiencies, and can be carried out by using a micronutrient-based powder (Sprinkles®), which enables families to 'fortify' their own foods, including complementary foods, safely and appropriately (SGHI, 2006).

The use of iron supplementation in areas endemic for malaria has been a standing controversy for the international public health community owing to concerns that iron therapy may exacerbate infections – and, in particular, malaria – given that malaria parasites require iron for their growth. A total of 2309 cases of malaria were reported in Tajikistan in 2005, although the number of cases has decreased significantly, from over 19,000 in

2000 to only 318 in 2008 (Sazawal *et al.*, 2006; WHO, 2006b); however, both malaria and malnutrition are present in Tajikistan.

According to the *Tajikistan Multiple Indicator Cluster Survey 2005* (known as MICS 2005; see SCS/UNICEF, 2006), in 2005 the prevalence of children that were underweight (moderately and severely) was 17%, with 4% classified as severely underweight; about 27% were stunted, while 7% were wasted. Children in Khatlon Oblast and Gorno-Badakhshan Autonomous Oblast (GBAO) were more likely to be underweight and stunted; children in Khatlon and those living in poor households were more likely to be exposed to global acute malnutrition (GAM) (about 14%) (SCS/UNICEF, 2006). In 2003, the national prevalence of anaemia (Hb < 11 g/dl) among children aged 6 to 59 months was 38%, with higher rates among children aged 6 to 23 months (SCS/UNICEF, 2006). In Khatlon, anaemia prevalence was 50%, and in GBAO it was 55%, with severe cases of anaemia coexisting (3% in GBAO) with more moderate cases (UNICEF, 2004). Iron deficiency was present in 54% of children with moderate and severe anaemia (UNICEF, 2004). Both iron deficiency anaemia and growth retardation are still major concerns among infants and young children in Tajikistan, especially in the highly deprived and remote rural areas – such as Khatlon and GBAO (WFP, 2005).

Based on this background information, the present study was designed to implement an integrated food-based strategy for improving complementary feeding (CF) and nutritional status of infants and children aged from 6 to 24 months of age in two regions of Tajikistan: Khatlon and GBAO. The objective was to evaluate the efficacy of age-specific Food-based Complementary Feeding Recommendations (FBCFRs) and the long-term effectiveness and feasibility of an in-home fortification using micronutrient sprinkles (Sprinkles®), with the purpose of optimizing CF and reducing anaemia in children from 6 to 24 months of age (Zlotkin *et al.*, 2001, 2003a,b, 2004a,b). The project was supported by the Ministry of Health of the Republic of Tajikistan as part of a national public health campaign to optimize CF patterns.

Subjects and Methods

Study location

The study was conducted between November 2007 and April 2009 in two regions of Tajikistan: Khatlon and GBAO. Within the territory of these regions, 20 villages were selected, ten of which were located in the districts of Rushon, Shugnon and Roshtqala in GBAO and the other ten in Bokhtar, Muminobod and Shurobod districts in Khatlon. In this specific context, but nevertheless comparable with other environments, poor diet was clearly identified as a key cause of iron deficiency. Infants' diets generally contained an insufficient amount of animal source foods (ASFs) at a low frequency of consumption (UNICEF, 2004); concurrently, non-haem iron was likely to be inadequately bioavailable as a result of the consumption of inhibitors of iron absorption, such as black tea, along with the absence of enhancers, such as fresh fruit or vegetables, besides the early introduction of cow's milk (UNICEF, 2004).

The picture is enriched by data on the rate of breastfeeding among infants under 4 months of age, which, in 2005, was slightly above 36% (SCS/UNICEF, 2006). The percentage of children aged less than 6 months who were exclusively breastfed was even lower, at about 25%. Exclusive breastfeeding was higher among children in GBAO (51%). At age 6–9 months, 15% of children received breast milk and solid or semi-solid foods. By the age of 12 to 15 months, roughly 75% of young children were still breast-fed, while about 33% received breast milk up to 20–23 months. In GBAO, children, male infants and those living in the poorest households were most likely to continue receiving breast milk. However, only 7% of children aged from 6 to 11 months could be considered adequately fed. Among all infants aged from 0 to 11 months, adequate CF rises to a still-low 16%, mainly because of the higher proportion of breastfed children (SCS/UNICEF, 2006).

Study subjects

To select subjects for this study, approximately 500 children in 20 selected clusters (villages) were screened in November and December 2007. Because anaemic infants and young children (IYC) were the target population for the study, blood Hb levels and nutritional status were assessed during the screening phase. IYC with an Hb concentration >7 g/dl and <11 g/dl, and aged from 6 to 12 months, were eligible to enter the study. Exclusion criteria were: the presence of severe clinical malnutrition (weight-for-height Z-score, or WHZ, < –3), Hb level < 7 g/dl, severe chronic illness and congenital abnormalities; in addition, children receiving iron supplementations or enrolled in a therapeutic feeding programme were also excluded. The study was a 12 month pilot trial in anaemic IYC from 6 to 24 months of age who were allocated to one of two intervention groups.

The study design was explained to the Tajik health authorities at regional and district levels, and had the support of the Tajik Ministry of Health. Community health workers were informed about the study objectives and trained on the screening procedures. During the screening, mothers and infant caretakers living in the villages were asked to bring their infants to the health centres, and the 12 month project was carefully explained to all mothers. An individual signed informed consent was obtained from all mothers of the participants before starting the measurements, and each mother was informed about her right to stop the interview, screening and project at any stage. Infants underwent a series of measurements to evaluate their nutritional status at the beginning of the study; measurements included an Hb test, anthropometric measurements, dietary assessment and clinical examination. The baseline assessment also investigated household socio-economic characteristics, as well as water, sanitation, hygiene practices and the conditions of dwellings.

Study design

The study was designed as a 12 month pilot trial in anaemic IYC 6–12 months of age. A two-stage cluster sampling methodology was carried out to implement the trial. During the first stage of this, 20 clusters (villages) were selected using the probability proportional to population size (PPS) methodology and were randomly assigned to one of the two intervention groups: Group A, to receive FBCFRs and Group B to receive FBCFRs plus Sprinkles®. At the second stage, 30 eligible households were selected from each cluster, and the recruited children (n = 209) were randomly assigned either to Group A (n = 104) or to Group B (n = 105).

The Project

Formulation of Food-Based Complementary Feeding Recommendations (FBCFRs)

Using the linear programming (LP) approach, effective, cost-affordable and age-specific FBCFRs were drafted for Tajikistan based on the nutrient requirements of infants and children between 6 and 24 months; existing complementary feeding (CF) patterns, iron-rich locally available foods and traditional recipes were identified as well (see Briend *et al.*, 2003; Ferguson *et al.*, 2004, 2006; Allen *et al.*, 2006; also *Optimization of Complementary Feeding Recommendations through Linear Programming (LP) in Tajikistan*, WHO/UNICEF unpublished report, 2007), and were incorporated within the dietary recommendations developed for this study.

Recommendations were formulated with the goal of optimizing knowledge and infant feeding practices for three different age groups: 6–8, 9–11 and 12–23 months. The FBCFRs offered clear and comprehensive guidance to promote proper nutrition behaviour among mothers.

The main points were to:

- timely introduce ASFs (meat, egg, dairy products) legumes, fresh fruit and vegetables into the diets of infants;
- discourage the early introduction of black tea (heavily consumed by the Tajik population and commonly given to infants), which prevents the absorption of iron;
- increase the consumption of iron-rich foods;

- make use of age-specific food baskets that include the daily consumption of fruit, vegetables, cereals, milk and *kefir* (home-made yogurt) as basic daily ingredients;
- combine ingredients properly; and
- guarantee a balanced daily distribution of meals, including snacks.

All mothers received nutritionally adequate and practical dietary counselling on a monthly basis according to the age group and breastfeeding status of their child; portion sizes were expressed in standardized home measures (e.g. the typical Tajik cup – the *piola*, teaspoon and tablespoon). Mothers and caretakers were also provided with weekly cards to document the amount, type and frequency of foods given to their children. These weekly cards were used to assess their compliance with the study and, as a consequence, its feasibility.

The in-home fortification programme was implemented in ten of the 20 clusters selected in the first-stage sampling: Group B (in-home fortification intervention) received the same FBCFRs plus 30 Sprinkles® sachets each month. Sprinkles® are sachets containing a blend of micronutrients in powder form, which are easily added to foods prepared at home. The product was developed by the Sprinkles Global Health Initiative (SGHI) to prevent and treat micronutrient deficiencies among young children and other vulnerable groups at risk (SGHI, 2006). The consumption of Sprinkles® consisted of the daily intake of a standard Nutritional Anaemia Formulation sachet, properly mixed with the meal. The composition of one sachet is: 12.5 mg iron, 5 mg zinc, 300 µg vitamin A, 160 µg folic acid and 30 mg vitamin C (SGHI, 2006).

Caretakers received two types of toolkit every month:

- The Group A (FBCFR) toolkit contained: FBCFRs provided on paper, with illustrations, and specific for the age group concerned (6–8, 9–11 and 12–23 months) and for breastfeeding status; a pictorial guide illustrating the food items and quantities; and four weekly record cards to facilitate the assessment of compliance.

- Group B (FBCFRs plus Sprinkles®) received the same toolkit as Group A, plus 30 sachets of Sprinkles® micronutrient powder and a brochure illustrating the use of Sprinkles®. Feeding recommendations for this group included the daily use of micronutrient powder.

Nutrition education

Nutrition education and capacity-building represented a key component of the study, as inadequate diet is one of the main contributing factors to micronutrient malnutrition among children in Tajikistan (UNICEF, 2004; also D'Acapito, P., Mistura, L., Adrianopoli, M., Ferrari, M. and Maiani, G. (2007) *Optimized Feeding Recommendations and in-home Fortification in Two Regions of Tajikistan (Khatlon and Gorno-Badakhshan). A Pilot Project for the WHO/UNICEF*, Rome, Complementary Feeding Initiative: Trial Protocol. Unpublished protocol). It was essential to act with an integrated approach to tackle the immediate causes of this specific type of malnutrition. The intention behind the inclusion of nutrition education was to optimize infant nutrition in terms of the knowledge and behaviour of mothers, while taking into consideration the environmental contexts in which these mothers lived (households and communities). The study aimed to extend the basic concepts of child nutrition and infant care in this broader social framework. Therefore, the selected population was assisted by health workers, who were trained in infant feeding principles and, in addition, discussion groups with mothers of selected children also welcomed other community members in several villages. Health workers were responsible for advising mothers on a monthly basis using interactive approaches, such as cooking demonstrations and group discussions. Interactive approaches and techniques were introduced to increase the mothers' motivation to feed their offspring properly, and to improve the quality of their infants' dietary intakes, as key activities in reducing micronutrient deficiency, especially in situations where families have limited resources.

Activities to promote improved nutrition practices were supported by pictorial material with illustrations and photos that was produced for this study (an example is given in Fig. 18.1). The photos showed locally available foods, along with recommended quantities, which were represented using Tajik household utensils. Practical dietary indications, such as breastfeeding, food preparation and the use of Sprinkles®, were clearly illustrated, as well as the appropriate daily and weekly food utilization and consumption (Zlotkin *et al.*, 2003b). Standardized illustrations and photos were shown in all the documentation for mothers, which included the FBCFRs in pictorial form, an 'atlas' (guide) with pictures and captions, and the compliance sheets. In order to standardize all visual information, the same photos and illustrations were included in the teaching material for health workers, who received the FBCFRs in pictorial form, along with information on the FBCFRs in written form.

A child's nutritional status is strongly correlated with the mother's education. If the mother has difficulty reading or interpreting nutritional recommendations provided in written form, it is very unlikely that she will comply with recommendations; in contrast, the expressive power of a picture, designed to represent commonly used foods and tools, facilitates the transmission of the message, which then becomes easy to understand.

Focus group discussions

Monthly monitoring activities also included discussion groups with mothers at the health centre (D'Acapito *et al.*, 2007; see last section for details) to strengthen contact with the field staff and refresh the general understanding of the project's aims. Discussions were also an occasion to boost the mothers' health and nutrition knowledge; health workers were available to answer questions and to clarify misconceptions. The discussion groups represented the bases for setting up focus group discussions to investigate possible challenges of the project implementation. Focus groups were led by health workers

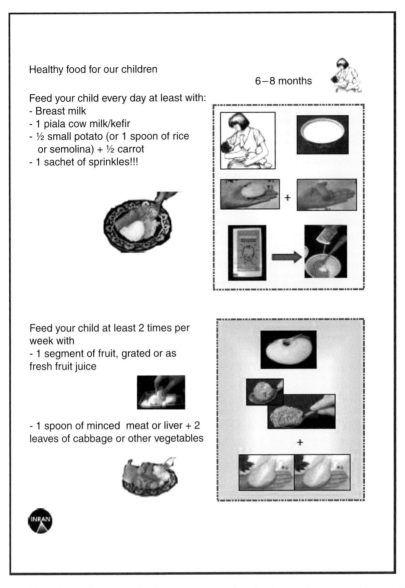

Fig. 18.1. Food-based complementary feeding recommendations in pictorial form as used in an in-home fortification project for anaemic children in Tajikistan. Age group: 6–8 months. Breastfeeding status: breastfed. Photo: Altero Aguzzi, Italian National Research Institute on Food and Nutrition (INRAN).

who had background knowledge and experience in participatory appraisal methodologies, and discussions were based on a question line adapted to the Tajik rural context and made use of field level livelihood analysis tools (FAO, 2001). The aim of the focus group discussions was to identify potential constraints in following the recommendations and using the Sprinkles®, and to explore possible opportunities and solutions together with the mothers.

Data Collection

Questionnaires on breastfeeding practices, frequency of feeding and household socio-economic characteristics were administered at baseline. Enrolled children underwent a series of measurements at baseline, which were then repeated at the three follow-ups (3, 6 and 12 months after baseline); these included measurement of blood Hb concentrations, iron status, anthropometric measurements and dietary assessment. Every month, data on morbidity and any Sprinkles® side effects, and on project compliance were collected (Tielsch *et al.*, 2006). All methods of assessment and measurement were standardized so that all infants, irrespective of their group assignment, were monitored for the outcome(s) in an identical manner.

The training of field staff and standardization of all techniques took place at baseline before data collection. Further training sessions were delivered before the first and second follow-ups to reinforce the knowledge of field staff on dietary assessment and nutrition education activities. Additional assistance was also provided to nurses on anthropometric measurements and techniques for the collection of capillary blood samples.

Structured interviews with mothers were conducted on a monthly basis to collect information about the diet of their children. Questionnaires were formulated to gather data on: (i) Sprinkles® consumption (quantity and frequency); (ii) morbidity recall and potential side effects, infectious diseases and other illnesses, using a recall of 2 weeks; (iii) compliance with FBCFRs; and (iv) 24 h dietary recall.

Dietary assessment

A dietary assessment was performed throughout the study using combined techniques to estimate food intakes, dietary diversity and compliance with FBCFRs. A Food Frequency questionnaire (FFQ) was administered at the beginning of the study as a baseline dietary diversity assessment. Mothers were asked about their children's food frequency intakes on a daily, weekly and monthly basis. Food items were then grouped into seven categories, as defined by WHO *et al.* (2008) for IYC: (i) grains, roots and

tubers; (ii) legumes and nuts; (iii) dairy products; (iv) ASFs (meat, fish, poultry and offal); (v) eggs; (vi) vitamin A-rich fruit and vegetables; and (vii) other fruit and vegetables. Intake frequencies – referring to the month preceding the interview – aggregated accordingly.

Compliance with FBCFRs was assessed by means of a pictorial booklet in which food and food preparation pictures were combined in such a way as to visually reproduce food recommendations and standardized amounts/portion sizes. Mothers were asked to simply tick, on a daily basis, the food consumed by the child. To help mothers with food combinations and portion sizes, the same pictures – showing locally available foods and typical Tajik cups and plates – were used during the nutrition education sessions and cooking demonstrations. Different sets of combined picture recommendations were produced in accordance with age group, breastfeeding status and Sprinkles® intake. This kind of approach, in which written recommendations were unnecessary, was chosen in order to reduce the risk of low compliance due to poor education of the mothers.

On a monthly basis, the compliance forms compiled by the mothers were collected and a 24 h dietary recall was carried out. Dietary recalls were mainly used to validate compliance with the FBCFRs (in both qualitative and quantitative terms) and to assess daily feeding practices. Furthermore, the 24 h dietary recall analysis made it possible to obtain observations of dietary diversity throughout the study.

Haemoglobin

In all children between 6 to 24 months, capillary blood samples were collected to measure their anaemia status. A field haemoglobin analyser (Hemocue™) was used to assess Hb to the nearest 0.1 g/dl. Hemocue controls used a control cuvette. The instruments were used only if the reading was within ± 0.3 g/dl of the cuvette factory value. The Hemocue liquid control was run on each Hemocue after checking the control cuvette.

Anthropometric measures

All anthropometric measurements were conducted by the field staff at each follow-up using standardized techniques. Anthropometric measurements were taken for children from 6 to 24 months old. Weight was determined using an electronic digital scale (UNICEF cat. no. 01-410-15) measuring to the nearest 100 g for children or the nearest 20 g for infants. Infants were weighed with an adult and their weight was determined as the difference between the combined weight and the adult's weight. Recumbent length was measured in children under 2 years using an Infant–Child–Adult Height Board. To reflect the proper measurement for height, 0.7 was subtracted from the length value. For children over 2 years old, standing height was measured (WHO, 2006a). Anthropometric measurements were converted into Z-scores of the index weight-for-length, using the 2006 WHO growth standards (WHO, 2006a).

Data Analysis

The Student's t-test was used to evaluate the significance of differences between mean values of selected indicators between Group A and Group B. Analysis of variance (Anova) for repeated measurements and post hoc comparison was performed to test the differences between means of the main parameters of the haemoglobin and anthropometric measurements. The anthropometric index WHZ was calculated using WHO Anthro software to assess the growth performance (WHO, 2006a). All statistical analyses were performed using the SPSS statistical software package for Microsoft Windows (Version 12.00, SPSS Inc., Chicago, Illinois).

24 hour dietary recall

All data derived from the 24 hour dietary recall were entered into the NutriSurvey software (an English translation of a commercial German software (EBISpro) which is available free for non-commercial use; see http://www.nutrisurvey.de/lp/background_info.htm) and processed to estimate the dietary profiles of the subjects. The NutriSurvey software was used as the main food composition reference. The composition of buckwheat, cooked carrot, cooked onion, kaki, beef sausage, sour cream, sunflower seed oil and bread was derived from the USDA (US Department of Agriculture) National Nutrient Database for Standard Reference (http://www.ars.usda.gov/main/site_main.htm?modecode=12-35-45-00). The composition of commercially available porridge and *kefir* were based on the nutritional facts label of standard porridge and *kefir*.

An estimation of dietary diversity was not originally planned in this study but, on the basis of the data obtained from the 24 h dietary recall, the infants' dietary diversity was observed during the analysis phase. The consumption of food items was recorded by the 24 h dietary recall questionnaire. The types of food consumed were aggregated during processing of these data into the seven food groups specified for IYC by WHO *et al.* (2008), and already identified for this study (see Dietary assessment section above), which indicated the number of food groups consumed daily. The number of food groups consumed by any child over the past 24 h was then simply calculated. Data from the first dietary assessment were compared with data from the last one, and may serve as support to the nutritional adequacy data.

Anaemia

The severity of anaemia levels was classified according to the blood Hb concentration. The cut-off points used for the classification refer to the WHO definition of anaemia (WHO, 2001) and are based on blood Hb concentrations expressed in g/dl.

In order to estimate correctly the Hb levels in villages at higher altitudes, the correction procedure of the International Nutritional Anemia Consultative Group was used (Nestel and INACG, 2002).

Results

The initial number of recruited children ($n = 209$), distributed in both groups (104 in

Group A and 105 in Group B) decreased throughout the 12 month study. Figure 18.2 shows that 209 children were recruited at the beginning of the study and underwent the complete baseline assessment; among them, 157 were monitored at the first follow-up (3 months), 156 at the second (6 months) and 147 children at the final follow-up (12 months). However, only 107 children (58 in Group A and 49 in Group B) out of the original 209 attended all the three follow-ups, and so only their complete nutritional and health profile was available over the 12 month period for a longitudinal analysis. This chapter aims to illustrate the longitudinal results collected from children who were enrolled at baseline and who then completed all three follow-up measurements (*n* = 107: 58 in Group A and 49 in Group B).

Several factors determined the absence of children during the monitoring phase as determined from key informants, such as village health workers, neighbours and relatives, who were consulted to provide an explanation of the possible reasons. Migration and change of workplace by heads of household were considered the principal causes for withdrawing from the study, while temporary drop-outs were attributable mainly to the short-term absence of the family from the village, or to the sickness of mothers and children.

At baseline, the groups did not differ significantly in blood Hb concentrations. Table 18.1 gives the nutritional indicators of the sample at baseline.

The baseline scenario, compared with data from the three follow-ups, is illustrated in Table 18.2, which includes both the

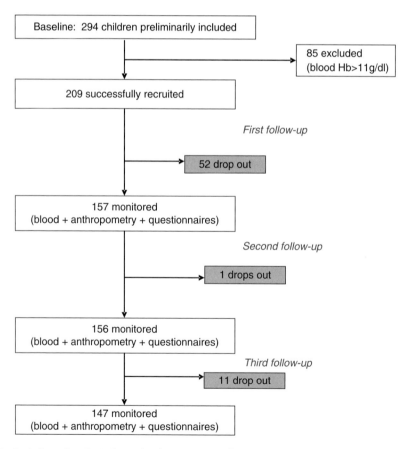

Fig. 18.2. Study flow chart for in-home fortification project for anaemic children aged 6–12 months in Tajikistan. Hb, haemoglobin.

anthropometric and Hb data. The sample is divided into the two intervention groups to which the children were assigned (A: FBCFRs; B: FBCFRs plus Sprinkles®). Body weight and length (height) are significantly lower in Group A than in Group B at baseline, although this difference does not affect the intra-sample characteristics, because moderate malnutrition did not imply an exclusion of children at baseline. The Hb concentrations are slightly higher in Group A at baseline, but the difference is not statistically significant, thus confirming the homogeneity of Hb levels in the selected sample.

The prevalence of moderate acute malnutrition (WHZ -2 to -3) was 12% in both groups at baseline and decreased to 2% at the third follow-up. This suggests that the implementation of CF in this target group has contributed positively to the children's growth. Conversely, it is important to emphasize the statistically significant increase of mean Hb levels in both groups, in particular considering that all recruited children were anaemic at baseline (>7 g/dl and <11 g/dl). Figure 18.3 shows the prevalence of anaemic children by intervention group at each follow-up.

The number of anaemic children dropped dramatically at the first follow-up in both groups; this result clearly implies the successful outcome of both studies during the first 3 months of the project. Hb levels were significantly different between groups in all three follow-ups, and were higher in Group B. In Group A, longitudinal differences were observed between the baseline and the first and second follow-ups, while in Group B significant differences were seen between the baseline and the second follow-up, suggesting that both interventions were also effective at the time of the second follow-up.

Findings on morbidity and side effects suggested that episodes of diarrhoea occurred more frequently among children in Group A. There were similar results for respiratory illness, severe vomiting and visits to physicians.

The analysis performed on nutritional adequacy provides evidence of the impact of

Table 18.1. Baseline characteristics of subjects in an in-home fortification project in Tajikistan. Group A to receive FBCFRs (Food-Based Complementary Feeding Recommendations) only; Group B to receive FBCFRs + Sprinkles®.

Characteristic	Group A	Group B
No. of subjects	104	105
Males:females (%)	45:55	61:39
Weight-for-height Z-score	-0.4 ± 1.0^a	-0.0 ± 1.0^a
Blood haemoglobin (Hb) (g/dl)	9.9 ± 0.7	9.94 ± 0.7

[a]Student's *t*-test between groups: *P* value <0.05.

Table 18.2. Changes in anthropometric and biochemical (blood haemoglobin) variables in an in-home fortification project in Tajikistan, by group at baseline and each follow-up. Group A received FBCFRs (Food-Based Complementary Feeding Recommendations) only; Group B received FBCFRs + Sprinkles®.

	Group A	Group B
No. of subjects:	58	49
Weight for height Z-score (WHZ)[a]		
Baseline	-0.5 ± 1.0a	-0.2 ± 1.1e
Follow-up I (3 months)	-0.3 ± 0.9b	-0.1 ± 0.8f
Follow-up II (6 months)	-0.8 ± 0.9c	-0.5 ± 1.3g
Follow-up III (12 months)	-0.2 ± 0.9d	-0.0 ± 0.8h
Haemoglobin (Hb, g/dl)[a]		
Baseline	9.9 ± 0.7i	9.8 ± 0.8n
Follow-up I	10.4 ± 1.0i[b]	12.2 ± 1.8n,o[b]
Follow-up II	9.8 ± 1.2m[b]	10.4 ± 1.4o,p[b]
Follow-up III	10.5 ± 1.2i[b]	11.0 ± 1.5n,p[b]

[a]One-way ANOVA for repeated measures: values in the same columns (i.e. for Group A or for Group B) with different letters are significantly different, *P* value <0.05.
[b]Student's *t*-test between groups: *P* value <0.05.

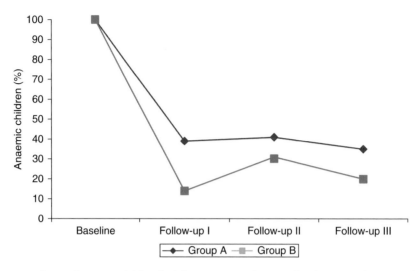

Fig. 18.3. Prevalence of anaemic children by follow up 3, 6 and 12 months after a complementary feeding intervention in an in-home fortification project for anaemic children aged 6–12 months in Tajikistan. Group A, FBCFRs (Food-Based Complementary Feeding Recommendations) only; Group B, FBCFRs + Sprinkles®.

the feeding recommendations. The mean adequacy, compared with the recommended nutrient intakes (RNIs), for each nutrient, by follow-up and by group, is illustrated in Table 18.3 (this analysis did not include data on the consumption of Sprinkles®). The definition of RNI used here is equivalent to that of the recommended daily allowance (RDA) used by the Standing Committee on the Scientific Evaluation of Dietary Reference Intakes of the Food and Nutrition Board (FNB) of the Institute of Medicine of the US National Academy of Sciences (FNB, 1997; WHO/FAO, 2002).

The adequacy of diet energy content and of the majority of micronutrients fell within the recommended range in both groups at all follow-ups. The energy intake between groups did not show differences at the baseline or at the different follow-ups; however, intakes of thiamine, folic acid and iron were all below the RNIs for both groups and in all follow-ups. Iron intake was still poor; it was weakly correlated with fish, meat and cereal consumption, while *mosh* (pulses), lentils, chickpeas, beans and chicken eggs were the foods that principally contributed to the intake of iron. Statistical analysis found no significant differences in nutrient intakes by group or by follow-up. The intake of zinc was high at the first follow-up and maintained a

good level at the second and third follow-ups in Group A; in Group B the intake of zinc was lower at the first follow-up, but there was an increase in the second and third follow-ups. A considerable increase was also observed in the intake of vitamin C at the second follow-up in both groups; acceptable levels were sustained at the third follow-up in both groups. The observed intakes of zinc suggest that ASFs were actually introduced into infants' diets; these results, along with the increased intake of vitamins C and A, suggest that all factors contributing to iron absorption have been optimized.

It should be noted that the goal of the FBCFRs was not to have solely food-based RNIs; these were determined primarily with the aim of proposing feasible food recommendations. The FBCFRs were based on the concept that children eat food, not nutrients. In fact, increasing the amount of food in order to meet micronutrient requirements would also have led to an exponential increase in energy and protein intake, thereby making the customary child's diet unfeasible. A second reason is linked to expectations of improvement: considering that the iron intake of Tajik children in the study areas was already low (UNICEF, 2004); an improvement such as that observed through this food-based

Table 18.3. Dietary adequacy as percentage RNI (recommended nutrient intake) in an in-home fortification project in Tajikistan, by group at each follow-up: I, 3 months; II, 6 months; III, 12 months. Group A received FBCFRs (Food-Based Complementary Feeding Recommendations) only; Group B received FBCFRs + Sprinkles®.

Nutrient/energy	Group A			Group B		
	Follow-up I	Follow-up II	Follow-up III	Follow-up I	Follow-up II	Follow-up III
Energy	132 ± 59	116 ± 58	99 ± 62	97 ± 31	136 ± 46	155 ± 34
Protein	302 ± 198	271 ± 176	234 ± 230	169 ± 104	286 ± 123	255 ± 92
Folic acid	58 ± 42	53 ± 38	43 ± 24	37 ± 16	58 ± 27	56 ± 21
Iron	54 ± 33	54 ± 60	46 ± 45	32 ± 17	51 ± 18	66 ± 74
Niacin equiv.	195 ± 129	167 ± 102	148 ± 130	121 ± 64	188 ± 71	148 ± 67
Pantothenic acid	127 ± 62	125 ± 70	101 ± 58	89 ± 44	143 ± 39	134 ± 78
Retinol equiv.	164 ± 119	88 ± 70	107 ± 76	98 ± 98	145 ± 124	148 ± 88
Riboflavin	141 ± 105	149 ± 77	117 ± 84	89 ± 77	156 ± 62	189 ± 76
Thiamine	78 ± 50	72 ± 73	56 ± 52	49 ± 31	67 ± 31	69 ± 92
Vitamin B_6	197 ± 142	163 ± 73	142 ± 70	147 ± 73	208 ± 69	156 ± 54
Vitamin B_{12}	341 ± 306	314 ± 227	281 ± 293	187 ± 189	304 ± 169	406 ± 174
Vitamin C	77 ± 54	105 ± 79	85 ± 71	72 ± 43	102 ± 49	90 ± 92
Zinc	107 ± 78	89 ± 62	80 ± 86	56 ± 39	92 ± 40	87 ± 39

intervention can already be considered an important step towards better nutrition.

Figures 18.4a and 18.4b show the dietary diversity in terms of number of food groups consumed by children (24 h dietary recall); these two figures compare the initial (baseline) assessment and the third (final) follow-up assessment. The aim was to assess whether mothers fed their children with more food groups, thus improving food diversity and, as a consequence, the quality of the diet in compliance with the FBCFR.

Based on observations from the 24 h dietary recalls, the number of food groups consumed in Group A increased at the third follow-up; therefore, it could be assumed that mothers from Group A have been more compliant with the recommendations than mothers from Group B (Fig. 18.4a,b). A key point emerging from focus groups in the villages of Group B might explain this result: during the discussion it was confirmed that the use of Sprinkles® was very much accepted among mothers but, at the same time, it emerged that the feeding recommendations were harder to put into practice. In contrast, mothers in Group A were conscious that only feeding recommendations could have an impact on the nutritional status of their children, which could be a strong motivation to follow feeding recommendations.

Conclusions

This study has demonstrated that in-home fortification of complementary foods using Sprinkles® (containing iron, zinc, vitamin A, folic acid and vitamin B), combined with FBCFRs (intervention B), had positive effects on infants with moderate anaemia, which was eradicated in 80% of children receiving FBCFRs + Sprinkles® at the end of the study, so that only 20% of children remained anaemic (see Fig. 18.3). As expected, micronutrient powders were well accepted by mothers owing to several advantages of the product, such as its easy preparation, the free distribution of sachets by health workers and the novelty factor. The high level of acceptance of Sprinkles® resulted in the majority of children receiving them reaching Hb levels >11 g/dl. A second important finding of this study was that similar effects (on Hb levels and dietary patterns) were achieved, at least in part, with the FBCFRs alone (intervention A).

The combined intervention used in this pilot project represented an integrated strategy aimed at optimizing infant feeding by covering issues such as nutrition, care and hygiene practices. This is of particular importance in rural Tajikistan, where the prevalence of iron deficiency and anaemia is high, especially

(a)

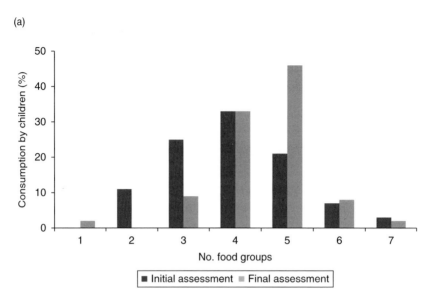

(b)

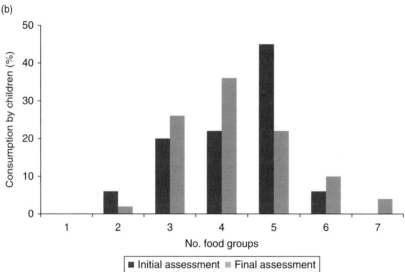

Fig. 18.4. Food group consumption by children in an in-home fortification project for anaemic children aged 6–12 months in Tajikistan: (a) number of food groups consumed at the initial assessment and at follow-up III (final assessment) in Group A (as % children), given FBCFRs (Food-Based Complementary Feeding Recommendations) only; and (b) number of food groups consumed at the initial assessment and at follow-up III (final assessment) in Group B (as % children), given FBCFRs + Sprinkles® micronutrients.

in young children, and is caused by inadequate diet and, in some cases, poor hygiene. Although Tajikistan has vast water resources, limited access to clean water, and a high prevalence of water-borne diseases, constitute a major public health problem and are one of the main causes of child malnutrition in the country (SCS/UNICEF, 2006).

An important conclusion from the study is that in-home fortification represents an appropriate intermediate solution when there is a risk (or occurrence) of micronutrient deficiencies. However, given the fact that micronutrient powders are not food, and cannot be consumed without food, the use of effective and affordable food-based recommendations, based on feasible combinations of locally available foods, should be strongly encouraged, taking existing food patterns and portion sizes into account. This pilot confirms the necessity of field-testing dietary recommendations, which helped to evaluate potential difficulties in the implementation, feasibility and sustainability of feeding recommendations. It was clear that health workers played a crucial role in nutrition education. Building the capacity and skills of health workers in infant feeding is an optimal way to ensure consistency of recommendations and, as a consequence, improve the nutritional knowledge and motivation of mothers.

As observed in this study, the consumption of legumes and pulses, a highly nutritious food group and good source of vitamins and minerals, contributed largely to the infants' iron requirement; in fact, legumes are a popular food and form part of the Tajik regular diet. The increased availability of these products – as well as animal source foods – in local markets and cultivated/raised at home would give an impetus to the consumption of locally produced micronutrient-rich foods. In the Tajik rural context, interventions related to livestock, the management of pastoral risks, water management and winter preparedness would encourage the production of iron-rich vegetables and support livestock breeding. This could ensure access to nutritious foods for food-insecure households that might not be able to afford them otherwise.

In conclusion, food-based approaches, when adequately supported by multi-sectoral interventions, can effectively enable people to make appropriate food choices, thus improving their diets and addressing specific micronutrient deficiencies.

Acknowledgements

We would like to thank the WHO Tajikistan Country Office, Aga Khan Development Network and UNICEF Tajikistan Country Office for their support in the implementation of this project, and the US Centers for Disease Control and Prevention (CDC) for the financial support and inputs during the protocol development and implementation phase.

The Aga Khan Health Service (Aga Khan Development Network, Tajikistan) is particularly acknowledged for cooperation provided during the field activities in the GBAO and Khatlon Regions. Thanks are also extended to the INRAN (Italian National Research Institute on Food and Nutrition) Unit of Human Nutrition, in particular to Dr Eugenia Venneria and Dr Jara Valtuena Santamaria for their contribution in the analyses of serum samples. We also acknowledge Dr Altero Aguzzi from INRAN, who took all the photos used for the educational material, which formed the basis of the nutrition education activities. Finally, we would like to give a special thank you to Dr Francesco Branca of WHO, Geneva, who contributed significantly from the beginning of the study. All authors reviewed, commented on and approved the manuscript.

References

Allen, L., de Benoist, B., Dary, O. and Hurrell, R. (eds) (2006) *Guidelines on Food Fortification with Micronutrients*. World Health Organization, Geneva, Switzerland and Food and Agriculture Organization of the United Nations, Rome (available at: http://whqlibdoc.who.int/publications/2006/9241594012_eng.pdf) (accessed 17 June 2013).

Briend, A., Darmon, N., Ferguson, E. and Erhardt, J.G. (2003) Linear programming: a mathematical tool for analyzing and optimizing children's diets during the complementary feeding period. *Journal of Pediatric Gastroenterology and Nutrition* 1, 12–22.

de Benoist, B., McLean, E., Egli, I. and Cogswell, M. (eds) (2008) *Worldwide Prevalence of Anaemia 1993–2005: WHO Global Database on Anaemia*. World Health Organization, Geneva, Switzerland. Available at: http://whqlibdoc.who.int/publications/2008/9789241596657_eng.pdf (accessed 18 June 2013).

FAO (2001) *Socio-Economic and Gender Analysis Programme (SEAGA): Field Level Handbook*. Food and Agriculture Organization of the United Nations, Rome.

Ferguson, E.L., Darmon, N., Briend, A. and Premachandra, I.M. (2004) Food-based dietary guidelines can be developed and tested using linear programming analysis. *Journal of Nutrition* 134, 951–957.

Ferguson, E.L., Darmon, N., Fahmida, U., Fitriyanti, S., Harper, T.B. and Premachandra, I.M. (2006) Design of optimal food-based complementary feeding recommendations and identification of key "problem nutrients" using goal programming. *Journal of Nutrition* 136, 2399–2404.

FNB (1997) *Dietary Reference Intakes for Calcium, Phosphorus, Magnesium, Vitamin D, and Fluoride*. Standing Committee on the Scientific Evaluation of Dietary Reference Intakes, Food and Nutrition Board, Institute of Medicine of the National Academies. National Academy Press, Washington, DC.

Nestel, P. and INACG (2002) Adjusting hemoglobin values in program surveys. International Nutritional Anaemia Consultative Group (INACG) Steering Committee, Washington, DC. Available at: http://pdf.usaid.gov/pdf_docs/PNACQ927.pdf (accessed 18 June 2013).

Sazawal, S., Black, R.E., Ramsan, M., Chwaya, H.M., Stoltzfus, R.J., Dutta, A., Dhingra, U., Kabole, I., Deb, S., Othman, M.K. and Kabole, F.M. (2006) Effects of routine prophylactic supplementation with iron and folic acid on admission to hospital and mortality in preschool children in a high malaria transmission setting: community-based, randomised, placebo-controlled trial. *The Lancet* 367, 133–143.

SCS/UNICEF (2006) *Tajikistan Multiple Indicator Cluster Survey 2005*. State Committee on Statistics of the Republic of Tajikistan/United Nations Children's Fund, Dushanbe.

SGHI (2006) *Micronutrient Sprinkles for Use in Infants and Young Children: Guidelines on Recommendations for Use, Procurement, and Program Monitoring and Evaluation*. Sprinkles Global Health Initiative, Toronto, Ontario, Canada. Available at: http://sghi.org/resource_centre/GuidelinesGen2008.pdf (accessed 18 June 2013).

Tielsch, J.M., Khatry, S., Stoltzfus, R.J., Katz, J., LeClerq, S.C., Adhikari, R., Mullany, L.C., Shresta, S. and Black, R.E. (2006) Effect of routine prophylactic supplementation with iron and folic acid on pre-school child mortality in southern Nepal: community-based, cluster-randomised, placebo-controlled trial. *The Lancet* 367, 144–152.

UNICEF (2004) *Micronutrients Status Survey in Tajikistan, 2003*. UNICEF (United Nations Children's Fund) Tajikistan Country Office, Dushanbe.

WFP (2005) *Household Food Security and Vulnerability Survey in Rural Tajikistan, November 2004*. ODAV(VAM) Report, Vulnerability Analysis and Mapping Branch, World Food Programme, Rome.

WHO (2000) *The World Health Report 2000 – Health Systems: Improving Performance*. World Health Organization, Geneva, Switzerland.

WHO (2001) *Iron Deficiency Anaemia: Assessment, Prevention and Control*. World Health Organization, Geneva, Switzerland.

WHO (2006a) *Multicentre Growth Reference Study Group. WHO Child Growth Standards: Length/height-for-age, Weight-for-age, Weight-for-length, Weight-for-height and Body Mass Index-for-age: Methods and Development*. World Health Organization, Geneva, Switzerland.

WHO (2006b) *Iron Supplementation of Young Children in Regions Where Malaria Transmission is Intense and Infectious Disease Highly Prevalent*. Joint statement, World Health Organization, Geneva, Switzerland with United Nations Children's Fund, New York.

WHO/FAO (2002) *Human Vitamin and Mineral Requirements. Report of a Joint FAO/WHO Expert Consultation. Bangkok, Thailand*. World Health Organization, Geneva, Switzerland and Food and Agriculture Organization of the United Nations, Rome.

WHO/UNICEF (2003) *Global Strategy for Infant and Young Child Feeding*. United Nations Children's Fund and World Health Organization, Geneva, Switzerland.

WHO/UNICEF (2004) *Focusing on Anaemia. Towards an Integrated Approach for Effective Anaemia Control. Joint WHO/UNICEF Statement*. United Nations Children's Fund and World Health Organization, Geneva, Switzerland.

WHO, UNICEF, USAID, AED, UCDavis and IFPRI (2008) *Indicators for Assessing Infant and Young Child Feeding Practices. Part I: Definitions; Part II: Measurement; Part III: Country Profiles. Conclusions of a Global Consensus Meeting held 6–8 November 2007 in Washington D.C., USA*. World Health Organization, US Agency for International Development, Academy for Educational Development, University of California Davis and International Food Policy Research Institute. Published by WHO, Geneva, Switzerland.

Zlotkin, S., Arthur, P., Antwi, K.Y. and Yeung, G. (2001) Treatment of anaemia with microencapsulated ferrous fumarate plus ascorbic acid supplied as sprinkles to complementary (weaning) foods. *The American Journal of Clinical Nutrition* 74, 791–795.

Zlotkin, S., Antwi, K.Y., Schauer, C. and Yeung, G. (2003a) Use of microencapsulated iron (II) fumarate sprinkles to prevent recurrence of anaemia in infants and young children at high risk. *Bulletin of the World Health Organization* 81, 108–115.

Zlotkin, S., Arthur, P., Schauer, C., Antwi, K.Y., Yeung, G. and Piekarz, A. (2003b) Home-fortification with iron and zinc sprinkles or iron sprinkles alone successfully treat anaemia in infants and young children. *Journal of Nutrition* 133, 1075–1080.

Zlotkin, S., Christofides, A., Schauer, C., Asante, K.P. and Owusu-Agyei, S. (2004a) Home fortification using sprinkles containing 12.5 mg of iron successfully treats anaemia in Ghanaian infants and young children. *The FASEB Journal* 18, 343:2 [abstract].

Zlotkin, S.H., Christofides, A.L., Hyder, S.M., Schauer, C.S., Tondeur, M.C. and Sharieff, W. (2004b) Controlling iron deficiency anaemia through the use of home-fortified complementary foods. *The Indian Journal of Pediatrics* 71, 1015–1019.

19 Towards Long-term Nutrition Security: The Role of Agriculture in Dietary Diversity

Brian Thompson* and Janice Meerman
*Food and Agriculture Organization of the
United Nations, Rome, Italy*

Summary

A major obstacle to securing investments in agriculture and food-based approaches for improving nutrition is providing proof of efficacy. Do food-based approaches lead to reductions in malnutrition? To answer this question we need to develop a credible evidence base that articulates the links in the chain between agricultural policy, food production, access and intake, and nutritional status. This chapter reports on recent research that throws some light on the links between agriculture and dietary diversity, both key in this chain. Findings are presented from Bangladesh, where a study looked at the nutrient composition of rice cultivars; from Kenya and Tanzania, where research was conducted on how crop diversity is related to diet quality; and from Malawi, Kenya and Uganda, where the nutritional diversity of cropping systems was studied. The concept of the 'nutrition gap' – the gap between what foods are grown and available and what foods are needed for a healthy diet – is introduced. The nutrition gap is a useful concept that illustrates the importance of dietary diversity and the better appreciation of how traditional food security models may fall short in their efforts to reduce malnutrition. Increased production of staple crops is typically the main goal and driver of these models. Improvements in nutrition are seen more as a function of purchasing power and increased total energy supply, which is assumed to follow automatically from reductions in income poverty. Narrowing the nutrition gap requires moving past this model to one that includes food *and* nutrition security. The latter is focused on, inter alia, increasing the consumption of a diversified and high-quality diet, as opposed to just increasing total energy consumption. The chapter provides examples of nutrition-sensitive agriculture and food-based strategies and interventions that can be used to improve dietary diversity within specific agro-ecological zones, and for particular food typologies. Taken together, the evidence and examples illustrate the significant and crucial role that agriculture can play in improving dietary diversity and nutrition in poor country contexts.

Introduction

A major obstacle to securing investments in agriculture and food-based approaches for improving nutrition is providing proof of efficacy. Developing a credible evidence base that articulates the links in the chain between agricultural policy, food production, access and intake, and nutritional status is essential to meeting this challenge. This chapter presents research findings on the links between agriculture and dietary diversity, both key in this chain and of particular relevance in poor rural contexts where malnutrition rates are

---

*Contact: brian.thompson@fao.org

often high. It provides examples of nutrition-sensitive agriculture and food-based strategies and interventions that can be used to improve dietary diversity within specific agro-ecological zones and for particular food typologies. Taken together, the evidence and examples illustrate the role that agriculture can play in improving dietary diversity and nutrition in poor country contexts. The chapter is arranged in three main sections: Dietary Diversity and Nutrition; Dietary Diversity and Agriculture; and How Can Agriculture Improve Dietary Diversity? Narrowing the Nutrition Gap for Specific Food Typologies. These are followed by a conclusion. A brief outline of the chapter is given below.

Dietary Diversity and Nutrition: After a preliminary discussion of why traditional food security models often fall short of reducing malnutrition, the concepts of nutrition security and 'narrowing the nutrition gap' are introduced and the key role of dietary diversity in these concepts is discussed. Although the association between dietary diversity and nutrition outcomes seems self-evident, the precise degree and manner in which the former has an impact on the latter remains unclear. Nevertheless, there are numerous studies providing strong evidence that dietary diversity plays an unequivocal role in determining nutritional status. Dietary diversity has been shown to be a good predictor of the micronutrient content of the diet, with the nutritional quality of the diet improving as a larger diversity of food items and food groups are consumed; it has also been shown to be significantly associated with positive nutrition outcomes, such as reduced stunting rates.

Dietary Diversity and Agriculture: There is no proven link between improved diversification of production systems and improved dietary diversity, but there is a growing body of evidence suggestive of an association between greater crop diversity, improved dietary diversity and improved nutrition. Selected findings from this evidence base are presented, namely research on the nutrient composition of rice cultivars in Bangladesh, research on how crop diversity in Kenya and Tanzania is related to diet

quality, and research on the nutritional diversity of cropping systems in Malawi, Kenya and Uganda.

How Can Agriculture Improve Dietary Diversity? Narrowing the Nutrition Gap for Specific Food Typologies: Potential management and policy strategies for integrating dietary diversity goals into agriculture and for narrowing nutritional gaps across a range of agro-ecological settings are presented. These strategies focus on improving crop/livestock diversity and/or purchasing power by:

- increasing small-scale production of micronutrient-rich foods for own/local consumption;
- increasing commercial production of micronutrient-rich foods;
- promoting preservation techniques to maintain micronutrient levels in commonly eaten foods and reduce postharvest losses; and
- selecting and breeding plants to increase micronutrient levels.

Intervention examples for each strategy are provided. The examples are framed according to specific food typology and agro-ecological zone:

- Rain-fed roots and tubers in West Africa.
- Irrigated/rain-fed rice in South and South-east Asia.
- Rain-fed cereals in Central and East Africa.
- Irrigated/rain-fed maize and beans in Central America.

Education and/or social marketing activities that aim to increase consumption of micronutrient-rich foods are featured as essential to the success of most examples.

Conclusion: The study concludes by emphasizing the potential that nutrition-sensitive agriculture and food-based approaches have for improving dietary diversity and nutrition. Policy recommendations for increasing political commitment to agriculture's role in reducing malnutrition are briefly presented as a necessary complement to what has been the paper's main focus – which is to present selected findings and examples of specific interventions from a growing evidence base.

Dietary Diversity and Nutrition

Why traditional food security models fall short: increasing production of staple crops is not enough to accelerate reductions in malnutrition

Agricultural development programmes that aim to address food security by increasing production of staple crops are, by themselves, often not enough to accelerate reductions in hunger and malnutrition. Increased staple crop production may result in increased energy availability but this, on its own, does not guarantee comparable improvements in nutrition outcomes. Similarly, direct reductions in income poverty and improved purchasing power do not generally result in proportional reductions in malnutrition. Although higher incomes do improve nutrition outcomes, they tend to do so at unacceptably slow rates. For example, a doubling of GNP (gross national production) per capita in developing countries has been shown to reduce child underweight rates by only 9% (Haddad et al., 2003). Further, data from many countries show persistently high undernutrition rates in regions and households where staple crop production is high and food availability is good (Haddad et al., 2003).

Malnutrition can occur despite increased food availability and higher incomes for a number of reasons, including poor maternal and child feeding practices, inequitable household food allocation, inadequate sanitation, poor or non-existent health services and lack of access to drinkable water. In addition to these immediate and underlying determinants, a leading cause of persistent malnutrition is low dietary diversity, that is, poor quality and variety of food in the diet.

Low dietary diversity can occur in a variety of contexts, including those where food availability is good and purchasing power is sufficient. It is typically expressed as a monotonous diet that is too high in carbohydrates and too low in protein, fat and micronutrients. This intake pattern is not uncommon in many parts of the developing world, even among households that can afford to eat better, and it eventually results in malnutrition, even in situations where total dietary energy supply (DES) may be adequate. Nutrition-related anaemia, and iron, zinc and vitamin A deficiencies, are examples of 'hidden hunger', malnutrition that can occur in individuals who are consuming enough total energy but not enough macronutrient- and micronutrient-rich foods such as meat, fish, eggs, dairy, legumes, fruits and vegetables. In less secure households, where incomes and DES are low, malnutrition resulting from inadequate calorific intake will be exacerbated by poor dietary diversity. In both cases, increasing consumption of a diversity of nutrient-rich foods is crucial to improved nutrition outcomes.

Nutrition security and narrowing the 'nutrition gap'

To improve the chance that increases in staple crop production and purchasing power do lead to accelerated reductions in malnutrition, agricultural development programmes must focus on nutrition security in addition to food security. Achieving nutrition security requires the consumption of a diet that is adequately diversified in terms of macronutrients and micronutrients, as well as a sanitary environment, adequate health services and proper care and feeding practices. While food security may increase the total quantity of energy available for consumption, only nutrition security can guarantee the quality and diversity of food that is necessary for protecting and promoting good nutritional status and health. Just as improving food security can be thought of in terms of narrowing the gap between current and potential production yields, improving nutrition security can be thought of in terms of narrowing the 'nutrition gap' between current food intake patterns and intake patterns that are optimal in terms of macronutrient and micronutrient content. Narrowing the nutrition gap requires improving dietary diversity through increasing the availability of and access to the foods that are necessary for a healthy diet, and increasing actual intake of those foods.

The example of optimized food intake presented in diagrammatic form at the top of Fig. 19.1 shows how various food groups can be combined (optimized) to ensure both food security (adequate energy intake) and nutrition security (adequate macronutrient and micronutrient intake). In contrast, the DES data for Ghana and Ethiopia, at the bottom of Fig. 19.1, indicate monotonous carbohydrate-heavy diets low in protein, fat and micronutrients. Narrowing the nutrition gap requires increasing dietary diversity to correct this imbalance.

Evidence base

There is strong evidence for the positive impact of dietary diversity on nutritional status. First, increased dietary diversity has been shown to be a good predictor of the micronutrient content of the diet, with nutritional quality of the diet improving as a larger diversity of food items and food groups is consumed (Shimbo *et al.*, 1994; Hatloy *et al.*, 1998; Steyn *et al.*, 2006; Waijers *et al.*, 2007; Moursi *et al.*, 2008). Moursi *et al.* (2008) found that dietary diversity scores were predictive of dietary micronutrient density, and hence dietary quality, among children aged 6 to 23 months in urban Madagascar. Similarly, Steyn *et al.* (2006) assessed whether food variety (mean number of different food items consumed) and dietary diversity scores were good predictors of nutrient adequacy in South African children. They found that both food variety and dietary diversity showed

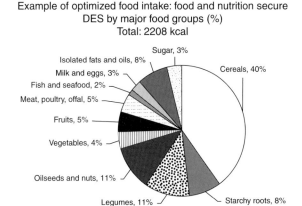

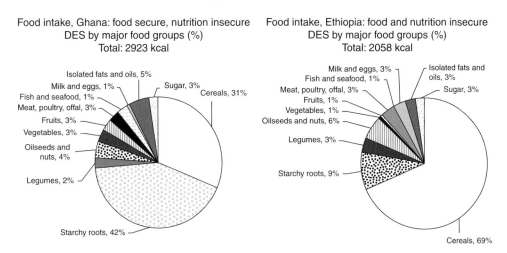

Fig. 19.1. An example of the 'nutrition gap'. Total dietary energy supply (DES) by major food groups in Ethiopia and Ghana (bottom) are compared with a model of optimized intake (top). From Author.

high and significant positive correlations with nutrient adequacy (see Fig. 19.2).

Secondly, dietary diversity has been significantly associated with improved child growth, namely reduced stunting, wasting and underweight (Kant et al., 1993; IFPRI, 1998; Arimond and Ruel, 2004; Steyn et al., 2006). Steyn et al. (2006) found significant correlations between height-for-age Z-score (stunting; HAZ), weight-for-height Z-score (wasting; WHZ) and weight-for-age Z-score (underweight; WAZ)

and dietary diversity in South African children, indicating a strong relationship between dietary diversity and child growth (see Fig. 19.3). In a more far-reaching study, Arimond and Ruel (2004) used data from 11 countries in Africa, Asia and Latin America to assess the relationship between dietary diversity and stunting.[1] In all but one country, improved dietary diversity was found to be significantly associated with improved height-for-age Z-scores.

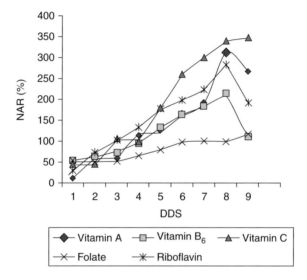

Fig. 19.2. Ratio between dietary diversity score (DDS) and mean nutrient adequacy ratio (NAR). From Steyn et al. (2006).

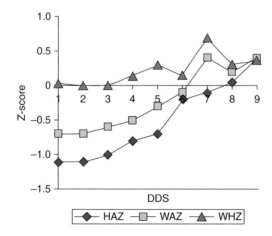

Fig. 19.3. Ratio between dietary diversity score (DDS) and child growth: HAZ, height-for-age Z-score; WAZ, weight-for-age Z-score; WHZ, weight-for-height Z-score. From Steyn et al. (2006).

Child growth – stunting, wasting and underweight – is commonly used both in assessing nutritional status in children under 5 years old, and as a proxy for the nutritional status of populations as a whole. In sum, a substantial body of evidence now exists regarding the validity of using dietary diversity to predict nutrient adequacy.

Dietary Diversity and Agriculture

There is no proven link between the improved diversification of production systems and improved dietary diversity, but there are a number of findings suggestive of an association between greater crop diversity, improved dietary diversity and improved nutrition. A growing body of evidence points to the positive impact that the production of nutrient-rich foods can have on quality and variety of intake. The evidence base is diverse and ranges from meta-analyses to original research conducted at the farm or village level. Selected findings from three specific studies are briefly discussed below.

Nutrient composition of rice (and other crop) cultivars in Bangladesh (Kennedy *et al.*, 2005)

This study developed two 'plant genetic diversity' (PGD) indicators to assess which cultivars within the same crop species were consumed by households in central Bangladesh ($n = 313$). The first indicator disaggregated crop species into individual varieties or cultivars. Rice, for example, was disaggregated into 38 different varieties. The second indicator was used to identify germplasm type based on the degree of modification present in each cultivar. Each cultivar was classed as 'modern/high-yielding', 'locally improved', 'traditional/rustic' or 'unknown'.

For rice consumption, the study found that the vast majority of households surveyed ate modern/high-yielding cultivars and that almost all households consumed rice more than once a day. Daily consumption of pulses was much less ($n = 119$). The consumption of

green leafy vegetables, which have great potential to improve dietary quality due to their high nutrient content (see next main section: 'How Can Agriculture Improve Dietary Diversity? Narrowing the Nutrition Gap for Specific Food Typologies'), was also low. Although over 50 varieties of green leafy vegetables were mentioned by farmers and over 17 varieties were identified during household interviews as food sources, this category was, on average, consumed by less than half of the sample.

The implications of the PGD indicators for dietary diversity and nutrition are multiple. First and foremost, they have the potential to increase the precision and specificity of household dietary diversity surveys. Knowing that a household has consumed rice X times in the past week is one thing; knowing that a household has consumed X variety of rice X times in the past week is something else entirely. From a nutrition perspective, the latter is preferable because different cultivars within the same crop species can vary considerably in terms of nutrient composition. Understanding which cultivars are being consumed and which are not increases understanding of nutrient intake.

Moreover, in situations where a large number of households report frequent consumption of a crop variety that is relatively low in nutrients, there are clear implications in terms of food and agriculture-based nutrition programmes. It becomes much easier to advocate narrowing the 'nutrition gap' through increased production and consumption of high-nutrient varieties when there is strong evidence that current production systems and consumption patterns are nutritionally deficient.[2]

Furthermore, PGD indicators can be used to quantify the depth of household knowledge of different crops. For example, the Kennedy *et al.* (2006) study found that most respondents were unable to identify which pulse germplasm type they were eating. Although this does not have any immediate nutritional implications, it does serve as a proxy for local knowledge, or lack thereof, of specific crops. Local knowledge, in turn, can be a good indicator of current food preferences. For the study described here, this appears to have been the case.

As already noted, pulse consumption was low in this study and, indeed, both pulse production and consumption have been declining in Bangladesh. Given that pulses are high in certain amino acids that are limited in rice, which is what – in most cases – they appear to have been replaced by, this trend does not bode well for dietary diversity or nutrition (see next main section for further discussion of pulse production).

Promotion of traditional African vegetables in Kenya and Tanzania: a case study of an intervention representing emerging imperatives in global nutrition (Herforth, 2010)

Conducted within the context of an agricultural programme promoting the production, marketing and consumption of traditional African vegetables (TAVs), one of this study's aims was to examine the association between crop diversity and dietary diversity among smallholders in East Africa. Some 338 households in Kiambu District of Central Province, Kenya, and in Arusha Region, northern Tanzania, were surveyed at baseline and 1 year later. Data were collected on agricultural production, marketing, nutrition knowledge and attitudes, medicinal uses of TAVs, dietary intake, preschool child weight and household demographics. In both countries, crop diversity was significantly and positively associated with dietary variety (individual foods consumed), and in Tanzania crop diversity was also positively associated with dietary diversity (food groups).

What is more, the medicinal use of vegetables, for example as a treatment for anaemia, was widely reported, though knowledge of the micronutrient content of vegetables was not. This second finding points to the importance of building on existing knowledge and practices to increase participation in and the sustainability of behaviour change communication programmes (discussed further in next main section).

This study also provides an in-depth discussion of promoting specific crop varieties within local contexts. Like Kennedy et al. (2005), Herforth cites the importance of promoting cultivars with higher bioavailable amounts of specific nutrients. However, strong emphasis is also placed on, inter alia, consideration of consumption preference, agronomic potential (e.g. length of production cycle, yields and pest resistance) and market demand.

Herforth also presents data showing that varietal diversity – that is, the production of more than one cultivar at once – may be better than producing single varieties at meeting multiple nutritional needs. The point is made that nutrients do not vary unilaterally across crop cultivars. For example, out of four amaranth varieties, the variety highest in iron was found to be lowest in vitamin C, which is, incidentally, an iron absorption enhancer. In fact, each amaranth variety is shown to have a comparative advantage in one or more nutrients, but not in all.

This and many other findings are used to argue for the potentially positive nutrition impact of varietal diversity. For instance, households in Arusha that grew more amaranth varieties were found to also eat amaranth more frequently, even after controlling for the total volume of amaranth harvested. A number of hypotheses are provided for why this is so, including that of continuous availability – more varieties produced leads to more varieties available at a given point in time – and the fact that more varieties means that more palates (of adults and children alike) can be pleased at once.

Herforth points out that some of the findings could simply be interpreted as meaning that some households like TAVs more than others. Nevertheless, the fact that no one single variety stands out as superior across all nutrient categories remains. The production and consumption of a cultivar that is especially high in a specific nutrient may be appropriate when a particular deficiency is being targeted, but in terms of maximizing overall nutrition, the promotion of varietal diversity within a given crop may lead to increases in total quantity consumed as well as to improved nutrient intake.

Assessing nutritional diversity of cropping systems in sub-Saharan Africa (Remans et al., 2011)

This study used a novel indicator, 'nutritional functional diversity' (FD) to assess the nutritional diversity of cropping systems across 170 farms in Millennium village clusters in Malawi (Mwandama, in southern Zomba District), western Kenya (Sauri, in Nyanza Province) and south-western Uganda (Ruhiira, in Isingiro District), and to explore the associations between crop diversity and nutrition. Data were collected on edible plant species, food security, dietary diversity and micronutrient deficiencies. Scores for nutritional FD were calculated for each farm assessing the crop system's total nutrient content, macronutrient and micronutrient content, and mineral content. Findings included:

- a strong positive correlation between the number of edible species grown and nutrient availability at farm level; and
- a strong negative correlation between low nutritional FD scores and dietary diversity at village level. In other words, data collected across all three villages indicated that low scores in nutritional FD at the village level occurred in conjunction with poor dietary diversity.

These findings are similar to those of Herforth in that they make a case for varietal diversity. Here too, it seems that species availability may be associated with improved diversity of intake.

However, in addition to evidence in support of varietal diversity, the study also found that, despite the correlation between edible species grown and nutrient availability at farm level, two farms with the same number of species had radically different nutritional FD scores (see arrows in Fig. 19.4a). This difference is explained by trait analysis. Both farms grew maize, cassava, beans, bananas, pigeon peas and mangoes, but the higher scoring farm also grew pumpkins, mulberries and groundnuts, its lower scoring counterpart grew avocados, peaches and blackjack (a vegetable).[3] The difference in nutrient content between these additional crops was presented as the explanation for the surprisingly disparate

nutritional FD scores. Although the sample size is far too small to be statistically significant, this finding does have important, albeit obvious, implications for narrowing the nutrition gap. Even when crop diversity appears to be sufficient in terms of number, the nutritional diversity provided by those crops may still be low. Moreover, despite the importance of varietal diversity, there may be one or two key crops, in this case mulberries and pumpkins, which have particular potential for boosting the nutrient content of a given production system.

This study also makes the point that even in villages where most households are subsistence farmers, the average proportion of food consumed from own production is around 50%. The importance of the food system, including local markets, is emphasized within this context, as well as the fact that a significant correlation was found between the number and value of food items bought and sold at local markets and household food security and dietary diversity indicators at each of the three study areas.

Even though not explicitly mentioned by the authors, this type of finding provides support for the idea that crop diversity is essential to healthy local markets as well as to local incomes because it smooths price volatility. In a situation where everyone is growing only one or two crops, demand remains weak and profits low. Conversely, if a drought or other shock results in a major shortage, prices can become prohibitive for much of the local community, with negative consequences in terms of food and nutrition security.

How Can Agriculture Improve Dietary Diversity? Narrowing the Nutrition Gap for Specific Food Typologies

Assuming that agriculture can play a role in improving dietary diversity, what can be done within the sector to narrow nutritional gaps in dietary patterns across a variety of agro-ecological zones, production systems and food typologies? To answer this question, pathways in food systems for dietary

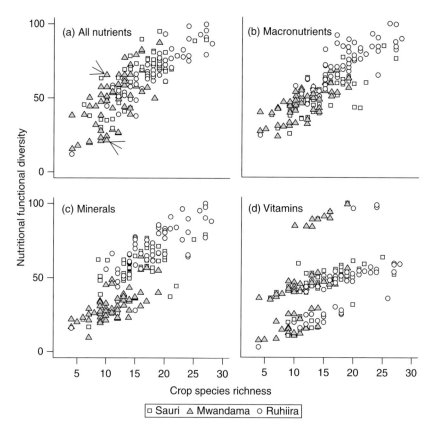

Fig. 19.4. Nutritional functional diversity (FD) scores are positively associated with the number of edible species grown at farm level ('crop species richness') in village clusters in Kenya (Sauri), Malawi (Mwandama) and Uganda (Ruhiira). The arrows in (a) indicate two farms with the same number of species but radically different nutritional FD scores. From Remans *et al.* (2011).

diversity must be identified. Table 19.1 includes some major impact pathways and their functions.

Crop and livestock diversity and purchasing power are two areas that, perhaps to a greater degree than the other pathways in the table, can be addressed directly via interventions based wholly within the agricultural sector. Some of the most important of these interventions are:

- increasing small-scale production of micronutrient-rich foods for own/local consumption;
- increasing commercial production of micronutrient-rich foods;
- promoting preservation techniques to maintain micronutrient levels in commonly

eaten foods and to reduce postharvest losses; and
- selecting and breeding plants to increase micronutrient levels.

This section provides examples of interventions for these strategies. Each focuses on ways to boost production and/or consumption of high-quality foods in one of a series of 'typical' agriculture-based food typologies based on geographical area.[4] It is important to note that within each of the areas described, intake patterns differ according to a host of factors, and the following examples should be qualified as only broadly representative of commonly consumed diets in a given region. Their primary purpose is not to catalogue all of the intake patterns in a particular area, but rather to illustrate

Table 19.1. Some major impact pathways in food systems for dietary diversity.

Pathway	Functions
Crop and livestock diversity	Affects immediate availability of macronutrients and micronutrients for producer households
	Affects purchasing power
Purchasing power, especially for women	Is essential to access
	Is essential for avoidance of post-shock, harmful coping mechanisms
	Resources and income flows that women control have been shown to have disproportionately positive impacts on health and food and nutrition security
Cultural norms	Affects food allocation and dietary diversity at household and community levels
Infrastructure	Essential to market access: even if purchasing power is adequate, lack of roads, railways and other basic transportation infrastructure constrains access to markets
	Lack of cold storage or other preservation facilities increases postharvest losses of perishable, nutrient-rich produce
Stability of supply and the relative prices of available food	Affects consumer preferences and hence quality/quantity of intake

how poor dietary diversity occurs in a wide variety of contexts and to provide examples of ways to improve the situation.

Many of these interventions, although framed according to specific food typologies, can be applied to a range of countries, agroecological zones and dietary patterns. Each food typology includes a number of specific country examples.

Rain-fed roots and tubers in West Africa – Burkina Faso, Côte d'Ivoire, Ghana and Nigeria

One of the most important staple food crops in West Africa is cassava. Hardy and drought resistant, cassava maintains acceptable yields on low-fertility soils year round and is of great importance for subsistence farmers throughout the region. Yams, potatoes, sweet potatoes and taro are other staple foods grown in this area. All of these tubers are high in carbohydrate. Diets in this region also include bananas, plantains, rice, maize, sorghum, groundnuts and a variety of vegetables. Meals typically consist of a starchy staple (e.g. cassava-based *gari or foufou*) and sauce, the latter including a variety of ingredients, most commonly groundnuts and/or vegetables.

The consumption of animal source foods (ASFs) in western Africa can be low, especially among the rural poor. Bushmeat and insects, small livestock and poultry (for both meat and dairy) and fish are eaten, but quantities are often small. As a result, protein intake may be low in many root- and tuber-based West African diets, especially when cassava is the main food source. Cassava roots are very low in protein, with 0.8 g/100 g edible weight (Wargiono *et al.*, 2002), compared with 6.4 g for rice; both maize and wheat have 9 g protein/100 g edible weight (FAO, 1992). While yams and most other roots and tubers have higher protein contents than cassava, their nutritional composition is also inadequate to ensure nutrition security if not accompanied by sufficient protein-rich foods, such as ASFs and pulses.

In addition to low protein intake, this food typology may also be lacking in adequate amounts of fat and essential micronutrients, including vitamin A, iodine, zinc and iron. For instance, 12 countries from the region either had vitamin A deficiency of 10% or more, and/or iron deficiency anaemia of 20% or more, in 2007 (World Bank, 2006a). Moreover, even in those West African countries where DES is adequate, macronutrient and micronutrient deficiencies may persist.

In Ghana, for instance, DES meets population requirements, but contributions to DES by protein and fats are lower than recommended (FAO, 2009a). This situation clearly illustrates the difference between food security and 'food and nutrition security' (see Fig. 19.1). Without sufficient diversification, adequate calories rarely result in acceptable rates of declines in malnutrition.

Improving the protein content of cassava would be one very important way that agriculture could narrow the nutrition gap in West Africa, as this crop is one of the most commonly consumed staples in the region. To date, high-protein genotypes have been identified; the current challenge is to increase endogenous proteins within common varieties (Beach, 2009).

Encouraging the consumption of cooked cassava leaves also has potential for improving nutrient intake in areas of West Africa where they are not considered to be a conventional food source. Cassava leaves are high in protein, vitamins A and C, and calcium. Especially noteworthy is the combination of vitamin C and calcium, as the former increases bioavailability of the latter. Furthermore, cassava leaves are available year round, unlike a number of other vegetables that are commonly consumed in West Africa. Finally, encouraging cassava leaf consumption in this region could be extremely cost-effective. It uses an existing resource which is already widely available, even in remote areas, and can be harvested at weekly intervals from plants that are as young as 5 months old (Nweke, 2004). In some cases, the only inputs necessary would be a communication strategy to increase awareness of the leaves as a potential food source, combined with education on processing procedures that eliminate toxicity (e.g. a three-step process of soaking, pounding and boiling to remove cyanogens from the leaves). Depending on the state of extension services and social marketing capacity, the promotion of increased consumption of cassava leaves could have very high returns on investment.

Vitamin A deficiency (VAD) rates are high in many West African countries. Stimulating the production and consumption of red palm oil (RPO), which is extremely

high in vitamin A, is one way to reduce VAD and, at the same time, generate income in the region. A pilot study in Burkina Faso showed that schoolchildren whose lunches were supplemented with 15 ml RPO three times a week showed significant improvements in serum retinol (vitamin A) levels (Zeba et al., 2006). From a nutrition and public health perspective, meals supplemented with RPO are a sustainable, food-based alternative to vitamin A supplements. From an agricultural perspective, palm oil plantations and the extraction and commercial distribution of RPO have income-generating potential, especially for women, who are typically the ones involved in this industry. Increasing women's purchasing power is fundamental to improving nutrition, as the resources and income flows that women control have been shown to have disproportionately positive impacts on health and food and nutrition security (World Bank, 2007). A national strategy that combines a public health campaign to increase the consumption of RPO, in conjunction with incentives based in the agricultural sector to increase RPO production, could narrow the nutrition gap through direct changes in intake and potentially increased purchasing power.

Irrigated/rain-fed rice in South and South-east Asia – Bangladesh, Cambodia, Indonesia, Laos, Sri Lanka and Vietnam

Rice-based food typologies are common throughout South and South-east Asia (as well as other parts of the developing world; see Box 19.1). Consumption patterns vary between and within countries, but most diets consist primarily of rice supplemented to varying degrees with vegetables, pulses, ASFs and some fruits. Fat and oil intake is often low, especially among low-income groups. For many households, especially rural households, DES is predominantly derived from carbohydrates. Based on data from FAO's Food Balance Sheets, 77% of total DES in Laos came from rice in 2002 (FAO, 2003a). In Bangladesh, 73% of DES was derived from rice in 2003. For Cambodia, the amount was 68%; for Indonesia it was 80%

Box 19.1. Global rice consumption and research priorities.

Rice remains the most important staple throughout the developing world. It provides more calories than any other food to low and low–middle income countries, and is critical to global food security. Moreover, rice consumption is projected to increase through to at least 2025, even though total per capita global food consumption has stabilized. Africa is likely to be an important driver of this growth (Pandey *et al.*, 2010).

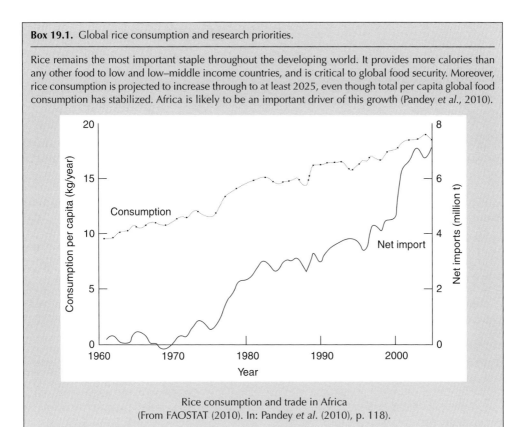

Rice consumption and trade in Africa
(From FAOSTAT (2010). In: Pandey *et al.* (2010), p. 118).

(FAOSTAT, 2004). These are aggregate figures; it is highly likely that the numbers for lower income quintiles are substantially higher.

Rice research priorities currently include efforts to increase yield and yield stability as well as resistance to the effects of climate change. Improving nutrient content is also a priority (Pandey *et al.*, 2010). From a nutrition perspective, the latter is of particular interest. Selective breeding to improve nutrient content is one of the agriculture-based interventions highlighted throughout this chapter. Although it does not increase dietary diversity per se, selective breeding of staple crops aims to increase total nutrient intake and can be an important complement to crop and dietary diversification programmes. This approach holds particular potential in communities where rice or other staple monocropping is deeply entrenched.

Reducing the negative environmental effects that rice cultivation can have is also a research priority (Pandey *et al.*, 2010). One way to achieve this goal, while simultaneously increasing the nutritional diversity of the production system, is through integrated horticulture/aquaculture or VAC projects, as discussed below. This strategy is particularly well suited to wet rice cultivation, as sustainable fish and shrimp production can occur in paddies after rice crops are harvested.

Even though malnutrition in Asia as a whole is decreasing, South Asia still has some of the highest prevalence rates of malnutrition in the world (IFPRI, 2010). Serious challenges also remain in South-east Asia (IFPRI, 2010). For instance, stunting prevalence rates in Cambodia, Laos and Vietnam were 37%, 40% and 36%, respectively, over the period 2000–2007 (UNICEF, 2010). In addition, the estimated prevalence of iron deficiency anaemia for women and children is high throughout the region, and up to 80% for children under 5 years old (MI, 2009). The monotonous diets described above are one of the reasons for these persistent high rates of malnutrition.

Rice production cycles vary according to country and region, but most areas where rice is grown have dry seasons during which non-paddy rice crops can be harvested. Facilitating the cultivation of dry season crops can be especially important in areas where rice mono-cropping is common, as monocropping can increase vulnerability to production-based, cyclical patterns of food insecurity. For example, Kennedy *et al.* (2005), discussed above, found that in Bangladesh, the cultivation of lentils, peas and other pulses has declined, partly because rice is a more lucrative crop, but also because the growing season of pulse crops is longer than that of rice, and because many pulses require more inputs and maintenance than rice crops.

Introduction or reintroduction of nutritious, low-input, short-duration crops might, therefore, be appropriate for improving the availability of and access to a more diversified diet. Mung beans, for example, are high in protein, and particularly in lysine, the limiting amino acid of most cereal grains, and also in iron, B vitamins, folate, vitamin C and a number of other nutrients. Mung beans were traditionally grown by the poor but have become less popular owing to the reasons cited above. Recent improvements in the nutritional content of mung beans, and in their pest and disease resistance and maturation cycle, could facilitate their reintroduction (Spielman and Pandya-Lorch, 2009). Additional selling points include a short production cycle (approximately 60 days), minimal moisture requirements and improved soil fertility via nitrogen fixation.

Soybean production for local consumption is another option. Although often promoted as a commodity crop for global markets, soybean cultivation can also be encouraged among smallholders to diversify production and capture positive rotation effects. Soybeans are high in protein and are a good source of poly- and mono-unsaturated fats, as well as of omega-3 fatty acids. Mustard is also an alternative: in addition to having highly nutritious and edible leaves, this plant's hardy oilseeds could increase fat intake. Mustard is appropriate for many rice-based food typologies,

particularly those that are rain fed and hence drought prone.

Interventions that increase the availability of nutritious crops are an important first step in improving nutrition security, but do not, in and of themselves, guarantee improved outcomes at the individual or household level. The cassava-based interventions described above focused on a staple food that is already commonly consumed in West Africa. In contrast, the introduction of a food that may not be especially popular or common (e.g. soybeans in Bangladesh) must be accompanied by social marketing and education efforts to encourage consumption. This is because the target population may not be open to the introduction of new foods – even those that are nutritious and practical – from a production perspective. Furthermore, traditional dietary habits may work against good nutritional advice and/or may further reduce the nutritional value of foods (e.g. food taboos, or cooking rice in excessive water as opposed to using absorption methods).

Thus, extension-based social marketing and education services play a crucial role in creating awareness and promoting behavioural change. However, in many countries, agricultural extension, especially nutrition education services, are underfunded or absent. Investing in these services is imperative to the second step in narrowing the nutrition gap, which is to increase the actual intake of foods necessary for a healthy and balanced diet. In South and South-east Asia, where preferences for polished rice, cooking habits and cultural beliefs may exacerbate malnutrition, extension-based nutrition services are badly needed both to improve existing habits and to promote healthy new ones.

Integrated horticulture/aquaculture projects are one way to improve household access to ASFs, fruits and vegetables. In many areas of South and South-east Asia, they also fit into traditional production strategies. In Vietnam, for example, the integration of the home lot, garden, livestock and fishpond, or VAC system (garden, pond, animal pen; originally from the three Vietnamese words *Vuon* for garden, *Ao* for pond and *Chuong* for cattle shed), has been officially promoted since the 1980s as part of a more general policy to improve crop diversification and nutrition security (Hop, 2003). VAC farms typically include a pond stocked with fish placed close to the home, livestock or poultry pens situated near or over the pond to provide an immediate source of organic fertilization and gardens that include both annual and perennial crops for year-round food provision, as well as products for market; garden waste may also be used for pond fertilization (Fig. 19.5). The promotion of VAC in Vietnam is believed to have had a positive impact on the country's nutrition outcomes. Vietnam's National Nutrition Survey 2000 showed marked improvements from 1987 in terms of the consumption of ASFs and fruits and vegetables and, while this progress is undoubtedly due to many different factors, VAC is considered to have played an important role (Hop, 2003).

Although the VAC system is specific to Vietnam, integrated horticulture/aquaculture projects are appropriate for a wide array of agro-ecological zones and have great potential throughout South and South-east Asia (FAO/IIRR/WorldFish Center,

2001). Fruit and vegetable cultivation on fish pond embankments, the growing of short-cycle species in seasonal ponds and ditches, integrated fish–duck, fish–chicken or fish–pig farming, and rice–fish farming, are all examples. From a nutrition perspective, these strategies are exemplary in that they address deficits in ASFs and fruits and vegetables simultaneously. For example, even a small amount of haem iron (found only in ASFs) consumed with a meal where most of the iron is non-haem (i.e. plant-derived), will enhance absorption of the iron in the meal. The addition of a small amount of fish or meat (e.g. 30 g) to a meal containing non-haem iron will result in much greater absorption of iron (Thompson, 2007). If this meal contains vitamin C-rich fruits or vegetables, iron absorption will be further enhanced. In all regions, integrated horticulture and aquaculture projects increase the probability of more balanced meals being consumed on a more regular basis. In South and South-east Asia, where iron deficiency anaemia is especially pronounced, such projects present culturally acceptable and viable opportunities to increase the dietary availability of iron and other essential micronutrients.

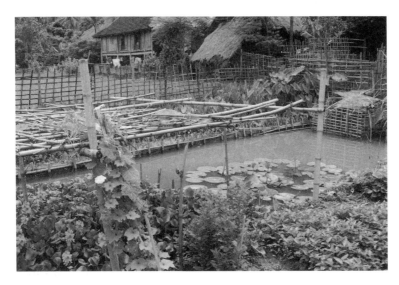

Fig. 19.5. Integrating farming activities such as horticulture and aquaculture provides multiple nutritional and other benefits for household members in the uplands of northern Vietnam. Photo: M. Halwart/Fisheries and Aquaculture Department, Food and Agriculture Organization of the United Nations, Rome.

Rain-fed cereals in Central and East Africa – Central African Republic, Chad, Democratic Republic of Congo, Kenya, Malawi and Tanzania

The most common cereals used as staples in many areas of Central and East Africa include sorghum, millet, rice and maize. Other foods grown and consumed in this region include cassava, other starchy roots and pulses. Fruits and vegetables are also cultivated, but production may be limited as a result of little or no access to water, seeds and other inputs, time constraints and lack of knowledge of horticultural techniques. Livestock production in Central Africa is the lowest on the continent owing in part to endemic trypanosomiasis, which causes anaemia, emaciation, decreased milk yields and death in non-resistant breeds of cattle and other livestock (ILCA/ILRAD, 1988). Though livestock production in parts of East Africa may be high relative to that in Central Africa, it remains underdeveloped, especially in terms of small ruminants and other options that do not require economies of scale.

Typical diets in Central and East Africa consist primarily of a cereal-based porridge or paste (e.g. *nsima* in Malawi, *ugali* in Kenya) complemented by a meat- or fish-based sauce, or by a relish that could include meat, fish and/or a variety of vegetables or legumes. Such meals are usually eaten twice a day. Fruits may also be consumed, but intakes are highly seasonal and may also be limited in terms of access (e.g. budget constraints, poor transportation infrastructure). Like the food typologies described above, diets are often lacking in micronutrients and macronutrients, and may also be inadequate in terms of energy content. Intake patterns may be especially deficient in areas where conflict and political unrest have weakened infrastructure and reduced production.

For example, based on data from food balance sheets, total energy intake in the Democratic Republic of Congo (DRC) was 1605 kcal in 2003 (FAOSTAT, 2003), with as much as 76% of the calories coming from cereals and starchy roots. It is unlikely that these very poor and monotonous diets will have improved much in recent years. Even in more

politically stable states, dietary diversity can be extremely poor. In Malawi, for instance, cereals and starchy roots provide more than three quarters of the available calories (FAOSTAT, 2008), with ASFs and fruits and vegetables providing only 3% and 4%, respectively. Even though lack of diversity in the Malawian diet is especially pronounced, and most certainly contributes to the particularly high rates of stunting (47% in 2009);[5] stunting rates are high or very high throughout much of Central and East Africa (UNICEF, 2009; Government of Malawi, 2011). Micronutrient deficiencies are also common. Thirteen countries in this region had prevalence of vitamin A deficiency above 10% and/or a 20% prevalence of iron deficiency anaemia in 2007 (Haddad *et al.*, 2003).

Increasing small-scale production of micronutrient-rich foods at the community or household level is one way to improve crop diversity and increase the availability of fruits and vegetables. However, implementation is contingent on, inter alia, water availability, soil quality and seed availability. In many parts of Central and East Africa, these factors are in limited supply. Keyhole gardens, which are simple to implement and require minimal inputs, are one solution in such contexts. These gardens can be built in places where it is difficult to grow gardens (rocky areas, shallow arid/or compacted soils, etc.), and are often placed near the entrance of houses to facilitate watering with household waste water. As keyhole gardens are self-contained and can be built close to the home, they are good options where violence prevents smallholders from travelling to and from their fields and can keep a close eye on their produce to prevent theft. Keyhole gardens can maintain their soil fertility for 5 to 7 years, produce food all year round even under harsh temperatures and are prolific, supporting production of at least five varieties of vegetables at a time (FAO, 2009b). The gardens have a simple drip-irrigation system based on a lined basket, which is placed in the centre of the garden and disperses water throughout (Fig. 19.6); the system uses significantly less water than do more conventional gardens.

As mentioned above, trypanosomiasis is one of the constraints facing the livestock

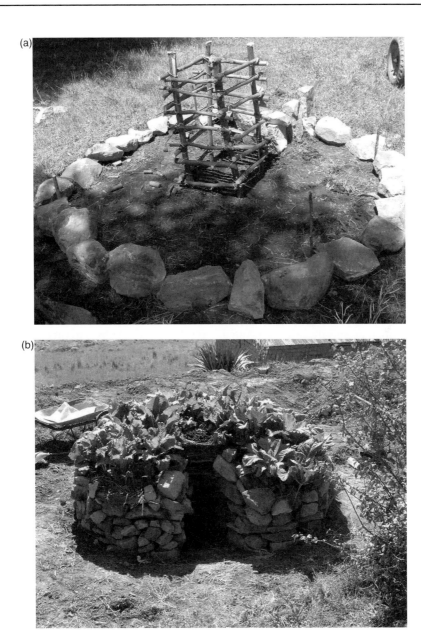

Fig. 19.6. A keyhole garden: (a) initial construction, including an (unlined) irrigation basket; and (b) after the construction has been finished and planted. Photo courtesy of FAO (2013).

sector in Central Africa and, while animal production is higher in East Africa, there are also opportunities for smallholders in this region to increase their output of poultry and small ruminants. Cross-breeding to improve hybrid vigour, increase resistance to trypanosomiasis and increase meat and dairy yields is one way to improve production, though the sustainability of this strategy is an issue as it requires constant maintenance of breeding stock as well as the regular and costly reintroduction of non-indigenous species.

A solution better suited to smallholders, especially those facing budget constraints, is to increase the productivity of existing local animals. Introducing improved housing and supplementary feeding through improved extension services can go a long way to reducing what are often extremely high losses among small ruminants and poultry. For example, in areas where mortality rates for poultry are high, chickens and their eggs are raised more to earn income rather than for home consumption. Farmers often allow the majority of their eggs to hatch in order to maintain the flock as an asset base, thus reducing the opportunities to improve dietary intake through direct egg consumption. If poultry mortality rates can be reduced through improved housing and supplementary feeding, as opposed to simply letting chickens forage, the risk to the farmer in maintaining the flock will be reduced, allowing for the increased consumption of eggs. From a nutrition perspective, supplementing Central and East African diets with regular egg consumption could increase intake of protein, fat and vitamin A.

As most crops are seasonal, production surpluses are often lost as a result of poor harvesting practices and inadequate processing, packaging, storage and preservation techniques. Postharvest losses can be especially high for micronutrient-rich foods, which are highly perishable and lose substantial amounts of vitamin C and carotenoids after a few days. Although postharvest losses of perishables are high throughout the developing world, they are especially high in sub-Saharan Africa (Aworh, 2008).

Large-scale reductions in postharvest losses require improvements in infrastructure (e.g. cold chain refrigeration, road construction and repairs) that are beyond the scope of this chapter. However, strategies to reduce postharvest losses that are rudimentary, low-cost and appropriate for smallholders do exist. For example, the solar drying of β-carotene rich fruits and vegetables (e.g. mangoes, pumpkins and orange-fleshed sweet potatoes) can preserve vitamin A levels for up to 6 months. Simple solar dryers can also be used for green leafy vegetables such as amaranth, which is common in both East and Central Africa, and is high in iron, folic acid and vitamin C. Basic techniques,

such as growing root crops in raised beds or mounds to avoid damaging the roots during harvest, can make a difference, especially among cereal-based food systems where roots and tubers may be stored to eat as supplementary staples in lean seasons between grain harvests (FAO, 1989).

Irrigated/rain-fed maize and beans in Central America – El Salvador, Guatemala, Honduras and Nicaragua

Maize and beans are grown and eaten throughout Central America. Together with sugar, these staples provide the bulk of energy supplies for most households. In Guatemala, for example, in 2003 almost 90% of DES was cereal (primarily maize), beans and sugar (FAO, 2003b). Maize may be eaten in the form of tortillas, beans are typically mashed into a paste or cooked as a soup or stew, and copious amounts of sugar are added to weak coffee, or sometimes to a thin, maize porridge (atol). These items may be complemented by a cow's milk cheese (queso blanco), eggs, plantains, avocados, bananas, carrots, chillies, onions, tomatoes and/or leafy greens. However, in many cases, meals are lacking in diversity and inadequate in terms of fat, ASF-based protein and micronutrients. Meat is often too expensive for regular consumption, especially among low-income and indigenous groups, and fruits and vegetables may be consumed in insufficient quantities to ensure nutrition security.

The lack of dietary diversity contributes to high rates of malnutrition in much of Central America, namely El Salvador, Guatemala, Honduras and Nicaragua. In these countries, malnutrition rates are comparable to those found in sub-Saharan Africa and South Asia. Guatemala has the third highest stunting rate in the world, and in El Salvador, Honduras and Nicaragua, approximately one out of every three children under 5 years old is stunted (World Bank, 2006b; UNICEF, 2009). Micronutrient deficiencies also persist in many areas. For instance, in Guatemala, 16% of preschool-aged children are deficient in vitamin A and 38% are anaemic (de Benoist et al., 2008; WHO, 2009).

Fish farming is increasing throughout the developing world, although the fish raised are primarily for export and not generally consumed by the local population. As many aquaculture ventures displace indigenous species that may be a traditional food source for local populations, the consumption of indigenous fish species may decline, resulting in an overall decrease in intakes of ASFs. Moreover, even when farmed species are consumed by local populations, net micronutrient intake can still decrease, as many small, indigenous fish are actually higher in micronutrients than popular farmed varieties (Roos *et al.*, 2007). This is especially true when indigenous species are consumed whole, owing to the high calcium content of the bones (see Table 19.2). Encouraging continued consumption of indigenous fish species, sometimes considered 'trash' in comparison with farmed varieties, could increase micronutrient intake and may also encourage efforts to design ecologically friendly, polyculture fish farms that include both commercial and indigenous species. This intervention is of relevance to many areas of Central America, where a majority of fish farms raise tilapia and other species for export.

Currently, many areas of Central America are primarily engaged in maize monocropping. Reintroduction of the *milpa* system, which promotes the intercropping of maize, beans and vegetables, is a traditional way to increase crop diversity that can improve dietary diversity, especially if accompanied by extension-based nutrition education services to promote healthy diets. Similarly, the use of greenhouses to increase production of cabbages, sweet potatoes, tomatoes and fruit has been successful in Guatemala and could be introduced into other countries in the area (FAO, 2009c). Again, a nutrition education component would be essential to increase the actual consumption of the fruits and vegetables.

Conclusion

Health-based approaches to nutrition such as vitamin supplementation, home-based fortification (Sprinkles®) and the use of ready-to use-therapeutic foods are generally singular, discrete and clearly defined; they are relatively easy to implement and it is also relatively easy to assess their impact. They have also been proven to be cost-effective across a variety of contexts.

In contrast, agriculture and food-based approaches are designed to address more complex problems related to poverty and to access to foods and other essential goods and services that are required for nutrition security. Consequently, they are generally not as straightforward to design, are more cumbersome to implement and, given the multiplicity of confounding factors involved, are difficult to evaluate, and it is difficult to assess their effectiveness and to claim attribution.

Progress in promoting and implementing food-based strategies to achieve sustainable improvements in nutritional status has, therefore, been slow. They were overlooked in the past as governments, researchers, the donor community and health-oriented organizations preferred approaches for overcoming malnutrition that had rapid start-up times and produced quick and measurable results. In terms of policy, agriculture-based nutrition programmes have not been especially attractive to politicians, who remain focused on the political imperative of achieving self-sufficiency in staple foods. Smallholders, extension agents and other stakeholders rarely have much nutrition training or knowledge,

Table 19.2. Selected micronutrient contents (per 100 g edible portion) of darkina (*Esomus danricus*), a 'trash fish', compared with nutrient contents of two commonly farmed varieties (carp and tilapia), with recommended daily intake (RDI) for each nutrient. From Nutrient information from Joegir Toppe, Food and Agriculture Organization of the United Nations, Rome (2009).

	Fish species			
Nutrient content	Carp	Tilapia	Darkina	RDI
Calcium (Ca), mg	41	10	800	1000
Iron (Fe), mg	1.24	0.56	12.0	12
Zinc (Zn), mg	1.48	0.33	4.0	9
Vitamin A, μg RAE[a]	9	0	890	900

[a]RAE, retinol activity equivalent.

and may have competing incentives, especially if the proposed interventions come at the expense of time spent on other important activities. Finally, the long and complicated causal chain that exists between agricultural policy, production systems, access, intake and nutritional status makes proof of efficacy a major challenge.

However, providing evidence of how agriculture-based interventions can improve nutrition outcomes is essential to increasing agriculture's visibility on national and international nutrition agendas. Furthermore, narrowing the nutrition gap – the gap between what foods are grown and available and what foods are needed for a healthy diet – can only occur when national policy makers and members of the international development community recognize the essential role that nutrition-sensitive agriculture and food-based approaches can play in reducing malnutrition.

In addition to building a strong evidence base, this requires incorporating explicit nutrition objectives and considerations into agricultural research agendas and agriculture development policies and programmes, building the capacity of institutions and individuals at country level, and promoting nutrition security at regional and global levels. While not discussed in this chapter, these goals are essential to building political commitment to and operational capacity for reducing malnutrition through agriculture-based programmes. Taken together with what this chapter has focused on – the growing body of evidence suggestive of an association between greater crop diversity, improved dietary diversity and improved nutrition, as well as examples of what actually needs to happen on the ground – realization of these goals should make agriculture's potential contributions to improving diets and raising levels of nutrition more of a reality.

Given that much of the developing world remains agriculture based, and that many of the most malnourished populations depend upon this sector for their livelihoods, the importance of nutrition-sensitive agriculture and food-based approaches is clear. Such approaches are viable, cost-effective, long-term and sustainable solutions for improving diets and raising levels of nutrition – and assisting communities and households to feed and nourish themselves adequately is the sustainable way forward.

Acknowledgements

Many thanks to Rosaline Remans and Anna Herforth for generously sharing their data and findings, as well as to Stefano Gavotti for advice regarding PESA Centroamérica and the *milpa* system, Remi Nono Womdim for the discussion on pulse/rice intercropping, Simon Mack for information on livestock production in Central and East Africa, and Jogeir Toppe and Iddya Karunasagar for advice on integrating nutrition into aquaculture projects. Many thanks also to staff of the Nutrition Division at FAO, including Marie-Claude Dop, Gina Kennedy, Terri Ballard, Ellen Muehlhoff, Florence Egal, Chiara Deligia and Maylis Razes.

Notes

[1] Benin, Cambodia, Colombia, Ethiopia, Haiti, Malawi, Mali, Nepal, Peru, Rwanda and Zimbabwe.

[2] Assuming that the production systems are, at least partially, designed for own/local consumption.

[3] *Bidens pilosa*, family *Asteraceae*.

[4] Countries selected as per the FAO (Food and Agriculture Organization of the United Nations) regional classification system. Available via the FAO Country Office Information Network at: http://coin.fao.org/coin (accessed 19 June 2013).

[5] Based on the World Health Organization (WHO) classification for assessing severity of malnutrition in children 0 to 5 years of age where stunting is <20% (low), 20–29% (medium), 30-39% (high) or ≥40% (very high).

References

Arimond, M. and Ruel, M.T. (2004) Dietary diversity is associated with child nutritional status: evidence from 11 demographic and health surveys. *Journal of Nutrition* 134, 2579–2585.
Aworh, O.C. (2008) The role of traditional food processing techniques in national development: the West African experience. In: Robertson, G.L. and Lupien, J.R. (eds) *Using Food Science and Technology to Improve Nutrition and Promote National Development: Selected Case Studies*. International Union of Food Science and Technology (IUFoST), Oakville, Ontario, Canada, Chapter 3. Available at: http://www.iufost.org/iufostftp/IUFoST_Case%20Studies-1.pdf (accessed 19 June 2013).
Beach, L. (2009) *Perspectives for Enhancing Protein Content in Cassava*. USAID (US Agency for International Development), Washington, DC.
de Benoist, B., McLean, E., Egli, I. and Cogswell, M. (eds) (2008) *Worldwide Prevalence of Anaemia 1993–2005: WHO Global Database on Anaemia*. World Health Organization, Geneva, Switzerland. Available at: http://whqlibdoc.who.int/publications/2008/9789241596657_eng.pdf (accessed 18 June 2013).
FAO (1989) *Prevention of Post-harvest Losses: Fruits, Vegetables and Root Crops, a Training Manual*. Food and Agriculture Organization of the United Nations, Rome.
FAO (1992) *Food Composition Table for Use in East Asia*. Food and Agriculture Organization of the United Nations, Rome.
FAO (2003a) *Nutrition Country Profile – Laos*. Food and Agriculture Organization of the United Nations, Rome.
FAO (2003b) *Nutrition Country Profile – Guatemala*. Food and Agriculture Organization of the United Nations, Rome.
FAO (2009a) *Nutrition Country Profile – Ghana*. Food and Agriculture Organization of the United Nations, Rome.
FAO (2009b) *Food Security, Nutrition and Livelihoods: Lessons from the Field.. Keyhole Gardens in Lesotho, Project Title: Protecting and Improving Food and Nutrition Security of Orphans and HIV/AIDS-affected Children (GCP/RAF/388/GER)*. Food and Agriculture Organization of the United Nations, Rome. Available at: http://www.fao.org/ag/agn/nutrition/docs/FSNL%20Fact%20sheet_Keyhole%20gardens.pdf (accessed 20 June 2013).
FAO (2013) Keyhole gardens for better nutrition and livelihoods. TECA (Technologies and practices for small agricultural producers), Food and Agriculture Organization of the United Nations, Rome. Available at: http://teca.fao.org/technology/keyhole-gardens-better-nutrition-and-livelihoods#sthash.OxwrKF4s.dpuf (accessed 28 June 2013).
FAO/IIRR/WorldFish Center (2001) *Integrated Agriculture–aquaculture: A Primer*. FAO Fisheries Technical Paper 407, Food and Agriculture Organization of the United Nations, Rome/International Institute of Rural Reconstruction, Cavite, Philippines/WorldFish Center (formerly International Center for Living Aquatic Resources Management), Penang, Malaysia. Available at: http://www.fao.org/docrep/005/Y1187E/y1187e00.htm#TopOfPage (accessed 20 June 2013).
FAOSTAT (2003) FAOSTAT Food balance sheets: Democratic Republic of Congo. Food and Agriculture Organization of the United Nations, Rome.
FAOSTAT (2004) FAOSTAT Food balance sheets: Bangladesh, Cambodia, Indonesia, Sri Lanka. Food and Agriculture Organization of the United Nations, Rome.
FAOSTAT (2008) FAOSTAT Food balance sheets: Malawi. Food and Agriculture Organization of the United Nations, Rome.
Government of Malawi (2011) *Malawi Demographic and Health Survey, 2010. Preliminary Report*. National Statistics Office, Zomba, Malawi and MEASURE DHS, ICF Macro, Calverton, Maryland.
Haddad, L., Alderman, H., Appleton, S., Song, L. and Yohannes, Y. (2003) Reducing child malnutrition: how far does income growth take us? *The World Bank Economic Review* 17, 107–131.
Hatloy, A., Torheim, L. and Oshaug, A. (1998) Food variety – a good indicator of nutritional adequacy of the diet? A case study from an urban area in Mali, West Africa. *European Journal of Clinical Nutrition* 52, 891–898.
Herforth, A. (2010) Promotion of traditional African vegetables in Kenya and Tanzania: a case study of an intervention representing emerging imperatives in global nutrition. Dissertation, Cornell University, Ithaca, New York.
Hop, L. (2003) Programs to improve production and consumption of animal source foods and malnutrition in Vietnam. *Journal of Nutrition* 133, 4006S–4009S.

IFPRI (1998) *Commercial Vegetable and Polyculture Fish Production in Bangladesh: Their Impacts on Income, Household Resource Allocation and Nutrition. Vols. 1 and 2.* International Food Policy Research Institute, Washington, DC.

IFPRI (2010) *2010 Global Hunger Index. The Challenge of Hunger: Focus on the Crisis of Undernutrition.* International Food Policy Research Institute, Washington, DC.

ILCA/ILRAD (1988) *Livestock Production in Tsetse Affected Areas of Africa: Proceedings of a Meeting Held in Nairobi, Kenya from the 23rd to 27th November 1987.* International Livestock Centre for Africa/ International Laboratory for Research on Animal Diseases, Nairobi.

Kant, A., Schatzkin, A., Harris, T., Ziegler, R. and Black, G. (1993) Dietary diversity and subsequent mortality in the First National Health and Nutrition Examination Survey Epidemiologic follow-up study. *The American Journal of Clinical Nutrition* 57, 434–440.

Kennedy, G., Islam, O., Eyzaguirre, P. and Kennedy, S. (2005) Field testing of plant genetic diversity indicators for nutrition surveys: rice-based diet of rural Bangladesh as a model. *Journal of Food Composition and Analysis* 18, 255–268.

MI (2009) Micronutrient Initiative: Asia. Available at: http://www.micronutrient.org/english/view.asp?x=548 (accessed 19 June 2013).

Moursi, M.M., Arimond, M., Dewey, K.G., Trèche, S., Ruel, M.T. and Delpeuch, F. (2008) Dietary diversity is a good predictor of the micronutrient density of the diet of 6- to 23-month-old children in Madagascar. *Journal of Nutrition* 138, 2448–2453.

Nweke, F. (2004) *New Challenges in the Cassava Transformation of Ghana and Nigeria.* EPTD Discussion Paper No. 118, Environment and Production Technology Division, International Food Policy Research Institute, Washington, DC.

Pandey, S., Byerlee, D., Dawe, D., Doberman, A., Mohanty, S., Rozelle, S. and Hardy, B. (eds) (2010) *Rice in the Global Economy: Strategic Research and Policy Issues for Food Security.* IRRI (International Rice Research Institute), Los Baños, Philippines. Available at: http://irri.org/index.php?option=com_k2&view=item&id=9504:rice-economy&lang=en (accessed 19 June 2013).

Remans, R. *et al.* (2011) Assessing nutritional diversity of cropping systems in African villages. *PLoS ONE* 6(6): e21235. doi:10.1371/journal.pone.0021235.

Roos, N., Wahab, A., Reza Hossain, M.A. and Haraksingh Thilsted, S. (2007) Linking human nutrition and fisheries: incorporating micronutrient-dense, small indigenous fish species in carp polyculture production in Bangladesh. *Food and Nutrition Bulletin* 28, S280–S293.

Shimbo, S., Kimura, K., Imai, Y., Yasumoto, K., Yamamoto, K., Kawamura, S., Watanabe, T., Iwami, O., Nakatsuka, H. and Masayuki, I. (1994) Number of food items as an indicator of nutrient intake. *Ecology of Food and Nutrition* 32, 197–206.

Spielman, D.J. and Pandya-Lorch, R. (eds) (2009) *Millions Fed: Proven Successes in Agricultural Development.* International Food Policy Research Institute (IFPRI), Washington, DC.

Steyn, N.P., Nela, J.H., Nantel, G., Kennedy, G. and Labadariosa, D. (2006) Food variety and dietary diversity scores in children: are they good indicators of dietary adequacy? *Public Health Nutrition* 9, 644–650.

Thompson, B. (2007) Chapter 20: Food-based approaches for combating iron deficiency. In: Kraemer, K. and Zimmermann, M.B. (eds) *Nutritional Anemia.* Sight and Life Press, Basel, Switzerland, pp. 337–358. Available at: http://www.dsm.com/content/dam/dsm/cworld/en_US/documents/sal-nutritional-anemia-book.pdf (accessed 19 June 2013).

UNICEF (2009) *The State of the World's Children 2009: Maternal and Newborn Health.* United Nations Children's Fund, New York.

UNICEF (2010) Information by country: East Asia and the Pacific. United Nations Children's Fund, New York. Available at: http://www.unicef.org/infobycountry/eastasia.html (accessed 19 June 2013).

Waijers, P.M.C.M., Feskens, E.J.M. and Ocke, M.C. (2007) A critical review of predefined diet quality scores. *British Journal of Nutrition* 97, 219–231.

Wargiono, N., Richana, N. and Hidajat, A. (2002) Contribution of cassava leaves used as a vegetable to improve human nutrition in Indonesia. In: Howeler, R.H. (ed.) *Cassava Research and Development in Asia: Exploring New Opportunities for an Ancient Crop. Proceedings of the Seventh Regional Workshop held in Bangkok, Thailand. Oct 28-Nov 1, 2002.* Centro Internacional de Agricultura Tropical (CIAT), Cali, Colombia, pp. 466–471. Available at: http://ciat-library.ciat.cgiar.org:8080/jspui/bitstream/123456789/2194/1/cassava_research_development_asia.pdf (accessed 19 June 2013).

WHO (2009) *Global Prevalence of Vitamin A Deficiency in Populations at Risk 1995–2005. WHO Global Database on Vitamin A Deficiency.* Available at: http://whqlibdoc.who.int/publications/2009/9789241598019_eng.pdf (accessed 19 June 2013).

World Bank (2006a) *Repositioning Nutrition as Central to Development: A Strategy for Large-Scale Action*. World Bank, Washington, DC. Available at: http://siteresources.worldbank.org/NUTRITION/Resources/281846-1131636806329/NutritionStrategy.pdf (accessed 19 June 2013).

World Bank (2006b) Fighting Malnutrition in Central America. Available at: http://go.worldbank.org/K5QV2HEUR0 (accessed 19 June 2013).

World Bank (2007) *From Agriculture to Nutrition: Pathways, Synergies and Outcomes*. Agriculture and Rural Development Department, World Bank, Washington, DC. Available at: http://typo3.fao.org/fileadmin/user_upload/eufao-fsi4dm/doc-training/bk_wb_report.pdf (accessed 19 June 2013).

Zeba, A., Prevel, Y.M., Some, I.T. and Delisle, H.F. (2006) The positive impact of red palm oil in school meals on vitamin A status: study in Burkina Faso. *Nutrition Journal* 5, 17.

20 Building Nutritional Self-reliance

George Kent*

University of Hawaii, Honolulu, Hawaii, USA

Summary

Nutritional self-reliance refers to the capacity of individuals and communities to make their own good decisions relating to their nutrition. The issue is important because some nutrition interventions weaken the abilities and motivations of people to provide for themselves. This disempowerment can result from the ways in which commodities are provided, and also from the ways in which information is assembled and decisions are made. Agencies should favour programmes that strengthen people's capacity to define, analyse and act on their own problems, and thus help to build individual and community self-reliance with regard to nutrition.

Introduction

Nutrition programmes are commonly evaluated on the basis of their impacts on anthropometric measures such as children's stunting, underweight and birth weight. However, nutrition programmes for children or families sometimes weaken the abilities and motivations of people to provide for themselves, especially when those programmes last too long. Interventions to deal with malnutrition should be assessed not only in anthropometric terms, but also in terms of their impact on nutritional self-reliance – the capacity of individuals and communities to make their own good decisions relating to their nutrition.

The concern is particularly serious in feeding programmes. Local nutritional self-reliance can be weakened whether the products delivered are ordinary foods or whether they are those that are specially formulated to combat particular nutritional deficiencies – products such as vitamin A capsules or protein biscuits. The risk of overdependence on outsiders is higher with specially formulated products.

The central concern is not whether the *products* are made locally, but whether the *decisions* are made locally. The emphasis is on self-reliance, not self-sufficiency. As these terms are understood here, self-reliance emphasizes local control, while self-sufficiency refers to local production to meet local needs. Self-reliance allows for trade and other kinds of interactions with others according to the community's best judgement about what would be good for its members. Self-reliance emphasizes self-rule and autonomy, while self-sufficiency emphasizes economic independence and autarky.

*Contact: kent@hawaii.edu

Self-reliance means openness to interaction with others, as that is judged to be beneficial. Self-sufficiency leans towards foregoing interaction with others (Kent, 2010, 2011).

The difference becomes clear when we look at fast-food franchises. They might reflect local self-sufficiency in the sense that their supplies are produced locally, but they would not show local self-reliance if a distant corporate office determined all their policies. Building self-reliance means building independence. The idea is captured in an update to an old adage, attributed to J.D. Chiarro: 'Give a man a fish, and he eats for a day. Teach a man to fish, and you no longer own him'.

The idea of local self-reliance is not new, but more needs to be done to clarify ways in which agencies at higher levels, both nationally and internationally, could help to build local self-reliance more systematically. This study illustrates ways in which agencies at higher levels could help to build nutritional self-reliance within communities.

Commodities

Pressures that undermine nutritional self-reliance arise in many different contexts. One major concern is the promotion of special products for dealing with malnutrition. An example is given by an appeal for funds by Save the Children, which said its 'low-cost, highly effective health programmes give gravely imperiled girls and boys the help they need to survive by providing:

- vitamin A supplements to prevent blindness and early death;
- antibiotics to treat infections;
- oral rehydration therapy to treat dehydration; and
- vaccines to prevent common diseases like malaria'.

This list suggests that special products are needed to help children survive. All of them can be useful, but there is no mention here of how parents and communities might be involved, or how they might be helped to do more for their children. There is no hint of what might happen when outsiders stop supplying these products. Save the Children should

acknowledge what it knows very well: that addressing nutrition problems involves more than just delivering medicines. In some cases, the need for such products can be sharply reduced through better use of ordinary local foods and better care and health services.

The Save the Children list is just one indicator of a growing tendency to treat malnutrition as a medical problem. Severe malnutrition *is* an illness and should be treated medically. Extraordinary measures may be needed to restore the person, child or adult, to a normal life, although such measures, usually prescribed and delivered by outsiders, sometimes at great expense, should be viewed as temporary and as just that – extraordinary measures. They should be designed to get people back to normal and not to become normal. They should not create dependency on outside decision makers and outside funders.

In sudden-onset emergencies, hunger must be prevented immediately. There is a place for feeding programmes. However, chronic malnutrition in all its many forms should be addressed in broad social, political and economic terms, and not only in clinical terms. Treating an issue as a medical problem when it does not need to be treated in that way disempowers people. For example, suggesting that capsules must be used to treat vitamin A deficiency, without at the same time showing how to make better use of local foods to deal with the problem, is disempowering (Latham, 2010).

The *medicalization* of nutrition issues is closely linked to *commodification*, the tendency to view malnutrition as something that can be addressed by supplying new commodities, especially processed foods. The issues are illustrated by the debate over 'Plumpy'Nut', a peanut-based food specially designed to treat severe acute malnutrition in young children. Jeffrey Sachs and colleagues argue that it should not be oversold:

Plumpy'Nut is not a miracle cure for global hunger or for global malnutrition. Plumpy'Nut addresses only one kind of hunger – acute episodes of extreme food deprivation or illness, the kind mainly associated with famines and conflicts. Plumpy'Nut is not designed for the other major kind of hunger, notably chronic hunger due to long-term poor diets. Nor is it designed to fight long-term malnutrition that is due to various kinds of chronic micronutrient deficiencies, such as iron, zinc and vitamin A deficiencies. ... Of the billion or so people in our world suffering from undernourishment, Plumpy'Nut is appropriate only for a small fraction. Most of the chronically undernourished need not a solution to acute undernutrition through food aid but regular access to a long-term, balanced healthy diet.

(Sachs *et al.*, 2010)

The World Food Programme (WFP) has become a major promoter of such products, as illustrated by its Project Laser Beam:

This five-year, $50 million initiative in Bangladesh and Indonesia will combat undernutrition through changes in food, hygiene and behaviour. Launched in 2009, it is a WFP-led initiative working with Fortune 500 companies and others in the private sector as well as three United Nations agencies – WFP, UNICEF and WHO. The aim is to harness the power of global, regional and local businesses. WFP's founding partners are Unilever, Kraft Foods, DSM and the Global Alliance for Improved Nutrition.

As an initial step, the Boston Consulting Group conducted a gap analysis in Bangladesh to determine the underlying causes of malnutrition in the country and potential solutions. Heinz also provided funding to allow WFP to conduct nutrition mapping in Bangladesh to assist WFP in developing its country specific nutrition strategy.

Project Laser Beam (PLB) will employ the many nutritional solutions already available in the marketplace, ensuring they are accessible to those in need. When gaps in products and services are identified, PLB will call on partners to step into the breach to develop new ones for the fight against child hunger in other countries. Special nutritious foods for children under two are desperately needed, yet there is a lack of products or services on the market. PLB aims to systematically employ current tools while creating a stimulating environment in which innovations become real.

(WFP, 2010a, p. 14)

Several corporations are set to sharply increase their sales of food commodities based on health claims (Cave, 2010). For example,

PepsiCo says its new Global Nutrition Group 'is part of our long-term strategy to grow our nutrition business from about US$10 billion in revenues today to US$30 billion by 2020' (PepsiCo, 2010; quoted in Nutraceuticals World, 2010). On nutraceuticals, Lucas and Jack (2010) say that 'Nutraceuticals are a step up from the fortified foods market, which is expected to be worth $175bn worldwide'. Such products may be useful under some conditions, but because of the profit incentive, they are likely to be promoted excessively. Better breastfeeding, good health services and ordinary foods are likely to meet children's needs more effectively and more economically, especially over the long run.

The risks involved in the promotion of these commodities by well-funded international agencies and the business interests behind them are well illustrated by WFP's promotion of Plumpy'Doz:

WFP delivered *Plumpy'Doz* to children in Ouagadougou and Bobo Dioulasso through an innovative voucher system. In 2009, 360 metric tons of the ready-to-use, nutritious food supplement were distributed to more than 40,000 children under two – 20,237 girls and 20,089 boys. Health centres in these locations report better nutrition among children who have received the specialized product, a paste supplement made from vegetable fat, peanut butter, sugar and milk. Burkinabe children, who have grown fond of the supplement, have nicknamed it "chocolate".

(WFP, 2010a, p. 28)

These vouchers might be a way of distributing free samples, in anticipation of marketing these products as a new kind of treat.

Some companies, such as Nutriset (the maker of both Plumpy'Nut and Plumpy'Doz), have promoted local production of these special foods, but outsiders generally control these operations as franchises. They do little to build local nutritional self-reliance. Indeed, they may do the opposite by creating doubts about whether ordinary family foods could meet the family's needs as well as the more exotic processed products that come in from the outside.

While special medicines might be needed to *treat* nutritional problems as therapy, in most cases the *prevention* of such problems should rely on familiar local foods. Studies that demonstrate the efficacy of medical treatments as a means of prevention (e.g. Isanaka *et al.*, 2009; Rotondi and Khobzi, 2010) frequently fail to ask whether the same preventive effect might have been achieved with better use of ordinary foods. Some studies do consider the locally available options. For example, a study in a rural and poor district of Burkina Faso showed that improving gruel for children through better use of familiar local foods was just as effective as using micronutrient fortification (Ouédraogo *et al.*, 2010).

Special products from outside the community should be considered if they produce real benefits that cannot be obtained with local foods, although outside suppliers of commodities are likely to have interests that go beyond concern for the health and well-being of the community. These concerns have to be balanced against the health benefits derived from use of the products. The possibilities for gaining the same benefits with local foods should be explored. The final decision about what to use should come from within the community.

There is no reason to resist commercialization as such. Those of us who live on store-bought foods should not insist that others must produce their own food. However, there are risks – for high-income as well as low-income people – that should be assessed in specific local conditions. We should be concerned about the following:

1. Health claims for particular foods may be exaggerated. This is especially true for fortified foods.
2. There are many ways in which processed commercial foods can be bad for consumers' health.
3. There are some safety risks with commercial foods that are unlikely to occur with non-commercial foods.
4. The idea that commercial foods are always more convenient may be overstated. Apples and carrots are ready to eat.
5. The purchase of processed foods from outside the local community means there is an outflow of funds that instead might have circulated locally, benefiting neighbours.

6. While some manufacturers of food products operate with high integrity, others may be primarily concerned with profits and sacrifice the well-being of consumers.
7. There is a need for caution about possible overdependence on foods from outside suppliers. People might have difficulties if the supply were to be cut off or if the prices increased sharply.
8. The commodity-centred approach to dealing with malnutrition can deflect attention away from the political, economic and social reforms needed to address problems of malnutrition at their source.

Nutrition Status Information

The preceding section pointed out that commodity-centred interventions often have the effect of shifting decision making about nutrition issues to agencies outside the community. Similar things can happen when outsiders dominate the management of information relating to nutrition.

Consider, for example, the many efforts to collect information on nutrition status. One of the most prominent is the FAO (Food and Agriculture Organization of the United Nations) programme FIVIMS, the Food Insecurity and Vulnerability Information Management System. Decision makers at country, regional and global levels need reliable and timely information on the incidence and causes of food insecurity, malnutrition and vulnerability for improved policy and programme formulation, targeting and monitoring of the progress of interventions aimed at reducing poverty and hunger. Cross-sectoral food security analysis helps to strengthen the understanding of why people are food-insecure, malnourished or hungry. In line with the broad definition of food security, FAO supports its analysis along four key dimensions: availability, access, stability and utilization (FAO, 2010d).

Certainly, people working in agencies at country, regional and global levels need good information on which to base their decisions, but so do people in the community. However, the FIVIMS programme gives little attention to the ways in which people in the community might be supported with better information. Perhaps FIVIMS could devise ways to provide useful information to local communities so that they could make better decisions themselves. Perhaps it could advise on ways to support people in communities in collecting and analysing their own information.

Large-scale studies that evaluate the impact of nutrition programmes are usually designed to guide decision making by outsiders and serve the intended beneficiaries of the programmes only indirectly. When a World Bank study asks: 'What can we learn from nutrition impact evaluations?' the *we* does not include people in the communities being studied (World Bank, 2010). The findings are designed for use by technical specialists in the capital cities or in agencies based outside the country. Often the issues are defined in technical terms that are unfamiliar to people in the community. The data are rarely shared in any systematic way with the people who supposedly benefit from their collection.

The same issues arise in an exercise called *Mapping Food Security Actions and Resources Flows at a Country Level* (CFS Secretariat *et al.*, 2010), managed primarily by international agencies, including the Committee on World Food Security (CFS). A document from this exercise explains:

> The main objective of the proposed mapping tool is to provide multiple users with an improved capacity to make better informed decisions about how best to design national and regional policies, strategies and programmes and to allocate resources to achieve food security and nutrition objectives. The users include governments and their associated institutions, representatives of civil society, private sector organizations and other development partners that participate in country-led processes and are involved in promoting efforts to reduce hunger and malnutrition.
>
> (CFS Secretariat *et al.*, 2010, p. 2)

The mapping exercise appears to be based on the assumption that decisions would be made at national, regional and global levels, and not at the local level. Maps and other kinds of data collection activities usually are means for enabling others outside the community to make decisions affecting the community.

FIVIMS could develop a similar tool designed to provide data to communities that want to improve their nutrition situation locally. Even though people generally have a good idea of what goes on around them, data and maps of some kinds could help them to make better decisions concerning their own well-being. People at the community level would probably be happy to share their findings with outsiders who offer to organize such resources. However, problems can arise if outsiders simply assume that they should be the ones who make decisions affecting the community.

Dietary Self-reliance

The issue of self-reliance becomes very personal when it comes to decisions about the diet. It is generally agreed that people should be free to decide what they and their children should eat, but we also agree that governments have an important role in protecting us from dangerous products and helping us to understand what is good for us.

Within these broad outlines, there is much room for debate. Should governments prohibit certain foods they judge to be bad for us, perhaps because they are too fattening, too salty or too sugary? What control should governments have over food supplements and the fortified foods?

Similar issues arise on the role of non-governmental organizations (NGOs). They cannot prohibit or command anything, but they can give strong advice. Some people dismiss advisory groups such as the Center for Science in the Public Interest in Washington, DC as self-appointed 'food police' and suggest that they should not be given any attention at all.

There are no easy answers, but many different parties are proposing guidelines. The Codex Alimentarius Commission, a joint project of FAO and WHO (World Health Organization), regularly prepares guidelines on food, and many of them are adopted by national governments in their national laws and regulations. While the Codex focuses on the composition of foods, other guidelines are concerned with the conditions under which they are marketed. The International Code of Marketing of Breastmilk Substitutes, adopted by the World Health Assembly in 1981, provides guidance designed to limit the ways in which infant formula and food products for young children are promoted. Many nations have incorporated that guidance into their national laws. The Global Alliance for Improved Nutrition, GAIN, has published a Working Paper on using the code to guide marketing of complementary foods for young children (Quinn *et al.*, 2010). FAO's work on biodiversity has led to a call for a Code of Conduct for Sustainable Diets, also modelled on the International Code of Marketing of Breastmilk Substitutes (Burlingame, 2010). A group in Asia has advanced the Colombo Declaration on Infant and Young Child Feeding (IBFAN Asia, 2009). A recent essay calls for guidelines for Ready-to-Use Therapeutic foods, (RUFTs) based primarily on concern that such products could interfere with good breastfeeding practices (Latham *et al.*, 2011).

Rules and guidelines should be based on solid nutritional science, but often they are also influenced by special interest groups such as food producers, processors and sellers, and also by advocates of particular diets. People have strong opinions about these matters. The prevailing view is that families and local authorities, not national or global agencies, should make dietary decisions. Of course, families and local authorities should be well informed about the best current understandings of nutrition science specialists. Rather than assuming the authority to make detailed dietary decisions themselves, higher level agencies should help to inform local agencies and families so that they can make their own decisions. This is much better than having authorities issue directives to lower levels.

Strengthening dietary self-reliance is crucially important as a means of resisting pressures to eat in ways that serve the interests of others. As David Kessler, former commissioner of the US Food and Drug Administration (FDA) put it: 'While a combination of human biology, personal experience and a determined industry may explain why we overeat, we still have the ability to make

choices about whether we allow this triumvirate to dominate our behavior' (Kessler, 2009).

Concerns about who should make dietary decisions are well illustrated by the debate in India over the use of eggs in school meals. It came to a head when the Chief Minister of Madhya Pradesh 'vetoed his own government's proposal to include eggs in the mid-day meal programme, saying vegetarian food had everything the human body required and there was no need for the state's 66,000 anganwadis to change their menu' (Kidwai, 2010). Despite the fact that almost half of India's children are malnourished, three ministers opposed the proposal to include eggs, saying 'eggs would encourage non-vegetarianism'.

In India, the diverse diet that would have evolved naturally became skewed as a result of government policy. India's diet has been overloaded with cereals (Shatrugna, 2009), because they are the cheapest and most available form of calories:

> So in a country where vegetarians are a definite minority, we now plan our daily meals based on…a Brahminical notion of an 'easily available, balanced diet', and the cultural production of modern India as vegetarian. This was fine for the upper castes rich, who had the luxury of eating 3–4 kinds of vegetables and other supplements like nuts, oil etc., along with their rice, but for the poor, this meant serious lack of vital sources of energy. So if the poor man got his plate of rice and three rotis a day, he was expected to be happy and satisfied. The result? We survived, but barely.
>
> (Vena Shatrugna, quoted in Anand, 2008)

The result has been serious malnutrition among children throughout India. Children can do well with vegetarian diets, but not just any vegetarian diet. Children who do not consume animal products of any kind must have carefully composed, diverse diets. Poor children in India rarely get that. Indeed, because the food subsidy programmes focus on providing grains, children get too much grain and too little of the other foods they need. The simplest ways to compensate for the deficiency would be to include small amounts of animal products such as milk and eggs and, where it is acceptable, meat.

Why should the composition of meals be decided at high levels of government? Government can reasonably require that school meals include particular nutrients (energy, protein, various micronutrients), but leave it up to local officials to decide how those requirements are to be met. Many of the requirements could be met from local food sources.

As adults, we would find it insulting to have someone else decide what we should eat. There is a need to respect the dignity of communities, families and children as well. With the help of good nutrition education, parents and their children should be presented with good alternatives and they should be encouraged to make good nutritional choices themselves.

Subsidies for Nutrition Interventions

Any nutrition project that involves free or heavily subsidized products from outside agencies tends to subvert local decision making. This matters because subsidies are often designed to support producer interests more than consumer interests (Moss, 2010). If the product is offered free or with a heavy subsidy, along with the promoters' arguments in its favour, the outsiders would dominate the decision making. By paying for the product, the outsiders in effect bribe people to take what they offer.

In principle, one could imagine outside agencies providing funds directly to the community and offering the product separately, at a reasonable cost. If the people were well informed and made their own informed choice of the product, their role in decision making would be fully honoured.

This issue arises in high-income as well as low-income countries. The US Department of Agriculture's Special Supplemental Nutrition Program for Women, Infants and Children, commonly known as WIC, provides about half the infant formula used in the country, at no cost to their families (Oliveira et al., 2010). Many of them take the formula not only because it is free but also because it appears that the government

endorses its use (Kent, 2006). The situation would be quite different if families were instead provided with small amounts of money. They could at the same time be provided with science-based information, through WIC and other agencies, that compared the health impacts of formula feeding and breastfeeding. Having the families rather than the government decide how the money should be used would build the families' nutritional self-reliance.

This concern about subsidies can also arise with unprocessed products such as milk and eggs. If an outside agency decides milk and eggs should be provided with school meals, and gives the schools and the communities no voice and no choice, then local nutritional self-reliance would be weakened.

Empowering Interventions

Some nutrition programmes focus on maximizing the amount of assistance that is provided. Long-term programmes should instead focus on minimizing the need for assistance, reducing the demand for it, rather than increasing the supply.

Empowerment means increasing one's capacity to define, analyse and act on one's own problems. An empowering programme is one that steadily reduces the beneficiaries' need for it. It builds the capacity of individuals and communities to make their own good decisions on their nutrition.

There are several different approaches that agencies at national and global levels could take to help build nutritional self-reliance in communities. One approach is to make use of time limits for assistance. This was a key element of the welfare reforms in the USA in 1996. Under these reforms, it was established that individuals could benefit from particular programmes only for a limited number of years. What had been known as the welfare programme came to be known as Temporary Assistance for Needy Families (TANF), with emphasis on the *temporary*.

Similarly, instead of being based on long-term or open-ended commitments, international food aid could be designed around short-term programmes with well-designed exit strategies. For example, programmes for providing vitamin A capsules could be time limited and tied directly to programmes for increasing the production and consumption of appropriate local foods.

Time limitations should be accompanied by capacity building through educational programmes of various kinds. Capacity is defined as 'the ability of people, organizations and society as a whole to manage their affairs successfully. Capacity development is the process of unleashing, strengthening and maintaining of such capacity' (FAO, 2010a). This definition is based on the work of the Organization for Economic Co-operation and Development (OECD/DAC), and reflects a broad consensus of opinion (FAO, 2010a). Baillie *et al.* (2008) further discuss this topic in putting forward a conceptual framework for capacity building in public health nutrition practice.

Many communities are not well prepared to make important decisions relating to the nutrition of their people. Thus, there may be good reasons for outsiders to take the lead in making such decisions, but only for a time. The outsiders should see that part of their job is to enhance the capacity of people in the community so that after a while the outsiders' intervention is no longer needed.

To illustrate this approach, school meal programmes supported by the WFP could be established with the clear understanding from the outset that WFP's involvement would be time limited, and the joint task of WFP and the community during this period would be to plan a smooth exit process. WFP resources and management would be phased out and local resources phased in. The transition programme would build people's ability to take charge.

The concept of an 'enabling environment' is central to this approach. Feeding programmes should be accompanied by efforts to create enabling conditions that would allow people to provide for themselves. The core of capacity building at any level is education designed to empower.

Capacities need to be strengthened not only for agencies of national governments but also for sub-national governments, communities, families and individuals. Unfortunately, some advocates of capacity building seem to assume that those at higher levels always know what needs to be known, and need to teach what they know to people at lower levels. In some cases, it might be better if the higher levels simply facilitated peer-to-peer teaching and learning. For example, spaces could be created in which neighbours could share their knowledge of household food production. In many cases, those at the higher levels have much to learn. Under a well-facilitated dialogue process involving people at every level, all of them would be likely to learn a great deal.

Interventions that reduce people's range of choices are generally disempowering and likely to provoke resistance. Banning unhealthy food often raises complaints about interference with freedom of choice. In terms of building nutritional self-reliance, it is better to offer more good options rather than to prohibit bad ones. Policy makers should promote good foods and provide information that will strengthen people's capacity to make good dietary choices – make the healthy choice the easy choice.

Capacity-building efforts can focus on building knowledge and skills directly related to nutrition, but general education is helpful as well. Education for women has a strong positive impact on children's nutritional status, even when that education is not specifically about nutrition (Burchi and De Muro, 2009). The nutritional self-reliance of families and communities is likely to grow with improved general education for women, especially primary education.

The rights approach, centred on the human right to adequate food, has made important advances around the world (Kent, 2005; FAO, 2010c). However, many of its supposed beneficiaries do not know their rights and many of those who are supposed to carry the correlative duties do not know their obligations. Even if rights holders do know their rights, they might not know what to do to ensure that they are realized. When fully implemented, the rights approach enhances people's control over their own nutrition situations.

Some people interpret the right to food primarily in terms of entitlements to free or subsidized food. This is the dominant view in India's Right to Food Campaign (Right to Food Campaign, 2010). The campaign says little about what needy people might do for themselves. An alternative perspective is that the primary legal obligation of the state is to *facilitate* by establishing enabling conditions under which people can provide for themselves (Kent, 2005, 2010). The obligation of the state to *provide* food directly applies only when people are unable to provide for themselves through no fault of their own.

The idea that outsiders should facilitate needy people in providing for themselves was clearly articulated by a poor Haitian farmer:

> Here's what Jonas Deronzil has to say to the U.S. Government: "your policies are bad. Help us produce, don't give us food. We're not lazy. We have water. We have land, especially in the Artibonite. Give us seeds, give us material. Don't give us rice, we don't need it. Our country can produce rice. If we're short, we'll let them know. There's a lot of things I'd like to tell the American Government but I don't know where to find them. But if I could find the Americans, I'd tell them that.
>
> (Bell and Deronzil, 2010)

In the realm of managing information, communities should be supported in assembling and analysing their own nutrition data. Instead of enhancing the capacity of outsiders to make decisions that affect nutrition in the community, some resources could instead be used to enhance the information collection, analysis and decision-making capacity of people in the community.

There is a need to go beyond the management of pieces of information and also to encourage local analysis of the nutrition situation. The possibilities are illustrated by Alexandra Praun's work in Central America (Praun, 1982). *Promotores* or facilitators were trained to work with local groups, leading discussions on matters such as:

1. The nutrition situation in the locality.
2. Why do children die?
3. Why don't we have enough food?
4. The foods in the community.
5. Local food preparation.
6. The local food taboos and traditions.
7. The agricultural services in the region.

8. The health services in the region.
9. The food aid programmes in the region.
10. The communal/home garden situation.
11. The chicken, rabbit and pig farms situation.

To illustrate, the theme 'nutrition situation in our locality' was explored through a set of questions concerning local food prices, food availability, local production, family diet, common child sicknesses, budget used for food, and so on. The appropriate questions would naturally be different in different circumstances. They would not be addressed mechanically, as in some sort of examination, but would be used to stimulate an open-ended joint analysis of the local food situation (Praun, 1982).

In another case, in the Dominican Republic, a women's nutrition training course was established:

> Some 62 women started attending the course – structured along Paulo Freire's lines – which examined nutrition not only in technical terms but also in the social, political and economic context of the women's lives. They studied the nutritional situation of their own region and of the entire country. They also made surveys in their own neighbourhoods to assess the nutritional problems of their families, friends and neighbours, and to work out ways of dealing with them.
>
> (Hilsum, 1983)

As a result, the women, calling themselves Women of the South, developed detailed critiques of the export orientation of the country's agriculture and of their own excessive dependence on food aid; they launched a number of projects for food production and distribution; and they undertook a systematic programme of self-evaluation of their efforts (Hilsum, 1983).

The strengthening of communities can help to improve their nutrition status. Community-based strategies have proven effective, as in Lalitpur, India, where women from the village were facilitated in forming mother support groups (Kushwaha, 2010). Another study in India showed that 'a community-based programme that trains village health workers can have long-lasting impacts on child mortality' (Mann *et al.*, 2010).

FAO has a programme specifically desig-ned to support community-based action: the Participatory Nutrition Programme, under FAO's Nutrition Division (Thompson, 2000; Ismail, 2003, 2005). FAO describes the community-based approach as follows:

> Community-centred approaches for improving nutrition build capabilities and empower communities to effectively demand services and productive resources and at the same time support local initiatives for implementing food and nutrition programmes. This involves increasing the participation of communities in the design, implementation and monitoring of development programmes and interventions. Achieving household food and nutrition security requires co-ordination among local institutions that can or should support food-insecure groups.
>
> (FAO, 2010b)

Thus, the programme recognizes the need to build nutritional self-reliance at the commu-nity level.

In many places, there is no lead agency that gives sustained and comprehensive attention to nutrition. Community-based analysis and recommendations should be led by a specific agency with a clear mandate to give attention to the full range of nutrition issues. Existing village councils might do the job, or newly created food policy councils could provide the locus for community-based consultation relating to nutrition issues (Harper *et al.*, 2009; Mata'afa, 2009; Sagapolutele, 2009; Lukens, 2010; Kent 2011). These councils could facilitate constructive dialogue on local concerns and strengthen their communities as they stimulate improve-ments in specific policies. They could join their voices together to address higher levels of governance. The work of such councils should be facilitated by agencies at higher levels.

Evidence for the Effectiveness of Efforts to Build Nutritional Self-reliance

What evidence would demonstrate the value and effectiveness of efforts to build nutri-tional self-reliance? Methods should be devel-oping for assessing both initiatives from within the communities and interventions from outside.

The premise here is that strengthening nutritional self-reliance is inherently a posi-tive thing. Any action that does this should be endorsed, provided there are no countervail-ing harms that outweigh the benefits.

To some extent, the merits of any nutrition-related intervention can be judged on the basis of its character, even before the assessment of actual impacts 'on the ground'. For example, a project that helps people in any locality to jointly reflect on their nutrition concerns would score well. An intervention plan that involves talking with the people who are supposed to benefit would be better than one that does not. As such, the Food Aid Convention would score poorly because it is periodically renegoti-ated by the donor countries, with no involve-ment of the receiving countries (FAC, 2010; Harvey *et al.*, 2010).

A project that provides people with cap-sules to combat a particular type of malnutri-tion and is wholly funded and implemented by people outside the 'target' community would score poorly. The capsules might yield immediate nutritional benefits that outweigh that weakness, but on the dimension of build-ing nutritional self-reliance, the programme would score poorly.

There are no established measures of nutritional self-reliance, but sensible judge-ments can be made. The degree of nutritional self-reliance can be understood as the degree to which people, acting alone and in commu-nity, make their own decisions affecting what they are going to eat. This can be understood as a continuum. At one extreme, outsiders make all the decisions, with no consultation with those who will get the food – in the way that might occur in a prison or a refugee camp; in some cases, people might be treated as if they were livestock in a feedlot. At the other extreme, people make all their own decisions. They might draw in products and information from outside the community, but they base their choices on what they see as being in their own interests.

It would be useful to have good meas-ures of the level of nutritional self-reliance in any community. However, it might be more important to be able to estimate the extent to which interventions from outside the community are likely to strengthen or weaken its nutritional self-reliance. These judgements could be made systematically. To illustrate, given a list of nutrition projects with a brief description of each, a panel of judges who have familiarized themselves with the concept should be able to rank those projects on how likely they are to make a positive or negative impact on nutritional self-reliance. Is the project likely to shift the locus of decision making toward or away from the community? Guidelines could be developed to improve the validity and reliability of the judgements made.

Increased nutritional self-reliance is likely to be associated with improved nutritional status, but that should not be assumed to be true in every case. The strength of that linkage is really an empirical question, one that would depend on local circumstances. It would be useful to collect case studies of local initiatives and also of interventions from outside that have helped to build local nutritional self-reliance, and to examine how that and other factors interrelate and affect nutrition status.

If people are not well informed and well motivated on their nutrition, perhaps because their main source of information is advertisements for highly processed foods, increasing their capacity to make their own decisions is not likely to lead to improvements in their nutrition status. If people are addicted to bad food and not motivated to improve their health, they will be less likely to be affected by new scientific information about the qualities of different foods. Factors such as the quality of information and the motivations of the people can be viewed as intervening variables that influence the strength of the linkage between nutritional self-reliance and nutrition status.

The basic conclusion here does not require further evidence. There are many different ways in which outsiders can be helpful to communities with regard to their nutrition (Harvey et al., 2010; WFP, 2010b). Some forms of assistance can be disempowering because they only provide short-term relief, make bad situations more tolerable and have outsiders dominate the decision making. In those situations, the gift of assistance tends to stimulate demands for more assistance.

In contrast, assistance that is empowering helps people to address their nutrition concerns individually and together with their neighbours, building their nutritional self-reliance and reducing their need for assistance over time. Outside agencies can help to build nutritional self-reliance by recognizing the difference and favouring the more empowering approaches.

References

Anand, S. (2008) Why is modern India vegetarian? *Out-Caste*, Friday, March 21, 2008. Available at: http://out-caste.blogspot.com/2008/03/why-is-modern-india-vegetarian.html (accessed 21 June 2013).

Baillie, E., Bjarnholt, C., Gruber, M. and Hughes, R. (2008) A capacity-building conceptual framework for public health nutrition practice. *Public Health Nutrition* 12, 1031–1038. Available at: http://journals.cambridge.org/action/displayAbstract?fromPage=online&aid=5885972 (accessed 21 June 2013).

Bell, B. and Deronzil, D. (2010) Haiti: don't give us food, help us produce. *Toward Freedom*, Monday, 20 September 2010, 19:00. Available at: http://www.towardfreedom.com/home/americas/2114-haiti-dont-give-us-good-help-us-produce (accessed 21 June 2013).

Burchi, F. and De Muro, P. (2009) *Reducing Children's Food Insecurity Through Primary Education for Rural Mothers: The Case of Mozambique.* University Roma Tre and Food and Agriculture Organization of the United Nations, Rome. Available at: http://www.fao.org/sd/erp/documents2009/FAO-RomaTreFINALREPORT2.pdf (accessed 21 June 2013).

Burlingame, B. (2010) ...and sustainable diets. [Letter] *World Nutrition* 1, 164–165. Available at: http://www.wphna.org/wn_vitA_responsejuly2010.asp (accessed 21 June 2013).

Cave, A. (2010) Nestlé chief Peter Bulcke aims to teach the world about nutrition. *The Telegraph*, London, 8:00AM BST 03 October 2010. Available at: http://www.telegraph.co.uk/finance/newsbysector/

retailandconsumer/8038634/Nestle-chief-Peter-Bulcke-aims-to-teach-the-world-about-nutrition.html (accessed 21 June 2013).

CFS Secretariat, UN High-Level Task Force, OXFAM and ActionAid (2010) *Mapping Food Security Actions at Country Level: A Draft Concept Note. Prepared by a Task Team Comprised of the CFS Secretariat (FAO, IFAD, WFP), UN High-Level Task Force, OXFAM and ActionAid.* United Nations Committee on World Food Security, Rome. Available: at: http://www.donorplatform.org/index2.php?option=com_resource&task=show_file&id=2670 (accessed 21 June 2013).

FAC (2010) About the FAC. Food Aid Convention. London, UK. Available at: http://www.foodaidconvention.org/en/index/aboutthefac.aspx (accessed 21 June 2013).

FAO (2010a) Capacity Development Portal. Food and Agriculture Organization of the United Nations, Rome. Available at: http://www.fao.org/capacitydevelopment/en/ (accessed 21 June 2013).

FAO (2010b) Household food security & community nutrition: participatory nutrition. Food and Agriculture Organization of the United Nations, Rome. Available at: http://www.fao.org/ag/agn/nutrition/household_community_en.stm (accessed 21 June 2013).

FAO (2010c) The Right to Food: the human right to adequate food. Food and Agriculture Organization of the United Nations, Rome. Available at: http://www.fao.org/righttofood/index_en.htm (accessed 21 June 2013).

FAO (2010d) Food Insecurity and Vulnerability Information and Mapping Systems (FIVIMS). Food and Agriculture Organization of the United Nations, Rome. Available at: http://www.fao.org/knowledge/documents-detail/en/c/115824/?type=list (accessed 21 June 2013).

Harper, A., Shattuck, A., Holt-Giménez, E., Alkon, A. and Lambrick, F. (2009) *Food Policy Councils: Lessons Learned.* Development Report No. 21, Institute for Food and Development Policy, Oakland, California. Available at: http://www.foodfirst.org/en/foodpolicycouncils-lessons (accessed 21 June 2013).

Harvey, P., Proudlock, K., Clay, E., Riley, B. and Jaspars, S. (2010) *Food Aid and Food Assistance in Emergency and Transitional Contexts: A Review of Current Thinking.* HPG Synthesis Paper, Humanitarian Policy Group, Overseas Development Institute, London. Available at: http://www.odi.org.uk/sites/odi.org.uk/files/odi-assets/publications-opinion-files/6036.pdf (accessed 21 June 2013).

Hilsum, L. (1983) Nutrition education and social change: a women's movement in the Dominican Republic. In: Morley, D., Rohde, J.E. and Williams, G. (eds) *Practicing Health for All.* Oxford University Press, New York, pp. 114–132.

IBFAN (2009) *Colombo Declaration on Infant and Young Child Feeding. One Asia Breastfeeding Partners Forum 6, held in Colombo, Sri Lanka from November 18 to 21, 2009.* IBFAN (The International Baby Food Action Network) Asia, Delhi and Sarvodaya, Colombo, Sri Lanka. Available at: http://www.ibfan.org/art/colombo.pdf (accessed 21 June 2013).

Isanaka, S., Nombela, N., Djibo, A., Poupard, M., Van Beckhoven, D.V., Gaboulaud, V., Guerin, P.J. and Grais, R.F. (2009) Effect of preventive supplementation with ready-to-use therapeutic food on the nutritional status, mortality, and morbidity of children aged 6 to 60 months in Niger. *JAMA* 301, 277–285. Available at: http://jama.jamanetwork.com/article.aspx?articleid=183241 (accessed 21 June 2013).

Ismail, S., Immink, M., Mazar, I. and Nantel, G. (2003) *Community-based Food and Nutrition Programmes. What Makes them Successful? A Review and Analysis of Experience.* Food and Agriculture Organization of the United Nations, Rome. Available at: http://www.fao.org/docrep/006/Y5030E/Y5030E00.HTM (accessed 21 June 2013).

Ismail, S., Immink, M. and Nantel, G. (2005) *Improving Nutrition Programmes: An Assessment Tool for Action (Revised Edition).* Food and Agriculture Organization of the United Nations, Rome. Available at: ftp://ftp.fao.org/docrep/fao/009/a0244e/a0244e00.pdf (accessed 21 June 2013).

Kent, G. (2005) *Freedom from Want: The Human Right to Adequate Food.* Georgetown University Press, Washington, DC. Available at: http://press.georgetown.edu/sites/default/files/978-1-58901-055-0%20w%20CC%20license.pdf (accessed 21 June 2013).

Kent, G. (2006) WIC's promotion of infant formula in the United States. International Breastfeeding Journal 1(8), 1–14. Available at: http://www.internationalbreastfeedingjournal.com/content/1/1/8 (accessed 21 June 2013).

Kent, G. (2010) *Swaraj* against hunger. *Gandhi Marg* 32, 149–168. Available at: http://www2.hawaii.edu/~kent/SwarajAgainstHunger.pdf (accessed 21 June 2013).

Kent, G. (2011) *Ending Hunger Worldwide.* Paradigm Publishers, Boulder, Colorado.

Kessler, D.A. (2009) *The End of Overeating: Taking Control of the Insatiable American Appetite.* Rodale, New York.

Kidwai, R. (2010) Eggs? Chauhan says no – CM rejects govt proposal for mid-day meal menu. *The Telegraph*, Calcutta, India, Saturday, September 25, 2010. Available at: http://www.telegraphindia.com/1100925/jsp/nation/story_12980245.jsp (accessed 21 June 2013).

Kushwaha, K.P. (2010) *Reaching the Under 2s: Universalising Delivery of Nutrition Interventions in District Lalitpur, Uttar Pradesh.* Department of Pediatrics, BRD Medical College, Gorakhpur, Uttar Pradesh, India. Available at: http://www.bpni.org/BFHI/Reaching-the-under-2S-Universalising-Delivery-of-Nutrition-Interventions-in-Lalitpur-UP.pdf (accessed 4 July 2013).

Latham, M. (2010) The Great Vitamin A Fiasco. *World Nutrition* 1, 12–45. Available at: http://www.wphna.org/downloads/10-05%20WN%20commentary%20Latham.pdf (accessed 21 June 2013).

Latham, M., Jonsson, U., Sterken, E. and Kent, G. (2011) RUTF stuff: Can the children be saved with fortified peanut paste? *World Nutrition* 2, 62–85. Available at: http://www.wphna.org/2011_feb_wn3_comm_RUTF.htm (accessed 21 June 2013).

Lucas, L. and Jack, A. (2010) Food and pharma prove a rich mix. *Financial Times*, London, 12 October 2010. Available at: http://www.ft.com/cms/s/0/1f41bf6c-d62f-11df-81f0-00144feabdc0.html#axzz2WrRFg92r (accessed 21 June 2013).

Lukens, A. (2010) Democratizing food: Hawai'i's future food systems. *Honolulu Weekly*, 24 November 2010. Available at: http://honoluluweekly.com/feature/2010/11/democratizing-food/ (accessed 21 June 2013).

Mann, V., Eble, A., Frost, F., Premkumar, R. and Boone, P. (2010) Retrospective comparative evaluation of the lasting impact of a community-based primary health care programme on under-5 mortality in villages around Jamkhed, India. *Bulletin of the World Health Organization* 88, 727–736. Available at: http://www.who.int/entity/bulletin/volumes/88/10/09-064469.pdf (accessed 21 June 2013).

Mata'afa, T. (2009) A.S. Food Security Conference: 'Steer Your Own Canoe,' says UHM's Dr Kent. *Samoa News Home*, 19 February 2009.

Moss, M. (2010) While warning about fat, U.S. pushes cheese sales. *New York Times*, 6 November 2010. Available at: http://www.nytimes.com/2010/11/07/us/07fat.html?_r=1andnl=todaysheadlinesandemc=tha1 (accessed 21 June 2013).

Nutraceuticals World (2010) *Nutraceuticals World.* Available at: http://www.nutraceuticalsworld.com/ (accessed 21 June 2013).

Oliveira, V., Frazão, E. and Smallwood, D. (2010) *Rising Infant Formula Costs to the WIC Program: Recent Trends in Rebates and Wholesale Prices.* Economic Research Report No. 93, Economic Research Service, US Department of Agriculture, Washington, DC. Available at: http://www.ers.usda.gov/media/136568/err93_1_.pdf (accessed 21 June 2013).

Ouédraogo, H.Z., Traoré, T., Zèba, A.N., Dramaix-Wilmet, M., Nennart, P. and Donnen, P. (2010) Effect of an improved local ingredient-based complementary food fortified or not with iron and selected multiple micronutrients on Hb concentration. *Public Health Nutrition* 13, 1923–1930. Available at: http://journals.cambridge.org/action/displayAbstract?fromPage=online&aid=7914921 (accessed 21 June 2013).

PepsiCo (2010) PepsiCo establishes global nutrition group. *Nutraceuticals World*, 8 October 2010. Available at: http://www.nutraceuticalsworld.com/contents/view/29588 (accessed 21 June 2013).

Praun, A. (1982) Nutrition education: development or alienation? *Human Nutrition: Applied Nutrition* 36A, 28–34.

Quinn, V., Zehner, E., Schofield, D., Guyon, A. and Hoffman, S. (2010) *Maternal, Infant and Young Child Nutrition (MIYCN) Working Group: Using the Code of Marketing of Breast-milk Substitutes to Guide the Marketing of Complementary Foods to Protect Optimal Feeding Practices.* GAIN Working Paper No. 3, Global Alliance for Improved Nutrition, Geneva, Switzerland. Available at: http://www.gainhealth.org/sites/www.gainhealth.org/files/working%20paper%203LR_with_insert.pdf (accessed 21 June 2013).

Right to Food Campaign (2010) New Delhi. Available at: http://www.righttofoodindia.org/ (accessed 21 June 2013).

Rotondi, M.A. and Khobzi, N. (2010) Vitamin A supplementation and neonatal mortality in the developing world: a meta-regression of cluster-randomized trials. *Bulletin of the World Health Organization* 8, 641–716. Available at: http://www.who.int/entity/bulletin/volumes/88/9/09-068080/en/index.html (accessed 21 June 2013).

Sachs, J., Fanzo, J. and Sachs, S. (2010) Saying "Nuts" to Hunger. *Huffington Post*, 6 September 2010. Available at: http://www.huffingtonpost.com/jeffrey-sachs/saying-nuts-to-hunger_b_706798.html (accessed 21 June 2013).

Sagapolutele, F. (2009) Governor establishes food policy council by executive order. *Samoanews Home* Available at: http://papgren.blogspot.com/search?q=SAGAPOLUTELE (accessed 21 June 2013).

Shatrugna, V. (2009) Exclusive cereal dependence. *Down to Earth*, New Delhi, 15–30 September 2009. Available at: http://www.downtoearth.org.in/node/3859 (accessed 21 June 2013).

Thompson, B. (2000) Community-centred food-based strategies for alleviating and preventing malnutrition. In: Tolba, M.K. (ed.) *Our Fragile World: Challenges and Opportunities for Sustainable Development*. EOLSS, Oxford, UK. Also online as chapter in: *Impacts of Agriculture on Human Health and Nutrition – Vol. I, Encyclopedia of Food and Agricultural Sciences, Engineering and Technology Resources, Encyclopedia of Life Support Systems (EOLSS)*. Available at: http://www.eolss.net/Sample-Chapters/C10/E5-21-02.pdf (accessed 21 June 2013).

WFP (2010a) *Fighting Hunger Worldwide: Annual Report 2010*. World Food Programme, Rome. Available at: http://documents.wfp.org/stellent/groups/public/documents/communications/wfp220666.pdf (accessed 21 June 2013).

WFP (2010b) *Revolution: From Food Aid to Food Assistance – Innovations in Overcoming Hunger*. World Food Programme, Rome. Available at: http://www.wfp.org/content/revolution-food-aid-food-assistance-innovations-overcoming-hunger (accessed 21 June 2013).

World Bank (2010) *What Can We Learn from Nutrition Impact Evaluations? Lessons from a Review of Interventions to Reduce Child Malnutrition in Developing Countries*. Independent Evaluation Group, World Bank, Washington, DC. Available at: http://siteresources.worldbank.org/EXTWBASSHEANUTPOP/Resources/Nutrition_eval.pdf (accessed 21 June 2013).

Contribution of FAO Departments and Divisions Towards Improving Food and Nutrition Security and Promoting Agriculture and Food-based Approaches Sensitive to Nutrition

Part IV of the Proceedings assembles contributions prepared by the Departments and Divisions of the Food and Agriculture Organization of the United Nations (FAO), giving examples of how nutrition issues and considerations are being mainstreamed into FAO's work, thus improving diets and raising levels of nutrition.

Contributions from the Agriculture and Consumer Protection Department (AG):

21 Measurement of Dietary Diversity for Monitoring the Impact of Food-based Approaches
Nutrition and Consumer Protection Division (AGN), Agriculture and Consumer Protection Department (AG)

22 Nutrition Education and Food Security Interventions to Improve Complementary Feeding in Cambodia
Nutrition and Consumer Protection Division (AGN), Agriculture and Consumer Protection Department (AG)

23 Activities of the Animal Production and Health Division (AGA) of FAO to Improve Food and Nutrition Security
Animal Production and Health Division (AGA), Agriculture and Consumer Protection Department (AG)

24 The Role of the Plant Production and Protection Division (AGP) of FAO in Supporting Crop Diversification for Sustainable Diets and Nutrition
Plant Production and Protection Division (AGP), Agriculture and Consumer Protection Department (AG)

25 Impact of the Work of the Rural Infrastructure and Agro-Industries Division (AGS) of FAO on Improving Food and Nutrition Security
Rural Infrastructure and Agro-Industries Division (AGS), Agriculture and Consumer Protection Department (AG)

Contributions from the Economic and Social Development Department (ES):

26 Work of the Agricultural Development Economics Division (ESA) of FAO on Nutrition
Agricultural Development Economics Division (ESA), Economic and Social Development Department (ES)

27 Towards an Improved Framework for Measuring Undernourishment
Statistics Division (ESS), Economic and Social Development Department (ES)

28 Gender Dimensions of Food and Nutrition Security: Women's Roles in

21 Measurement of Dietary Diversity for Monitoring the Impact of Food-based Approaches

Nutrition and Consumer Protection Division (AGN),*† Agriculture and Consumer Protection Department (AG)

Food and Agriculture Organization of the United Nations, Rome, Italy

---

Summary

Monotonous diets based mainly on energy-dense, but micronutrient-poor starchy staples are common in food-insecure areas and contribute to the burden of malnutrition, particularly to inadequate micronutrient intake. Food-based strategies have been recommended as the first priority to meet micronutrient needs. An essential element to food-based approaches involves dietary diversification – or the consumption of a wide variety of foods across nutritionally distinct food groups. Increased dietary diversity is associated with increased household access to food as well as increased individual probability of adequate micronutrient intake. Dietary diversity is measured as the number of individual food groups consumed over a given reference period. FAO has developed guidelines on the use of a standardized tool for measuring dietary diversity that can be administered at either the household or individual level. The tool uses an open recall method to gather information on all the foods and drinks consumed by the household or individual over the previous 24 h. The foods and drinks mentioned by the respondent are then recorded into one of 16 standardized food groups. Data collected using the dietary diversity tool can then be analysed in several different ways to provide a picture of dietary patterns within a community as well as among vulnerable groups. Examples of analytical approaches and programmatic uses are drawn from studies in Mozambique and Tanzania. These examples illustrate how information collected from the dietary diversity tool can be used to inform baseline assessment, programme design and monitoring and evaluation.

Introduction

Micronutrient malnutrition, i.e. vitamin and mineral deficiencies, affects one third of the population worldwide (Mason *et al.*, 2001). Monotonous diets based on starchy staples lack essential micronutrients and contribute to the burden of malnutrition and micronutrient deficiencies. Food-based strategies have been recommended as the first priority to meet micronutrient needs (Allen, 2008). An essential element of food-based approaches involves dietary diversification – the consumption of a wide variety of foods across nutritionally distinct food groups – as a way to meet recommended intakes of nutrients. As conventional

---

*Contributors: Gina Kennedy, Maylis Razes, Terri Ballard and Marie Claude Dop
†Contact: g.kennedy@cgiar.org

quantitative dietary assessment surveys are costly and cumbersome to conduct and analyse, there is great interest in using simple proxies of intake that can be measured quickly and easily and that validly reflect nutrient intake. This was the rationale for developing dietary diversity measurement tools as proxies for quantitative dietary intake.

Definition and Measurement of Dietary Diversity

Dietary diversity is defined as the number of individual food items or food groups consumed over a given period of time (Ruel, 2003). It can be measured at the household or individual level through the use of a questionnaire. Most often it is measured by counting the number of food groups rather than food items consumed. The type and number of food groups included in the questionnaire and subsequent analysis may vary, depending on the intended purpose and level of measurement. At the household level, dietary diversity is usually considered as a measure of access to food (e.g. of household capacity to access costly food groups), while at individual level it reflects dietary quality, mainly micronutrient adequacy, of the diet. The reference period can vary, but is most often the previous day or week (WFP, 2009; FAO, 2011).

Scientific Evidence for the Use of Dietary Diversity Scores

Over the past decade there have been three large multi-country validation studies and many smaller studies that have looked at the association between dietary diversity and food security and/or micronutrient adequacy of the diet.

Hoddinott and Yohannes (2002), for example, studied the association between household dietary diversity scores and dietary energy availability in ten countries. Increasing household dietary diversity significantly improved energy availability. The study results suggest that dietary diversity

scores have potential for monitoring changes in dietary energy availability, particularly when resources are lacking for quantitative measurements.

A second multi-country study of the diets of children aged 6–23 months from ten sites was undertaken to test the association between dietary diversity and mean micronutrient density adequacy of complementary foods. Significant positive correlations were observed in all age groups and in all countries except one (Working Group on Infant and Young Child Feeding Indicators, 2007).

Recently, the association between dietary diversity and micronutrient adequacy of the diets of women of reproductive age was assessed in five countries. Dietary diversity was significantly associated with micronutrient adequacy at all sites (Arimond et al., 2010). Other studies carried out in individual countries and across diverse age groups have also shown positive correlations between dietary diversity scores and micronutrient adequacy ratios (Hatloy et al., 1998; Mirmiran et al., 2004, 2006; Steyn et al., 2006; Kennedy et al., 2007).

In conclusion, dietary diversity scores have been shown to be valid proxy indicators for dietary energy availability at household level and for the micronutrient adequacy of the diets of young children and women of reproductive age.

FAO's Dietary Diversity Guidelines

FAO (Food and Agriculture Organization of the United Nations) has published operational guidelines for measuring dietary diversity in a standardized way, based on a tool originally developed by the USAID (US Agency for International Development)-supported Food and Nutrition Technical Assistance Project (FANTA) (Swindale and Bilinsky, 2006; FAO, 2011). The FAO data collection tool uses an open recall method to gather information on all foods and drinks consumed by the household or individual over the previous 24 h. The foods and drinks recalled by the respondent are then recorded into one of 16 standardized food groups. Probing is used to capture the consumption of any food groups not mentioned in the open recall.

The FAO guidelines describe how to adapt the tool to local food systems and also recommend the following ways of reporting information collected on dietary diversity:

- Dietary diversity scores are simple counts of the number of food groups consumed at individual or household level. The two dietary diversity scores recommended by FAO are the Household Dietary Diversity Score (HDDS), which is based on 12 food groups, and the Women's Dietary Diversity Score (WDDS), which is based on nine food groups. Mean scores can be compared across population subgroups and over time.
- Dietary profiles based on food groups consumed by a majority of individuals/ households categorized in subgroups of the population (for instance by tertile of dietary diversity score) can be compared to provide insights on consumption patterns across these subgroups.
- The percentage of individuals or households consuming food groups or combinations of nutrient-dense food groups (such as food groups rich in Vitamin A) can be analysed.

Case Studies that Illustrate Potential Uses of Dietary Diversity as a Food and Nutrition Security Indicator

Examples of analyses drawn from Mozambique and Tanzania show the potential uses of dietary diversity to inform the design, targeting, monitoring and evaluation of food and nutrition security interventions and programmes. These are described below.

The dietary diversity questionnaire was included in a baseline and follow-up assessment of a food and nutrition project carried out in central Mozambique in the districts of Chibabava (Sofala Province) and Gondola (Mancina Province) (FAO, 2008). Baseline assessment was conducted in November–December 2006 during the pre-harvest season and the follow-up in July 2007 after the maize harvest. The assessments covered a total of 300 households.

Dietary diversity scores were low across both seasons and districts (a mean of 3.9 food groups out of 12). Figure 21.1 shows dietary profiles by tertile of the dietary diversity score during the pre-harvest season in both districts combined. In the lowest tertile (households consuming fewer than four food groups) the majority of households consumed 'cereals', 'green leafy vegetables' and 'vitamin A rich fruit (survey carried out in the

Food groups consumed by >50% of households by DD tercile
(Mozambique hungry season)

Lowest DD <4	Medium DD 4–5	High DD >5
Cereals	Cereals	Cereals
Green leafy vegetables	Green leafy vegetables	Green leafy vegetables
Vitamin A-rich fruit	Vitamin-A rich fruit	Vitamin A-rich fruit
	Oil	Oil
		Other vegetables
		Fish
		Legumes, nuts and seeds

Fig. 21.1. Food groups added to the diet as diversity score increases in central Mozambique: combined results from studies in two areas (Chibabava and Gondola districts) in 2006–2007. DD, dietary diversity. From FAO (2008).

mango season)' while in the highest tertile the majority of households also consumed items from the food groups 'oil', 'other vegetables', 'fish' and 'legumes/nuts/seeds'.

Figures 21.2 and 21.3 show data from the two surveys for the district of Chibabava. These figures illustrate how the measurement of dietary diversity can be used to monitor changes in dietary patterns over time. Figure 21.2 shows percentage of households consuming legumes/nuts/seeds for the two survey periods stratified by food security status as measured by the FANTA Household Food Insecurity Access Scale (HFIAS) (Coates *et al.*, 2007). During the first survey, which corresponded to the pre-harvest period, the percentage of households consuming legumes/nuts/seeds was higher in the food-insecure households than in the others. The percentage of food-insecure households consuming legumes/nuts/seeds dropped by 80% between seasons, while in the food-secure households it increased slightly. This indicates

that economic access to legumes, nuts and seeds was most likely to have been the cause of decline in consumption in the food-insecure households. Figure 21.3 shows the percentage of households consuming fish over the two survey periods, similarly stratified by food security status. The percentage of households consuming fish dropped during the postharvest period in both food-secure and food-insecure groups, although the decline was greater in the food-insecure group, indicating a problem of availability – and not just of access – for this food group. The severe floods that Chibabava experienced before the second survey round caused a decline in fish stocks.

Dietary diversity was measured in a baseline assessment survey of 628 households in slum areas of urban Tanzania in 2008. Mean HDDS varied by wealth tertile of household food insecurity (as measured by HFIAS), ranging from a mean of 6.0 in the most food-insecure to a mean of 7.2 in the

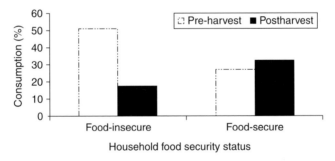

Fig. 21.2. Monitoring the consumption of legume/nuts/seeds in Chibabava District in central Mozambique in 2006–2007 by household food security status as measured by the FANTA (Food and Nutrition Technical Assistance) Household Food Insecurity Access Scale (HFIAS). From FAO (2008).

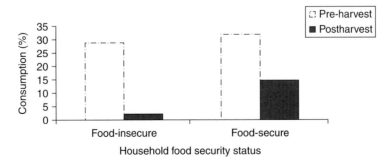

Fig. 21.3. Monitoring the consumption of fish in Chibabava District in central Mozambique in 2006–2007 by household food security status as measured by the FANTA (Food and Nutrition Technical Assistance) Household Food Insecurity Access Scale (HFIAS). From FAO (2008).

most food-secure group (Razès, M. and Dop, M.C. (2010) *Report of the Re-analysis of the Tanzania Urban Food and Nutrition Security Survey*. Unpublished report from Nutrition Division, FAO, Rome) (Fig. 21.4). Figure 21.5 shows the percentage of Tanzanian households consuming micronutrient-rich food groups by wealth tertile.

In the wealthiest group, twice as many households consumed the food groups of 'meat/ offal', 'milk' and 'fruit' as in the least wealthy group.

These two case studies show how dietary diversity can be used to assess diets in terms of mean dietary diversity and percentage of households consuming nutritionally important

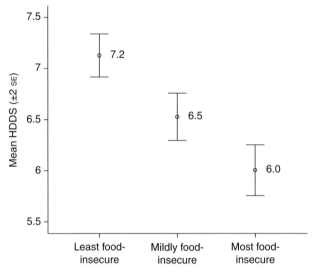

Fig. 21.4. Mean Household Dietary Diversity Score (HDDS) in slum areas of urban Tanzania in 2008 by food insecurity tertile as measured by the FANTA (Food and Nutrition Technical Assistance) Household Food Insecurity Access Scale (HFIAS). From Razès, M. and Dop, M.C. (2010) *Report of the Re-analysis of the Tanzania Urban Food and Nutrition Security Survey*. Unpublished report from Nutrition Division, FAO, Rome.

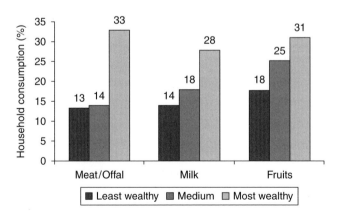

Fig. 21.5. Household consumption of micronutrient-rich food groups in slum areas of urban Tanzania in 2008 by wealth tertile. From Razès, M. and Dop, M.C. (2010) *Report of the Re-analysis of the Tanzania Urban Food and Nutrition Security Survey*. Unpublished report from Nutrition Division, FAO, Rome.

food groups. An analysis of dietary diversity by subgroups of a population allows the setting of measurable targets for improvement for the group with the lowest dietary diversity. For example, in Mozambique the dietary profile of the higher tertile of dietary diversity can be used as a target to be reached by all households. For urban Tanzania, a target would be to increase the percentage of poorest households consuming micronutrient-rich food groups to reach the level of that of the wealthier households. In particular, an important objective of programmes could be to increase consumption of animal foods in poor households.

When consecutive assessments have been conducted, it is possible to assess seasonal differences with the objective of developing agricultural and food-security interventions to compensate for seasonal decreases in dietary diversity. Moreover, information on dietary diversity in two or more time periods is useful for helping decision makers to understand the effects of both normal seasonal variation and of shock variations on dietary consumption. This information will enable them to define and plan actions to improve access to important food groups, such as legumes/nuts/seeds and fish, as shown in the Mozambican example.

Use of dietary diversity scores has several statistical limitations. Both the HDDS and the WDDS are based on a small number of food groups (12 for HDDS and nine for WDDS). This narrow range in the scores limits the ability to detect changes or differences in the mean score, particularly when the sample size is small. Except for infants and young children (WHO, 2010), there is no universally recognized cut-off point above or below which households or individuals can be classified as having adequate or inadequate dietary diversity. Additionally, at household level, the tool does not capture out-of-home food consumption, thus potentially leading to an underestimation of household dietary diversity in urban areas and among populations where out-of-home food consumption is common. At individual level, the indicator does not suffer from this limitation. Given these limitations, it is strongly recommended not to use the dietary diversity measure as a stand-alone tool. It should be integrated into broader survey instruments and the results triangulated with other characteristics of interest, such as wealth or food security status, in order to obtain a holistic picture of the food and nutrition security situation in a community.

Collecting information on dietary diversity should be of interest to any programme or initiative where a primary or secondary objective is to improve the diet of the beneficiary population. Dietary diversity data are useful for evaluating the impact of food and nutrition security programmes. Other sectors that could usefully incorporate this information into their monitoring and evaluation systems include agriculture, fisheries and forestry. Dietary diversity can also be used to help evaluate programmes that address cross-cutting issues such as biodiversity, gender equality, HIV/AIDS or the Right to Food, where improving the quality of diets is an important outcome.

References

Allen, L. (2008) To what extent can food-based approaches improve micronutrient status? *Asia Pacific Journal of Clinical Nutrition* 17(S1), 103–105.

Arimond, M., Wiesmann, D., Becquey E., Carriquiry, A., Daniels, M., Deitchler, M., Fanou-Fogny, N., Joseph, M., Kennedy, G., Martin-Prevel, Y. and Torheim, L.E. (2010) Simple food group diversity indicators predict micronutrient adequacy of women's diets in 5 diverse, resource-poor settings. *Journal of Nutrition* 140, 2059S–2069S.

Coates, J., Swindale, A. and Bilinsky, P. (2007) *Household Food Insecurity Access Scale (HFIAS) for Measurement of Food Access: Indicator Guide, Version 3*. Food and Nutrition Technical Assistance II Project (FANTA-II Project), Academy for Educational Development (AED), Washington, DC. Available at: http://pdf. usaid.gov/pdf_docs/PNADK896.pdf (accessed 24 June 2013).

FAO (2008) *Report on use of the Household Food Insecurity Access Scale and Household Dietary Diversity Score in Two Survey Rounds in Manica and Sofala Provinces, Mozambique, 2006–2007. FAO Food Security Project*

GCP/MOZ/079/BEL. Version 2, FAO May 2008. Food and Agriculture Organization of the United Nations, Rome. Available at: http://www.foodsec.org/fileadmin/user_upload/eufao-fsi4dm/docs/moz_diet.pdf (accessed 24 June 2013).

FAO (2011) *Guidelines for Measuring Household and Individual Dietary Diversity*. Food and Agriculture Organization of the United Nations, Rome. Available at: http://www.fao.org/docrep/014/i1983e/i1983e00.pdf (accessed 24 June 2013).

Hatloy, A., Torheim, L. and Oshaug, A. (1998) Food variety – a good indicator of nutritional adequacy of the diet? A case study from an urban area in Mali, West Africa. *European Journal of Clinical Nutrition* 52, 891–898.

Hoddinott, J. and Yohannes, Y. (2002) *Dietary Diversity as a Food Security Indicator*. Food and Nutrition Technical Assistance Project (FANTA Project), Academy for Educational Development (AED), Washington, DC. Available at: http://pdf.usaid.gov/pdf_docs/PNACQ758.pdf (accessed 24 June 2013).

Kennedy, G., Pedro, M.R., Seghieri, C., Nantel, G. and Brouwer, I. (2007) Dietary diversity score is a useful indicator of micronutrient intake in non-breast-feeding Filipino children. *Journal of Nutrition* 137, 1–6.

Mason, J., Lofti, M., Dalmiya, N., Sethuraman, K. and Deitchler, M. (2001) *The Micronutrient Report: Current Progress and Trends in the Control of Vitamin A, Iodine, and Iron Deficiencies*. Micronutrient Initiative, Ottawa, Ontario, Canada. Available at: http://www.micronutrient.org/resources/publications/mn_report.pdf (accessed 24 June 2013).

Mirmiran, P., Azadbakht, L., Esmaillzadeh, A. and Azizi, F. (2004) Dietary diversity score in adolescents – a good indicator of the nutritional adequacy of diets: Tehran lipid and glucose study. *Asia Pacific Journal of Clinical Nutrition* 13, 56–60.

Mirmiran, P., Azadbakht, L. and Azizi, F. (2006) Dietary diversity among food groups: an indicator of specific nutrient adequacy in Tehranian women. *Journal of the American College of Nutrition* 25, 354–361.

Ruel, M.T. (2003) Operationalizing dietary diversity: a review of measurement issues and research priorities. *Journal of Nutrition* 133, 3911S–3926S.

Steyn, N.P., Nel, J.H., Nantel, G., Kennedy, G. and Labadarios, D. (2006) Food variety and dietary diversity scores in children: are they good indicators of dietary adequacy? *Public Health Nutrition* 9, 644–650.

Swindale, A. and Bilinsky, P. (2006) *Household Dietary Diversity Score (HDDS) for Measurement of Household Food Access: Indicator Guide, Version 2*. Food and Nutrition Technical Assistance Project, (FANTA), Academy for Educational Development (AED), Washington, DC. Available at: http://www.fantaproject.org/downloads/pdfs/HDDS_v2_Sep06.pdf (accessed 24 June 2013).

Working Group on Infant and Young Child Feeding Indicators (2007) *Developing and Validating Simple Indicators of Dietary Quality and Energy Intake of Infants and Young Children in Developing Countries: Additional Analysis of 10 data sets*. Food and Nutrition Technical Assistance (FANTA) Project, Academy for Educational Development (AED), Washington, DC. Available at: http://www.fantaproject.org/downloads/pdfs/IYCF_Datasets_Sep07.pdf (accessed 24 June 2013).

WFP (2009) *Comprehensive Food Security & Vulnerability Analysis Guidelines*. World Food Programme, Rome. Available at: http://documents.wfp.org/stellent/groups/public/documents/manual_guide_proced/wfp203202.pdf (accessed 24 June 2013).

WHO (2010) *Indicators for Assessing Infant and Young Child Feeding Practices: Part I Definitions*. World Health Organization, Geneva, Switzerland. Available at: http://whqlibdoc.who.int/publications/2008/9789241596664_eng.pdf (accessed 24 June 2013).

22 Nutrition Education and Food Security Interventions to Improve Complementary Feeding in Cambodia

Nutrition and Consumer Protection Division (AGN),*† Agriculture and Consumer Protection Department (AG)

Food and Agriculture Organization of the United Nations, Rome, Italy

------

Summary

Improving child feeding during the first 2 years of life is crucial for preventing and reducing chronic undernutrition and micronutrient deficiencies. This project aimed to improve food security (FS) and dietary diversity, with focus on infant and young child feeding between the ages of 6 and 23 months, in vulnerable rural households in Cambodia. It covered 356 households in nine provinces. Integrated with targeted FS actions, the formative research technique 'Trials of improved practices' (TIPS) was used to test the acceptability and feasibility of complementary feeding recipes, and involved families in making the best possible use of locally available resources, with emphasis on animal source foods, fruits and vegetables, and a little oil for improved child feeding. A total of 15 nutritionally improved recipes (rice based or sweet potato/taro based, enriched with a variety of readily available local foods) were developed. Approximately 70% of households achieved better dietary diversity using locally available foods 3–5 times a week. Items in a child's diet increased from two to three food items to ten or more. Other notable achievements included the acquisition of knowledge and skills by mothers and caregivers, and information sharing with non-participants, suggesting a good potential for peer education by TIPs participants. The improved recipes and recommendations were disseminated to 9000 households during the period January to 30 April 2011 through community nutrition promoters trained by the project. The results support the need for combining dietary counselling with targeted FS actions aimed at increasing nutrient-dense local foods.

Background

The burden of undernutrition continues to be high in many developing countries. Approximately 600,000 deaths of under 5 year olds can be prevented by ensuring optimal complementary feeding (CF) (UNICEF, 2011). According to the Cambodian Demographic Health Survey (CDHS) 2010, 28.3% of children under 5 years old are underweight (more than 11 times the rate of a healthy population), and 39.9% of children are stunted (16 times higher than a healthy population). The CDHS results suggest that the sustained high food prices following the 2008 food price crisis may have caused

------

*Contributors: Ellen Muehlhoff, Ramani Wijesinha-Bettoni, Charity Dirorimwe and Koungry Ly
†Contact: ellen.muehlhoff@fao.org

stagnation in the improvement of both under-weight and stunting.

The critical window of opportunity for preventing undernutrition and micronutrient deficiencies is while a mother is pregnant and during a child's first 2 years of life (UNICEF, 2009). After this, it may be difficult to reverse the effects of poor nutrition on stunting, and some of the functional deficits may be permanent. Low-quality CF combined with inappropriate feeding practices and a lack of reliable information during this period have been identified as fundamental causes contributing to childhood nutritional inadequacy (Hotz and Gibson, 2005; Shi and Zhang, 2011; UNICEF, 2011). Growing attention is now given to the role of agriculture in improving nutrition, with recent programmes including the EU (European Union) Food Facility; the USAID (US Agency for International Development) Feed the Future initiative and the World Bank's Scaling Up Nutrition (SUN) Framework. Recent work in Malawi also supports the need for linking agricultural interventions with nutrition interventions (Bezner-Kerr et al., 2011).

CF interventions include nutritional education on CF practices, fortification or supplementation with micronutrients and various processing/preparation techniques for enhanced nutrient density and bioavailability. There is no single 'best approach' that can be universally applied, although in areas with a high prevalence of food insecurity, interventions that include the provision of additional food – and not just education – may be more effective (Dewey and Adu-Afarwuah, 2008). Educational interventions that include a strong emphasis on feeding nutrient-rich animal source foods may be more likely to show an effect on child growth. A food-based approach that promotes the use of a variety of nutrient-rich local foods may be more effective than programmes targeting individual nutrient deficiencies (Dewey and Adu-Afarwuah, 2008). Such an approach can be more sustainable in the longer term than programmes that rely on donor funding and the distribution of micronutrients or food supplements alone, as they are designed to empower local populations and limit dependency on external resources.

Educational interventions can effectively improve CF practices and thereby enhance child nutrition and growth (Shi and Zhang, 2011). The most effective educational interventions use a carefully selected, small number of specific key messages about practices that can feasibly be adopted by the target population, rather than general advice on child feeding (Dewey and Adu-Afarwuah, 2008). Ideally, the messages chosen should be based on a needs assessment and formative research with the target group in order to identify the practices most in need of improvement and amenable to change. Successful interventions are also culturally sensitive, accessible and integrated with local resources, as well as affordable and convenient for local families (Shi and Zhang, 2011). Researchers need to obtain a good understanding of how local people prepare CF and whether year-round local food supplies are sufficient to meet nutrient requirements. If possible, other family members and the community should be involved in order to create a supportive environment for facilitating and maintaining behaviour change (Shi and Zhang, 2011). It may also be necessary to pay attention to gender bias in interventions that require behaviour modification for improving child feeding practices (Bhandari et al., 2004). The costs to households and the public health system are further issues that should be considered.

Trials of Improved Practices (TIPs) Methodology

The Trials of Improved Practices (TIPs) methodology is a formative research technique used in programmes that promote behaviour change and was first used in the 1970s in nutrition programme design (Dickin et al., 1997; Manoff Group, 2005). TIPs are based on a process that uses several interactive information-gathering methods with mothers/key participants in a programme. The research follows an iterative process of trial and evaluation within the family setting. Figure 22.1 shows the steps involved in the TIPs implementation phase. The rest of this chapter describes an application of the TIPS methodology in Cambodia.

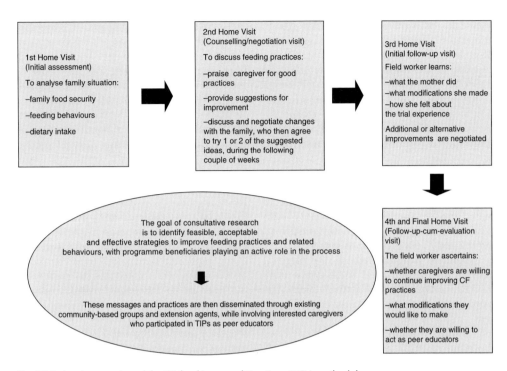

Fig. 22.1. Implementation of the Trials of Improved Practices (TIPs) methodology.

Description of Activities

Context and coverage

The FAO (Food and Agriculture Organization of the United Nations)/EU Food Facility (EUFF) Project 'Improving the Food Security of Farming Families Affected by Volatile Food Prices GCP/CMB/033/EC' (December 2009–June 2011) was aimed at improving food security (FS) through increased rice, vegetable and fish production in targeted households. The nutritional objectives of the project were to improve dietary diversity and family feeding practices, with a focus on infant and young child feeding (IYCF) between the ages of 6 and 23 months to prevent and address child undernutrition.

The TIPs field work was conducted in 356 households in nine provinces in Cambodia, covering two districts per province and two villages per district (Table 22.1).

Table 22.1. Sample sizes for a Trials of Improved Practices (TIPs) project with a focus on infant and young child feeding in 356 households in nine provinces in Cambodia.

Age group (months)	No. households		
	Southern provinces	Northern provinces	Total
0–6	26	44	70
7–8	48	35	83
9–11	45	52	97
12–24	39	67	106
Total	158	198	356

The TIPS process

Preparatory phase

Before conducting the TIPS field work, an Assessment and Counselling Guide was developed, agriculture extension, nutrition, health and community development staff were trained (99 facilitators from the

Ministries of Agriculture, Women's Affairs and Health) and the locations and age groups of children were identified. The facilitators received a 5 day training course that included the following: basic nutrition; IYCF recipe development (which included food preparation practicals and evaluating the acceptability of the IYCF dishes); the development of seasonal food availability and gender-based activity calendars; home-based nutrition counselling; and the process of implementing TIPs. The recipes used at this stage were from a provisional list developed by the national team after focus group discussions with households (HHs) in a few communities during the early TIPs preparatory phase.

Families with children in the targeted age groups were invited for a community mobilization (CM) meeting, after which interested families were enrolled for the TIPs process. A final selection was made after taking into account the socio-economic diversity of the community and, where possible, including families with visibly sick and/or malnourished children.

The CM also included a dialogue with the community on the types of foods produced or collected from nature, and the seasons when foods are available. This led to the development of a 'Seasonal food availability calendar (SFAC)' in four of the villages (Fig. 22.2), which allows the preparation of balanced CF and family meals based on seasonal food availability. The SFACs serve as a tool for creating awareness of FS and the nutritional challenges faced by target communities, provide opportunities for focused community action planning and facilitate stronger links between community action planning for FS enhancement and nutrition improvement initiatives.

Implementation phase

The TIPS implementation phase consisted of three home visits per household. During the initial visit, a dietary assessment was made and seasonal food availability and accessibility recorded. Based on the household assessment, a total of 15 rice-based, sweet potato/taro-based CF recipes enriched with a variety of readily available local foods

were developed. The basic CF recipes consisted of starchy food + (fish or eggs or groundnuts or meat) + green leafy vegetables + a small quantity of oil. Some of the issues considered at this stage included the WHO (World Health Organization) 'Indicators to assess adequacy of CF practices', which include a minimum list of food groups (≥4 food groups), seven recommended food groups, minimum age-appropriate meal frequency, the quantity of ingredients to use and the volume of cooked food. The latter was determined using both the WHO recommendations (WHO, 2000; PAHO/WHO, 2003) and an FAO-developed method for assessing the quantities of main ingredient (uncooked food consisting of cereal or sweet potato/taro) to use for one meal per child. The recipes were introduced to the households through community-based cooking sessions and were subsequently tested for acceptability and feasibility in home settings for 2 months (see below). In addition to the recipes, caregivers were strongly encouraged to complement the recipes with mashed fresh fruit/vegetables daily and to give CF with foods of animal origin at least two to three times a week.

During the second visit, feeding practices and problems were discussed. This included identifying and praising good practices already used, suggesting improvements for inappropriate practices – such as giving plain rice porridge with salt or with monosodium glutamate added (in relatively better-off HHs), and persuading the mother to select a few ideas to try out.

During the third visit, the feeding trials were evaluated to assess the extent to which households had adopted the nutritionally improved recipes, and to determine the constraints to adopting the practices and the motivating factors that encourage households to continue the improved practices. The motivating factors reported included child development benefits such as children being more alert and active, plus increasing in weight; children eating more and sleeping well; positive comments from neighbours who had observed improvements in children; and encouragement from health staff at outreach and clinic visits.

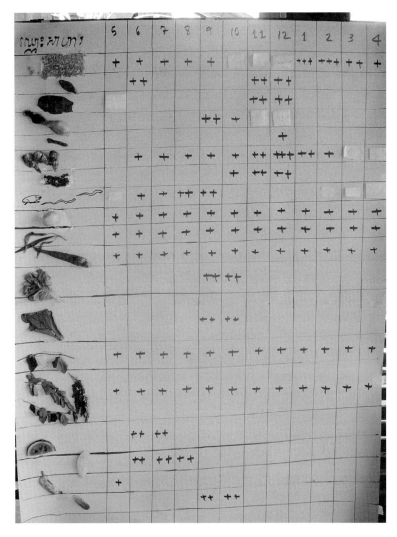

Fig. 22.2. A seasonal food availability calendar (SFAC) developed in the preparatory phase of the Trials of Improved Practices (TIPs) process in a study in Cambodia. The months are given in the top row of the figure. Availability is indicated by plus signs, with +++ indicating the peak season for a particular food.

Evaluation and dissemination phase

In this phase, the most acceptable and feasible CF practices and recipes resulting from the TIPs formative research were identified to be used for wider dissemination to the community. These recommendations were rolled out to 9000 households during the period January to 30 April 2011 through community nutrition promoters trained by the project.

Description of Results

The initial household assessment visit indicated that 78% of children under 6 months old were exclusively breastfed. Common feeding problems in this age group included giving water when the child was sick or too hot, and giving condensed milk or formula milk when the mother was not producing enough milk. The dietary variety was found to be poor for children aged 6–23 months (Fig. 22.3).

After the implementation of TIPs, there was a marked increase in the number of caregivers adding other food items such as fish or meat to plain *borbor* (a rice 'soup' or 'porridge') (Fig. 22.4). Other notable achievements are shown in Table 22.2. Some of the key challenges identified, together with possible solutions are shown in Table 22.3.

This project clearly demonstrates that significant changes in children's and families'

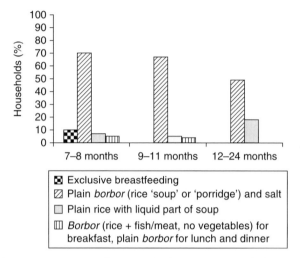

Fig. 22.3. Households participating in complementary feeding (CF) practices before the implementation of the Trials of Improved Practices (TIPs) process in a study of infants and young children in Cambodia.

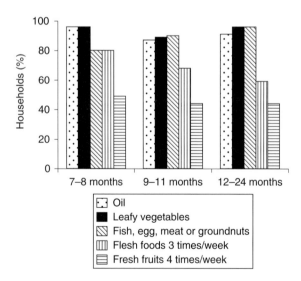

Fig. 22.4. Households participating in complementary feeding (CF) practices after the implementation of the Trials of Improved Practices (TIPs) process in a study of infants and young children in Cambodia. The process included participation in community mobilization cooking demonstrations and dietary counselling by TIPs facilitators. Data are presented on the percentages of households adding food items to *borbor* (plain rice 'soup' or 'porridge'); items included flesh foods (fish, meat) and leafy vegetables (morning glory – *Convolvulaceae* sp., ivy gourd, amaranth, etc.).

Table 22.2. Positive results on complementary feeding (CF) practices resulting from implementation of the Trials of Improved Practices (TIPs) process in a study of infants and young children in Cambodia.

Achievement	Evidence/other information
Families are keenly interested to learn about good diets and child feeding using local foods	Qualitative evidence
Greater dietary diversity, using local foods	Approximately 70% of households achieved better dietary diversity using available foods 3–5 times a week. Items in a child's diet increased from 2–3 food items to 12 or more
Total contribution of CF to child's diet met WHO (World Health Organization) recommendations for energy, protein, fat and vitamin A and zinc for children aged 6–11 months	In the majority of recipes, 30–45% of the energy came from fats and oils and 12–15% from proteins. Each recipe provides 37%, 54% and 67% of RDA (recommended dietary allowance) for energy for children aged 6-8, 9–11 and 12–24 months, respectively
Acquisition of knowledge and skills by mothers and caregivers	Most mothers showed a good understanding of the proportions of rice to fish or meat and the amount of oil and leafy vegetables to add when preparing CF relative to the recommended amounts
Empowerment of mothers	Development of skills and confidence of mothers via dietary counselling and participatory cooking demonstrations held at the initial community mobilization meeting
Information sharing with non-participants: good potential for peer education by TIPs households	Some caregivers voluntarily encouraged 1–2 friends, neighbours or relatives to adopt CF practices
Mothers continued feeding improved CFs, even after TIPs completed	Mothers changed their cooking and purchasing patterns
Promoting local food resources can be an effective strategy for improving child feeding, preventing and addressing moderate malnutrition	Mothers of sick/malnourished children tried a wider variety of recipes and were enthusiastic to continue

diets can be achieved using a comprehensive food-based approach. Furthermore, families were empowered to feed their children and themselves using locally available food sources, which is a sustainable approach. Some mothers applied the concept and even developed their own recipes to provide more diversity for their children.

Finally, the success of the project can be attributed to three key features: (i) institutional collaboration – dedication and commitment from government partners in three line ministries (Women's Affairs, Agriculture and Health); (ii) the fact that it was built on existing community-based organizations, which are useful as a platform for wider dissemination of positive nutrition messages and for fostering behavioural changes for longer term sustainability by creating support networks at community level; and (iii) community mobilization

meetings (which involved cooking demonstrations) and led to increased awareness of locally available foods and the adoption of improved cooking technology, such as fuel-efficient stoves.

Future Plans

Although the available evidence suggests that household food security combined with intensive nutrition education can translate into improvements in dietary intake, nutritional status and child growth, further rigorous scientific research that records dietary intake, child growth and micronutrient status, and measures the impact on child growth is needed. Such evidence will be particularly important for future programmes and policy development to confidently advocate for food and dietary strategies to address child undernutrition.

Table 22.3. Challenges and possible solutions in complementary feeding (CF) practices resulting from implementation of the Trials of Improved Practices (TIPs) process in a study of infants and young children in Cambodia.

Challenges	Possible solutions
Major constraints families face are seasonal food availability and affordable sources of micronutrient-rich foods (particularly fish, aquatic species and fresh fruit)	Combine dietary counselling with targeted and responsive food security (FS) actions aimed at increasing locally available, nutrient dense foods, as in the following proposals: although the aquaculture component of the current project benefits households with access to fish ponds, future programmes should also focus on developing poultry production; the current agricultural component included vegetables but not fruit production. Future programmes should include early maturing fruit trees, such as papaya
Families complained of time constraints in preparing improved CF on a daily basis, particular in seasons where mothers are busy working on the rice fields	The possibility of supplying parents with ready-to-eat foods (or RUTFs) prepared locally, using locally available ingredients, needs to be carefully considered for future programmes
Meeting the zinc requirements (for children aged 12–24 months) and iron requirements for all children ≤24 months remains a challenge	The production of and access to fish and aquatic species, poultry and fresh fruits needs to be improved
	Complementary solutions are needed, including fortification of appropriate foods with nutrients that are the most limiting in children's diets
How to successfully scale up the intervention	Messages chosen for broad dissemination will need modification to be specific to the setting (Daelmans et al., 2009)
	It is necessary to make use of existing delivery platforms and local communication channels to implement the interventions and ensure greater sustainability over time (Dewey and Adu-Afarwuah, 2008; Daelmans et al., 2009; Shi and Zhang, 2011)
Having well-trained field staff will be crucial for success	Provide longer training in basic nutrition and simpler TIPs tools for field staff
	Provide refresher training

The German government has funded a research project (GCP/INT/108/GER) to study the impact of CF interventions for children 6–23 months of age in two countries, Malawi and Cambodia, starting in January 2011 over the next 4 years. The research will be conducted within the context of existing FAO FS and nutrition programmes in these countries, in partnership with the Justus-Liebig-University of Giessen, Germany.

The objectives of this project are to document: (i) the effectiveness of TIPs for generating sustainable feeding recommendations and recipes that result in better dietary intakes and nutritional status; (ii) the extent to which locally available and affordable foods can meet the nutritional requirements of children aged 6–23 months; (iii) the effectiveness and impact of combining behaviour change communication with crop and dietary diversification; and (iv) the extent to which improved complementary feeding practices will be sustained over time and can be replicated and scaled up through local delivery and support mechanisms. The research findings will be widely disseminated and contribute to informing nutrition policy and programme design in developing countries.

References

Bezner-Kerr, R., Berti, P.R. and Shumba, L. (2011) Effects of a participatory agriculture and nutrition education project on child growth in northern Malawi. *Public Health Nutrition* 14, 1466–1472.

Bhandari, N., Mazumder, S., Bahl, S., Martines, J., Black, R.E., Bhan, M.K. and Infant Feeding Study Group (2004) An educational intervention to promote appropriate complementary feeding practices and physical growth in infants and young children in rural Haryana, India. *Journal of Nutrition* 134, 2342–2348.

Daelmans, B., Mangasaryan, N., Martines, J., Saadeh, R., Casanovas, C. and Arabi, M. (2009) Strengthening actions to improve feeding of infants and young children 6 to 23 months of age: Summary of a recent World Health Organization/UNICEF technical meeting, Geneva, 6–9 October 2008. *Food and Nutrition Bulletin* 30(2 Suppl.), S236–S238.

Dewey, K.G. and Adu-Afarwuah, S. (2008) Systematic review of the efficacy and effectiveness of complementary feeding interventions in developing countries. *Maternal and Child Nutrition* 4(Suppl. 1), 24–85.

Dickin, K., Griffiths, M. and Piwoz, E. (1997) *Designing by Dialogue: A Program Planner's Guide to Consultative Research for Improving Young Child Feeding: Support for Analysis and Research in Africa*. Prepared by the Manoff Group and Academy for Educational Development (AED) with support by the USAID Bureau for Africa's Health and Human Resources Analysis for Africa (HHRAA) Project through the Support for Analysis and Research in Africa (SARA) contract AOT-0483-C-2178-00. Available from SARA, AED, Washington, DC. Available at: http://www.globalhealthcommunication.org/tool_docs/58/designing_by_dialogue_-_full_text.pdf (accessed 24 June 2012).

Hotz, C. and Gibson, R. (2005) Participatory nutrition education and adoption of new feeding practices are associated with improved adequacy of complementary diets among rural Malawian children: a pilot study. *European Journal of Clinical Nutrition* 59, 226–237.

Manoff Group (2005) *Trials of Improved Practices (TIPs): Giving Participants a Voice in Program Design*. Washington, DC. Available at: http://www.manoffgroup.com/resources/summarytips.pdf (accessed 24 June 2012).

PAHO/WHO (2003) *Guiding Principles for Complementary Feeding of the Breastfed Child*. Pan American Health Organization, Washington, DC and World Health Organization, Geneva, Switzerland. Available at: http://www.who.int/nutrition/publications/guiding_principles_compfeeding_breastfed.pdf (accessed 24 June 2012).

Shi, L. and Zhang, J. (2011) Recent evidence of the effectiveness of educational interventions for improving complementary feeding practices in developing countries *Journal of Tropical Pediatrics* 57, 91–98.

UNICEF (2009) *Tracking Progress on Child and Maternal Nutrition: A Survival and Development Priority*. United Nations Children's Fund, New York. Available at: http://www.unicef.pt/docs/Progress_on_Child_and_Maternal_Nutrition_EN_110309.pdf (accessed 24 June 2012).

UNICEF (2011) Nutrition: Complementary Feeding. United Nations Children's Fund, New York. Available at: http://www.unicef.org/nutrition/index_24826.html (accessed 24 June 2012).

WHO (2000) *Complementary Feeding. Family Foods for Breastfed Children*. World Health Organization, Geneva, Switzerland. Available at: http://whqlibdoc.who.int/hq/2000/WHO_NHD_00.1.pdf (accessed 24 June 2012).

23 Activities of the Animal Production and Health Division (AGA) of FAO to Improve Food and Nutrition Security

**Animal Production and Health Division (AGA),*† Agriculture and
Consumer Protection Department (AG)**
Food and Agriculture Organization of the United Nations, Rome, Italy

---

Summary

Livestock have multiple important roles and functions, including their direct contribution to food availability and access for smallholders. Livestock products are major sources of protein, micronutrients (iron, zinc, calcium, vitamins B_{12}, A and riboflavin) and fats. They are particularly important for poorly nourished people and infants in developing countries. At a global level, the livestock sector is undergoing unprecedented changes due to increased demands for foods derived from animals, especially in the urban areas of the rapidly growing economies. This is placing increasing pressures on natural resources. The changes in the livestock sector have significantly outpaced the capacity of governments and societies to provide the necessary policy and regulatory framework. The Animal Production and Health Division of FAO takes an active role in identifying the drivers of the sector as well as the risks and policy options for enhancing food security and peoples' livelihoods and health while, at the same time, protecting the environment.

Introduction

The Food and Agriculture Organization of the United Nations (FAO) published its flagship *The State of Food and Agriculture: Livestock in the Balance* in 2009 (also known as the SOFA report; FAO, 2009). New challenges faced by the global food and agriculture sector due to demographic and dietary changes, climate change, bioenergy developments and natural resource constraints are extensively addressed therein. The livestock sector has developed as one of the most dynamic parts of the agricultural economy. Globally, the sector has been undergoing unprecedented changes due to the booming demand for foods derived from animals, especially in the urban areas of the rapidly growing economies. The 'livestock revolution' reflects the increase in production and consumption of animals and their products, increasingly produced by commercial livestock production and the associated food chains. At the same time, millions of rural people still keep livestock in traditional production systems, where they support livelihoods and household food security.

The rapid growth and transformation of the livestock sector has often taken place in

---

*Contributors: Katinka de Balogh, Daniela Battaglia and Samuel Zombou
†Contact: katinka.debalogh@fao.org

an institutional void. The speed of change has significantly outpaced the capacity of governments and societies to provide the necessary policy and regulatory framework to ensure an appropriate balance between the provision of private and public goods. The result has been systemic failures, apparent in widespread environmental damage and threats to human and animal health, and in social exclusion. The Animal Production and Health Division of FAO takes an active role in identifying the drivers of the sector as well as the risks and policy options for enhancing food security and people's livelihoods and health, while protecting the environment.

Change in the Livestock Sector

Rapid growth and technological innovation have led to structural changes in the livestock sector, including: a move from smallholder mixed farms towards large-scale specialized industrial production systems; a shift in the geographic locus of demand and supply to the developing world; and an increasing emphasis on global sourcing and marketing. These changes have implications for the ability of the livestock sector to expand production sustainably in ways that promote food security, poverty reduction and public health.

Consumption trends and drivers of proteins of animal origin in the world

The consumption of livestock products has increased rapidly in developing countries over the past decades. Since the early 1960s, the consumption of milk per capita in developing countries has almost doubled, meat consumption has more than tripled and egg consumption has increased fivefold. This has translated into considerable growth in global per capita intake of energy derived from livestock products, but with significant regional differences. Consumption has increased in all regions except sub-Saharan Africa. Also, the former centrally planned economies of Eastern Europe and Central Asia saw major declines around 1990. The greatest increases have occurred in East and South-east Asia and in Latin America and the Caribbean.

The growing demand for livestock products in a number of developing countries has been driven by economic growth, rising per capita incomes and urbanization. In recent decades, the global economy has experienced an unparalleled expansion, with per capita incomes rising rapidly. These rises, together with population growth and urbanization, are the driving forces behind a growing demand for meat products in developing countries. To meet rising demand, global annual meat production is expected to expand from the present 228 million tonnes (mt) to 463 mt by 2050, with cattle population estimated to grow from 1.5 billion to 2.6 billion and that of goats and sheep from 1.7 billion to 2.7 billion.

Production trends and drivers of proteins of animal origin in the world

Developing countries have responded to the growing demand for livestock products by rapidly increasing production. Between 1961 and 2007, the greatest growth in meat production occurred in East and South-east Asia, followed by Latin America and the Caribbean. Most of the expansion in egg production was in East and South-east Asia, while in South Asia milk production dominated.

Supply-side factors have enabled expansion in livestock production. Cheap inputs, technological change and efficiency gains in recent decades have resulted in declining prices for livestock products. This has improved access to animal-based foods even for those consumers whose incomes have not risen.

Favourable long-term trends in input prices (e.g. feed grain and fuel) have played an important role. Declining grain prices have contributed to increased use of grains as feed and downward trends in transportation costs have facilitated the movement not only of livestock products but also of feed. Recent

increases in grain and energy prices may signal the end of the era of cheap inputs.

Proteins of Animal Origin Contributing to Human Nutrition and Health

Globally, livestock contributes 15% of total
food energy and 25% of dietary protein.
Products from livestock provide essential
micronutrients that are not easily obtained
from plant food products.

Consumption varies very much in different countries, and in less developed economies, the deficit of highly valuable protein of
animal origin, and its consequences in terms
of human health and development, are still
unacceptable. In *The Hungry Planet: What the
World Eats* (Menzel and D'Alusio, 2005), Peter
Menzel presents food consumption data
and photographs from 24 different countries
(30 families) over a 5 year period; 25 of these
photographs have been reproduced on the
Time web site (see Menzel, 2008). Families
representative of each country are depicted
with the food normally consumed in the
course of a week. This illustrates the great
variability of weekly expenditure on food
in different parts of the world.

Livestock products are major sources of
protein, micronutrients (iron, zinc, calcium,
vitamins B_{12}, A and riboflavin) and fats. They
are especially important for poorly nourished
people and infants in developing countries.
Globally, ~4-5 billion people in the world are
deficient in iron. This and other important
nutrients (e.g. vitamin B_{12} and A, zinc and calcium), are readily available in meat, milk and
eggs, but they are not so easily obtained from
plant foods. Negative health outcomes associated with inadequate intake of these nutrients include anaemia, stunted child growth,
rickets, impaired cognitive abilities, blindness, neuromuscular deficits and – in severe
cases – death.

Liver and eggs are an important source
of vitamin A; they help to prevent blindness
or poor vision due to poor nutrition and contribute to building a strong immune system.
Zinc, which is readily available from red
meat and the darker parts of chicken meat, is

essential for strengthening the immune system, providing protection and promoting
recovery from infectious diseases, including
diarrhoea.

Current consumption patterns of animal
source foods in much of the developed world
exceed nutritional needs, and increase the
risk of heart disease, certain types of cancer,
stroke and diabetes.

Contribution of Animal Production to Livelihoods, Food Security and Poverty Reduction

Contribution of animal production to livelihoods

Livestock are central to the livelihoods of the
poor. Over a billion poor people depend on
livestock for their livelihoods and 60% of rural
households keep livestock. Livestock have
multiple important roles and functions, including: the provision of employment to the farmer
and family members; their roles as a store of
wealth and as a form of insurance; their contribution to gender equality by generating
opportunities for women; their contribution
to recycling waste products and residues
from cropping or agro-industries; their role in
improving the structure and fertility of soil;
and their role in controlling insects and weeds.
Livestock manure can also serve as an energy
source for cooking and in contributing to food
security. Livestock also have a cultural significance – ownership may form the basis for the
observation of religious customs or for establishing the status of the farmer.

Strong demand for animal food products
offers significant opportunities for livestock
to contribute to economic growth and poverty reduction. However, many smallholders
are facing several challenges in remaining
competitive with larger, more intensive production systems. FAO recommends that
smallholders be supported in taking advantage of the opportunities provided by an
expanding livestock sector and in managing
the risks associated with increasing competition. Broader rural development strategies

creating off-farm jobs should help those that may be unable to adapt and compete in a rapidly modernizing sector. According to the 2009 SOFA report, policy makers also need to recognize and protect the safety net function of livestock for the very poor.

Contribution of animal production to food security

Malnutrition remains a persistent problem in many developing countries. The latest FAO statistics indicate that nearly a billion people in the world are undernourished.

Livestock contribute directly to food availability and access for smallholders, often in complex ways. Smallholders sometimes consume their home production directly, but they often choose to sell high-value eggs or milk in order to buy lower cost staple foods. The indirect role of livestock in supporting food security through income growth and poverty reduction is crucial to overall development efforts.

Contribution of animal production to poverty reduction

Most rural households, including the very poor, keep livestock. Expanding markets for livestock products would appear to offer opportunities for improving the incomes of the many rural poor who depend on livestock for their livelihoods. However, while the growth and transformation of the sector have created opportunities, the degree to which these can be harnessed by people living in poverty and in marginalized areas is not clear.

Animal Production and Environmental Health

Animal production, environment and climate change

Livestock production is placing increasing pressures on natural resources – land, air, water and biodiversity. Corrective action is needed to encourage the provision of public goods such as valuable ecosystem services and environmental protection. This will involve addressing policy and market failures and developing and applying appropriate incentives and penalties. Livestock contribute to and are victims of climate change. The sector can play a key role in mitigating climate change. For example, adoption of improved technologies, encouraged by appropriate economic incentives, can lead to reduced emissions of greenhouse gases by livestock.

Animal health

Some animal health services are public goods in that they protect human and animal public health and thus benefit society as a whole. Animal diseases reduce production and productivity, disrupt local and national economies, threaten human health and exacerbate poverty. Animal health systems have been neglected in many parts of the world, leading to institutional weaknesses and information gaps as well as to inadequate investments in animal health-related public goods. Producers at every level, including poor livestock keepers, must be engaged in the prevention of animal disease.

Animal Production and the Animal Health Division of FAO

The mission of the Division (http://www.fao.org/ag/againfo/home/en/index.htm) is to assist FAO members to take full advantage of the contribution that the rapidly growing and transforming livestock sector can make towards the achievement of the Millennium Development Goals (MDGs). In addition, facilitating the participation of smallholder livestock farmers in the increasingly competitive market for livestock commodities can contribute to food security, improved human nutrition and the safeguarding of animal and public health, the maintenance of animal genetic diversity and the minimization of the environmental impact of livestock production. Such participation can also respond to various other societal needs, such as gender equity, animal welfare, occupational health and safety, etc. The Division works closely with governments, producers and the civil society to increase the productivity of animal source foods, enhance veterinary public health and food safety, tackle environmental and climate change, support animal welfare and protect natural resources. Themes that are addressed relate to animal production (income generation, livelihood) and reducing animal-related human health risks.

References

FAO (2009) *The State of Food and Agriculture: Livestock in the Balance*. Food and Agriculture Organization, Rome. Available at: http://www.fao.org/docrep/012/i0680e/i0680e00.htm (accessed 24 June 2013).

Menzel, P. (2005) What the World Eats. Part I, Part II. What's on family dinner tables around the globe? Photographs by Peter Menzel from the book *"Hungry Planet"*. *Time* Photos. Available at: http://www.time.com/time/photogallery/0,29307,1626519,00.html and http://www.time.com/time/photogallery/0,29307,1645016,00.html (accessed 24 June 2013).

Menzel, P. and D'Aluisio, F. (2005) *The Hungry Planet: What the World Eats*. Material World Books, Napa and Ten Speed Press, Berkeley, California.

24 The Role of the Plant Production and Protection Division (AGP) of FAO in Supporting Crop Diversification for Sustainable Diets and Nutrition

Plant Production and Protection Division (AGP),*† Agriculture and Consumer Protection Department (AG)
Food and Agriculture Organization of the United Nations, Rome, Italy

---

Summary

FAO's Plant Production and Protection Division (AGP) works to strengthen global food security by promoting sustainable crop production intensification (SCPI), which aims at producing more from an area of land while at the same time conserving resources, reducing negative impacts on the environment and enhancing natural capital and the flow of ecosystem services. The basic concept is the integration and harmonization of appropriate crop production practices, technologies and policies in order to increase crop productivity in a sustainable manner, thereby meeting the key Millennium Development Goals of reducing hunger and preserving natural resources and the environment for future generations. AGP also supports crop diversification for sustainable diets, nutritional health and income generation, and supports the global food economy through the implementation of international treaties. The focus of AGP's activities is to enhance and strengthen: (i) effective and strategic decisions that increase crop production using an ecosystem approach and nutrition-sensitive crop diversification; (ii) national capacities to monitor and to respond effectively to transboundary and other important outbreak pests; (iii) policies and technologies appropriate to needs of members to reduce negative impact of pesticides; and (iv) conservation and sustainable use of plant genetic resources with strong linkages between conservation, plant breeding and seed sector development. Most of AGP's activities related to supporting improved diets and increased nutrition in developing countries focus on horticulture and high-value crops. That said, there are active linkages among AGP teams that facilitate interdisciplinary activities. AGP collaborates closely with other FAO Divisions and external partners in interdisciplinary activities, such as nutrition, food quality and safety, post-harvest processes, food losses and waste, economics and policy.

---

*Contributors: NeBambi Lutaladio, Marjon Fredrix, Alison Hodder, Remi NonoWomdim and Wilfried Baudoin
†Contact: nebambi.lutaladio@fao.org

Description of the Activities of the Division

Overview of AGP operations

AGP technical operations support the achievement of FAO's Strategic Objective A, Sustainable intensification of crop production, which is composed of four Organizational Results (ORs):

- A1 – Policies and strategies on sustainable crop production intensification and diversification at national and regional levels.
- A2 – Risks from outbreaks of transboundary plant pests and diseases sustainably reduced at national, regional and global levels.
- A3 – Risks from pesticides sustainably reduced at national, regional and global levels.
- A4 – Effective policies and enabled capacities for better management of plant genetic resources for food and agriculture, including seed systems at national and regional levels.

In the new FAO strategic framework, AGP's work related to improving diets and improving nutrition – in the context of crop production and food security – is included in OR-A1 under two Organizational Outputs, namely:

- A01G201 – Evidence-based support tools and instruments for sustainable crop production intensification, through an ecosystem approach.
- A01G202 – Enhanced capacity of members to implement sustainable crop production intensification and diversification strategies for health and improved livelihoods.

The Division's work is summarized in a publication that describes its role that was published in 2012 (FAO, 2012a).

Current efforts place emphasis on smallholder production units for: (i) promoting high-value horticultural crops for health, nutrition and income in rural, urban and peri-urban areas in line with quality and safety standards; (ii) developing and testing policy tools and approaches to assist countries in developing their horticulture sector; and (iii) supporting 'Growing Greener Cities' strategies to address the challenges of rapid urbanization by promoting horticulture-based activities as a contribution to improved food and nutrition security, sustainable diets and nutritionally diverse crops, and better livelihoods for the urban population.

Diversification of smallholder crop production is a crucial step in agricultural development. Broadening production to include horticulture and high-value crops allows smallholders to diversify sources of food in local diets and enter domestic markets for higher value products. It also strengthens resilience to economic and climate risks. Diversified production can help to improve nutrition, strengthen livelihoods, create opportunities for local agro-processing, generate employment along the value chain and stimulate rural economic development.

As part of an FAO nutrition-sensitive food systems approach, FAO programmes for crop diversification include among their goals improvements in the nutritional health status of low-income households through increased production of nutrient-rich foods for both direct consumption and generation of the income needed to procure the amount and variety of food that families need. Among nutritionally vulnerable households, especially those with limited land, one of the most effective diversification strategies is homestead food production. By employing household labour intensively on small vegetable gardens and fruit tree plots, homestead production improves the quality of family nutrient intake, while allowing women to fulfil domestic and childcare roles. With extension support, facilitated access to land, credit and markets, and economies of scale achieved through the organization of women in groups, homestead programmes can also generate incomes that women control, leading to better child nutrition and health, sustainable livelihoods and community development.

Growing horticultural crops increases the supply of fresh, nutritious produce and improves poor peoples' economic access to food when their household production reduces their food bills and when growers earn a living from sales. Access to nutritious food is a key dimension of food security. In Africa and Asia, urban households spend up to 80% of their food budgets on cheap 'convenience' foods that are often deficient in vitamins and minerals. Horticultural foods, such as fruits, vegetables and nuts, are important for the daily diet and are among the richest natural sources of micronutrients – they provide dietary fibre, vegetable proteins and other bioactive components.

However, in developing countries, daily fruit and vegetables consumption is just 20–50% of the Food and Agriculture Organization of the United Nations/World Health Organization (FAO/WHO) recommendations. An FAO/WHO expert consultation in 2004 on diet, nutrition and the prevention of chronic diseases recommended a daily intake of no less than 400 g of fruit and vegetables (excluding potatoes and other starchy tubers) to prevent heart disease, cancer, diabetes and obesity (FAO/WHO, 2005). That level of intake can also prevent morbidity and mortality caused by micronutrient deficiencies, including birth defects, mental and physical retardation, weakened immune systems, blindness and even death. Dietary diversification through horticulture-based food intake, therefore, is a sustainable approach to fighting micronutrient malnutrition in both developed and developing countries.

AGP activities relating to sustainable diets, nutritional health and improved livelihoods

Growing Greener Cities – contributing to urban food and nutrition security

Towns and cities in the world's developing countries are growing on an unprecedented scale. Poor urban households spend up to 80% of their income on food. That makes them highly vulnerable when food prices rise or their incomes fall.

To help developing countries meet the challenges of massive and rapid urbanization, FAO/AGP launched a multidisciplinary initiative, 'Growing Greener Cities' (GGC),

under its Programme for Urban and Peri-urban Horticulture (UPH) (FAO, 2010a, 2013). This initiative aims at ensuring the access of urban populations to safe, good-quality horticultural produce and to healthy and secure environments. GGC helps governments and city administrations to optimize policies, institutional frameworks and support services for UPH, to improve production and marketing systems and to enhance the horticulture value chain.

Urban and peri-urban horticulture helps developing cities to meet challenges related to sustainable diets and nutrition. First, it boosts the physical supply of fresh, nutritious produce that is available year round. Secondly, it improves the economic access of the urban poor to food when their household production of fruit and vegetables reduces their food bills and when growers earn a living from sales.

A survey has been conducted that compiled information from some 40 countries for the first status report on UPH in Africa: *Growing Greener Cities in Africa: First Status Report on Urban and Peri-urban Horticulture in Africa* (FAO, 2012b). This document is a decision support tool that will assist countries in optimizing policies, institutional frameworks and support services for UPH. It was produced as part of the GGC initiative supported by policy makers in Africa.

Promotion of fruit and vegetables initiative for health

The 'Global Fruit and Vegetables for Health Initiative' (GF&VH Initiative) and the 'Kobe Framework for Action' were established by FAO and WHO in 2004 to guide the development of cost-effective and effective interventions for the promotion of adequate consumption of fruit and vegetables for health (FAO/WHO, 2005). These have led to a series of regional workshops to promote and support implementation of fruit and vegetable programmes at national or subnational levels in developing countries.

In this process, national or local production capacities, traditional agricultural and dietary practices, prevailing patterns of nutrition, the health status of the population and existing fruit and vegetable promotion programmes are being taken into consideration.

The framework includes the following general principles:

- Availability.
- Accessibility.
- Affordability.
- Acceptability – quality, taste, safety, type of food, cultural sensitivity.
- Equity – including the underprivileged.

These serve to appropriately tailor fruit and vegetable promotion programmes to target group(s).

In 2011, an initiative for Promotion of Fruit and Vegetables for Health (PROFAV) was endorsed by 22 English-speaking African countries in order to promote nutrition-sensitive agriculture and a horticultural crop-based approach for improving diets (PROFAV, 2011). The initiative aims at mapping existing national policies and programmes, documenting production and consumption, supporting programme development and strengthening cooperation among health, education and agriculture sectors. Under PROFAV, the integration of efforts involving stakeholders in the horticulture, nutrition, health and education sectors is considered essential for the effective promotion of fruit and vegetables (F&V) for health. There is also need for joint efforts between the public and private sectors in commercializing and modernizing horticulture. While promotion of F&V has long been part of general nutrition education, there is now a need to focus on promoting their availability and consumption. The importance of advocacy, information and community education in changing negative attitudes to the consumption of F&V is now well recognized.

School gardens

School gardens are found in many countries, in different forms and sizes, and with varying aims. In most cases, the school garden is an area of land within the school grounds or nearby. Vegetables, flowers, medicinal plants, trees, bushes and many other plants are usually grown. Occasionally, small animals – such as ducks, rabbits, chickens, goats and even fish – are also kept. In cities where schools have limited space or lack open space, the school garden can consist of plants grown in containers. Although the term 'school garden' embraces a variety of gardening and agricultural elements, these gardens usually have two things in common:

- Schoolchildren actively help parents and other interested community members in creating and maintaining the garden.
- Schoolchildren use the garden – for learning, for recreation and by eating what is harvested.

School gardens are a proven means of promoting child nutrition. They familiarize children with horticulture, provide fresh fruit and vegetables for healthy school meals, help teachers to develop nutrition courses and, when replicated at home, improve family nutrition as well. Over the past 10 years, FAO/AGP, in collaboration with FAO's Nutrition Division (AGN), has provided tools, seeds and training to establish thousands of school gardens in more than 30 countries.

Impact Indicators and Highlights of Achievements

The Growing Greener Cities for urban and peri-urban horticulture initiative

Brief descriptions are given of three GGH for UPH initiatives:

- A project for development of UPH in five cities in the Democratic Republic of Congo (DRC) is helping to grow 150,000 t of vegetables a year, supply fresh, nutritious produce to 11.5 million urban residents, build sustainable livelihoods for 16,000 small-scale market gardeners, and generate jobs and income for 60,000 people in the horticulture value chain (FAO, 2010b).
- Based on the information disseminated and exchange of experiences gained in multiple cities, several countries have perceived the need to formulate a GGC strategy in order to secure the integration

of UPH into city development plans (e.g. Botswana, Egypt, Afghanistan, Madagascar and Tanzania) and expressed a need for assistance. Countries that have already formulated a GGC strategy and related action plan have strengthened their institutional frameworks by establishing national UPH units at the level of the Ministry of Agriculture, and at the decentralized level in municipalities, e.g. the DRC, Rwanda, Burundi.

- Donor funding has been mobilized to support GGC–UPH initiatives, also through decentralized cooperation (e.g. Italy for Rwanda and Senegal; France for Madagascar and Egypt; Spain and the United Nations Development Programme (UNDP) for Mozambique and Afghanistan; the African Development Bank for DRC and the World Bank for Congo).

The Fruit and Vegetable Health Initiative: strengthening capacities

An outline is given of three initiatives under the GF&VH programme:

- Cameroon and Niger have adopted policies and strategies on crop diversification, including National Horticulture Master Plans. In Central and South America, the exchange of experience and lessons learned in seven countries served as the basis for defining models to assist other countries in the implementation of urban and peri-urban agriculture/horticulture programmes.
- Several countries are in the process of establishing multidisciplinary platforms (agriculture, health/nutrition and education) and formulating a National Horticulture Development Master Plan with emphasis on the role of fruit and vegetables in a sustainable diet for health, and with due attention to gender dimensions.
- The exchange of expertise and networking among developing countries has allowed the strengthening of national capacities (e.g. Bolivia and Mozambique;

Egypt and Afghanistan; DRC and Burundi; and DRC and Guinea) with inputs from scientific institutions and universities (e.g. Polytechnic of Milan in Senegal; University of Bologna in Côte d'Ivoire).

School, home, community and micro-gardens

Three of these projects are described:

- In the El Alto municipality of La Paz, AGP supported a micro-gardens programme for low-income families. Some 1500 households were trained in the organic cultivation of fruits, vegetables and herbs in small low-cost greenhouse units measuring 40 m^2. The units provide fresh vegetables all year round for home consumption and sale through neighbourhood markets. The result was a general improvement in child nutrition and family savings (averaging US$30/month), which were spent on eggs and meat.
- A project launched in 2010 in Nicaragua aims to create in and around the capital, Managua, 500 micro-gardens and 12 demonstration and training centres in neighbourhoods and schools. In collaboration with Nicaragua's Institute of Agricultural Technology, it provides drip irrigation systems and training in intensive vegetable production for low-income beneficiaries, which are expected to number 9500. To ensure the sustainability of the project, beneficiaries will also be trained in operating and maintaining UPH infrastructure, including low-cost greenhouses and tunnel seedling nurseries, and in monitoring the quality of rainwater collected for use in irrigation.
- In collaboration with the Ministry of Agriculture in Senegal, FAO/AGP has helped to introduce micro-garden technology and start community gardening centres in low-income areas of Dakar and the neighbouring city of Pikine. More than 4000 urban residents, most of them women, have started micro-gardens,

which produce on average 30 kg/m^2 of vegetables a year, enough to satisfy family needs and provide a surplus for sale. In 2008, the micro-gardens programme won UN-HABITAT's Dubai Award for Best Practice to Improve the Living Environment. The US$30,000 prize is being used to consolidate and expand the programme.

Future Plans

AGP will continue to work on the three action areas outlined above. Further discussions with AGN will be useful to identify how current work on sustainable diets and nutrition security can be integrated more efficiently and be better reflected in the three areas, as well as in other AGP initiatives. To have an impact on nutrition, AGP needs to work with AGN to identify deficits in local diets and micronutrient intakes, and understand the motivations and constraints that determine household consumption decisions.

In summary, future activities on crop diversification should have a specific focus on sustainable diets in the context of nutrition-sensitive agriculture and the development of normative guidelines, tools and indicators to characterize and measure sustainable diets in different agro-ecological zones. Following the success of international meetings in Cameroon, Senegal and Tanzania, global initiatives in horticulture will continue, in partnership with WHO and regional bodies such as NEPAD (The New Partnership for Africa's Development), on rural, urban and peri-urban horticulture and on the relationship between production and nutritional outcomes.

References

FAO (2010a) *Growing Greener Cities*. Food and Agriculture Organization, Rome. Available at: http://www.fao.org/ag/agp/greenercities/pdf/GGC-en.pdf (accessed 25 June 2013).

FAO (2010b) *Growing Greener Cities in the Democratic Republic of the Congo*. Food and Agriculture Organization, Rome. Available at: http://www.fao.org/docrep/013/i1901e/i1901e00.pdf (accessed 25 June 2013).

FAO (2012a) *Crop Diversification for Sustainable Diets and Nutrition: The Role of FAO's Plant Production and Protection Division*. Food and Agriculture Organization, Rome. Available at: http://www.fao.org/ag/agp/greenercities/pdf/CDSDN.pdf (accessed 25 June 2013).

FAO (2012b) *Growing Greener Cities in Africa: First Status Report on Urban and Peri-urban Horticulture in Africa*. Food and Agriculture Organization, Rome. Available at: http://www.fao.org/docrep/016/i3002e/i3002e.pdf (accessed 25 June 2013).

FAO (2013) *Urban and Peri-urban Horticulture: Projects*. Available at: http://www.fao.org/ag/agp/greenercities/en/projects/index.html (accessed 25 June 2013).

FAO/WHO (2005) *Fruit and Vegetables for Health. Report of a Joint FAO/WHO Workshop, 1–3 September 2004, Kobe, Japan*. World Health Organization, Geneva, Switzerland and Food and Agriculture Organization, Rome. Available at: http://www.fao.org/ag/magazine/FAO-WHO-FV.pdf (accessed 25 June 2013).

PROFAV (2011) *PROFAV 2011: Promotion of Fruit and Vegetables for Health. Anglophone Africa Regional Workshop on Promotion of Fruit and Vegetables for Health, Mount Meru Hotel, Arusha, Tanzania, 26–30 September, 2011: General Report, Conclusions and Recommendations*. Food and Agriculture Organization, Rome. Available at: ftp://ftp.fao.org/ag/agp/docs/PROFAV_Arusha_092011.pdf (accessed 25 June 2013).

25 Impact of the Work of the Rural Infrastructure and Agro-Industries Division (AGS) of FAO on Improving Food and Nutrition Security

Rural Infrastructure and Agro-Industries Division (AGS),*[†]
Agriculture and Consumer Protection Department (AG)
Food and Agriculture Organization of the United Nations, Rome, Italy

---

Summary

Halving the number of people who suffer from hunger by 2015 is a key challenge of the Millennium Development Goals (MDGs). In efforts to achieve this goal, emphasis has been placed by many development programmes on promoting agro-enterprise development, product value addition and food processing. The Rural Infrastructure and Agro-Industries Division (AGS) of FAO has long adopted this approach. It works in collaboration with members to address their specific needs related to food and agro-industry development through the provision of advisory support, technical information and capacity-building activities. This may be illustrated with a recently ended project in Swaziland entitled 'Promotion of Community Based Agro-Processing'. The project sought to build the capacity of rural communities to process safe, nutritious, quality food products, with the objective of enhancing their food and nutrition security and increasing their incomes. The project built the capacity of Home Economics Extension staff from the Ministry of Agriculture to support and train women's groups in the country's rural development areas (RDAs) in community level food processing (see Figs 25.1 and 25.2). The groups were trained to produce a range of products including jam, juice, bottled fruits, dried vegetables, the local condiment *atchar* and soup mix (see Figs 25.3 and 25.4). Some of the products are marketed jointly and some used for home consumption. It was evident that products with a strong local demand and high nutritional value, such as the soup mix developed, condiment recipes and dried vegetables were the most successful. They helped to improve the food security and nutrition of the communities as well as generating income for the women's groups involved in processing.

Focus of the Work of the Rural Infrastructure and Agro-Industries Division (AGS)

The Rural Infrastructure and Agro-Industries Division (AGS) of FAO (Food and Agriculture Organization of the United Nations) aims to assist farmers and agribusiness in developing managerial and technical skills for supporting production, postharvest processes, infrastructure, marketing and financial operations related to developing and improving

---

*Contributors: Stephanie Gallat and Komivi Sodoke
[†]Contact: ags-director@fao.org

311

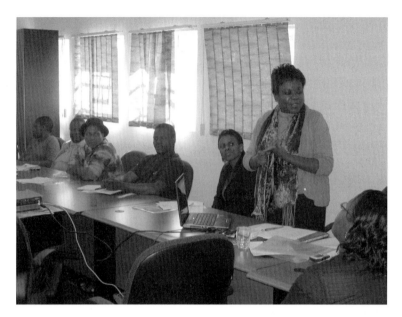

Fig. 25.1. Capacity building: theoretical session of Home Economics Extension staff from the Ministry of Agriculture of Swaziland, May 2008. Photo courtesy of FAO/Gallatova.

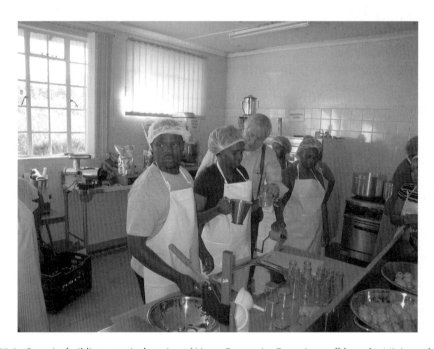

Fig. 25.2. Capacity building: practical session of Home Economics Extension staff from the Ministry of Agriculture of Swaziland, May 2008. Photo courtesy of FAO/Gallatova.

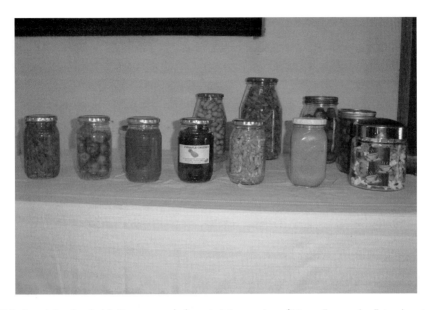

Fig. 25.3. Jam, juice, bottled fruits processed after a training session of Home Economics Extension staff from the Ministry of Agriculture of Swaziland, May 2008. Photo courtesy of FAO/Gallatova.

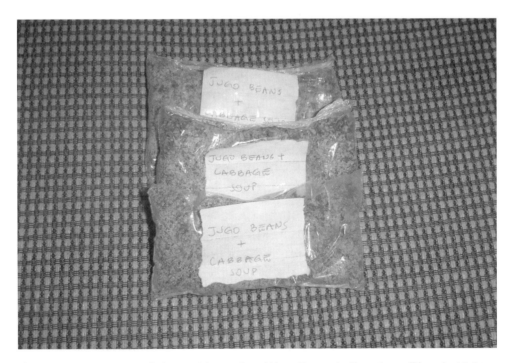

Fig. 25.4. Soup mix processed after a training session of Home Economics Extension staff from the Ministry of Agriculture of Swaziland, May 2008. Photo courtesy of FAO/Gallatova.

efficiency, competitiveness and profitability of agricultural and food enterprises.

Up to June 2012 the Division was composed of four groups: the Agribusiness and Finance Group, the Agro-Food Industries Group, the Market Linkages and Value Chains Group and the Infrastructure and Engineering Services Unit. From June 2012, the Infrastructure and Engineering Services Unit was disbanded and its work transferred to a different Divison. The work of the remaining three groups is described in the following sections.

The Agribusiness and Finance Group

The Agribusiness and Finance Group provides technical guidance and supports policy and institutional responses of FAO members to the challenges of agribusiness development, farm commercialization and rural financial systems (see Fig. 25.5).

The Agro-Food Industries Group

The Agro-Food Industries Group reinforces the capacity of the public sector to work with the private sector to develop competitive agro-food industries and augment their contribution to increased productivity and competitiveness of the agricultural sector and rural development through value addition and increased employment (see Fig. 25.6).

The Market Linkages and Value Chains Group

The Market Linkages and Value Chains Group reinforces public sector capacity to work with the private sector and civil society organizations in order to develop value chains for primary and fresh products, with particular attention to strengthening farmer–market–agribusiness linkages (see Fig. 25.7).

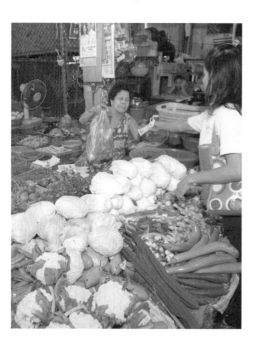

Fig. 25.5. Picture depicting or symbolizing the key areas of support provided by the Agribusiness and Finance Group of the Rural Infrastructure and Agro-Industries Division (AGS), FAO. Photo courtesy of FAO/Dan White.

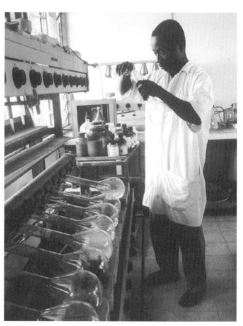

Fig. 25.6. Picture depicting or symbolizing key areas of support provided by the Agro-Food Industries Group of the Rural Infrastructure and Agro-Industries Division (AGS), FAO. Photo courtesy of FAO/Pietro Cenini.

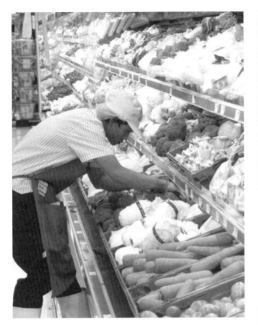

Fig. 25.7. Picture depicting or symbolizing key areas of support of the Market Linkages and Value Chains Group of the Rural Infrastructure and Agro-Industries Division (AGS), FAO. Photo courtesy of FAO/Dan White.

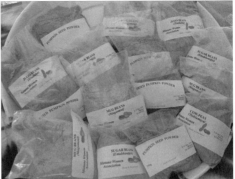

Fig. 25.8. Value-added food products – pumpkin powder, bean powder – jugo beans, sugar beans, mungo beans – processed and commercialized by women's associations in Swaziland. Photo courtesy of FAO/Gallatova.

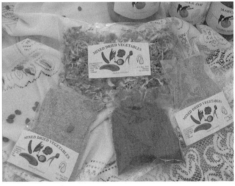

Fig. 25.9. Value-added food products – mixed dried vegetables – processed and commercialized by women's associations in Swaziland. Photo courtesy of FAO/Gallatova.

Impact of AGS Work in Food and Nutrition Security

Key areas of work for AGS are the development of agro-enterprise and the promotion of food processing and value addition. Depending on the size and level of commercialization, agro-enterprises can be classified as micro (home-based), small or medium. All can contribute to improved nutrition and food security through creating employment in off-farm activities (such as handling, processing, packaging, storage and transportation), increasing incomes through the commercialization of value-added products (see Figs. 25.8 and 25.9) and improving the living standards of farmers and processors.

The development and strengthening of microenterprises can contribute to a sustainable improvement of food and nutrition security at household level. Food preservation ensures greater availability of foods throughout the year, including in lean seasons, and particularly of seasonal and perishable crops such as fruits and vegetables that provide essential micronutrients to the diet, and are particularly crucial for the diet and nutritional status of children, pregnant women, HIV-affected persons and other vulnerable groups.

Case Study on the Promotion of Small-scale Community-based Agro-processing in Swaziland

Description and context of the project

This project aimed at strengthening the capacities of Home Economics Officers (HEOs) from the Ministry of Agriculture and Cooperatives to support and train women's groups in the country's rural development areas (RDAs) in home-based, community-level food processing activities (see FAO, 2008; Fig. 25.10).

Community-based processing cannot compete with commercial, professionally managed companies in terms of quality, volume and marketing. However, the project provided important lessons on the key factors that contribute to successful community food processing.

Swaziland has a high prevalence of HIV/AIDS and the Ministry of Health encourages the consumption of nutritious, easily digestible foods. Convenience is also important; due to the impact of HIV/AIDS, communities are increasingly searching for labour-saving technologies and processed foods that are quicker and easier to prepare. A popular and convenient product is instant soup mix imported from South Africa. However, the soup mix is expensive and contains preservatives and other additives that the Ministry of Health does not recommend for HIV/AIDS patients as they can lower immunity. Community processing groups have developed an additive free, convenient and highly nutritious alternative made only of dried green vegetables (Fig. 25.11) and ground beans (the grinding process is pictured in Fig. 25.12). The product (see Fig. 25.13) is affordable and extremely popular, and is starting to replace the soup mixes imported from South Africa.

It was very evident from the project that products with a strong local demand and high nutritional value (soup mixes, condiments and dried vegetables) were more successful than products intended for sale only on the commercial market (jam, juice, bottled fruit), where they had to compete with other, often

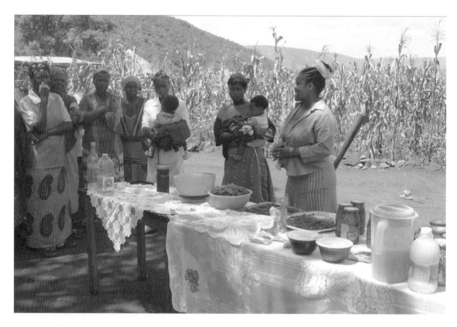

Fig. 25.10. Exhibition of community-level vegetable processing by a rural women's association in Swaziland. Photo courtesy of FAO/Gallatova.

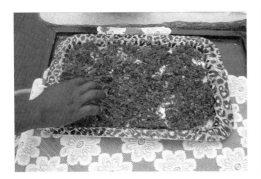

Fig. 25.11. One of the main production phases (the bleaching and drying of vegetables) in the processing of a new instant soup mix developed by community groups in Swaziland. Photo courtesy of FAO/ Gallatova.

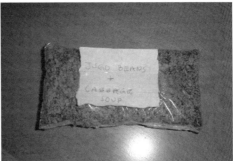

Fig. 25.13. An instant soup mix made by community groups in Swaziland: the final product. Photo courtesy of FAO/Gallatova.

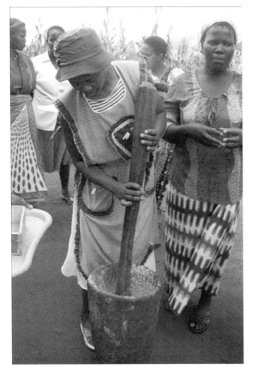

Fig. 25.12. Another of the main production phases (the grinding of beans) in the processing of a new instant soup mix developed by community groups in Swaziland. Photo courtesy of FAO/Gallatova.

imported, products and clearly lacked a competitive advantage. The instant soup mix described above (Fig. 25.14) is an example of a product made by community groups with a

strong local demand which has not only improved the nutrition of the communities, but also generated much needed income to support their families.

Lessons learned

This project is an example of actions currently undertaken by the Rural Infrastructure and Agro-Industries Division to improve food and nutrition security. From it, many lessons were drawn:

- In order for projects in food and nutrition security to be successful, it is important to conduct a feasibility study to ascertain the scale and level of technology that is really needed, and then support them with adequate training and technical advice. For micro-level enterprises, sophisticated and larger scale technologies are often not appropriate and lead to inefficient utilization and inability of groups to pay back loans.
- Micro- and small-scale enterprises can prepare nutritious processed foods with relatively few resources (material and financial).
- In order to be successful, products should be widely appreciated and consumed by the community and used for home consumption as well as for income generation.

Constraints

In the case of soup mixes, improvements need to be made if production is to be scaled up and quality improved. For example:

- Better drying techniques for vegetables are needed: an improved solar drier would improve the colour and vitamin content of the vegetables.
- A mechanized mill for grinding beans would enhance efficiency because the present method using a pestle and mortar is laborious and slow and would present the main bottleneck if production is scaled up.
- Improved packaging and labelling would be desirable: at present, a good product is spoiled by poor-quality packaging and unattractive and inaccurate labelling. Improved packaging would enhance the shelf life and quality of the product and make it more attractive to buyers.

Many of these issues, and others, are covered by Fellows (1997), who provides comprehensive guidelines on small-scale fruit and vegetable processing, and by Palipane and Rolle (2008), who discuss good practices for assuring the postharvest quality of exotic tree fruit crops in Jamaica.

Future Plans

Some of the key focus areas of AGS work in the 2012–2013 biennium (FAO, 2011) relating to improving food and nutrition security include:

1. Support for postharvest loss-reduction programmes: strategies and priorities for reducing losses all along the value chain; guidance on management practices and technologies to reduce losses; technical support for field programmes (see, for example, FAO, 2013).
2. Support for the small and medium agro-processing enterprise (SMAE) development programme through capacity building; programmes to enhance competitiveness will receive greater attention (see, for example, Santacoloma et al. 2009 and Tartanac et al., 2010).
3. Support of emergency recovery programmes in areas such as enterprise development through guidance on rebuilding sustainable livelihoods through agro-enterprise development.
4. Collaboration with the World Food Programme (WFP) on the Purchase for Progress programme is expected to become an important area of action.

References

FAO (2008) Project *TCP/SWA/3101 'Promotion of Small-scale Community-based Agro-processing'*. Internal document, Food and Agriculture Organization, Rome.

FAO (2011) *The Director-General's Medium Term Plan 2010–13 (Reviewed) and Programme of Work and Budget 2012–13*. Food and Agriculture Organization, Rome, pp. 99, 106, 123. Available at: http://www.fao.org/docrep/meeting/021/ma061e.pdf (accessed 12 July 2013).

FAO (2013) INPhO: Information Network on Post-harvest Operations. Available at: http://www.fao.org/inpho (accessed 25 June 2013).

Fellows, P. (1997) *Guidelines for Small-scale Fruit and Vegetable Processors*. FAO Agricultural Services Bulletin No. 127, Food and Agriculture Organization, Rome. Available at: http://www.fao.org/docrep/w6864e/w6864e00.HTM (accessed 25 June 2013).

Palipane, K.B. and Rolle, R. (2008) *Good Practice for Assuring the Post-harvest Quality of Exotic Tree Fruit Crops Produced in Jamaica: A Technical Guide*. Food and Agriculture Organization, Rome. Available at: http://www.fao.org/fileadmin/user_upload/ags/publications/exotic_fruit_book_web.pdf (accessed 25 June 2013).

Santacoloma, P., Röttger, A. and Tartanac, F. (eds) (2009) *Course on Agribusiness Management for Producers' Associations* [Five modules]. Food and Agriculture Organization, Rome. Available at: http://www.fao.org/capacitydevelopment/pubres/results/zh/?target=2&infotype=79 (accessed 25 June 2013).

Tartanac, F., Santacoloma, P. and Röttger, A. (eds) (2010) *Formation en Gestion d'Enterprises Associatives Rurales en Agroalimentaire*. Version adaptée pour l'Afrique francophone. Matériel de Formation en Gestion, Commercialisation et Finances Agricoles de la FAO 10, Food and Agriculture Organization, Rome. Available at: http://www.fao.org/docrep/013/i1936f/i1936f00.htm (accessed 25 June 2013).

26 Work of the Agricultural Development Economics Division (ESA) of FAO on Nutrition

Agricultural Development Economics Division (ESA),*† Economic and Social Development Department (ES)
Food and Agriculture Organization of the United Nations, Rome, Italy

Summary

The Agricultural Development Economics Division (ESA) of FAO carries out various types of work on food and nutrition security. ESA engages in five main types of activities: conducting economic research and analysis; providing analytical tools; producing publications; providing advisory services; and organizing international fora. Examples of each of these types of work are described here as they relate to food and nutrition security.

Introduction

The Agricultural Development Economics Division (ESA)[1] of the Food and Agriculture Organization of the United Nations (FAO) engages in five main types of activities: economic research and analysis; analytical tools; publications; advisory services; and international fora. For each of these areas of work, ESA collaborates with colleagues in the Nutrition Division (AGN) and throughout FAO, as well as with staff of other organizations.

Economic Research and Analysis

The Division is well known for its economic research and analysis on agriculture as related to food security and nutrition,[2] poverty and equity, agricultural trade, natural resource economics, government policy and strategies for poverty reduction. Major research initiatives include those on smallholders in transition,[3] and on long-term global perspectives of food and agriculture.[4]

The work on smallholders aims at promoting the understanding of the changing role of rural income-generating activities and agriculture for poverty reduction, development and improved food security, drawing on the Rural Income Generating Activities (RIGA) databases,[5] and on other sources. RIGA provides a publicly available database on sources of income, compiled using 32 household surveys covering 18 countries in Africa, Asia, Eastern Europe and Latin America. One of the key innovations of the

---

*Contributor: Sarah Lowder
†Contact: terri.rancy@fao.org

RIGA database is that, where available, it provides panel data on households. This affords researchers the rare opportunity to examine changes in a single household's income over time and to do so with nationally representative data sets. To date, work with the RIGA database has allowed researchers from various organizations to undertake analyses on a variety of subjects, such as the impact of high food prices on urban and rural households, and the impact of agriculture and rural incomes from other sectors on food security.

The Division's research and analysis also includes analysis of the long-term challenges facing global food and agriculture, including growth in demand, climate change, pressure on natural resources, changes in technology and the prevalence of undernourishment.

Analytical Tools

The ESA provides or contributes to monitoring and analytical tools such as the Integrated Food Security Phase Classification (IPC),[6] Food Security and Nutrition Analysis Unit (FSNAU),[7] the Food Insecurity and Vulnerability Information Mapping System (FIVIMS), the global stunting map, methodologies for calculating undernourishment figures and other work.

The Agriculture and Consumer Protection Department (AG) and ESA are Co-Lead Technical Units of the FSNAU in Somalia, a well-established and well-respected unit covering food security and nutrition in the protracted crisis in Somalia. The FSNAU is the main source of information and analysis on the food security and nutrition situation in Somalia used by the international community as well as for local stakeholders' response to the emergency situation. Regular FSNAU reports are the central source of information for an emergency response programme that totals US$500–600 million annually.

The first version of the IPC was developed by the FSNAU, and the revised guidance, *IPC Technical Manual Version 2.0: Evidence and Standards for Better Food Security Decisions*, was issued in 2012.[8] IPC is a tool that is now used for food security and nutrition analysis and planning in over a dozen countries of

sub-Saharan Africa and also in a few Asian countries (e.g. Tajikistan), with the potential for application in developing countries throughout the world. It provides a standardized scale that integrates food security, nutrition and livelihood information into a clear statement about the nature and severity of a crisis and implications for strategic response.

Publications

The ESA is in charge of several publications, including two of FAO's flagship publications, *The State of Food and Agriculture* (SOFA),[9] and *The State of Food Insecurity* (SOFI).[10]

SOFA is FAO's main flagship publication, and has been produced since 1947 in response to the Director-General being tasked with reporting to the biennial FAO Conference on the state of food and agriculture. The report contains a comprehensive, yet easily accessible, overview of trends in food and agriculture, including the presentation of FAO figures on undernourishment, which are discussed in relation to information on its causes. Each year it also examines a specific topic of major relevance to agriculture and food security.

The 2009 issue of SOFA was dedicated to the livestock sector, including its role in nutrition. SOFA 2010–2011 is entitled *Women in Agriculture: Closing the Gender Gap for Development*. It provides comprehensive data and analysis documenting and assessing the costs of the gender gap faced by rural women in access to land, livestock, education, financial services, extension, fertilizers, tools and employment opportunities. The report provides compelling empirical estimates of the production and food security gains that could be achieved simply by closing the gender gap in agricultural input use. The report incorporates sex-disaggregated information on food security and nutrition, including measures of malnutrition from well-known international data sets and a wide literature review.

SOFI, published since 1999, raises awareness about global hunger issues, examines underlying causes of hunger and malnutrition and monitors progress towards hunger reduction targets established at the 1996 World Food Summit and the Millennium

Summit. It reports the widely used under-nourishment figures produced by FAO.

The 2010 issue reported that:

- the number of undernourished people in the world remains unacceptably high at 925 million in 2010, despite its first decline in 15 years;
- this decline is largely attributable to a more favourable economic environment in 2010 and the fall in both international and domestic food prices since 2008;
- a total of 925 million people were under-nourished in 2010 compared with 1023 billion in 2009; and
- however, the number of hungry people was higher in 2010 than before the food and economic crises of 2008–2009.

Advisory Services

The ESA provides advisory services on national and regional policy on food and nutrition security as well as on the Right to Food. Examples include services provided in Bangladesh and the Caribbean.

Since 2005, FAO and other partners have provided advisory services to the Government of Bangladesh through the National Food Policy Capacity Strengthening Programme (NFPCSP). Through the NFPCSP, the government has drafted a new National Food Policy, a Plan of Action and a Country Investment Plan for Food Security. Such policies and pro-gramme planning in Bangladesh now take a comprehensive and cross-sectoral approach to food security that includes addressing human nutrition, rather than being exclu-sively focused on food availability, as pro-grammes did in the past. The National Plan of Action for Food Security includes nutrition interventions such as:

- emphasis on balanced diets and a supply of sufficient nutritious food for vulner-able groups;
- food supplementation and fortification (vitamin A, iron–folate supplementation and iodized salt); and
- promotion and protection of breastfeed-ing and complementary feeding.

By providing technical inputs FAO sup-ported the drafting of a Regional Food and Nutrition Security Policy (RFNSP) for the Caribbean region. This involved extensive consultation among stakeholders, including Member States of the Caribbean Community (CARICOM). The policy was approved by the Ministers for Agriculture of countries in the Caribbean in October 2010. Several priority action areas were identified. Of special inter-est to nutrition is the promotion of healthy diets, particularly through nutrition educa-tion in the schools.

International Fora

Finally, the Division organizes and services international fora for global policy on food and nutrition security. These include the Committee on World Food Security,[11] the Alliance Against Hunger and Malnutrition,[12] and the Global Forum on Food Security and Nutrition.[13]

The Committee on World Food Security (CFS) was established in 1974 and reformed in 2009 to be more inclusive, participative and responsive to key issues affecting food security and nutrition at country, regional and global levels. Access to neutral, expert advice, and outreach to all stakeholders has been improved through a High-Level Panel of Experts on Food Security and Nutrition, an Advisory Group that includes participants from a wide-range of stakeholder organizations, and a CSO (civil society organization) Global Mechanism. The vision of the new CFS is to be the most inclusive international and intergovernmental platform for all stakeholders to work together to ensure food security and nutrition for all. The first session of the reformed CFS was held in October 2010. It included the launching of the 2010 SOFI, as well as policy round tables on the following themes:

- Food security in protracted crises (the SOFI 2010 theme).
- Land tenure and international invest-ment in agriculture.
- Managing vulnerability and risk.

Also central to the 2010 CFS Session were deliberations on a global strategic framework for food security and nutrition, as well as country, regional and global initiatives on food security and nutrition, including a mapping of food security actions at the country level.

The Alliance Against Hunger and Malnutrition was created in 2003 in response to the Rome Declaration of the *World Food Summit: Five Years Later* by FAO, IFAD, WFP and Bioversity International.[14] A global partnership, the Alliance brings together local, regional, national and international institutions with the aim of promoting policy dialogue in the fight against hunger. Since its inception, the Alliance has facilitated the establishment of national and regional alliances throughout the world. The Alliance facilitates efforts of its global partners and of national alliances to bring together civil society, the private sector and governments, all aimed at building political will to reduce hunger and malnutrition.

The Global Forum on Food Security and Nutrition (FSN forum) provides an informal, virtual international forum that is accessible to many through the Internet. The FSN forum has more than 2600 members from 140 countries representing UN organizations, non-governmental organizations (NGOs), universities, governments and researchers. Many field practitioners are active in the forum, thus bringing practical knowledge to the discussion. The FSN forum has hosted 62 online discussions on a number of topics, many of which focus on nutrition, such as:

- Food security and nutrition security: what is the problem and what is the difference?
- Putting people first: nutrition, a key to integrated programming for poverty reduction?

Conclusions

This chapter has provided an overview of the food and nutrition security work of the ESA division of the FAO as presented at the International Symposium on Food and Nutrition Security: Food-based Approaches for Improving Diets and Raising Levels of Nutrition, held at FAO Headquarters, Rome, in December 2010. ESA's work has changed somewhat since the symposium, as the division is, of course, constantly evolving in response to needs expressed by FAO member states, the organization itself and the international community.[15] Since December 2010, the ESA has started work on some new activities relevant to food and nutrition security, such as dedicating its annual flagship publication, SOFI 2013, to the subject of food systems for better nutrition.

Notes

[1] For more information, please see: http://www.fao.org/economic/esa/en/ (accessed 25 June 2013).

[2] Throughout this chapter the terms food security, food security and nutrition, and food and nutrition security are used interchangeably.

[3] For more information, please see: http://www.fao.org/economic/riga/en/ (accessed 25 June 2013).

[4] For more information, please see: http://www.fao.org/economic/esa/esag/en/ (accessed 25 June 2013).

[5] For more information, please see: http://www.fao.org/economic/riga/riga-database/en/ (accessed 25 June 2013).

[6] For more information, please see: http://www.ipcinfo.org/ (accessed 25 June 2013).

[7] For more information, please see: http://www.fsnau.org/ (accessed 25 June 2013).

[8] For more information, please see: http://www.ipcinfo.org/ipcinfo-detail-forms/ipcinfo-resource-detail0/en/c/162270/ (accessed 25 June 2013).

[9] For more information, please see: http://www.fao.org/publications/sofa/en/ (accessed 25 June 2013).

[10] For more information, please see: http://www.fao.org/publications/sofi/en/ (accessed 25 June 2013).

[11] For more information, please see: www.fao.org/cfs (accessed 25 June 2013).

[12] For more information, please see: http://www.theaahm.org/ (accessed 25 June 2013).

[13] For more information, please see: http://www.fao.org/fsnforum/ (accessed 25 June 2013).

[14] For more information, please see: http://www.fao.org/worldfoodsummit/english/index.html (accessed 25 June 2013).

[15] The most complete and up-to-date overview of the work of the Division is available at: http://www.fao.org/economic/esa/en/ (accessed 25 June 2013).

27 Towards an Improved Framework for Measuring Undernourishment

Statistics Division (ESS),*† Economic and Social Development Department (ES)
Food and Agriculture Organization of the United Nations, Rome, Italy

———————————

Summary

The FAO Statistics Division (ESS) currently estimates the prevalence of undernourishment using a probabilistic model that is composed of three key data elements. The first is the dietary energy supply (DES), i.e. the daily calories available per person, which serves as the mean of a log-normal distribution; the second is the coefficient of variation (CV), i.e. a measure of the dispersion in the distribution of calorific energy; and the third is a threshold measure of the minimum dietary energy requirements (MDER) of a representative individual. Current efforts aim to: (i) improve data quality, coverage and conversion factors for the compilation of food balance sheets (FBS); (ii) update and expand measures that capture the distribution of food availability; and (iii) gauge more accurately the minimum dietary energy requirement in a given population. The ESS is responsible for the compilation of FBS and efforts have been undertaken by the Division to harness more precise information on food availability at the national level. These involve improved data collection methods, a focus on data quality and capacity-building initiatives with counterpart national statistical agencies. The ESS is currently implementing improvements in methodology with initiatives to gather, process and disseminate data in a more timely and accurate manner to improve the satisfaction of users worldwide.

Background and Objectives

This chapter reviews ongoing efforts and future plans to improve the Food and Agriculture Organization of the United Nations (FAO) methodology for measuring undernourishment. These efforts follow, inter alia, the recommendations of the 'Independent External Evaluation (IEE) of FAO' published in 2007,[1] which suggested that 'considerably greater priority should be given to the provision of basic data and statistics' and more generally that the 'time has come for a total re-examination of the statistical needs for the 21st century and how they can best be met'. Monitoring progress in hunger reduction is contingent on accurate, reliable and timely data, and on robust methods that measure the prevalence of hunger food insecurity and vulnerability.

FAO currently estimates the prevalence of undernourishment using a probabilistic model. The model is informed by three key data elements. The first is the dietary energy supply (DES), i.e. the daily calories available per person, which serves as the mean of a log-normal distribution; the second is the coefficient

*Contributors: Josef Schmidhuber, Adam Prakash and Gladys Moreno García
†Contact: ess-director@fao.org

© FAO 2014. *Improving Diets and Nutrition: Food-based Approaches*
(eds B. Thompson and L. Amoroso)

of variation (CV), i.e. a measure of the dispersion in the distribution of food calorific energy; and the third is a threshold measure of the minimum dietary energy requirements (MDER) of a representative individual.

The specific contribution of this note to these goals entails the description of current efforts to: (i) improve data quality, coverage and conversion factors for the compilation of food balance sheets (FBS); (ii) update and expand measures that capture the distribution of food availability; and (iii) gauge more accurately the minimum dietary energy requirement in a given population.

Dietary Energy Supply

Proposals have been made to measure the prevalence of undernourishment (PU) based on empirical food energy supplies derived from survey data. While sound in principle, such an approach is not feasible given the obligation to produce estimates in a timely and continuous manner for all countries, and also the relative paucity of available surveys. Hence, underpinning the framework for measuring undernourishment is the need for sound food balance sheet data.

The FAO Statistics Division (ESS) is responsible for the compilation of FBS, and efforts have been undertaken by the division to harness more precise information on food availability at the national level. These involve improved data collection methods, a focus on data quality and capacity-building initiatives with counterpart national statistical agencies. For instance:

- Reviewing the FAO data collection system and harmonizing the methodology adopted at national level to collect food and agriculture data in a way that would be consistent with internationally accepted definitions and classifications.
- Identifying new methods of data collection and data processing for the compilation of food and agriculture statistics.
- Promoting initiatives aimed at identifying the most efficient methods for integrating agricultural statistics into the respective National Statistic Development System.

- Creating networks between national and international statisticians involved with food and agricultural statistics.

Recognizing that food consumption over time is expected to be less variable than food availability, given the possibility of storage, approaches to determine actual food consumption can also be enhanced and corroborated by making use of household food expenditure and acquisition surveys from representative samples of the population, where they exist. Incorporating this information will also improve the estimation of the probable distribution of food consumption in the population.

Irrespective of where data are sourced is the need to convert consumption into dietary energy content in order to calculate the average DES. However, conversion factors may be difficult to obtain and are not easily generalized across food items. To address the accuracy in the methodology of converting foodstuffs to a DES equivalent, the ESS is currently reviewing and updating food composition tables for individual countries.

Distribution of Food Availability

The currently adopted assumption concerning the distribution of dietary calorie intake in the population is also under review. The guiding principles will be those of trying to define the most flexible yet parsimonious parametric model that closely fits observed reliable empirical distributions to correctly represent the distribution of access to food in a country, with special attention to modelling the tails of the distribution.

While the currently employed log-normal assumption fulfils parsimony, there is scope to improve the accuracy of the distribution's parameters – the mean (average DES) and the CV. Furthermore, given that these parameters vary with time, being especially responsive to changes in prices and household income, it is essential that they are updated as soon as new information becomes available. To this end, research is being conducted in exploring the relationship that exists between the CV of DES (in its income component) and per capita income, while controlling for income distribution. The aim of this endeavour is that estimates of undernourishment can then be produced when FBS or survey data are unavailable.

Minimum Dietary Energy Requirement

The appropriate cut-off point required to determine, in the probabilistic sense, the prevalence of undernourishment in the population is the minimum dietary energy requirement (MDER), which is interpreted as the minimum of the distribution of dietary energy requirement (DER) in a population. As individual requirements are not observable, there can be no basis for the direct estimate of the underlying distribution. Consequently, indirect estimation procedures are needed. Such procedures may be based on available information from nutrition experts, as obtained through nutrition surveys and clinical trials, and on knowledge of the demographic structure of the population.

FAO currently adopts the latter approach to indirectly estimate MDER by assuming an 'acceptable range' of DER in groups of individuals of the same sex and age, and using the observed sex–age composition in each country. The acceptable range assumption is based on the basal metabolic rate for the lowest acceptable body weight for that sex–age combination, adjusted for a minimal physical activity level compatible with a normal life. Estimated minimum DERs of each sex–age class are then aggregated at the country level using the proportion of the population in the corresponding sex–age groups as statistical weights. While no large variation is expected to exist between the metabolic rates of people in different countries within the same sex–age group (though differences across latitude could be important), the sex–age composition of the population does change over time, as does the estimated cut-off point.

Updating the MDER calculations includes updating the database on average physiological heights of a given population. FAO's Nutrition Division (AGN) is updating national height profiles, using data reported at the country level. Where empirical height data are not available, average heights will be estimated based on anthropometric models.

In conclusion, by implementing improvements in methodology in tandem with initiatives to gather, process and disseminate data in a more timely and accurate manner, FAO will maintain its position as the global leader in food security and agricultural statistics.

Note

[1] Available at: ftp://ftp.fao.org/docrep/fao/meeting/012/k0827erev1.pdf (accessed 25 June 2013).

28 Gender Dimensions of Food and Nutrition Security: Women's Roles in Ensuring the Success of Food-based Approaches

Gender, Equity and Rural Employment Division (ESW),[*†]
Economic and Social Development Department (ES)
Food and Agriculture Organization of the United Nations, Rome, Italy

─────────────

Summary

This chapter argues for the importance of considering gender as a central variable in food-based approaches to food and nutrition security, given women's key roles in household food preparation, allocation and distribution, timing, frequency and quantities, dietary choices, as well as in subsistence food production, which is the primary source of household access to food, especially among low-income populations with constrained access to market purchased food. The chapter discusses the importance of relying on the gender lens in designing food-based interventions for food and nutrition security because of the influence of gender in intergenerational and intra-generational nutritional outcomes. It illustrates the difference between food access and availability, and the greater vulnerability of women and children in extreme situations, such as seasonal food scarcity, food crises, climate change and complex emergencies. Concluding comments propose the integration of gender as crucial in food-based approaches to food and nutrition security, including two strengths of the Gender, Equity and Rural Employment Division (ESW) of FAO in this regard – capacity development and enhancing the evidence base on women's key roles in household food security.

Introduction

Food-based approaches to improving diets and nutritional status focus primarily on the household as the entry point for programme interventions and knowledge enhancement. The rationale for such a focus is because of the influence of household variables as key determinants of nutritional outcomes (Strauss and Thomas, 1995; Christiaensen and Alderman, 2001). Household level access to food, intra-household food distribution patterns and the utilization patterns of available food and other resources towards optimal nutritional gains render the household as the primary locus of influence for food security and nutrition. Less well documented, however, are the intra-household practices and relationships that affect the latter, including the roles and responsibilities assumed by different household members in the assurance of dietary quality and nutrition outcomes.

───────

*Contributor: Nandini Gunewardena
†Contact: esw-pact-team-list@fao.org

Gender roles are critical in this regard, given the key roles assumed by women in household food preparation, allocation, distribution, timing, frequency, quantities and dietary choices, as well as other related variables that bear critically on the nutrition outcomes of household members. As such, the lens of gender in analysing household food and nutrition can serve as a useful framework in designing food-based approaches to food and nutrition promotional interventions.

The gender lens can deepen our understanding of the three dimensions of food security by revealing the gender-specific differences, constraints and opportunities that influence household and community food availability, access and utilization. For example, analysis of caloric access and utilization differences by gender and age, varied nutrition requirements by gender and age and at various points in the life cycle (pregnancy, lactation, early childhood), and the cycle of undernutrition that hinges on women's reproductive health and nutritional status can all inform food-based approaches to nutrition security in a more precise and comprehensive manner. The gender lens can further illustrate the differences between access and availability. Even when food is available, there are other intervening factors that lead to disparities in food and nutrition security within the household, such as gender differences in access to food, household food allocation and distribution patterns, maternal knowledge of dietary composition (caloric and micronutrient content), child feeding practices (often influenced by customs and beliefs), and caregiving variations. Furthermore, gender differentials in access to food production inputs/ resources and access through the market, and women's predominance in low-yield and poorly remunerated subsistence agriculture, can significantly undermine household food and nutrition security. Therefore, analyses of the specific contributions that women make to household food and nutrition security that draw on the evidence base (gender-disaggregated data and information) is vital for better targeting and sustainable food and nutrition security outcomes. This chapter discusses why gender matters in food-based approaches to nutrition, the mandate of the Gender, Equity and Rural Employment Division (ESW) of FAO (Food and Agriculture Organization of the United Nations) in addressing food and nutrition security and some forward-looking strategies for gender integration in food-based approaches to food and nutrition security.

Why Gender Matters: Visibility and Vulnerability

In targeting food-based approaches to food and nutrition security, a consideration of the inverse relationship between visibility and vulnerability can offer insights on why gender matters in the success of interventions. The design of initiatives tailored to women as the primary caregivers responsible for household food consumption patterns and rates is one aspect of this equation. Recognition of the gender roles in household food preparation and distribution can enhance such initiatives by focusing on improving women's knowledge and practices. Projects can be designed with a consideration and aim of developing the capacity levels of local women. The manner in which time poverty (lack of time) intervenes to compromise the effectiveness of such initiatives is a third factor that merits consideration, given the complex array of tasks on which rural lives and livelihoods depend.

Insufficient accounting of these factors adds to the invisibility of gender roles within and between households and can, in turn, compromise the sound targeting of food and nutrition security measures. The dearth and gaps in data on gender differences in subsistence agriculture and household food production, including the related problem of undercounting and under-reporting, compounds the invisibility of women's contributions to agricultural production. The available data indicate that women comprise an average of 43% of the agricultural labour force in developing countries, ranging from 20% in Latin America to 50% in sub-Saharan Africa and East Asia (FAO, 2010). Reliable gender-disaggregated data and information can therefore enhance the design and outcome of food-based approaches to food and nutrition security.

Invisibility compounds vulnerability in a number of ways, apart from the basic issue of underestimating it. The intersection of poverty and vulnerability and their simultaneous impact on undernutrition is a key concern here. Recent research by Svedberg (2008) on child malnutrition in India, for instance, confirms the significance of poverty as a determinant of child malnutrition; this has also been found in related cross-country studies. Given the higher incidence of poverty among women, ascertained through the evidence on gender-based wage disparities, occupational hierarchies, underemployment, non-remunerated work and differential access to land, resources, agricultural inputs and services, the likelihood of a greater vulnerability to food and nutrition insecurities among women and children is high. Lower incomes, especially among female-headed households, can place them at greater risk of nutritional insecurity as dietary quality is sacrificed to calorific sufficiency. Women's greater vulnerability to malnutrition and food security thus has implications not only for themselves, but for all household members, given the key role that women assume in household food access and utilization. Moreover, women's responsibilities in community care translate such vulnerabilities across the community.

How Gender Matters in Intergenerational and Intra-generational Nutrition Status: The Life Cycle

It is well known that nutrition deficiencies begin in utero, where maternal malnutrition is a critical factor influencing fetal growth and, subsequently, the nutritional status of newborns and implications across the life cycle. As documented by UNICEF (1998), the immediate causes of child malnutrition can be attributed to the interaction of two household level variables – poor diet and infections – both of which are related to maternal health (including nutritional status), well-being and practices. Similarly, gender issues influence the underlying set of factors identified by UNICEF: household food security, care, environment (water use and sanitation practices) and gender relations. Gender matters in determining intergenerational and intra-generational nutritional status given the ways in which

gender-discriminatory practices compromise female nutritional status, and the confluence of factors associated with women's reproductive health. Evidence from Bangladesh (HHI 2001; WFP 2004), for example, has revealed that women's control of household resources can be considered as 'the single most important basic factor that determines malnutrition in Bangladesh' (WFP, 2004). Research has shown that women tend to meet the nutritional needs of children better than men, who are less likely to spend additional income on increased food consumption for children (Diskin, 1994). According to Amartya Sen (1988), 'there is a good deal of evidence from all over the world that food is often distributed very unequally within the family – with a distinct sex bias (against the female) and also an age bias (against the children)'. The lasting intergenerational effects of hunger and/or poor nutrition among women and girls have been documented by the United Nations Administrative Committee on Coordination/Sub-Committee on Nutrition (Pojda and Kelley, 2000), and established in at least one study on India (Ramalingaswami et al., 1996). The intergenerational cycle is complicated by malnourished women bearing low birth weight babies who tend to be immune compromised, with long-term implications for cognitive deficits, productivity losses and morbidity risks.

Similarly, the household-level effects of gender relations and gender roles have to do with the way that women's education and knowledge levels on health, sanitation and dietary quality have an impact on household nutrition security, both intergenerationally and intra-generationally. Svedberg (2008) reports female illiteracy as a significant factor, for example, in child underweight in India. Women's central role in household food allocation, decisions about individual food needs and child feeding practices (including diet, quantity, timing, frequency, etc., which are especially critical during the first 5 years of age when nutritional security is crucial for proper physical and cognitive development) are related factors that merit consideration. Furthermore, women's near-exclusive roles in food preparation, distribution and storage can affect household food safety and quality, while their key roles in child rearing and childcare ultimately have an impact on the overall health status of all household members, directly or indirectly. Given the association between infections and unsafe water, poor sanitation and hygiene practices – because they lead to leakage of calories even among adequately nourished children – women's near-exclusive roles in household water (i.e. in conveying, storing, using and distributing), and the confluence of low income and poverty as they translate into poor sanitation (facilities and practices), and thereby compromise household nutrition, must be considered.

Examples from sub-Saharan Africa (SSA), where the threat of desertification is very high, reveal that women travel 6–8 km daily each way to collect and transport water. In extreme situations, as in Ethiopia, women have been reported to walk over 25 km one way in search of water, awaking at dawn and returning after nightfall. In some parts of northern Ghana, women walk over 20 km a day to fetch 5 gallons of water a trip. Fetching and hauling water over long distances result in other risks for women, such as the opportunity costs of this activity and the health risks related to the strain and heavy loads, but also because women often drink from unsafe water sources along the way.

What Are the Ways in Which Gender Matters? Access and Availability

Yet another set of underlying factors that condition household food and nutrition security is gender disparities in access to agricultural services and resources, and gender-differentiated roles in agricultural production, postharvest processing and food storage, as well as market access to food (see Arimond et al., 2010, on the pathways between agricultural interventions and nutrition). As the State of Food and Agriculture 2010–11 discusses (FAO, 2010), lack of access to resources and services seriously hampers women's agricultural productivity and, in turn, household food security. Given the predominance of women in subsistence agriculture in developing countries – which contributes to the mainstay

of the diet of the rural poor – they represent a critical link in household production and consumption. Women's over-representation in low-wage or non-remunerated agricultural production (often referred to as the feminization of agriculture), and the resulting income limitations, have been identified as a constraining factor in market access. As a recent document from the International Food Policy Research Institute (IFPRI) notes: 'Empirical evidence shows that increasing women's control over land, physical assets and financial assets serves to raise agricultural productivity, improve child health and nutrition, and increase expenditures on education, contributing to overall poverty reduction' (Meinzen-Dick et al., 2011).

More general estimates allocate over 80% of agricultural production to the responsibility of women, including major decisions over seed selection, water, crops, animal husbandry and food storage. Women's decision making is also considered to increase as men opt for non-farm activities (i.e. non-agricultural wage employment, such as fishing, trades, self-employment, etc.), or migrate for work in urban areas or other regions/countries. In such situations, women are generally responsible for the continuous round of activities associated with household and community subsistence food production. The high incidence of female-headed households among the poor (estimated at some 70%) means that, in addition to their normal tasks, women undertake the central decisions regarding how to allocate land, labour and other resources between competing needs, in order to ensure household food and nutrition security. It is plausible then, that women and children in female-headed households are hit first and hardest by food crises.

When Gender Matters: Seasonal Scarcity, Food Crises and Climate Change

In situations of scarcity and crisis, including the recent food price crisis, as well as long-term trends such as climate change and complex emergencies, it is primarily women and children, especially from populations that are systematically disempowered by their class, race, ethnicity, caste and/or other marginal social locations who are at greater risk and more vulnerable to food and nutrition insecurity.

As documented by the World Food Programme (WFP, 2005), the first to reduce their food intake in a crisis are female and elderly members, who also take on manual labour to meet household food needs as the crisis deepens. According to one scholar, Pamela Sparr, women serve as the major 'social shock absorbers' (Sparr, 1992) in times of crisis, cushioning their families, households and communities, while bearing the brunt of deprivation themselves. For example, Bairagi (1986) reports that female children were more adversely affected by famine in rural Bangladesh than were boys, and Sen (1988) reports how women and girls were systematically disadvantaged in food relief efforts and access to relief supplies in the aftermath of flooding that destroyed crops and farmland in West Bengal, and in the 1991 Bangladesh cyclone.

A sombre example of extreme coping measures by women comes from Haiti, the poorest nation in the western hemisphere, where over half (52%) of the population fell below the poverty line even before the tragic earthquake of January 2010: pregnant women's consumption of 'mud cookies' – an edible clay found in Haiti's Central Plateau, considered to be a source of calcium – evidently the last resort of hunger pains in recent times. The tripling of fuel prices and 50% price increases in basic foods such as rice, beans, fruit and condensed milk in 2009 has been documented to have exacerbated the food insecurity of impoverished Haitians. Ultimately, food shortages take a bigger toll on women and girls for many reasons associated with subtle and overt gender discrimination – they tend often to be the last fed in poor households for both economic and cultural reasons.

Where climate change is concerned, women's extensive use of forest products for subsistence and their concomitant knowledge of seeds and species (Hoskins, 1983; Dankelman and Davidson, 1988), their extensive knowledge of local ecosystems, and the traditional practices that women have adopted based on this knowledge, contribute significantly to biodiversity conservation and environmental protection. Around the world, women actively manage forest resources and contribute to forest conservation and regeneration. In the Himalayan hills of Nepal and India, women have traditionally been central as decision makers on regeneration and in decisions about community rules of harvesting and product extraction. In tribal areas of India and Nepal, women whose livelihoods depend largely on the collection, sale and processing of non-timber forest products have historically made decisions about harvesting techniques that avoid rapid depletion and sustain production. In some places, women have better knowledge than men about the qualities, growing patterns and potential use of forest species and grasses than men. The extensive knowledge of indigenous women on plant species and their uses have been well documented (Norem et al., 1989). Yet women's knowledge tends to be overlooked, and they are poorly represented in decision making on environmental and development issues at the local, national and international arenas.

Where Gender Matters Can Be Addressed: Strategic Programme Interventions

ESW leads and coordinates the organization's work on gender integration and in ensuring gender equality in agriculture and rural development and food and nutrition security programmes. The Division is working to mainstream gender within all technical areas of FAO's mandate by advancing analytical work, raising awareness, building capacities, providing technical assistance and supporting the development of gender-disaggregated data in agricultural censuses.

ESW assumes a key role in generating the evidence base that provides a compelling rationale for why gender matters. For example, the Division supports the capacity development of national institutions to improve their understanding and analysis of rural vulnerabilities related to gender and social inequalities. Its analytical work attempts to capture gender differences in access to resources and inputs for food production, the gender-specific impact of epidemics (i.e. HIV/AIDS) on food and nutrition security, and gender-related constraints and challenges in agricultural productivity, rural development and food and nutrition security. Field programme activities supported by ESW staff focus on integrating gender in farmer field schools in several member countries, and in strengthening women's active engagement in rural institutions (farmer organizations). In sum, ESW is well positioned to serve in an advocacy and capacity-development role in gender-responsive food-based approaches to food and nutrition security strategies advanced by FAO's Nutrition Division (AGN).

In terms of the way forward, ESW can assume two strategic roles in enhancing food-based approaches to food and nutrition security: (i) support for enhancing and utilizing the evidence base to design project and programme implementation; and (ii) support for gender-sensitive policy reforms and programme design. In terms of the former, work currently under way in ESW includes several activities: guidance and support to member countries on inclusive rural institutions, knowledge building and capacity development on gender mainstreaming across sector-specific initiatives (particularly in agriculture), strategies to target FAO programmes and projects to vulnerable populations (including women), the monitoring and evaluation of gender mainstreaming efforts, and continuous efforts to strengthen the evidence base. Expansion and further strengthening of analytical efforts is necessary in order to deepen our understanding of the context-specific linkages between agricultural production, gender disparities and household-level effects on food and nutrition security, as argued by IFPRI (Meinzen-Dick *et al.*, 2011). In terms of policy support, ESW produces policy briefs that illustrate the significance of equitable and gender-sensitive rural policies that pave the way for proactive and protective measures toward safeguarding food and nutrition security.

References

Arimond, M., Hawkes, C., Ruel, M.T., Sifri, Z., Berti, P.R., Leroy, J.L., Low, J.W., Brown L.R. and Frongillo, E.A. (2011) Agricultural interventions and nutrition: lessons from the past and new evidence. In: Thompson, B. and Amoroso, L. (eds) *Combating Micronutrient Deficiencies: Food-based Approaches.* Food and Agriculture Organization of the United Nations, Rome and CAB International, Wallingford, UK, pp. 41–73.

Bairagi, R. (1986) Food crisis, nutrition, and female children in rural Bangladesh. *Population and Development Review* 12, 307–15.

Christiaensen, L. and Alderman, H. (2001) *Child Malnutrition in Ethiopia: Can Maternal Knowledge Augment the Role of Income?* Africa Region Working Paper Series No. 22, World Bank. Washington, DC.

Dankelman, I. and Davidson, J. (1988) *Women and Environment in the Third World: Alliance for the Future.* Earthscan, London.

Diskin, P. (1994) *Understanding Linkages Among Food Availability, Access, Consumption, and Nutrition in Africa: Empirical Findings and Issues from the Literature.* MSU International Development Working Paper No. 46, Michigan State University, East Lansing, Michigan.

FAO (2010) *The State of Food and Agriculture 2010–11. Women in Agriculture: Closing the Gender Gap for Development.* Food and Agriculture Organization of the United Nations, Rome.

HKI (2001) *When the Decision-maker is a Woman, Does it Make a Difference for the Nutritional Status of Mothers and Children?* Bangladesh Nutritional Surveillance Project Bulletin No. 8, Helen Keller International Bangladesh, Dhaka.

Hoskins, M. (1983) *Rural Women, Forest Outputs and Forestry Projects.* Food and Agriculture Organization of the United Nations, Rome.

Meinzen-Dick, R., Behrman, J., Menon, P. and Quisumbing, A. (2011) *Gender: A Key Dimension Linking Agricultural Programs to Improved Nutrition and Health.* 2020 Conference Brief 9, Leveraging Agriculture for Improving Nutrition and Health: Highlights from an International Conference. International Food Policy Research Institute (IFPRI), Washington, DC. Available at: http://www.ifpri.org/sites/default/files/publications/2020anhconfbr09.pdf (accessed 26 June 2013).

Norem, R.H., Yoder, R. and Martin, Y. (1989) Indigenous agricultural knowledge and gender issues in Third World agricultural development. In: Warren, D.M., Slikkerveer, L.J. and Titilola, S.O. (eds) *Indigenous Knowledge Systems. Implications for Agriculture and International Development*. Studies in Technology and Social Change No. 11, Technology and Social Change Program, Iowa State University, Ames, Iowa, pp. 91–100.

Pojda, J. and Kelley, L. (eds) (2000) *Low Birthweight A Report Based on the International Low Birthweight Symposium and Workshop held on 14–17 June 1999 at the International Centre for Diarrhoeal Disease Research in Dhaka,* Bangladesh. ACC/SCN Nutrition Policy Paper #18, Administrative Committee on Coordination/Sub-Committee on Nutrition, Geneva, Switzerland.

Ramalingaswami, V., Jonson, U. and Rohde, J. (1996) Commentary: The Asian enigma. In: *The Progress of Nations 1996*. United Nations Children's Fund (UNICEF), New York, pp. 11–17. Available at: http://www.unicef.org/pon96/nuenigma.htm (accessed 26 June 2013).

Sen, A. (1988) Family and food: sex bias in poverty. In: Srinivasan, T.N. and Bardhan, P.K. (eds) *Rural Poverty in South Asia*. Columbia University Press, New York, pp. 453-472.

Sparr, P. (ed.) (1992) *Mortgaging Women's Lives: Feminist Critiques of Structural Adjustment*. Zed Books, New York.

Strauss, J. and Thomas, D. (1995) Human resources: empirical modeling of household and family decisions. In: Behrman, J. and Srinivasan, T.N. (eds) *Handbook of Development Economics, Volume 3, Part A*. Elsevier, Maryland Heights, Missouri, pp. 1883–2005.

Svedberg, P. (2008) Why malnutrition in shining India persists (NFHS123rev3 text doc. /2008-11-25/ (revision for ISI conference). Paper prepared for [and presented to]: *4th Annual Conference on Economic Growth and Development, December 17–18, 2008, Indian Statistical Institute, New Delhi*. Available at: http://www.isid.ac.in/~pu/conference/dec_08_conf/Papers/PeterSvedberg.pdf (accessed 26 June 2013).

UNICEF (1998) *The State of the World's Children 1998: Focus on Nutrition*. Published for United Nations Children's Fund, New York by Oxford University Press, New York.

WFP (2004) Women's Nutritional Status. World Food Programme, Rome. Available at: http://www.food-securityatlas.org/bgd/country/utilization/womens-nutritional-status (accessed 26 June 2013).

WFP (2005) Bangladesh Poverty Map 2005. Food Security at a Glance: 7. Food Vulnerability. Available at: http://foodsecurityatlas.org/bgd/country/food-security-at-a-glance#section-6 (accessed 26 June 2013).

29 Food-based Approaches for Improving Diets and Raising Levels of Nutrition: The Fish Story

Fisheries and Aquaculture Department (FI)*†
Food and Agriculture Organization of the United Nations, Rome, Italy

---

Summary

Improving diets and raising levels of nutrition - in terms of animal protein, essential nutrients, and micro-nutrients - is a key aspect of food security for millions of people around the world. Fish have an important role in nutrition-sensitive agriculture and food-based approaches that sustainably improve diets and raise levels of nutrition in terms of animal protein, essential nutrients and micronutrients. This chapter highlights a number of ways in which the fisheries and aquaculture sector does this and provides examples based on some of the work of the FAO Fisheries and Aquaculture Department.

Introduction

The fisheries and aquaculture sector is crucial to food and nutrition security, poverty alleviation and general well-being, and its importance is growing: people have never consumed as much fish nor depended so much on the sector for their livelihoods. Fisheries and aquaculture play a key role in providing food for billions who benefit from an excellent source of affordable, high-quality animal protein and micronutrients that are particularly important for mothers-to-be and young children.

Improving Diets: The Contribution of Fish to Animal Protein Intake

For a billion people, fish contributes at least 30% of animal protein intake, and for almost 3 billion

people fish contributes at least 15% of animal protein intake.[1] In 2008, capture fisheries and aquaculture supplied the world with 115 million tonnes (mt) of fish for human consumption, with an all-time-high average of 17 kg per capita (FAO, 2010).[2] There are also countries in which the per capita supply of fish is over 25 kg/person a year and where fish provides a major part of the animal protein in peoples' diets.

In terms of animal protein, food fish represented 16.1% of total supply in 2007 (when the total global animal protein supply was reported as 29.8 kg per capita), followed by poultry (14.8%), pork (14.4%) and beef (12.1%). In the same year, fish accounted for about 6.1% of total protein consumed (Fig. 29.1). Moreover, fish is one of the primary sources of animal protein in developing countries, contributing about 18% of the total animal protein supply (Fig. 29.2).

---

*Contributors: Rebecca Metzner, Jogeir Toppe, Yvette DieiOuadi and Tina Farmer
†Contact: fi-inquiries@fao.org

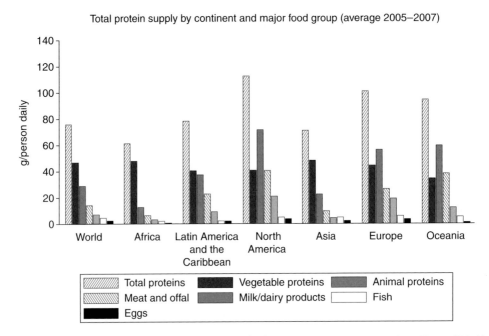

Fig. 29.1. Total protein supply by continent and major food group (2005–2007 average). From *State of World Fisheries and Aquaculture 2010*. Food and Agriculture Organization of the United Nations, Rome.

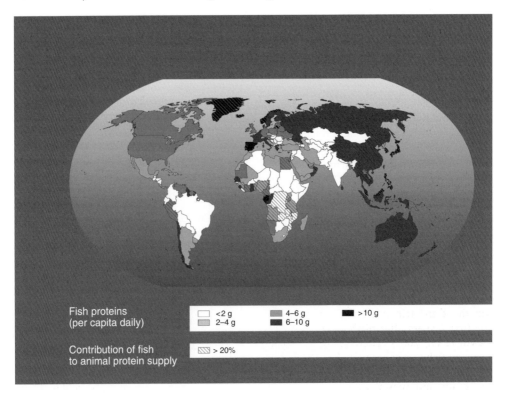

Fig. 29.2. Contribution of fish to animal protein supply (average 2005-2007). From *State of World Fisheries and Aquaculture 2010*. Food and Agriculture Organization of the United Nations, Rome.

The role of fish in ensuring food and nutrition security is not without challenges. As fish are among the most highly traded food commodities (nearly 40% of all production is exported), and with developing countries now accounting for 55% of world fish exports destined for human consumption in quantity terms, changes in fish stocks and fish trade have the potential to affect people's diets and nutrition. This means that the related issues of where, when and how fish are traded become extremely important in terms of ensuring food security and nutrition. The challenge is all the greater in poor areas where fish have been an affordable source of essential nutrients and in coastal populations where fish are a major source of animal protein and micronutrients.

Improving Nutritional Security: The Role of Fish as a Complete Nutritional Package

The contribution of fish as the most economical or affordable primary source of protein is all the more critical in the case of rural diets that may not be particularly diverse. Thus, it is vital to have this unique source of essential nutrients – not the least of which includes the long chained omega-3 fatty acids DHA[3] and EPA.[4]

Omega-3 fatty acids

There is increasing knowledge about the importance of long chained (LC) omega-3 fatty acids in brain and neural development in children, and also of their impact on mortality from coronary heart diseases (CHD) (FAO/WHO, 2011). DHA is a major building stone in the human brain and is mainly incorporated into the developing brain during the third trimester of pregnancy and the first 2 years after birth (Martinez, 1992; Lewin et al., 2005). There is an increasing focus on fish as a source of DHA and iodine, both essential for the early development of the brain and neural system, particularly because these nutrients are almost exclusively found in seafood.

In addition to the importance of the LC omega-3 fatty acids in brain and neural development in children, their role in reducing mortality from CHD is becoming more and more evident. A pooled analysis of 19 different studies showed a 36% risk reduction in CHD mortality with a daily consumption of 250 mg EPA + DHA (Mozaffarian and Rimm, 2006). The main sources of these fatty acids are fish and other seafood, and this underlines the importance of consuming fisheries products in all populations and all age groups.

Fish as more than proteins and omega-3

In addition to the benefits mentioned above, seafood provides more than proteins and omega-3 fatty acids. Fish provide a unique and complete source of micronutrients that are easily absorbed by the body, and this is extremely important when micronutrient deficiencies are affecting hundreds of millions of people, particularly women and children in the developing world.

- More than 250 million children worldwide are at risk of vitamin A deficiency.
- Two hundred million people have goitre, and 20 million are retarded as a result of iodine deficiency.
- Two billion people (over 30% of the world's population) are iron deficient.
- Eight hundred thousand child deaths a year are attributable to zinc deficiency (Table 29.1) (WHO, 2007, 2008, 2009).

One possible food-based approach in combating micronutrient deficiencies is increased access to and consumption of fisheries products. Increased consumption of fisheries products can be used to combat most of the major micronutrient deficiencies. Essential minerals, such as calcium, iodine, zinc, iron and selenium are widely found in fish products, particularly in fish bones and small species that are consumed whole. A very good source of iron and zinc, for example, is chanwa pileng (Esomus longimanus), a Cambodian fish; 20 g of this fish can cover the recommended daily intake of iron and zinc of a child. Moreover, seafood is almost the only natural source of iodine.

Table 29.1. Role of fish in resolving micronutrient deficiencies. From WHO (2007, 2008, 2009).

Micronutrient deficiency	Level of micronutrient/100 g edible part	Recommended daily intake for children

Iodine
    54 countries are still iodine deficient
    200 million people have goitre
    20 million people are retarded as a
        result of iodine deficiency
	Seafood is nearly the only natural food
	    source of iodine. There are 250 µg
	    iodine/100 g cod (*Gadus morhua*)
		120 µg

Iron
    Iron deficiency affects about 2 billion
        people (Halwart, 2006)
	Small-sized fish eaten whole are a good
	    iron source. There are 45 mg iron/100 g
	    chanwa pileng (*Esomus longimanus*)
		8.9 mg

Vitamin A
    250 million preschoolchildren are
        vitamin A deficient
	Small-sized fish eaten whole are a good
	    source of vitamin A. There are >2500 µg
	    RAE/100 g mola (*Amblypharyngodon
	    mola*)
		500 µg RAE[a]

Zinc
    800,000 child deaths/year are
        attributable to zinc deficiency
	Small-sized fish eaten whole are a good
	    source of zinc. There are 20 mg zinc/100 g
	    chanwa pileng (*Esomus longimanus*)
		3.7 mg

[a]RAE, retinol activity equivalents.

Vitamins such as vitamin A, D and the complex of B vitamins (particularly vitamin B_{12}) are found in significant amounts in different fish species. Species eaten whole are particularly good sources of vitamin A. Some small indigenous species, such as mola (*Amblypharyngodon mola*) from Bangladesh are particularly high in vitamin A, with >2500 µg RAE (retinol activity equivalents)/100 g fish (Roos *et al.*, 2007). Thus, 140 g of this fish could cover a child's weekly need of vitamin A.

Related FAO Fisheries and Aquaculture Department Activities

The cultivation of most rice crops in irrigated, rain-fed and deep-water systems offers a suitable environment for fish and other aquatic organisms. Over 90% of the world's rice cultivation - equivalent to approximately 134 million ha - is grown under flooded conditions. This not only provides habitat to a wide range of aquatic organisms, but also offers opportunities for their enhancement and culture. The sentence: 'There is rice in the fields, fish in the water' that is inscribed on a stone tablet from the Sukhothai[5] period reflects this combination that creates both abundance and sufficiency – a combination

that few other plant and animal combinations can match, and which it is more appropriate to culture together to improve nutrition and alleviate poverty (Halwart, 2006).

For more than 15 years, work on the development of sustainable aquaculture integrated practices in rural areas, such as rice–fish culture and integrated irrigation and fish farming (see Fig. 29.3), has been used as a way of enhancing fish consumption and reducing poverty among vulnerable farmers. Both normative and field activities have been carried out in many countries, including Mali, Benin, Sierra Leone, Burkina Faso, Cambodia and Laos (FAO/IIRR/WorldFish Center, 2001; FAO, 2008; Miller, 2009; Nurhasan *et al.*, 2010).

FAO's work with rice fish farming strategies has revealed that the number of aquatic rice field species is underestimated – and that almost 200 species are among those consumed. These supply a wide range of nutrients needed by the rural population, and cultivated species may be complemented by harvested species. This can be of particular significance for indigenous communities and for poor and vulnerable communities, especially in times of shortage of the main staples (see Box 29.1). Wild and gathered foods therefore provide important diversity, nutrition and food security.

The Fisheries and Aquaculture Department (FI) of FAO (Food and Agriculture Organization of the United Nations) also works on a vast range of activities related to improving the utilization and safety of fisheries products by providing technical advice and capacity building for:

(i) appropriate technologies for improved utilization; and (ii) better practices for hygienic fish handling, the use of ice, preservation, processing and marketing. There are both normative and applied products and activities in the development and dissemination of value-adding

(a)

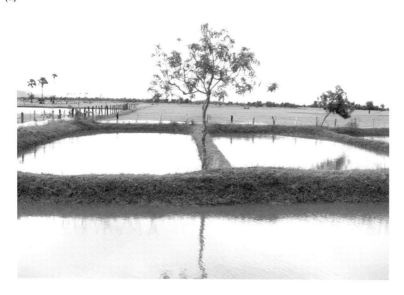

(b)

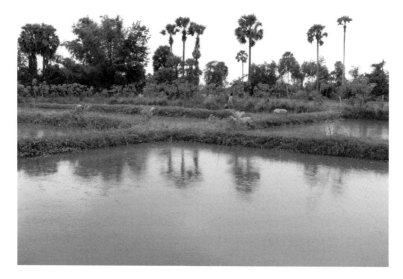

Fig. 29.3. Examples of integrated aquaculture approaches: (a) Mondulkri, Cambodia; (b) Stung Treng, Cambodia; (c) Dong Tao, Vietnam; (d) Hai Phong, Vietnam. Photos courtesy of R. Garcia Gomez.

(c)

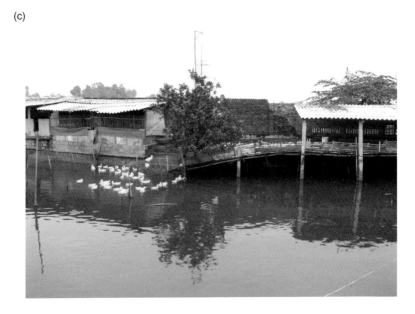

(d)

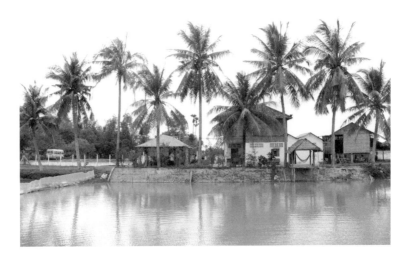

Fig. 29.3. Continued.

Box 29.1. Nutritional composition of aquatic species in Laotian rice field ecosystems.

In Laotian rice field ecosystems, aquatic animals consumed on a daily basis contained high amounts of protein (11.6–19.7% for fish, crustaceans, molluscs, amphibians and insects, and 3.3–7.8% for fermented fish) and a generally acceptable essential amino acid profile. They were also excellent sources of calcium, iron and zinc (Nurhasan *et al.*, 2010).

technologies, the reduction of postharvest losses and the development of affordable products. The FI also provides assistance for developing market structures and market information systems, and for identifying potential commercial partnerships.

To share this knowledge, the FI also works on promoting the health benefits of fish consumption, highlighting fish as a source of essential nutrients, and assists in the design of consumption promotion campaigns.

Looking Forward

Fish have an important role in nutrition-sensitive agriculture and food-based approaches that sustainably improve diets and raise levels of nutrition in terms of animal protein, essential nutrients and micronutrients.

Viable, cost-effective sustainable solutions to ensure food and nutrition security, combat micronutrient deficiencies, improve diets and raise levels of nutrition are essential, and the above examples of work highlight just a few of the ways in which the fisheries and aquaculture sector and the ongoing work of the FAO Fisheries and Aquaculture Department contribute to food and nutrition security. The approaches taken and work described also demonstrate how the fisheries and aquaculture sector is helping in reaching the nutrition-related Millennium Development Goals (MDGs), and supporting the right-to-food approach in preventing hunger and ensuring health and well-being, thereby fulfilling the vision of 'A world in which responsible and sustainable use of fisheries and aquaculture resources makes an appreciable contribution to human well-being, food security and poverty alleviation' (FAO, 2005).

Notes

[1]Note: All figures in this chapter refer to information and data as presented at the time of the symposium (December 2010). More recent and updated statistics are available on the FAO Fisheries and Aquaculture web site (http://www.fao.org/fishery/statistics/en). For the most recent version (2012) of the *State of World Fisheries and Aquaculture*, see http://www.fao.org/docrep/016/i2727e/i2727e00.htm (accessed 26 June 2013).
[2]Being a global figure, consumption per capita varies from less than 1 kg to over 100 kg consumed, depending on the area.
[3]Docosahexaenoic acid.
[4]Eicosapentaenoic acid.
[5]This Thai kingdom flourished some 700 years ago.

References

FAO (2005) *Fisheries and Aquaculture Department Vision Statement*. Food and Agriculture Organization of the United Nations, Rome.

FAO (2008) *FAO Aquaculture Newsletter (FAN) No. 40. Special Issue dedicated to COFI Sub-Committee on Aquaculture IV 06–10 October 2008, Puerto Varas, Chile*. Food and Agriculture Organization of the United Nations, Rome. Available at: http://www.fao.org/docrep/014/i0305e/i0305e00.htm (accessed 26 June 2013).

FAO (2010) *The State of World Fisheries and Aquaculture 2010*. Food and Agriculture Organization of the United Nations, Rome.

FAO/IIRR/WorldFish Center (2001) *Integrated Agriculture–aquaculture: A Primer*. FAO Fisheries Technical Paper 407, Food and Agriculture Organization of the United Nations, Rome/International Institute of Rural Reconstruction, Cavite, Philippines/WorldFish Center (formerly International Center for Living Aquatic Resources Management), Penang, Malaysia. Available at: http://www.fao.org/docrep/005/Y1187E/y1187e00.htm#TopOfPage (accessed 20 June 2013).

FAO/WHO (2011) *Report of the Joint FAO/WHO Expert Consultation on the Risks and Benefits of Fish Consumption, Rome, 25–29 January 2010*. FAO Fisheries and Aquaculture Report No. 978, Food and

Agriculture Organization of the United Nations, Rome. Available at: www.fao.org/docrep/014/ba0136e/ba0136e00.pdf (accessed 26 June 2013).

Halwart, M. (2006) Biodiversity and nutrition in rice-based aquatic ecosystems. *Journal of Food Composition and Analysis* 19, 747–751.

Lewin, G.A. *et al.* (2005) *Effects of Omega-3 Fatty Acids on Child and Maternal Health.* Summary, Evidence Report/Technology Assessment No. 118. Prepared by the University of Ottawa Evidence-based Practice Center under Contract No. 290-02-0021. AHRQ Publication No. 05-E025-2. Agency for Healthcare Research and Quality, Rockville, Maryland.

Martinez, M. (1992) Tissue levels of polyunsaturated fatty acids during early human development. *Journal of Pediatrics* 120, S129–S138.

Miller, J.W. (2009) *Farm Ponds for Water, Fish and Livelihoods.* FAO Diversification Booklet 13. Food and Agriculture Organization of the United Nations, Rome.

Mozaffarian, D. and Rimm, E.B. (2006) Fish intake, contaminants, and human health: evaluating the risks and the benefits. *JAMA* 296, 1885–1899.

Nurhasan, M., Maehre, H.K., Kjellevold Malde, M., Stormo, S.K., Halwart, M., James, D. and Elvevoll, E.O. (2010) Nutritional composition of aquatic species in Laotian rice field ecosystems. *Journal of Food Composition and Analysis* 23, 205–213.

Roos, N., Wahab, M.A., Chamnan, C. and Thilsted, S.H. (2007) The role of fish in food-based strategies to combat vitamin A and mineral deficiencies in developing countries. *Journal of Nutrition* 137, 1106–1109.

WHO (2007) *Assessment of Iodine Deficiency Disorders and Monitoring their Elimination.* World Health Organization, Geneva, Switzerland.

WHO (2008) *Worldwide Prevalence of Anaemia 1993–2005.* World Health Organization, Geneva, Switzerland.

WHO (2009) *Global Prevalence of Vitamin A Deficiency in Populations at Risk 1995–2005.* World Health Organization, Geneva, Switzerland.

30 Forestry in Improving Food Security and Nutrition

Forestry Department (FO)*†
*Food and Agriculture Organization of the
United Nations, Rome, Italy*

Summary

In the last two decades, there has been increasing interest in the role that forests play in food security and improved nutrition as a result of increased realization of the dependence of local people on forests and trees to meet important needs such as food and income. Forests and trees make a big contribution to improved diets and nutritional quality, by adding variety to diets, improving taste and palatability of staples and providing essential vitamins, protein and calories. They provide a large range of edible foods, such as seeds, fruits, leaves, roots, mushrooms and gums; they are habitat for wild animals, insects, rodents and fish; they provide fodder for livestock; and they provide fuelwood for food processing (Falconer and Arnold, 1991). The FAO Forestry Department provides to members legislative and policy support, capacity development and technical guidance on sustainable forest management, including trees outside forests, and on the sustainable management of wildlife within and outside protected areas. The aim of this work is to support improved livelihoods, including food security, nutrition and incomes of local people. There are some challenges related to policy environment, for example, lack of hard data on the contribution of non-wood forest products (NWFPs) to diets, and other governance constraints, that mask the visibility of forestry and its important role in national food security and nutrition policies and strategies.

Background

Forests and trees on farms are a source of food for more than a billion of the world's poorest people. For many small-scale farmers, trees are an integral part of their agricultural system, providing them with both cash and subsistence benefits. These benefits come from both trees that are planted or managed on their farms and from forest resources in communally managed, open-access or state-managed areas. The most direct way in which forests and trees contribute to food security is through their contribution to diets and nutrition. Fruits, seeds and roots of trees and other plants found in forests provide important nutrient and vitamin-rich supplements for rural households. They do this by adding variety to diets, improving the taste and palatability of staples and providing essential vitamins, protein and calories. Forest foods often form a small but critical

*Contributors: Fred Kafeero, Michelle Gauthier, Sophie Grouwels, Florian Steierer, Nora Berrahmouni and Paul Vantomme
†Contact: fo-adg@fao.org

part of an otherwise bland and nutritionally poor diet (FAO, 2011). Poor households, in particular, depend on non-wood forest products (NWFPs) for essential food and nutrition, medicine, fodder, fuel, thatch and construction materials and non-farm income.

The work of the Forestry Department of FAO (Food and Agriculture Organization of the United Nations) ranges from legislative and policy support to capacity development and technical support. It assists countries in developing income-generating tree and forest product enterprises, while also giving them greater incentive to sustainably manage and protect those resources. The work aims to improve livelihoods, and takes various different forms, including:

- FAO-led projects in remote rural areas, agroforestry in peri-urban and urban areas, and also in diverse ecological zones, including dense tropical forests, arid and semi-arid woodlands and mangroves.
- The FAO National Forest Monitoring and Assessment Programme, which undertakes national forest assessments that include specific information on trees outside forests, namely agroforestry systems and tree-based systems in urban environments.
- Developing practical guidelines that offer guidance to practitioners in setting up forestry interventions aimed at reducing poverty, including NWFPs for food and better nutrition (e.g. FAO, 2006).
- Developing guidance material for countries to undertake the systematic integration of agroforestry systems in rural and urban environments.
- Carrying out studies aimed at supporting FAO's 5-yearly Forest Resources Assessments to incorporate data on the reliance of local people on forests for food, income and poverty alleviation in a broader sense.
- Educating the policy makers, donors and senior officials from other sectors of development on the important role of forestry in improved nutrition and food security. In this respect, a policy brief on forestry, improved nutrition and food

security was launched in 2011 as part of the celebrations for The International Year of Forests.

Forestry for Better Nutrition

Many botanical and anthropological studies have documented edible forest products gathered by forest dwellers and non-forest dwellers alike (e.g. FAO 1983; Arnold et al., 1985; Malaisse and Parent, 1985; Gura, 1986). Agroforestry systems also integrate woody species into landscapes and allow for a sustainable and diversified production, and social, economic and environmental benefits (Leakey, 1996). Such systems contribute substantially to nutrition as a result of solutions that integrate food security (diversification of household production and family diet), public health (conservation of traditional medicinal plants) and social protection (source of other incomes).

FAO's field projects on dry-land forestry, NWFPs, community-based forest enterprise development, wildlife management and trees outside forests (including urban and peri-urban forestry) promote the use of forests and trees for income, food security and better nutrition. Within poor households, gender inequality in ownership and access to productive resources, such as land, causes women to rely heavily on NWFPs for income and nutrition.

Below are some specific examples of the contributions of forests and trees to improved nutrition.

Leaves

Wild leaves, either fresh or dried, are one of the most widely consumed forest foods. They are often used as the basis for soups, stews and relishes, which accompany carbohydrate staples such as rice or maize. This is important as it adds both flavour and nutritional value to diets. Wild leaves and leaves from planted trees in agroforestry systems can be excellent sources of vitamins A and C, protein and micronutrients such as calcium and iron that are commonly deficient in diets of nutritionally vulnerable communities. Common 'leaf vegetable' species eaten across different parts of Africa and rich in minerals and in vitamins A and C include *Gnetum africanum, Adansonia digitata, Cassia obtusifolia* and *Moringa oleifera.*

Fruits

Fruits are most commonly consumed raw as a snack or dietary supplement. Forest fruits are also widely used for making beverages, most notably beer. Fruits are especially good sources of minerals and vitamins, and sometimes contribute significant quantities of calories (Fig. 30.1).

A study by Campbell (1986) on the consumption of wild fruits in Zimbabwe, found that three species (*Diospyros mespiliformis, Strychnos cocculoides* and *Azanza garckeana*) were the most frequently consumed and also the most highly prized. In Senegal, wild fruit species such as *Boscia*, which fruits all year round, and *Sclerocarya*, which fruits at the end of the dry season, are most commonly used to meet the seasonal shortages of vitamins that occur at the beginning of the wet season. Agroforestry trees such as guava (*Psidium*

guajava), sugar apple (*Annona squamosa*), pawpaw (*Papaya* sp.) and mango (*Mangifera indica*) are important sources of vitamin C to many households (Fig. 30.2).

Seeds and nuts

Seeds and nuts generally provide important contributions to the diet through the addition of calories, oil and protein. Edible oil (fat) consumption is often low in developing countries and constitutes a major expense for the household (Truscott, 1986). In addition to the energy they provide, fats and oils from seeds and nuts are also important for the absorption of vitamins A, D, E and K. There are numerous examples of nutritionally important nuts and seeds gathered in forests, for example the nuts gathered from the Brazil nut tree (*Bertholletia excelsa*), pine nuts (from *Pinus pinea, P. edulis* and *P. koraiensis*), cola (*Cola edulis*) and chestnuts (*Castanea sativa*).

The shea tree (*Vitellaria paradoxa* and *V. nilotica*), which grows naturally across the West African Sahel region, is an important household resource in the savannah regions of Côte d'Ivoire, Ghana, Burkina Faso, Mali, Togo, Benin and Nigeria, where shea butter from the nuts is used as cooking oil/fat, as a condiment and for the topical treatment of

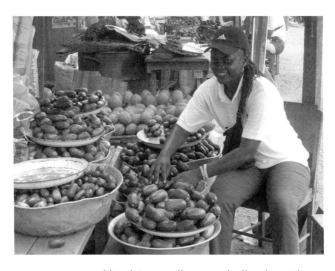

Fig. 30.1. Women in Democratic Republic of Congo collecting and selling fruits. Photo courtesy of Ndoye.

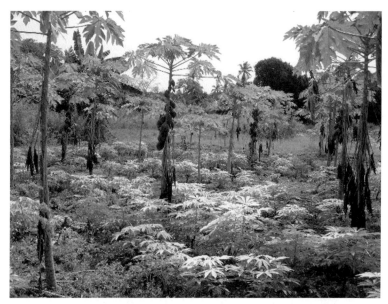

Fig. 30.2. Mixed cropping of papaya with cassava in the Maldives. Photo courtesy of S. Braatz.

various skin conditions. There are more than 500 million fruiting shea trees across the production belt, and FAO estimates that total shea nut production is approximately 600,000 metric tonnes (mt)/year (Ferris *et al.*, 2001).

Roots and tubers

A large variety of forest plants (climbers) have edible roots and tubers. These provide carbohydrates and some minerals. In Swaziland, Ogle and Grivetti (1985) found that approximately 10% of edible wild species commonly eaten were either bulbs or roots, although the only product/species used commonly was the bulbs of the soap aloe (*Aloe saponaria*).

Mushrooms

Mushrooms, gathered wild from forests and woodlands, are much liked in many cultures, and are added to sauces and relishes for flavouring (Box 30.1). In many cases, they provide substitutes for meat.

Honey

Trees in agroforestry systems and other plants growing in forests often play an important role in honey production as they provide year-round fodder for bees because they have different flowering times. In some cultures, honey is collected from wild colonies, although most honey is harvested from hives placed around farms or in neighbouring woodlands or forests. FAO has supported projects in Uganda and several West African countries to produce honey from forest ecosystems. Honey is an excellent source of sugar and is also an important ingredient in many traditional medicines (Fig. 30.3).

Gums and sap

Sap is frequently tapped for beverages and is often high in sugars and minerals. Gum is used as a food supplement and can also be a good source of energy. Both saps and gums have medicinal uses as well. The palmyra palm *(Borassus flabellifer)* is widely cultivated in southern India for its sap. Palm wine tapped from *Raphia hookeri* is popular in

Box 30.1. Mushroom collection in Siberia. From Vladyshevskiy *et al.* (2000).

For the indigenous people of northern and central Siberia, mushrooms are a non-wood forest product (NWFP), with up to 40% of families engaging in their collection. Eighteen species of mushrooms are collected from pine and birch forests across the region. The bulk of them are used for home consumption, but some people engage in processing and sale of mushrooms in local markets. Up to 100 kg of mushrooms/ha can be found in the most productive areas, although on average households collect no more than 5 kg of mushrooms a day.

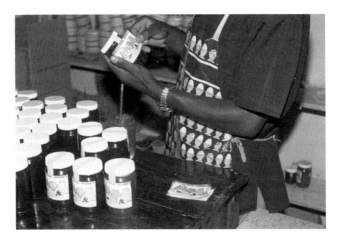

Fig. 30.3. Forest farmers in Uganda involved in the marketing of honey from forests. Photo courtesy of Roberto Faidutti.

West Africa as an important cultural beverage that is consumed in households several times a week (Falconer, 1989).

FAO projects in the arid zones promote the collection and processing of gum arabic (from *Acacia senegal*) for food and as a source of income for pastoralists.

Animal foods from forests and farm trees

Wild animals and fish are other important forest food products. Forested areas, mangroves and streams provide a habitat for many wild animal species and fish. The range of species consumed includes birds and their eggs, insects (Box 30.2), rodents, and other larger mammals.

For people living in close proximity to forests and fallow areas, wild animals are often an important part of their diet and, in some cases, supply the only source of animal protein. In West Africa, where the consumption of bushmeat is high, the most important game meat species are small animals (such as rodents) due to their natural abundance and unrestricted hunting. With the increasing threat to wildlife through illegal hunting, the Wildlife and Protected Area Management Team of FAO's Forestry Department are implementing a project in the Congo Basin to demonstrate that community-based conservation and management of wildlife can be a viable and most effective strategy for conserving the integrity of wildlife, forest ecosystems and biodiversity.

Fodder and browse for livestock

Many species of trees found on the farm, as well as those in forests and the associated shrubs and grasses, are used for animal feed, and provide protein, minerals and vitamins – either as browse or fodder. It has

---

Box 30.2. Forest caterpillars – an important contribution to local diets. From Durst *et al.* (2010).

Caterpillars are very common insects in the forests, can be easily gathered and are an abundant and popular food source in many parts of the world. They are an excellent source of nutrients – providing important contributions of fat and protein. Compared with meat or fish, caterpillars have higher protein and fat contents and provide more energy per unit. Research shows that 100 g of cooked insects provide more than 100% of the daily recommended requirements of vitamins and minerals.

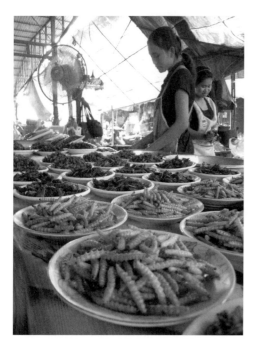

Fig. 30.4. Edible insects a source of food and income in Dong Makkhai market, Laos. Copyright: Arnold van Huis.

Fuel for cooking and processing of food

The main energy source for cooking and/or heating in most developing countries is fuelwood, and fuelwood and charcoal often represent the only domestically available and affordable sources of energy. As many dishes require cooking to make them digestible, fuelwood supplies indirectly affect the stability, quality and even the quantity of food consumed. Taste is another strong reason for using woody biomass for cooking – grilled or smoked dishes are important in diets in every society.

Fuelwood is an important aspect of food processing, which is in itself of central importance to nutritional stability as it serves to extend the supply of a food resource into a non-productive period. FAO's work on community forestry, agroforestry and trees outside forests therefore enhances access by local people to sustainable sources of fuelwood. This work also involves augmenting the energy efficiency of wood fuel and charcoal cooking systems, as well as improving the production of charcoal to abate the pressure on natural resources.

been estimated that 75% of the tree species (7000–10,000) of tropical Africa are used as browse (Wikens *et al.*, 1985). Fodder trees make a significant contribution to domestic livestock production which, in turn, influences milk and meat supply. Fodder contributes to maintaining draught animals and producing manure for organic fertilizer, thereby boosting agricultural production. Tree fodder may consist of leaves, small branches, seeds, pods and fruits, all of which supplement other feeds and which can be a crucial component of livestock diets during the dry season.

Generating income from forests and trees

Food insecurity is generally related to poverty and limited opportunities from employment or income generation. Where poor households are able to accrue some income, this is often directed towards improving food security. Trees on farms and forests, as well as NWFPs, have been shown across the world to provide important and often unrecognized sources of household income. In some cases, this comes from employment in forest industries or from the collection and sale of unprocessed tree and forest-derived products. The production of NWFPs for local markets can provide part-time, seasonal, occasional or full-time year-round employment, depending on the product, location and individual household. This flexibility makes NWFP-related activities particularly appealing to women, and enables them to combine collection and trade of these products with their other domestic duties and responsibilities.

Incomes can be substantially increased through the establishment of small or medium forest-based enterprises, which may secure better market access and share or add value to harvested products. Employment in forest industries, management and conservation provides jobs for around 10 million people worldwide, although this figure appears to have declined slightly in the recent past because of gains in labour productivity. Many countries report increased employment in management of protected areas. Given that most forestry employment takes place outside the formal sector, it is likely that official figures are an underestimation of their true contribution to rural livelihoods and national economies (FAO, 2011).

Conclusion

Although forests and trees outside forests make significant contributions to food security, improved quality of diets and the prevention of malnutrition in many parts of the world, this contribution is generally little known, especially outside the forest sector; so NWFPs are rarely taken into account in food security policies. The lack of data on the consumption of forest foods is equally responsible for the general under-reporting of the vital role that forests and trees play in improving local diets. It is necessary to raise the awareness of policy makers of the need for development programmes in food and nutrition that consider the contribution of NWFPs to local consumption patterns.

There is need for better inter-sectoral and inter-institutional coordination to foster the integration of agriculture, pastoralism, forestry, water, energy and other land-use sectors at policy, management and research levels. This would also increase the efficiency and effectiveness of FAO's normative work.

References

Arnold T.H., Wells, M.J. and Wehmeyer, A.S. (1985) Khoisan food plants: taxa with potential for future economic exploitation. In: Wickens, G.E., Goodin, J.R. and Field, D.V. (eds) *Plants for Arid Lands. Proceedings of Kew International Conference on Economic Plants for Arid Lands.* Allen and Unwin, London, pp. 69–86.

Campbell, B.M. (1986) The importance of wild fruits for peasant households in Zimbabwe. *Food and Nutrition* 12, 38–44.

Durst, P.B., Johnson, D.V., Leslie, R.N. and Shono, K. (eds) (2010) *Edible Forest Insects: Humans Bite Back!! Proceedings of a Workshop on Asia-Pacific Resources and their Potential for Development, 19–21 February 2008, Chiang Mai, Thailand.* RAP Publication 2010/2. FAO (Food and Agriculture Organization of the United Nations) Regional Office for Asia and the Pacific, Bangkok.

Falconer, J. (1989) *The Major Significance of "Minor" Forest Products: Local People's Uses and Values of Forests in the West African Humid Zone.* Community Forestry Note No. 6, Food and Agriculture Organization of the United Nations, Rome.

Falconer, J. and Arnold, J.E.M. (1991) *Household Food Security and Forestry – An Analysis of Socio-economic Issues.* Community Forestry Note No. 6, Food and Agriculture Organization of the United Nations, Rome.

FAO (1983) *Food and Fruit-bearing Species. Examples from East Africa.* FAO Forestry Paper No. 44/3, Food and Agriculture Organization of the United Nations, Rome.

FAO (2006) *Better Forestry, Less Poverty: A Practitioner's Guide.* FAO Forestry Paper No. 149, Food and Agriculture Organization of the United Nations, Rome.

FAO (2011) *Forests for Improved Nutrition and Food Security*. Food and Agriculture Organization of the United Nations, Rome.

Ferris, R.S.B., Collinson, C., Wanda, K., Jagwe, J. and Wright, P. (2001) *Evaluating the Marketing Opportunities for Shea Nut and Shea Nut Processed Products in Uganda*. Natural Resource Institute, Kampala, and FoodNet. Available at: http://www.foodnet.cgiar.org/Projects/Sheanut_Rep.pdf (accessed 26 June 2013).

Gura, S. (1986) A note on traditional food plants in East Africa: their value for nutrition and agriculture. *Food and Nutrition* 12, 18–26.

Leakey, R.R.B. (1996) Definition of agroforestry revisited. *Agroforestry Today* 8(1), 5–7.

Malaisse, F. and Parent, G. (1985) Edible wild vegetable products in the Zambian woodland area: a nutritional and ecological approach. *Ecology of Food and Nutrition* 18, 43–82.

Ogle, B.M. and Grivetti, L.E. (1985) Legacy of the chameleon edible wild plants in the kingdom of Swaziland, S. Africa. A cultural, ecological, nutritional study. *Ecology of Food and Nutrition* 16, 193–208.

Truscott, K. (1986) Socio-economic factors in food production and consumption. *Food and Nutrition* 12, 27–37.

Vladyshevskiy, D.V., Laletin, A.P. and Vladyshevskiy, A.D. (2000) *Role of wildlife and other non-wood forest products in food security in central Siberia*. Unasylva 51, 46–52.

Wickens, G.E., Field, D.V. and Goodin, J.R. (eds) (1985) *Plants for Arid Lands. Proceedings of Kew International Conference on Economic Plants for Arid Lands*. Allen and Unwin, London.

31 Legal and Institutional Aspects of Food and Nutrition Security

Development Law Service,*† Legal Office (LEG)
*Food and Agriculture Organization of the
United Nations, Rome, Italy*

Summary

The right to nutrition is implicitly recognized in a number of human rights instruments and explicitly so as far as children, pregnancy and lactation are concerned. The Voluntary Guidelines to support the progressive realization of the right to adequate food in the context of national food security (Right to Food Guidelines) adopted by the FAO Council in 2004 contain a number of references to nutrition. Human rights-based approaches imply the incorporation of participation, accountability, non-discrimination, transparency, human dignity, empowerment and the rule of law (PANTHER) principles into relevant nutrition programmes and legislation. Coordination among the institutions involved in food and nutrition security at the national level is a key challenge and can be met through framework law. A number of other sectoral laws also promote food and nutrition security.

Introduction

This chapter discusses the legal and institutional aspects of food and nutrition security from a human rights perspective. It explores the notion of nutrition as a human right by itself, and the rights that contribute to good nutrition, namely the right to adequate food, the right to health and the right to care.

The Right to Food Guidelines are explained and their contribution to nutrition highlighted. The meaning and implications of a human rights-based approach to food and nutrition are also summarized.

Finally, the main outlines of national legal and institutional frameworks for nutrition are briefly explored and the importance of inter-ministerial coordination highlighted.

Nutrition as a Human Right

Good nutrition according to common conceptual frameworks depends on access to food, health and care. International law recognizes each of these as a right in different ways, and also contains references to nutrition.

The right to adequate food, as part of the right to an adequate standard of living, and the fundamental right to be free from hunger, are recognized in article 11 of the

---

*Contributor: Margret Vidar
†Contact: devlaw@fao.org

International Covenant on Economic, Social and Cultural Rights (ICESCR, 1966).[1] The right includes elements of availability, access and adequacy. Adequacy relates to both the safety and nutritional value of the food as well as to its cultural acceptability.[2] The recognition of the right to be free from hunger specifies, inter alia, that state parties should take steps to disseminate principles of nutrition (article 11:2).

The right to safe drinking water, which is fundamental for good nutrition, is also recognized as part of the right to food and implicit in the right to health and the right to housing.[3] Nutrition is implicitly recognized in article 11, as this was meant, according to the drafters of the ICESCR, to have a broad and general meaning,[4] and also because the right to an adequate standard of living lists adequate food as one of the elements in an open and non-restrictive way. The Convention on the Rights of the Child (CRC, 1989)[5] recognizes in article 27 the right of the child to an adequate standard of living and lists among state parties' obligations assisting the parents with regard to nutrition.

The right to the highest attainable standard of physical and mental health is recognized in article 12 of the ICESCR. The Committee on Economic, Social and Cultural Rights (CESCR) has articulated that there are various interrelated and essential elements of the right to health, including availability, accessibility, acceptability and quality of the various determinants of health, and specified that access to clean drinking water and to sanitation are one of those elements.[6] This article can be said to recognize nutrition as a part of the right to health as, according to the CESCR, the right to health 'is not to be understood as the right to be healthy but extending to the underlying determinants of health such as an adequate supply of safe food, nutrition'.

The right to health is also recognized in article 24.2(c) of the CRC, which requires states to ensure both health and health services for children through provision of adequate nutrition. Furthermore, article 24.2(e) stipulates the obligations of states to ensure that children have access to education by disseminating basic knowledge of child health

and nutrition, the advantages of breastfeeding, hygiene and environmental sanitation and the prevention of accidents.

The Convention on the Elimination of All Forms of Discrimination Against Women (CEDAW, 1979)[7] recognizes a general right to non-discriminatory access to health services in article 12 and provides for specific reproductive rights, including nutrition rights during pregnancy and lactation.

'Care' refers to the physical assistance given by one person to another and also refers to the broader environment in which individuals live and enable them to care for themselves, such as adequate housing and education. The right to care in the sense of physical assistance has been spelt out in article 10 of the ICESCR for women, and care for children's nutritional needs is covered in articles 24 and 27 of the CRC. The right to adequate housing is part of article 11 of the ICESCR and the right to education is recognized, inter alia, in article 13 of the ICESCR.

While nutrition is not explicitly mentioned as a right in the key human rights instruments, it is understood to be implicit in the right to food and the right to health in the ICESCR and enjoys more explicit mention in the CRC and CEDAW.

Nutrition in the Right to Food Guidelines

The Voluntary Guidelines to support the progressive realization of the right to adequate food (Right to Food Guidelines) were adopted by consensus by the FAO Council in 2004,[8] and enjoy the support of all FAO members.

Guideline 10, entitled Nutrition, covers a number of issues relating to dietary diversity, eating habits and food preparation. It promotes the use of education, information and labelling against overconsumption or unbalanced diets. It also recommends the participation of stakeholders in production and consumption programmes and that micronutrient deficiencies should be addressed both through home and school gardens and fortification. The nutrition needs of HIV/AIDS sufferers and others are specifically highlighted. Guideline 10 promotes breastfeeding, including the International Code on Marketing of Breast-milk Substitutes and Protection against Misinformation about Infant Feeding. It refers to WHO (World Health Organization) and UNICEF (United Nations Children's Fund) guidelines at any given time for guidance on breastfeeding in the context of HIV/AIDS. It recommends parallel action in health, education and sanitary infrastructure for good nutrition. It also recommends that states and others address discrimination within households and respect cultural diversity with regard to food and nutrition.

Guideline 11 addresses food safety and consumer protection and highlights a number of relevant issues to this, which are not further described here.

Human Rights-based Approaches

Human rights principles are principles that relate to the process of implementing other rights, such as the rights to food, health and care and the right to nutrition. FAO generally refers to the seven PANTHER[9] principles in its illustration of human rights-based approaches.

Participation

In general, participation means the right to active, free and meaningful participation in decisions that affect a person. In the context of nutrition, the participation of the relevant sectors and of all stakeholders at community and household levels (both men and women) is needed for good nutrition planning and programme implementation. Parents should also be consulted and involved in the planning of services for children.

Accountability

In terms of accountability, public institutions and officials should be held accountable for their actions and failure to act. Furthermore, health workers who implement nutrition

programmes must also be held accountable for ensuring the provision of quality health care and treatment. In the context of nutrition, the nutrition situation (malnutrition rates) of a population is a good indicator of the realization of (or failure to achieve) the right to food and nutrition. To ensure accountability, the roles and responsibilities of different stakeholders participating in the nutrition strategy and programmes need to be clear. This requires an in-depth situation analysis of the causes of malnutrition, as they will determine which sectors should do what.

Non-discrimination

In general, no programme may discriminate on the basis of race, sex, religion, language or other such reason in its design or in its effect. In the context of nutrition, the analysis of malnutrition rates and causes can help to identify the needs of different population groups and the opportunities to address them. This requires disaggregated data (e.g. by gender, economic group, geographical area), but even if data are not available, analysis can be carried out through participatory assessment methods. Special emphasis should be put on reaching the most vulnerable people and attention must also be paid to intra-household distribution.

Transparency

Policies and programmes must be publicly available and accessible to beneficiaries. In the context of nutrition, special care should be taken to ensure that information is actively provided in local languages and through other media than the written word in order to reach illiterate people as well as those who are literate.

Human dignity

Everyone should be treated with respect and dignity simply because they are human beings. Nutrition interventions should therefore be implemented in a way that avoids long-term dependence on external or unsustainable sources of food. Feeding programmes should be respectful. Nutrition interventions should respect and value local cultural preferences, practices, knowledge and environment. At the same time, they should address cultural practices that have a negative impact on nutrition in a culturally sensitive way.

Empowerment

In general, people should have the knowledge and capacity to realize their own rights. Nutrition interventions should help people to make optimal use of their own resources (assets, skills and knowledge, etc.) to have good nutrition. This is a key for sustainability. Nutrition education plays a role in informing people about their nutritional needs and thus empowers them to improve their nutrition. Being able to know about and claim entitlement related to nutrition is also essential. For example, awareness building is needed in educational systems through the inclusion of nutrition in primary and secondary school curricula. In addition, community education (focusing on the vulnerable) can contribute to improving food and nutrition security at the local level.

Rule of law

In general, everyone, including state officials, is bound by the law of the land and may not act arbitrarily. Healthy nutrition is a human right and therefore demands the application of procedural rights. Nutrition interventions should be made on the basis of law, by people who have the legal responsibility and authority to carry them out, and provide for entitlements guaranteed by law and subject to redress in case of non-delivery.

National Legal and Institutional Frameworks

Food and nutrition security are by nature cross-sectoral issues that cannot be dealt with by one sector or ministry. Therefore, the Food and Agriculture Organization of the United Nations (FAO) promotes the establishment of inter-ministerial coordination mechanisms, preferably headed by the prime minister or president, to ensure a more coordinated action between agriculture, health, trade, transport and other key ministries of a country.

In recent years, food and nutrition security framework laws have been adopted in a steadily growing number of countries[10] to provide the legal basis for their coordination.[11] Many of these laws have been adopted in countries as part of implementing the right to adequate food, and in addition to establishing a mechanism and spelling out roles, these laws may do the following:

• Establish guiding principles, such as human rights principles.
• Recognize and spell out rights of citizens.
• Ensure civil society participation.
• Provide recourse for violations of rights.
• Set up a framework for monitoring.

In addition to general framework laws, a number of sectoral laws generally regulate aspects of nutrition security. Among these are food control laws for food safety and quality and laws on consumer information and protection against misinformation through marketing and labelling. Specific legislation exists in many countries to regulate the marketing of breast milk substitutes in accordance with the WHO Code of Conduct (1981)[12] on the matter. Legislation may also mandate the fortification of certain commodities, most commonly salt iodization.

Notes

[1]See http://www.ohchr.org/EN/ProfessionalInterest/Pages/CESCR.aspx (accessed 27 June 2013).
[2]Committee on Economic, Social and Cultural Rights (CESCR) (1999) General Comment 12: The right to adequate food. UN doc E/C.12/1999/5.
[3]Committee on Economic, Social and Cultural Rights (CESCR) (1999) General Comment 12: The right to adequate food. UN doc E/C.12/1999/5, and CESCR (2003) General Comment 15: The right to water. UN doc E/C.12/2002/11.

[4]Craven, M. (1995) The International Covenant on Economic, Social, and Cultural Rights: A Perspective on its Development. Clarendon Press, Oxford, UK, p. 301.

[5]See http://www.ohchr.org/EN/ProfessionalInterest/Pages/CRC.aspx (accessed 27 June 2013).

[6]Committee on Economic, Social and Cultural Rights (CESCR) (2000) General Comment No. 14: The Right to the highest attainable standard of health, UN doc E/C.12/2000/4.

[7]See http://www.un.org/womenwatch/daw/cedaw/text/econvention.htm#article12 (accessed 27 June 2013).

[8]Report of the Council of the FAO Hundred and Twenty-seventh Session (Rome, 22–27 November 2004), Appendix D. FAO doc CL 127/REP.

[9]PANTHER is an acronym standing for participation, accountability, non-discrimination, transparency, human dignity, empowerment and rule of law, coined by Margret Vidar of FAO. See FAO (2009) *Guide on Legislating for the Right to Food*. Right to Food Methodological Toolbox, Book 1, Food and Agriculture Organization of the United Nations, Rome.

[10]For instance: Brazil (Law no 11.236 of 2006 *Establishing the national food and nutrition security system*); Guatemala (law on national food and nutrition security system, decree no 32-2005 of 2005); and Indonesia (Food Act no 7/1996). Other countries, such as Mozambique and Uganda, have prepared drafts that are under discussion at the time of writing.

[11]For more information, see Knuth, L. and Vidar, M. (2010) *Constitutional and Legal Protection of the Right to Food around the World*. Right to Food Study, Food and Agriculture Organization of the United Nations, Rome.

[12]See http://www.who.int/nutrition/publications/code_english.pdf (accessed 27 June 2013).

32 Food and Agriculture-based Approaches to Safeguarding Nutrition Before, During and After Emergencies: The Experience of FAO

Emergency and Rehabilitation Division (TCE),[*†]
Technical Cooperation Department (TC)
Food and Agriculture Organization of the United Nations, Rome, Italy

---

Summary

Standard food-based approaches to nutrition in emergencies are dominated by food aid and emergency feeding programmes. However, agriculture has an important role to play as part of a more integrated package to tackle nutrition in emergencies. In order to maximize the impact of agriculture-based responses, two 'lenses' are important. First, a 'nutrition lens' to ensure that projects and programmes are designed, implemented and monitored with nutritional outcomes in mind. Secondly, a 'disaster risk management' lens, which highlights the importance of reducing the impact of disasters through risk reduction and recovery actions in addition to standard response actions. FAO is involved in a range of emergency projects with assumed or measured nutritional impacts, and is striving to apply both 'lenses' to its interventions in emergencies; however, there are a number of challenges. Meeting these challenges requires a combination of activities that include: nutrition awareness raising between FAO and the food security 'community'; incorporating nutrition-related objectives as well as required indicators for targeting and monitoring (e.g. dietary diversity for adults, diversity of complementary foods for children); building the evidence base on agriculture–nutrition linkages through improved monitoring and evaluation (M&E) and lesson sharing; advocating joint planning by agencies at country level using a shared conceptual and analytical framework for food and nutrition interventions; better articulation of Food Security and Nutrition clusters; and better enforcement of nutrition goals and mainstreaming in appeal programmes and project documents and monitoring. Support to sustainable food-based interventions in emergencies from a 'right to food' perspective is another area that requires a stronger focus.

Introduction

Food and agriculture-based approaches to improving nutrition in emergency contexts have not received the attention or emphasis that they deserve from the international community, academia or national governments. By 'food and agriculture-based' we include agricultural production (horticulture, crops, livestock, fisheries),[1] food processing and nutrition promotion, and exclude therapeutic and supplementary feeding and general food distribution (GFD).

It is important to present the case for food and agriculture-based approaches, while

---

*Contributors: Neil Marsland, Angela Hinrichs, Jackie Were, Laura Tiberi, Charlotte Dufour, Graiine Maloney and Fatouma Seid
†Contacts: neil.marsland@fao.org; tce-director@fao.org

acknowledging that there are a number of challenges. Addressing these challenges will require the documentation and dissemination of successful practices, strengthening of the capacity for designing, implementing and evaluating integrated food and nutrition security interventions, and more connectedness in planning and coordination between actors working within the spheres of agriculture and nutrition.

The Food and Agriculture Organization of the United Nations (FAO) has a key role to play in advocating for and strengthening country-level capacity to implement food and agriculture-based approaches in emergencies, and it has several relevant experiences and competencies on which to draw and from which to learn. The recent initiation of the Global Food Security cluster,[2] and increasing attention to nutrition in emergencies, provide good opportunities to intensify efforts to promote food and agriculture-based approaches to nutrition in emergency contexts.

Emergencies and Food

In emergencies, food intake may be compromised in a number ways, by:

- reduction of local food availability and household access to food (physical destruction, destruction of infrastructure);
- effects on food preparation practices and food safety due to lack of access to water, firewood, electricity;
- adverse effects on caring capacity and the feeding of young children;
- weakening or removal of previously existing coping strategies (e.g. migration, casual labour); and
- necessity for destructive and extreme coping options, e.g. family break-up, theft, prostitution, asset disposal.

In emergencies, most nutrition interventions focus on the treatment of acute malnutrition through therapeutic and supplementary feeding and GFD. When well designed and implemented these may indeed be vital for saving lives and preventing terminal asset depletion. However, they do not address the underlying causes of malnutrition, and may create unnecessary dependency and negatively affect self-esteem. They may also be very costly and may not be sustainable.

Complementing and replacing these approaches over time with well-designed and implemented food and agriculture-based responses would ensure sustainable improvements in the food and nutrition situation of affected households and communities. In order to maximize this benefit, food and agriculture-based responses should be designed, implemented and monitored using nutrition and disaster risk management (DRM) 'lenses'.

Nutrition and Disaster Risk Management (DRM) 'Lenses'

Applying a nutrition lens to agricultural interventions means that the design and monitoring of emergency agricultural projects needs to be done with an understanding of:

- which kinds of people are most at risk of malnutrition;
- what the causes of malnutrition are for these people; and
- how the proposed interventions will have an impact on their nutritional status.

Both intended and unintended consequences of emergency agricultural interventions should be evaluated in terms of potential impacts on nutrition at the design stage. Emergency responses should be designed and implemented in such a way as to protect, restore and enhance local food availability and household access to safe and nutritious foods, and to ensure that households have the knowledge and skills needed to make optimal use of this food.

Applying a nutrition lens also means using appropriate monitoring indicators. Dietary intake and diversity indicators – which provide a measure of household access to and consumption of diverse foods – are more appropriate than anthropometric measurements insofar as the latter are significantly affected by health status. Ideally, both anthropometry and dietary diversity indicators should be used together to improve understanding of specific impacts within a more general nutritional context.

The application of a nutrition lens within a DRM perspective widens the scope of nutrition interventions beyond the standard emergency response 'window' to include preparedness and transition/recovery phases. In terms of preparedness, this means that, for example, contingency planning for the food and agriculture sector should explicitly include actions that would reduce the risk of negative nutritional impacts and strengthen the resilience to possible shocks of households that are at risk of, or are affected by, malnutrition. This can be done by diversifying food production, improving food storage, diversifying livelihood strategies, and associating nutrition education with these interventions. Similarly, nutritional considerations should be mainstreamed not just into standard agricultural emergency responses but also into recovery and rehabilitation interventions through operations[3] designed to strengthen the resilience of local food systems and improve local feeding practices.

FAO and Food-based Approaches

FAO is striving to improve the nutritional impact of its food and agriculture-based interventions in emergencies by applying the nutrition lens within a DRM framework, as has just been described. FAO's experience has generated some interesting examples and success stories, and many lessons learned.

In Somalia, the FAO Food Security and Nutrition Analysis Unit (FSNAU) has developed a nutrition situation map based on an integrated analysis of the available nutrition information. The map clearly indicates the severity and magnitude of malnutrition in the country. This product, updated twice a year in parallel to the IPC (Integrated Food Security Phase Classification) household food access map (originally developed for use in Somalia by FSNAU),[3] helps to target food and agriculture interventions to those with different levels of nutritional vulnerability. The analysis also highlights the key drivers of the nutritional situation, including the role of public health (disease outbreaks,

poor water quality, etc.) and the role of food security, including dietary diversity.

In both Somalia and Indonesia, FAO has developed a Response Analysis Framework that requires practitioners from food, agriculture and nutrition sectors to come together and agree on the causes of nutritional problems using a shared conceptual framework. This joint problem identification lays a strong platform for coordinated responses across sectors and clusters. It gives agencies in the agricultural sector, inter alia, an understanding of how their actions and interventions are contributing to or could contribute to nutritional outcomes, and how this could be strengthened through inter-sectoral and inter-institutional collaboration.

In Niger, gendered livelihood support is yielding dividends in terms of improving access to food for family members. Several FAO projects are combining to provide off-season activities, the distribution of small ruminants and agricultural inputs, and the leasing of land and irrigation water, all targeting women. The empowerment of women through the appropriation of agricultural inputs, including land and water, has proved to be a key factor in reducing child malnutrition and vulnerability to food insecurity. The strengthening of household safety nets through the distribution of small ruminants to women allows them to have a productive role and contribute to the household economy. Women are reinvesting more than 50% of their income in improving household food access. The participation of mothers in social mobilization and agricultural production activities has contributed to strengthened social cohesion and improved nutritional practices.

In Gaza, 85% of traditional fishing grounds are now out of bounds due to restrictions imposed by the Israeli navy. As a result, per capita fish consumption has fallen from 5 kg/year in 2000 to 2.2 kg in 2009. Responding to this, FAO has introduced 100 aquaculture ponds in southern Gaza. The project will add an estimated 50 t of fish to the market in 2010, almost doubling the entire aquaculture sector's production in a year. It is planned to link the project with a fresh food voucher scheme, thereby ensuring that protein reaches the poorest and most food-insecure families.

In Afghanistan, FAO has been part of an innovative inter-agency and inter-sectoral collaboration to improve the nutrition of children and mothers affected by protracted crisis. Along with the United Nations Children's Fund (UNICEF), FAO has been co-chairing the Afghanistan Nutrition Cluster[4] since the activation of the cluster approach in the country in early 2008. While the close cooperation among major stakeholders has provided great opportunities for a more comprehensive approach to prevent and treat malnutrition, funding constraints have placed limits on collaboration. In response, the cluster applied for and was awarded funding from the Central Emergency Response Fund (CERF)[5] to implement an integrated and more sustainable approach to malnutrition. This approach provides food products for therapeutic and supplementary feeding linked to the promotion of improved complementary feeding for children and mothers, using locally available and affordable foods. Children and families identified as needing nutritional support also receive assistance for homestead food production (training, provision of simple agricultural inputs) and agricultural extension at clinic and community demonstration gardens.

Integrating nutrition into agricultural extension in a post-conflict recovery setting is a key aspect of the Junior Farmer Field and Life Schools (JFFLS) approach in northern Uganda. Children affected by conflict (either orphans or children separated from their families) work together with adult facilitators to integrate postharvest food utilization and processing skills with an understanding of basic nutrition and agricultural skills.

Various studies have investigated the impact of nutritional education on nutritional status. There is some evidence to suggest that nutrition education which provides simple messages tailored to low-income families has made an impact on caregiver child feeding practices and, subsequently, on child growth.[6] In certain kinds of emergency situations, providing nutrition education through community worker networks is possible and can have beneficial impacts. With this in mind, FAO has been training community workers in Zimbabwe in good nutrition and in the growing, processing and preparation of healthy food. The *Healthy Harvest* manual is being used as a mainstreaming tool in a variety of interventions promoted by the Department of Agricultural Research and Extension Services (AREX) in the Ministry of Agriculture in Zimbabwe as well as by the Ministry of Health and Child Welfare.

Key Challenges

There are several challenges to a more systematic mainstreaming of nutrition into agricultural interventions in emergencies. One critical issue in this regard is an inadequate evidence base. This is not just an FAO problem: the evaluation of food-based approaches has proved difficult and costly,[7] which is presumably a factor behind the lack of evidence. All other things being equal, improved diets *do* lead to improved nutritional status. However, the links between agricultural interventions, diets and nutritional status need to be much better documented and substantiated. One factor is that the design of project monitoring systems is often not suitable for demonstrating the relationship between nutrition and agriculture. Another issue is that many food-based approaches implemented at the local level by non-governmental organizations (NGOs) are part of a multi-sector intervention and hence it is difficult to compare the effect of food-based interventions with other components, such as water, sanitation and health (WASH).

A second and related challenge is that nutritional issues are often not even thought of in project design, implementation or monitoring. This is true of agencies and donors operating within an agricultural production or a household food security 'paradigm'. Here, it is assumed that increasing production on the one hand or increasing access to food at the household level on the other will automatically have beneficial nutritional outcomes.

Thirdly, even where they exist, food- and agriculture-based approaches with explicit nutritional objectives may be 'crowded out' of funding opportunities by therapeutic or supplementary feeding and GFD interventions at country level. This is due partly to the structure of humanitarian appeals and also to a general lack of awareness by agencies and donors of the potential of such approaches.

Fourthly, the fragmented humanitarian architecture at global and country levels does not facilitate joined-up thinking on nutrition issues. Examples like the cluster approach in Afghanistan mentioned earlier are rare: the nutrition cluster is normally concerned with public health and nutrient supplementation, the agriculture cluster is concerned with production and the food cluster is concerned with food aid. Food- and agriculture-based approaches to nutrition in emergencies often 'fall through the cracks'.

Ways Forward

In order to meet these challenges, the following steps are necessary. First, building up the evidence base is a high priority. One quick and cost-effective way to make progress on this is to include relevant indicators in the monitoring of food and agriculture-based projects. Of key significance are measures of food consumption and dietary diversity that can be directly attributed to the interventions. The Dietary Diversity Tool promoted by FAO is a simple tool that is useful for assessing impact of programmes on the nutritional quality of the diet.[8] At household level the tool is an indicator of access to food, but at individual level (e.g. in women) it is a proxy of the adequacy of micronutrient intake. While the tool was designed primarily to operate in the framework of programmes that address chronic food insecurity and malnutrition, it is also relevant in the context of emergency and recovery interventions.

Clearly, there is much to do to raise awareness of nutrition among food security and agricultural sector practitioners. Mainstreaming good practical publications into the work and thinking of practitioners is important in this regard. The FAO publication: *Protecting and Promoting Good Nutrition in Crisis and Recovery* (2005)[9] is one example of a very useful reference tool that needs to be more fully integrated into relevant capacity building and sensitization initiatives.

The introduction of food security clusters at global and national levels raises the prospect that food- and agriculture-based approaches to improving nutrition in emergencies will have a more stable and systematic institutional home. In order for this to happen, cluster leads and cluster member agencies will need to be sensitized and guided. More generally, nutrition should be looked at in a more holistic and less fragmented manner by the cluster system at country level, linked to and supported by the Food Security Cluster working with the Nutrition Cluster at the global level. This will require joint planning and problem identification processes oriented around a common, conceptual framework that integrates the various causes of malnutrition and allows each cluster to see clearly where it can play a role and where linkages to other clusters need to be made on the ground.[10]

Finally, donors and appeal processes should enforce nutrition mainstreaming as a matter of course in emergency food and agriculture projects. If done consistently, this will encourage clearer thinking about how food security and agriculture projects and programmes are contributing to nutritional objectives in emergencies.

Notes

[1]Including homestead production and productivity.
[2]For further information, see http://foodsecuritycluster.net/ (accessed 27 June 2013).
[3]For further information, see http://www.ipcinfo.org/ipcinfo-about/en/ (accessed 27 June 2013).
[4]Part of the Global Nutrition Cluster, commonly known as the GNC, which was established in 2006 as part of the Humanitarian Reform process. For further information see http://www.unicef.org/nutritioncluster/index_aboutgnc.html (accessed 27 June 2013).
[5]CERF is a humanitarian fund established by the United Nations to enable more timely and reliable humanitarian assistance to those affected by natural disasters and armed conflicts. One of the three objectives of the CERF is to strengthen core elements of humanitarian response in underfunded crises.

[6]Lartey, A. (2008) Maternal and child nutrition in sub-Saharan Africa: challenges and interventions. *The Proceedings of the Nutrition Society* 67, 105–108.

[7]O'Dea, J. (2010) Review of food-based routes to nutrition. Unpublished applied research brief: RAF Project, Food and Agriculture Organization of the United Nations, Rome.

[8]FAO (2010) *Guidelines for Measuring Household and Individual Dietary Diversity*, reprinted 2013. Food and Agriculture Organization of the United Nations, Rome. Available at: http://www.fao.org/docrep/014/i1983e/i1983e00.pdf (accessed 24 June 2013).

[9]FAO (2005) *Protecting and Promoting Good Nutrition in Crisis and Recovery: Resource Guide*. Food and Agriculture Organization of the United Nations, Rome. Available at: ftp://ftp.fao.org/docrep/fao/008/y5815e/y5815e00.pdf (accessed 24 June 2013).

[10]In this respect, lessons may be learned from bringing together the food, nutrition, agriculture and livelihoods clusters for a joint problem analysis for the Somalia 2011 CAP (consolidated appeal process) in August 2010. Also, lessons should be learned from the positive experiences in Afghanistan and other countries such as Pakistan, where FAO aims to mainstream food-based approaches to address malnutrition in the various agriculture relief and early recovery activities. Agriculture and the promotion of healthy diets is integrated into the recently developed Pakistan Integrated Nutrition Strategy (PINS).

33 Lessons from Support Given to the Implementation of Food Security Programmes in Over 100 Countries: The Feasibility of Integrated Food and Nutrition Security (F&NS) Approaches

Policy and Programme Development Support Division (TCS),*†
Technical Cooperation Department (TC)
Food and Agriculture Organization of the United Nations, Rome, Italy

---

Food security exists when all people, at all times have access to sufficient, safe and nutritious food to meet their dietary needs and food preferences for an active and healthy life.

World Food Summit Plan of Action, 13 November 1996.

Summary

FAO launched the Special Programme for Food Security (SPFS) in 1994 to assist member countries in their efforts to reduce the prevalence of hunger and malnutrition. Over a period of 14 years (1994–2008), the programme was implemented in 106 countries and mobilized US$890 million. Having learned from the experiences of the pilot phase, since 2001 FAO has been providing technical assistance in support of large-scale National and Regional Programmes for Food Security (NPFS and RPFS) designed, owned and implemented by national governments and regional economic integration organizations (REIOs) that target millions of food-insecure people. After a short description of the evolution of the FAO flagship programme for food and nutrition security (F&NS) in the changing world environment, the chapter highlights eight messages as lessons from past experiences, mainly focusing on: (i) the moral obligation of bringing well-known solutions and good practices to a scale commensurable to needs; (ii–iii) the need to go beyond food production and increased agricultural output and directly target the most marginal communities and vulnerable groups in terms of F&NS; (iv) adopting sustainability as a key principle of F&NS programmes; (v–vi) the feasibility and effectiveness of building effective partnerships for F&NS among agriculture, education and health sectors; (vii) inter-sectorial complementarity as a strength of integrated approach in F&NS; and (viii) mainstreaming F&NS approaches as an option to the creation of ad hoc programmes.

---

*Contributor: Stefano Gavotti
†Contact: spfs@fao.org

Introduction

The chapter gives a short description of the evolution of the Food and Agriculture Organization of the United Nations (FAO) flagship programme for food security according to the changing world environment, and presents a review of lessons learned. The intention is to demonstrate the effectiveness of designing and the feasibility of implementing food and nutrition security (F&NS) programmes that adopt a well-focused and comprehensive approach and directly build upon the complementarities and synergies that exist among the different pillars of F&NS. Examples are included from various countries, and there is an appendix that describes in more detail the implementation of a food security programme (PESA) in Mexico.

Background to the FAO Special Programme for Food Security (SPFS)

The development of the FAO Special Programme for Food Security (SPFS) can be summarized in the following points:

- FAO launched the SPFS in 1994 to assist its members in their efforts to reduce the prevalence of hunger and malnutrition. The SPFS was endorsed by the World Food Summit (WFS) in 1996 and its pilot phase was operational until the end of 2008. The strategy of that phase was to demonstrate through pilot projects how smallholder farmers could use low-cost technologies to raise their levels of production, improve productivity, diversify food production and thus ultimately improve their dietary intake.
- Over a period of 14 years (1994–2008), the SPFS pilot phase assisted 106 countries and helped to raise US$890 million. More than half of this amount was provided from the budgets of the developing countries involved and less than 10% from FAO's Regular Programme (including the Technical Cooperation Programme, TCP).
- Learning from the experiences of the SPFS pilot phase and other similar programmes, since 2001 FAO has been providing technical assistance to support large-scale National and Regional Programmes for Food Security (NPFS and RPFS). These are designed, owned and implemented by national governments and regional economic integration organizations (REIOs) themselves and are targeting millions of food-insecure people.
- Presently, 18 countries are implementing NPFS, and the NPFS documents are in different stages of formulation in 40 member countries. RPFS is operational within four regional organizations, namely the West African Economic and Monetary Union (UEMOA), The Economic Cooperation Organization (ECO), the Pacific Islands Forum (PIF) and the Caribbean Community Forum (CARICOM). RPFS complement NPFS and address cross-border issues, including management of water resources, food standards and safety, trans-boundary diseases and environmental issues.
- To maximize the scale and depth of impact, programmes aim to reach millions of people rather than thousands, and apply an approach of addressing simultaneously the different dimensions of food insecurity (not only food production, but also access to markets, nutrition and strong institutional frameworks for building food security at national and regional levels).
- The experience gained so far with NPFS and RPFS has shown that successful programmes benefit from political commitment at the highest level. The size of the budgets and the diversity of funding sources for the NPFS and RPFS that are already operational demonstrate that the level of commitment is high. Countries such as Nigeria, Mexico, Angola, Algeria, Chad, Jordan and Pakistan are already demonstrating their commitment by allocating their own budgetary resources to their own NPFS, and this has stimulated the interest of several funding partners.

SPFS was originally conceived as pilot demonstrations because very few resources were made available from the FAO Regular

Programme Budget. However, after only 5 years the programme was already able to mobilize more significant resources (in the order of several hundred million US dollars) from different sources, including from the internal budget, external donors and international financial institutions (IFIs). Through such resources, the programme could be scaled up in different countries and its scope broadened. Initially, the focus was mainly on small farmers' food production through improved water and crop management and small animal production, but progressively, attention was placed on income-generating activities, improved storage, marketing and value addition. The programme has also addressed the primary concerns of the most vulnerable by seeking alliances with social, safety-net programmes.

Lessons Learned

Lesson 1. Today 'piloting' is no longer a morally acceptable strategy for food security related initiatives

In spite of the good results that may be obtained with a small number of families/sites, unless a strategy is designed from the outset to reach large numbers, impact and sustainability will not be reached. This lesson was clearly identified by the programme's external evaluation in 2001–2002. FAO has shifted focus from the SPFS to the NPFS/RPFS National Investment Agriculture Programme (NIAP) in the framework of the Comprehensive Africa Agriculture Development Programme (CAADP).

Participating countries pushed FAO to scale up much faster than had first been planned from the initial findings and results of the SPFS. This has been the case with countries such as Nigeria and Mexico. In Mexico, the Secretariat of Agriculture, Livestock, Rural Development, Fisheries and Food (Secretaría de Agricultura, Ganadería, Desarrollo Rural, Pesca y Alimentación – SAGARPA) took the decision after the first 2 years to implement a decentralized project execution with the establishment of Rural Development Agencies (Agencias de Desarrollo Rural – ADRs). This was to provide for faster implementation than had been originally planned (in only 12 municipalities over six states), because SAGARPA considered that such a limited presence did not make any significant difference. So the governments of participating countries themselves decided the actual pace of scaling up according to the annual increase in allocation of resources.

Lesson 2. A food security programme cannot be confined to increasing agricultural output

The question of hunger is not one of production only, but also one of marginalization, deepening inequalities and social injustice. Increases in yields and production are a necessary condition for alleviating hunger and malnutrition, but not a sufficient one.
(O. De Schutter, 36th Session of the FAO Conference, November 2009)

Increasing speculation on land may take smallholder farmers off the land. Guaranteeing the Right to Food at a time of massive foreign direct investments in agriculture implies securing access to land for the cash-strapped poor. Land reforms must be accompanied by educational and financial/credit support. Improving food security means dealing with poor people's livelihoods and participatory approaches. Poor people – and women – are caught in a vicious circle of lack of resources and precariousness compounded by usury; their priorities are not limited to just producing more food. Other factors are just as important: domestic water; income generation to buy food and cover other basic needs, including paying school fees, getting energy or improved stoves for cooking; access to health services, hygiene and to basic education and literacy; secured land titles; and nutrition education. These factors often come out as priorities in participatory analyses, in other words, F&NS approaches are multidisciplinary programmes that should be discussed and solved possibly in alliance with specialized agencies other than the ministries of agriculture.

Lesson 3. Targeting and empowering vulnerable groups is an essential and prominent feature of food and nutrition security

Vulnerability and poverty is associated with isolation and marginality; as a consequence, F&NS programmes must break such isolation and offer medium- to long-term development perspectives translated through close support. Support cannot come from one-off investment projects; rather, it is an education and empowerment process, involving the promotion of grassroot institutions (self-help groups, farmer field schools, community-based organizations) that build poor people's capacity in many areas of livelihood and enable them to take informed decisions about their future.

Lesson 4. Sustainability is a key principle in food and nutrition security programmes

Participation, empowerment and capacity development for longer term sustainability are key principles that should guide F&NS programmes. The same principles do not always apply to food aid and humanitarian programmes. Instead of creating dependency on inputs external to the household, F&NS enhances self-reliance and initiative. Furthermore, sustainability can also be gradually injected into emergency and social programmes through F&NS (focus, approach). As far as technology options are concerned, these are primarily related to improved utilization of locally available, traditional knowledge and natural resources, rather than promoting the use of imported inputs (compost rather than fertilizer; local seed rather than hybrid or transgenic seed; local grains rather than concentrated animal feed).

Lesson 5: Food and nutrition security and education: a priority link

F&NS has more to do with changing the mindset of poor people and improving self-confidence, than just with transferring technologies, infrastructure and investments. For this reason, the most powerful interventions in F&NS are the ones directly targeted to children and school (school gardens linked to school feeding and nutrition education for the entire school community) and to women and children to improve the family livelihood; and to small farmers who wish to develop their managerial capacity, their ability to work in associations, in community based organizations, in small NGOs (nongovernmental organizations), and to negotiate with the local authorities on how best to jointly build F&NS. School gardens are also used to provide F&NS messages to the students, their teachers and parents. They are an excellent tool for nutrition education and are a practical means for building social capital, managerial capacity and leadership. An example of the setting up of a school garden programme in Nicaragua is given in Box 33.1.

Lesson 6. Agriculture and nutrition: the powerful link

Though the core of SPFS has been small-scale food production, the gradual increased capacity to deal with nutrition issues, often through young graduated students that assist the local team, has allowed a much better understanding of the baseline situation on nutrition and of the overall contribution of an F&NS programme to people's livelihoods, as has been exemplified by the food security programme in Mexico (PESA). Nutrition education messages are key for attracting women, facilitating the monitoring of results and evaluating the impact of F&NS initiatives. The results of an increased nutrition capacity at local level are often excellent in terms of the flow of communication that is established once agricultural technicians are trained in basic principles and can themselves monitor simple parameters to identify the progress of households in terms of dietary diversity, grain and water reserves, food quality and cooking habits, hygiene, etc. What are initially perceived as new challenges soon become active as new tools become available that provide a much clearer identity to any F&NS programme/project.

The nutrition strategy within SPFS has the clear objective of stimulating a greater commitment by the heads of households to produce

---

Box 33.1. Nicaragua: integrating food security in primary education.

Excellent work towards a growing partnership between agriculture and education sectors has been implemented in the framework of the FAO/SPFS (Food and Agriculture Organization of the United Nations Special Programme for Food Security) in Nicaragua.[1] This process started with the setting up of a few school gardens in Managua, including one at a school for disabled and blind children, with matching grants from the local municipality; it culminated after 3 years with the integration of nutrition education into the curriculum of the primary schools. Since 2005, one food security officer within the SPFS team has been assisting the Ministry of Education (MINED) on issues related to school gardens, integrated school feeding and the grafting of nutrition education into the curriculum, with a view to designing a comprehensive large-scale strategy. The use of the garden as a learning and social instrument to create nutrition awareness and citizenship (given the different age of the pupils involved) is one demonstration of the feasibility and richness of an integrated approach to food and nutrition security that FAO is promoting and that an increasing number of countries are adopting, despite the difficulties in coordinating interventions by different government sectors and the relative lengthy process involved.

Today, over 10,000 school centres and 15 Members of the Interuniversity Council on Food Sovereignty and Nutrition Security (Consejo Interuniversitario de Soberanía y Seguridad Alimentaria y Nutricional – CIUSSAN) participate actively in the implementation of national food and nutrition security (F&NS) and the Minister for Education is proud to announce that education through its own National Programme for Food Security (NPFS) is an important part of F&NS at national level. The MINED, together with FAO/SPFS, could greatly increase the estimated number of households that are directly affected by the activities of the project. Officials from the Ministry of Education (MINED) of Nicaragua have recommended that a Food and Nutrition Security Week (FNSW) be celebrated every year in all schools countrywide to commemorate World Food Day and to celebrate the contribution of the education sector to national food security and sovereignty.

[1]SPFS in Central America has been financed by AECID-Spain (the Spanish Agency for International Development Cooperation) since 1999.

---

food in their gardens for improving the quality and diversity of food of the families participating in the programme, thereby improving access to and availability of different types of food. More specific objectives usually refer to:

- Allowing a baseline assessment of the nutritional status of families and communities participating in the programme.
- Raising awareness among heads of families about possible weaknesses in their diet and the consequences for growth and health, especially of children under 5 years of age.
- Implementation of projects for food production in the garden, with families participating in the programme.
- Development of education programmes to explain the value and benefits of local foods for an improved and complete diet as well as for improving the hygiene and health of the households and communities that are participating in the programme.

The nutrition focus often facilitates the alliance of agriculture with the health and education sectors, mass media and policy

initiatives at regional level. An example is provided by the campaign *Come Sano* (Healthy Eating), which is jointly promoted in Central America by PESA, the Hunger Free Latin America and the Caribbean Initiative, and a number of regional radio networks. In Latin America, an example is 'Rural radio and FAO launch radio campaign "Healthy Eating" (*Onda Rural y FAO lanzan campaña radial "Come Sano"*)'[1] and in Guatemala 'A new subject matter for schoolchildren: growing and eating fresh food'.[2]

Lesson 7. Integrated approach to food and nutrition security: from complexity to complementarity

For an outsider, F&NS programmes may appear complex, while for poor people they should be simple and straightforward. This apparent complexity can be addressed through gradual approaches that appraise the context from the viewpoint of those who are food-insecure, and thereby empower them. Low-cost actions such as seeds and tool distribution linked to nutrition education and family/school/community gardens will be preferred (for instance 'start picking low-hanging fruits'). Complementary activities will be encouraged with all local actors that can provide pro-poor support. Experience shows that the best results are achieved when a programme/project tackles more than one dimension of F&SN simultaneously: food supply, access, utilization and long-term stability. However, this implies working at different levels (food producers, consumers, social programmes and policy/decision makers) and applying a multidisciplinary and multi-sectoral approach.

Breaking the habit of working in isolation and seeking partnership and alliances with actors pertaining to different sectors is a preferred way of operating for a typical F&NS programme. An illustration is the active participation of the private sector in the framework of the Brazilian National Council for Food Security and Nutrition (Conselho Nacional de Segurança Alimentar e Nutricional – CONSEA), which is the joint private public body that manages Fome Zero (Zero Hunger) – the local food purchase for redistribution to school feeding programmes as practised by the Food Purchase Programme (Programa de Aquisiçao de Alimentos – PAA) in Brazil. Another instance is the home-grown school feeding concept of FAO and the Purchase for Progress – P4P – of the World Food Programme (WFP). These are both typical examples that should be promoted elsewhere to take advantage of social programmes that result in direct stimulus to the local rural economy.

A multidisciplinary and multi-sectoral working mode identify and exploit the synergies generated by dealing simultaneously with more than one food security dimension. Linking agricultural production to nutrition education resulted in a more effective communication flow to a wider public instead of keeping limiting it to food producers and agricultural technicians. This has been the case with the SPFS projects in Central America where agricultural productivity messages have been complemented by campaigns on food quality, food habits and dietary diversity, hygiene and cooking recipes. Such messages are targeted to a much broader audience,

including urban groups, and serve as an intermediary between rural and urban sectors. They are, therefore, very effective in keeping awareness of the importance of family agriculture as a main actor of national F&NS. That is why nutrition education is a typical component of large-scale F&NS programmes, as can be seen in Mexico, Central America, Colombia and Ecuador. Further, it is a powerful tool for facilitating communication with women, who represent both a target and the most powerful actors in the fight for better nutrition.

Lesson 8. The institutionalization of food security and the formulation of specific programmes versus mainstreaming food and nutrition security principles, process and approaches

Many countries experience difficulties in the creation of a new institution, and in the funding of new programmes to deal with food security – which may prove counterproductive in the long run. Usually in a given country, agriculture and R&D programmes already exist that could be used to carry over the typical F&NS messages that have been described above to the largest audience (targeting, sustainability, complementarity, impact, evaluation), without the need to create duplication and possible friction among the existing institutions. An example of the process undertaken in Mexico in moving from an agriculture-focused intervention to the implementation of a public policy is presented in the appendix that follows this section of the chapter.

Taking a comprehensive approach to F&NS does not necessarily imply the creation of new programmes; it is, however, necessary to adopt a new working mode whereby the available forces are joined to provide a comprehensive solution through different sets of activities. A multi-sectoral approach in F&NS may represent a change compared with previous work habits, but it may be very effective in facilitating the building of political consensus at various levels, as is demonstrated by the rapid growth of PESA in Mexico.

Notes

[1]See http://www.pesacentroamerica.org/pesa_ca/come_sano.php (accessed 27 June 2013).
[2]See http://www.pesacentroamerica.org/Guatemala/noticias/huertos.php (accessed 27 June 2013).

Appendix: Mexico

Proyecto Estratégico para la Seguridad Alimentaria (PESA): from piloting food security interventions to implementing public policy in favour of smallholders in the most marginal rural areas of Mexico

Initially limited to operations in six states and 12 municipalities of Mexico, with a focus on helping selected groups of farmers boost food and agricultural production, from 2005 onwards, the scope of FAO assistance to the country via the SPFS programme rapidly broadened to support more ambitious national development objectives for food security, while also seeking more comprehensive geographical coverage. Using the UTF (Unilateral Trust Fund) modality, the Mexican authorities agreed to put catalytic resources at the disposal of FAO to assist with technical foci and capacity building at different levels in connection with a wide-ranging action programme being implemented by the Mexican Secretariat for Agriculture (SAGARPA). This programme was called Proyecto Estratégico para la Seguridad Alimentaria – PESA, or the Strategic Project for Food Security. The resulting ongoing SAGARPA/FAO project thus reflects the mutually beneficial and timely convergence of policy choices made by governments (stemming from a major assessment of the public extension system, including the lessons learned) and the preferred growth of the scope of interventions in support of food security at national and regional levels in interested countries.

The main innovative features of PESA are:

- A deliberate focus on the most marginal regions and vulnerable groups, which complements other SAGARPA programmes in the country.
- Participatory and multidisciplinary methods for solving food security problems with concrete actions at different levels (federal, state, municipal, local).
- The formulation of shared goals and use of a common logical framework, which facilitates dialogue between politicians and technicians in the various administrative territorial divisions of the country.
- An integrated approach to food security, including taking account of the varied interests of the whole family, starting from women; this approach allows for incremental and complementary improvements of living conditions, food production and dietary habits, and the organization of producers for marketing and processing. Confirmed best practices at community level are then used to influence decision making, policy formulation and planning at other levels.

This project can be presented as a showcase of the process undertaken to move from agriculture-focused interventions for food production with small-scale farmers to the implementation of a public policy. As recently stated in a food security forum by the SAGARPA Under-Secretary for Rural Development:

> Through PESA the Government of Mexico focuses on capacity development based on new rural extension work, with roles and profiles focusing on social and human aspects, to trigger a positive change in relations between individuals, groups and institutions involved in economic development and social development. By the capitalization of production units through support for investment in productive assets, new technologies, financing and organizational development, the government seeks to 'transform their challenges into opportunities and potential resources'. Over 80% of producers in the world are small scale, so that the future of nations is to work with them.

This is reflected by the increasing popularity of PESA, also evident in the application of funds from the Federal Expenditure Budget (PEF: Presupuesto de egresos de la Federación) in the last 5 years (2007–2011), which were obtained despite the prevailing difficult economic situation. The overall strategy of PESA is to be soon evaluated. Among the critical factors to be assessed is the flow of resources to the most marginal areas for productive types of investment. The evaluation will compare the flow of resources in the municipalities where the project has operated, starting in 2002; what is already known is the level of resources that the federal government has allocated from 2007 onwards for the implementation of projects in the framework of PESA strategy and methodology (approx. US$650 million); this has happened in response to a demand from members of parliament familiar with PESA in their own state of origin. In spite of the unfavourable economic trend, such resources have steadily grown, as shown in Table 33.1 below.

Besides PEF, the municipalities where PESA has been operating since 2002 have received funding from the major SAGARPA programmes, namely Alianza para el campo, PROCAMPO, SOPORTE, PRODUCE, Activos productivos, PATMIR, COUSSA, PROFEMOR, etc., as well as from other sources like SEDESOL, DIF, CDI, etc. It is clear that the FAO/SAGARPA project shows a substantial catalytic effect in redirecting government resources to the most marginal areas of the country.

At present, PESA operates in 15 (of the 32) states of Mexico, in 4183 local communities pertaining to 599 municipalities, including 105 of the 125 having a very low HDI (human development index). Over 120,000 poor families have benefited directly from locally based projects covering various aspects of production (soil and water management, poultry and small animal production, organic coffee, maize and beans) and improved livelihoods (e.g. more efficient stoves, better water harvesting and storage techniques, grain storage, vegetable gardens, nutrition education, marketing and ecotourism opportunities).

While very small in comparison, the UTF resources under the FAO project (around US$13 million from 2002 to 2010) have allowed for critical technical inputs and capacity-building activities to support the entire process. Operating through a central technical unit supplemented by decentralized staff at state level, technical and managerial support is provided to autonomous multidisciplinary groups (ADRs) that ensure a continuous flow of technical assistance to poor families in marginal communities, with strong backing from the FAO offices

Table 33.1. Allocation of SAGARPA (Secretariat of Agriculture, Livestock, Rural Development, Fisheries and Food) funds for Mexican Strategic Project for Food Security (PESA) from FAO/UTF[a] and the Federal Expenditure Budget.[b]

Year	FAO/UTF US$ (millions)	Federal Expenditure Budget for PESA type projects	
		Mexican pesos (millions)	US$ (millions) equiv.
2002	0.88		
2003	1.55		
2004	2.20		
2005	0.90		
2006	1.42		
2007		561	49
2008	1.21	1100	96
2009	2.27	1560	136
2010	2.66	1750	152
2011 (forecast)		2500	217
Total	13.09	7471	650

[a]FAO/UTF, Food and Agriculture Organization of the United Nations/Unilateral Trust Fund.
[b]PEF, Presupuesto Egresos Federales.

(country, regional and headquarters). In close consultation with national authorities, FAO has been able to bring its neutral and objective advice and its recognized advocacy capacities to bear on the formulation of the main social and technical dimensions of the programme.

Evaluation studies have described the main achievements of PESA as:

- It has demonstrated the potential to ensure self-identification of appropriate solutions to tackle complex food security problems.
- It has increased the availability of and access to food in highly marginal and poor areas.
- It has ensured a wide range of support services to rural areas where these services were not hitherto available.

34 Using Information Networks to Promote Improved Nutrition and Rural Development: FAO's Experience of Promoting School Milk Programmes

Policy and Programme Development Support Division (TCS),*†
Technical Cooperation Department (TC)
Food and Agriculture Organization of the United Nations, Rome, Italy

---

Summary

As a result of the lack of a mechanism to exchange information on school milk programmes among FAO members, FAO's Trade and Markets Division (EST) attempted to bridge this gap by using e-mail networks and an associated Internet site. Arising out of this process, 19 national and international conferences were organized dealing with the administration and financing of school milk programmes. E-fora members also agreed to celebrate a World School Milk Day. Following the first such day in 2000, the event is now celebrated in around 40 countries worldwide. School milk programmes predominantly rely on government support; however, there are a number of examples of programmes that operate without public financing. Children, and the food they eat, are influenced by an environment much wider than that of the school, although school-based programmes provide an excellent opportunity to promote milk consumption among children and, in so doing, establish a lifetime's habit.

FAO's Experience of Using Information Networks to Promote School Milk Programmes

In 1997, as a result of a number of requests received for information on school milk programmes, it became apparent that there was no forum for members of FAO (Food and Agriculture Organization of the United Nations) to exchange information on school milk. FAO's Trade and Markets Division (EST) attempted to bridge this gap by using e-mail networks and an associated Internet site.

As part of this process, FAO cooperated with national organizations in presenting a series of conferences on the provision of milk to children in school. The conferences focused on providing a forum for the exchange of information and experiences between professionals working with school milk programmes. The main focus of the programme was on the administration and financing of

---

*Contributor: Michael Griffin, Policy and Programme Development Support Division, ex Trade and Markets Division (EST), FAO
†Contact: school-milk-owner@fao.org

such programmes – based on the sharing of experiences from a range of countries. Between 1998 and 2006, conferences were held in South Africa (1998), the UK, Australia, Thailand, Austria, the Czech Republic, Colombia, Canada, Lebanon, Finland, China (2002), Mexico, Sweden, Iceland, Uruguay, the USA, China (2005), Uganda and South Africa (2006). As well as the conferences to which FAO was requested to lend its support, a number of others were held independently of FAO; many of these drew their inspiration from the organizers attending one of the FAO-assisted conferences in the countries listed above.

Underpinning the work on the conferences were e-mail fora (e-fora) that the Trade and Markets Division established to facilitate discussion and information exchange. Arising from e-fora discussions within the Division on the selection of a particular day on which school milk could be celebrated internationally, consensus was reached among members that World School Milk Day would be celebrated on the last Wednesday in September. The first such World School Milk Day was celebrated in 2000, and the day has since become an annual event celebrated in countries throughout the world. Its goal is to provide a particular day when attention is focused on school milk and thereby serves as a mechanism for its promotion. Importance is lent to the event by the fact that other countries are doing the same thing on the same day.

Background Information on School Milk Programmes

School milk programmes take many forms. Some programmes concentrate entirely on milk, whereas in others milk is only one of the elements involved. Funding varies considerably; in some cases, programmes are completely funded by the government, while in others funding is wholly private, and in many countries, there is a 'middle road', whereby funding consists of a mixture of public and private sources. Even in cases where the government is not directly involved in funding programmes, public policy, such as nutritional guidelines for school feeding, can have an important impact on the ability of school milk programmes to grow and prosper.

In some instances, programmes have been established under aid-funded assistance. While such assistance brings some benefits and can provide the necessary impetus to get a school milk programme up and operating, aid assistance is finite, and when it ends difficulties in sustaining the system using national resources frequently arise. In the past decade, programmes established in countries such as China, India, Saudi Arabia, Malaysia and Oman have provided an alternative scenario by starting up without any direct financial support from the government or from external agencies. In such cases, the system that eventually evolves is likely to be better in tune with domestic resources and therefore is more likely to be sustainable. In other cases, where limited government funds are available, an alternative approach may be to provide school milk to the poorest sections of the student population, leaving other sections of the programme to be self-financing. As already mentioned, the absence of direct government funding to the programme does not mean that government support in other areas, such as setting standards and providing guidelines on good nutritional practices, is not important.

By creating demand, school milk programmes can directly benefit dairy development. This is particularly true in countries with relatively undeveloped dairy industries. In such countries, school milk can serve as a vehicle to create a consumer base.

While school milk programmes predominantly rely on government support, a number of examples of programmes without a direct financial contribution from the government can be cited. Children, and the food they eat, are influenced by an environment much wider than that of the school, but school-based programmes do provide an excellent opportunity to promote milk consumption among children and, in so doing, establish a lifetime's habit.

Description of Programme Impact

A number of countries introduced school milk programmes as a result of the stimulus provided by attending one or more of the conferences in the FAO-assisted series. For example,

China, through delegates attending school milk conferences and via the networking facilitated by FAO, established a national school milk programme in 2000. The programme has had a strong positive impact on the development of milk production and, in addition to its nutritional role, has created jobs and increased incomes for Chinese dairy farmers. The Czech Republic and Poland both established national school milk programmes for primary schools as a result of delegates participating in the FAO conference series. In Colombia, local milk and dairy industry organizations hosted an FAO school milk conference in 2000. Arising out of this conference, authorities established a nationwide breakfast programme which today covers most of the country's school-aged children. The impetus for the national programme in Iran arose out of delegates participating in FAO conferences, and accessing ideas, information and experiences from other parts of the world; this was an important element in the establishment and development of the programme.

World School Milk Day is celebrated in approximately 40 countries each year. Promotion of the day and coordination of information exchange is carried out by the FAO Trade and Markets Division (EST). This Division also continues to support the work on school milk, maintaining e-fora – in the form of the School Milk List – that encompass members in 125 countries. In addition, the Division hosts a website for information exchange on school milk.[1]

Future Plans

The Trade and Markets Division will continue to moderate the e-fora and maintain the school milk Internet site. It is possible at some future point that the outcomes achieved to date could be amalgamated into FAO-wide work on school feeding.

Note

[1] http://www.fao.org/economic/est/est-commodities/dairy/school-milk/en/ (accessed 28 June 2013). To join The School Milk List – an e-forum to facilitate the exchange of information on developments relating to school milk programme, contact: fao-school-milk@fao.org

35 FAO Support to the Comprehensive Africa Agriculture Development Programme (CAADP) Process*

Regional Office for Africa and Investment Centre Division,†‡ Technical Cooperation Department
Food and Agriculture Organization of the United Nations, Rome, Italy

---

Summary

Over the last decade, FAO has served as a strategic partner to NEPAD (the New Partnership for Africa's Development) Planning and Coordination Agency (NPCA) and member countries in providing expertise for the design and implementation of the Comprehensive Africa Agriculture Development Programme (CAADP) which represents a vision for the restoration of agricultural growth, food security and the attainment of the MDGs (Millennium Development Goals) in Africa. CAADP is a strategic framework fully owned and led by African governments and stakeholders which guide country development efforts and partnerships in the agricultural sector. In a manner similar to the broader NEPAD agenda, it embodies the principles of peer review and dialogue, the adoption of best practices and mutual learning with the objective of raising the quality and consistency of country policies and strategies in the agricultural sector. FAO has been supporting the preparation of CAADP compacts and the formulation of national agricultural investment plans and programmes as well as their implementation. This chapter reviews the progress achieved in advancing the CAADP agenda in 2010–2013, and also examines current efforts to effectively link emergency responses to the current food security crises in the Horn of Africa and the Sahel to longer term investment plans and programmes that contribute to reducing structural vulnerabilities and improving resilience.

The Comprehensive Africa Agriculture Development Programme (CAADP): The Diagnosis

In most parts of the world, rates of hunger and malnutrition have fallen significantly in recent years, but in Africa these rates have shown little improvement. Africa has the highest proportion (one third) of people suffering from chronic hunger which, in sub-Saharan Africa, is as persistent as it is widespread. Between 1990 and 1992, and 2001 and 2003, the number of undernourished people increased from 169 million to

---

*This chapter has been updated from the presentation made at the *International Symposium on Food and Nutrition Security* held at FAO Headquarters in Rome in December 2010, based on a report presented to government delegations at the *FAO Regional Conference for Africa 2012* and further developments in 2013.
†Contributors: James Tefft, David Phiri, Guy Evers, Coumba Dieng, Alex Jones and Alberta Mascaretti
‡Contact: tcia-service@fao.org

206 million, and only 15 of the 39 countries for which data are reported reduced the number of the undernourished. Efforts to reduce hunger in the region have been hampered by a range of natural and human-induced disasters, including conflicts and the spread of HIV/AIDS. Widespread hunger and malnutrition in Africa determine and reflect deep poverty in the region. Almost two thirds of Africa's population is rural and thus is directly or indirectly dependent on agriculture for employment and sustenance. Sustained growth in agriculture is therefore crucial to cutting hunger and poverty in the region. Indeed, recent increases in overall GDP (gross domestic product) growth rates in parts of Africa track similar increases in agricultural GDP growth rates.

FAO Support to CAADP

CAADP was endorsed by African Ministers for Agriculture in June 2002 at the FAO (Food and Agriculture Organization of the United Nations) Regional Conference for Africa, and was subsequently adopted by African Heads of State and Government at their Summit in Maputo, Mozambique, in 2003. Following this endorsement and adoption, FAO has worked to support the African Union Commission (AUC) and the New Partnership for Africa's Development (NEPAD) Planning and Coordination Agency (NPCA) in translating the shared African-led CAADP vision for sustained, broad-based agricultural growth in Africa into concrete steps and actions at continental, regional and national levels.

To reach the agreed goal of average annual growth of 6% in agriculture, African Heads of State agreed in 2003 to commit at least 10% of national budgets to agricultural development within 5 years (Maputo Declaration of Agriculture and Food Security). The CAADP programme is designed around four key pillars: (i) extending the area under

sustainable land management and reliable water control systems; (ii) improving rural infrastructure and trade-related capacities for improved market access; (iii) increasing food supply and reducing hunger; and (iv) agricultural research, technology dissemination and adoption.

Between 2003 and 2008, despite significant efforts to solidify commitment to the programme's vision and principles, CAADP results on the ground were less than expected. In 2009, however, the G8 countries pledged at L'Aquila, Italy, to allocate US$22.2 billion in support of global food and nutrition security; of this, almost US$1 billion has been allocated to the Global Agriculture and Food Security Program (GAFSP). This pledge helped to jump-start the CAADP process. The hope of accessing a portion of these funds served as an incentive for member countries to accelerate the CAADP formulation process, so that by mid-2013, over 30 countries and three Regional Economic Communities (RECs) had successfully completed their CAADP Compacts.[1]

FAO has provided technical support for different aspects of the CAADP process in numerous countries. This has included: the preparation of background documents, contribution to peer review, and active participation in the country round tables that were organized to sign the Compacts in over 15 countries, contributions to the formulation of National Agricultural and Food Security Investment Plans (NAFSIP) in over 20 countries, and participation in the related business meetings.

Mainstreaming Fisheries, Forestry, Gender, Employment, Livestock and Nutrition into the CAADP Process

The calls for, and efforts to, 'mainstream' various sectors (e.g. fisheries, forestry, livestock) and issues (gender, employment and nutrition) into the CAADP process stemmed from the recognition that these sectors/issues have either not been fully elaborated in the CAADP Compacts or have been allocated relatively minimal budget in NAFSIP. In one country, for example, livestock programmes were not sufficiently developed and the budgetary allocation in the NAFSIP was significantly less (1% of the total value) than the livestock sector's contribution to agricultural GDP (14%).

In most cases, these omissions or underweighting can be attributed to the hurried manner in which many investment plans were formulated, e.g. in order to meet GAFSP submission deadlines. The limited number and capacity of sector experts who were actually involved in the formulation process also contributed to these imbalances and inconsistencies.

There is ample evidence to make the case for mainstreaming or incorporating livestock, forestry and fisheries into the CAADP process, given their important contributions to agricultural development. These sectors, together, account for approximately one third of Africa's agricultural GDP, with the bulk generated by the livestock sector. The contribution of the three sectors to sustainable agriculture is significant both economically and environmentally. More than 50% of Africa's arable land is cultivated under a variety of mixed farming systems, including mixed crop/livestock, agro-pastoral, pastoral and forest-based systems and coastal artisanal fishing.

Against this backdrop, FAO collaborated with the NPCA in 2006 to prepare a CAADP Companion Document. This document incorporated livestock in every CAADP pillar, with particular attention to the second pillar which is centred on 'improving infrastructure and trade-related capacities for market access'. The forestry component was modified to include four critical priority areas: (i) improvement of the policy, legislative and planning framework; (ii) strengthening the institutional structures to implement policies and legislation; (iii) increased investment, especially to

implement sustainable forest management and to enhance the availability of goods and services; and (iv) complementary investment for industrial development and supporting infrastructure. Finally, fishery sector mainstreaming focused on the integration of fisheries and aquaculture into the wider CAADP framework, emphasizing the benefits to African stakeholders of increased productivity, trade and improved environmental management.

On the nutrition side, interest in incorporating a nutrition dimension into the CAADP greatly increased following the increased attention to livelihoods and malnutrition during the 2008 food and financial crisis. This situation spurred the African Union (AU) to reaffirm its commitment to food and nutrition security within the context of CAADP Pillar 3, and established an annually observed Africa Day for Food and Nutrition Security (ADFNS). Furthermore, many African countries are joining the Scaling Up Nutrition (SUN) Movement, thereby committing to put the fight against malnutrition at the top of their political agendas.[2]

A nutrition review of CAADP investment plans found that nutrition objectives and activities were inconsistently incorporated and budgeted for in the majority of countries. Although some countries included nutrition in their overall CAADP framework by promoting dietary diversity, nutrition education and food safety, in most cases, the NAFSIPs remain insufficiently developed. The review further identified several areas where improvement is needed to prevent food and agriculture interventions from having negative impacts on nutrition, and to increase positive nutritional impacts. These areas included: strengthening inter-sectoral collaboration; improving nutrition assessments and the targeting of vulnerable households, women of reproductive age and children under 5 years old; diversifying production; fortifying food; and enhancing information management, in particular through more systematic monitoring and evaluation.

Building on the guidelines developed by the NPCA and on development partners' expertise, the NPCA initiated a series of multi-sectoral regional workshops to assist member countries in integrating nutrition objectives and activities within their NAIPs. The first workshop was held for West African countries in Dakar, in November 2011, and two other workshops were planned for 2012 and 2013 for East, Central and Southern Africa. FAO is providing technical and financial support to the NPCA Food and Nutrition Security unit for the workshop preparation, implementation and follow-up at regional and country level, as well as other activities, such as the organization of the ADFNS and support to Home-Grown School Feeding.

FAO also actively participated in a review of investment plans to determine how countries can more effectively address the evolving challenges of climate change. In this context, FAO is contributing to mainstreaming sustainable agriculture approaches (Climate Smart Agriculture) within investment plans and their implementation programmes. Additional funding to support the adoption of Climate Smart Agriculture is anticipated in the context of Rio+20.

Finally, FAO, in collaboration with other partners, is supporting the NPCA and RECs in enhancing the capacity of CAADP actors at country and regional levels, in particular for the formulation on NAFSIP and the implementation programmes.

GAFSP and FAO Support for CAADP

The Global Agriculture and Food Security Program (GAFSP)[3] is a Financial Intermediary Fund administered by the World Bank designed to address the underfunding of country and regional agriculture and food security strategic investment plans already being developed by countries. The total amount pledged by donors to GAFSP, equivalent to US$925 million, is allocated to the Public and Private Sector Windows. The resources received from the donors as of 30 June 2013 amount to the equivalent of US$970.2 million for the Public Sector Window. Donors include Australia, Canada, the Gates Foundation, the Republic of Korea, Spain and the USA. Ireland has contributed to the operating costs of the programme. To date, GAFSP has been the most visible funding instrument associated with CAADP; completion of a successful CAADP Compact, round table and national investment plan process is an absolute prerequisite for funding consideration by African countries under the GAFSP.

The focus of GAFSP is to improve the income and food security of poor people in developing countries through more and better country-led public and private sector investment aimed at strengthening sustainable smallholder food production by raising agricultural productivity, by linking farmers to domestic markets, by reducing risk and vulnerability, by improving non-farm rural livelihoods and through technical assistance. The objective of GAFSP grants is to fill the financing gaps in country and regional agriculture and food security strategies, targeting innovative and sustainable approaches that are directly linked to enhanced food security and poverty reduction, thereby contributing to the achievement of Millennium Development Goal (MDG) 1 to cut hunger and poverty by half by 2015. GAFSP supports only country-led initiatives, giving priority to those with evidence of stakeholder participation from project design to implementation.

By the end of 2013, 15 countries in Africa (out of a total of 26 recipients worldwide) had received GAFSP funding (totalling US$564 million) to implement priority programmes of their CAADP NAFSIPS, with FAO providing technical assistance to the GAFSP formulation process in seven of those countries.

Challenges for CAADP

The CAADP vision and guiding principles have galvanized attention on the importance of sustained levels of investment for sustainable agricultural productivity growth and improved food and nutrition security in Africa. In order to continue serving as a point of reference and as a coordinated framework for agricultural and food system development in the region, increased emphasis must be given to strengthening national and regional capacities for linking compacts and investment plans to policy and budget processes and innovative financing mechanisms. This section briefly discusses potential measures that could be considered in 2012–2013 as actions to energize the CAADP implementation process and create opportunities for translating investment plans and programmes into concrete actions on the ground.

The importance of domestic resource mobilization for the implementation of the CAADP Investment Plans

Having effectively formulated compacts, investment plans and programmes, the largest challenge facing most countries in CAADP implementation consists of mobilizing funds to finance the priority interventions. Although CAADP was designed and has evolved as a dynamic partnership of diverse stakeholders at continental, regional and national levels, effective implementation hinges first and foremost on the commitment and leadership of governments to determine priority public investments within which the government can allocate an adequate share of national budgetary resources.

Governments' own investments in CAADP programmes represent a critical step in the implementation process, serving as a concrete manifestation of their commitment to the process. Given today's tight fiscal environment, this call to invest public funds in CAADP priority programmes will inevitably require in-depth budgetary analysis to identify the best use of scarce fiscal resources, as well as concerted efforts to advocate and negotiate for the reallocation of government

funds. The establishment of effective, broad-based stakeholder alliances and capacity development to strengthen communication, advocacy and negotiation skills could assist CAADP Country Teams to garner political support and mobilize resources for financing CAADP programmes.

Although this call for domestic resource mobilization and investment may challenge the prevalent perception of CAADP as simply an opportunity to access development partner financing, member countries cannot underestimate the importance of government expenditure on critical public goods to catalyse future investment of producers, private sector actors and diverse external partners. For example, government investment to strengthen the legal framework for contract enforcement, to develop platforms for multi-actor dialogue or to develop rural infrastructure represent just a few of the many areas where public expenditure and institutional strengthening could help to catalyse private sector investment or address specific binding constraints.

In the policy or regulatory arena, the mobilization of private investment may also hinge on complementary government actions in many areas, including the development and enforcement of clear guidelines for public intervention in food markets, land tenure rules for foreign investment, guiding principles for public–private partnerships, or measures to ensure consistent application of trade agreements. Similarly, at regional level, public good investment, policy formulation or enforcement is needed to complement actions taken at national level. For example, the establishment and enforcement of uniform food safety norms and standards may make sense at the regional level. In many situations, both at national and regional levels, policies and regulations already exist; it is their systematic application and enforcement that need to be strengthened.

Strategic partnerships

The reallocation of government budgets to CAADP-aligned priority areas and the systematic implementation of key policies and regulations will require intensive engagement, lobbying and negotiating skills of diverse stakeholder coalitions and of a variety of state and non-state actors. Likewise, CAADP country teams may need to use similar approaches to more systematically link the CAADP framework to existing sector policy frameworks and programmes, innovative public–private partnerships or other emerging initiatives.

Building these innovative linkages or strategic partnerships with other policies, programmes and initiatives may provide opportunities to build on and benefit from existing processes, stakeholder alliances or existing political capital that could help drive the CAADP implementation process. Reciprocally, these other programmes and initiatives could benefit from the comprehensive framework and broad political support of the CAADP.

Each country's approach to creating strategic sector linkages and partnerships for enhanced CAADP implementation will need to be carefully crafted after taking into consideration the existing sociopolitical and institutional context, and identifying potential entry points to initiate action and opportunities for mutually beneficial alliances. This type of approach will ostensibly move from one that comprises series of sequential technical steps (such as those used to develop investment plans) to a more fluid, innovative one that joins the technical aspects to the policy, budgetary and political processes needed for effective implementation.

Action is required to ensure the support and collaboration of numerous line ministries, whether by greater alignment of CAADP plans to the prevailing sector policies and programmes that form the sectoral point of reference for the government, or by sustained collaboration with diverse actors at sub-national level who are involved in programme implementation. As many government programmes are often closely associated with major global or regional initiatives (e.g. SUN, the Special Programme for Aquaculture Development in Africa (SPADA), Save and Grow, etc.), a strategic partnership approach would strive to connect CAADP implementation to the products, services and funding that are available through them.

Similarly, at the regional level, member countries may want to explore opportunities for operationalizing their investment plans through new investment funds, such as the Regional Fund for Agriculture and Food (ECOWADF) of ECOWAS, a financing instrument to be established at the newly created Regional Agency for Agriculture and Food (RAAF).

Likewise, at the global level, member countries may see value in linking CAADP to emerging global initiatives such as Climate Smart Agriculture and price volatility, issues through which opportunities may exist for forming implementation alliances or accessing knowledge, funding and global political support for programme implementation. The increasing numbers of public–private partnership initiatives or diverse forms of South–South Cooperation are other logical choices for CAADP implementation partnership and potential access to innovative financing instruments.

To sustain the CAADP momentum during the coming years and to be successful in carrying out this facilitation, networking and advocacy role, CAADP Country Teams and stakeholders will undoubtedly need to improve their knowledge of complex policy, budgetary and political processes, and to strengthen their capacities in alliance building, negotiation and other skills that are needed to successfully manoeuvre through the complex technical and sociopolitical issues involved in effective implementation. Greater collaboration may also serve to unite under common purpose scarce human resources that are often spread too thin between similar but competing initiatives.

As there is limited knowledge on how to effectively move to implementation, country experiences will need to be documented and shared across countries in order to distil lessons of creative and effective actions taken by CAADP Country Teams. This peer learning process can already begin to identify and share best practices and showcase good examples of the last decade of experiences in formulating and implementing CAADP-related investment plans and programmes, which will be essential for sustaining the CAADP agenda.

Concluding Comments

In conclusion, moving forward, CAADP implementation will depend largely on the ability and commitment of member countries, RECs, the NPCA and development partners to develop sound and politically feasible processes that can translate CAADP NAFSIPs into tangible programmes that produce positive impacts on the livelihoods of the producers, pastoralists, fishermen and women of Africa.

Notes

[1] During the CAADP country round tables, key players come together to assess the realities of their own particular situation and develop a road map for going forward. This process leads to the identification of priority areas for investment through a 'CAADP Compact' agreement that is signed by all key partners.

[2] SUN countries include: Benin, Burkina, Ethiopia, the Gambia, Ghana, Madagascar, Mali, Mauritania, Mozambique, Namibia, Niger, Nigeria, Rwanda, Senegal, Sierra Leone, the United Republic of Tanzania, Uganda, Zambia and Zimbabwe.

[3] See http://www.gafspfund.org

36 Selected Findings and Recommendations from the Symposium

Brian Thompson and Leslie Amoroso*

Nutrition and Consumer Protection Division (AGN), Agriculture and Consumer Protection Department (AG), Food and Agriculture Organization of the United Nations, Rome, Italy

The following selected findings were prepared as a summary of the main conclusions and recommendations of the papers that were presented and of the discussions that took place during the *International Symposium on Food and Nutrition Security* held at FAO Headquarters in Rome, Italy, in December 2010. The symposium:

- *Regretted* that over the past 20–25 years food and agriculture-based initiatives for improving nutrition have been systematically neglected and underfunded.
- *Acknowledged* that food and agriculture serve as the foundation for nutrition and health.
- *Emphasized* that agriculture, including crops, livestock, fisheries and forestry activities, represents the broad field of activities concerned with the production, processing, storage, distribution and marketing of food and other commodities, along with related social, economic and environmental concerns.
- *Recognized* nutrition as a key link – the nexus – among agriculture, socio-economic development, food security and health.

- *Recognized* that the nutritional benefits of agricultural and food-based interventions arise from more than just the nutrient content of the foods consumed, and are mediated through a variety of social, economic and environmental factors.
- *Further recognized* the multifunctionality of agriculture, and that food and agriculture-based interventions result in multiple nutritional benefits rather than being limited to the benefits arising from nutrient-based interventions.
- *Highlighted* that focusing on the household with the intention of making it a viable social and economic unit able to meet the needs of all family members, multiplies the nutritional benefits of food and agriculture-based interventions.
- *Considered* that better dietary intakes and positive nutritional outcomes among poorly nourished populations can be achieved through better targeted, designed, implemented and evaluated policies, strategies, plans and programmes that recognize and capitalize on the linkages among agriculture, food safety, food security and nutrition.

*Contacts: brian.thompson@fao.org; leslie.amoroso@fao.org

- *Recognized* that food-based approaches address malnutrition at its source and have further social, cultural, economic and environmental benefits in being local solutions and bottom-up in nature and, therefore, are more likely to lead to long-term sustainable improvements in nutrition.
- *Further considered* that better designed, implemented and evaluated nutrition-sensitive food security and agricultural policies, strategies, plans and programmes, together with strengthened capacities in nutrition, have great potential to alleviate poverty and hunger, and to improve the food and nutrition situation in both urban and rural settings.
- *Emphasized* that food and nutrition security is a multifaceted concept, the realization of which requires the adoption of multidisciplinary, cross-cutting approaches to interventions. Common features of successful approaches to national policy, strategy, planning and programme development for improving food and nutrition security include:
  - a strong commitment to improving nutritional well-being and securing everyone's right to food;
  - a comprehensive understanding of food and nutrition security;
  - multi-sectoral actions targeted at the immediate, underlying and basic causes of malnutrition;
  - an appropriate mix of national, sectoral and community-focused interventions;
  - strong coordination, cooperation and joint planning among ministries – agriculture, nutrition, health and other sectors should work together and explore more closely synergies and how they could be better linked;
  - an emphasis on institutional capacity development and training at country level;
  - gender mainstreaming;
  - constructing and financing viable social protection programmes, including safety nets; and
  - viable partnerships between public and private sectors and between governmental and non-governmental organizations, and among national governments and other development assistance agencies.
- *Recognized* that women have a unique role as primary caregivers and producers and processors of food at the household level and are central to improving household food and nutrition security.
- *Stressed* that unless the basic and underlying causes of poverty, malnutrition, food insecurity, poor health and sanitation are tackled, success in reducing hunger and all forms of malnutrition is likely not to be achieved.
- *Recognized* the need for an engaged political process resulting in enhanced governance mechanisms and institutional frameworks for which nutrition sensitivity, inter-sectoriality and social participation are underlying principles.

In addition, the symposium recommended a focus on:

- Food and agriculture, not just on public health interventions such as breastfeeding, supplements and fortified foods, to improve nutrition.
- The nutritional quality, diversity and safety of food, and not just its quantity (energy) and adequacy.
- Consumption and utilization by the poor of adequate quantities of safe, good quality food for a nutritionally adequate diet, not just increasing production, raising incomes and improving access.
- Provision of a body of evidence that can document the impact that food and improved diets have on human health, growth and mental development. Demonstrating that agriculture-based interventions can improve nutrition outcomes is essential to increasing the visibility of agriculture on national and international nutrition agendas.
- Nutrition education, behaviour change and communication strategies, especially in view of the evidence that agricultural improvements alone do not necessarily lead to improvements in diets.

- Advocacy to help create the policy, institutional, social and physical environments that are conducive to ensuring access by all people to nutritionally adequate diets.
- Investing in crop and dietary diversity to narrow the 'nutrition gap' – the gap between what foods are grown and available and what foods are needed for a healthy diet. Narrowing the nutrition gap means improving the quality and diversity of the diet through increasing the availability of and access to the foods necessary for a healthy diet, and increasing the actual intake of those foods.
- Biofortification that provides micronutrient-rich plants for farmers to use for years to come and is therefore a feasible means of reaching malnourished populations in relatively remote rural areas, and delivering naturally fortified foods to people with limited access to commercially marketed fortified foods. This requires a one-time investment in plant breeding with no further financial outlays as would be required for traditional supplementation and fortification programmes.
- More effective articulation of nutrition objectives, concerns and considerations, and their better integration into the design and implementation of food security, agriculture and other sector development policies and initiatives to ensure: (i) that they are not detrimental to nutrition; and (ii) that potential opportunities to improve nutrition are identified and fully utilized.
- Incorporating nutrition-sensitive, agriculture- and food-based approaches into nutrition improvement policies and programmes.
- Technical support for the collection and analysis of evidence of the effectiveness of and impact that agriculture and food security interventions have for improving nutrition, as defined by access to improved dietary diversity, nutritional intakes and reductions in child undernutrition.
- Identifying best practices for improving nutrition-sensitive food- and agriculture-based approaches on a large scale and translating this knowledge into operational capacities within households, communities and governments, including policy guidance.
- Increased production, access to and consumption of an adequate quantity, quality and variety of food by the vulnerable and food-insecure.

The symposium also recommended the following specific actions:

- Analyse the magnitude and dimensions of malnutrition, who is affected, where they are affected and when to help identify causality and identify constraints and opportunities for interventions.
- Develop an evidence base through partnership and support for existing research initiatives.
- Document more systematically the importance of nutrition–agriculture–food security linkages, how nutrition adds value to food security and agriculture interventions, what contribution food-based approaches make to addressing nutrition problems and what the impact is of combined food security/agricultural and nutrition interventions on improving diets and nutritional levels.
- More research on impact indicators, including dietary intake, and on other less well documented but important outcomes such as labour and time benefits for women.
- Include impact evaluations as an intrinsic part of the process, factored in earlier on in the process. This requires a reliable monitoring and evaluation framework, and better communication of the lessons learned, as well as feedback from lessons learned into programme design.
- Provide more attention to the quality and diversity of the diet. Develop new plant varieties specifically for improving nutrition that have improved nutrient content, and better tolerance to low water availability – a major factor limiting crop yields, which is likely to become even more important with global warming; also, diversify the crop mix to reduce seasonality.

- Develop new agricultural practices that can increase production and farm incomes while conserving the environment.
- Incorporate explicit nutrition objectives and considerations into agricultural research agendas.
- Encourage technical experts in agricultural research and development, agricultural extension, fisheries and livestock to increase crop and dietary diversity for improved nutrition outcomes; assist farmers, including women farmers, to generate increased incomes and to effectively use such incomes for improved family nutrition, health and education, all of which are necessary for achieving the Millennium Development Goals.
- Provide a global overview on the extent to which nutrition is currently integrated into agriculture policies and programmes.
- Identify and mitigate risks posed by those agricultural policies and programmes that reduce household food security and increase malnutrition.
- Support policies for nutrition-sensitive food-based programmes, advocate for increased investments in them and strengthened institutions to help design and implement them.
- Develop training materials for the development of national and regional institutional and human capacities for better integrating nutrition into food security policies, strategies and programmes, and supporting their roll-out in selected countries.
- Raise the awareness of agricultural planners of the consequences of micronutrient deficiencies, and encourage them to advocate increases in the production and consumption of foods rich in the deficient nutrients.
- Give attention to agriculture- and food-based interventions that promote dietary diversity and the consumption of nutritionally enhanced foods.
- Give greater visibility to nutrition-sensitive agriculture through publications (e.g. special editions of FAO's *State of Food and Agriculture* (SOFA) and *State of Food Insecurity* (SOFI).
- Provide clear practical guidance on how to integrate nutrition objectives into agricultural policies and programmes, and how to leverage resources and investments for agriculture and build local institutional capacity.
- Reverse the decline in domestic and international funding for agriculture, food security and rural development in developing countries, and promote new investment to increase sustainable agricultural production and productivity, reduce poverty and work towards achieving food and nutrition security for all.
- Protect and promote nutrition in times of crisis, and incorporate nutrition objectives into emergency responses that support coping mechanisms, safeguard livelihoods and strengthen resilience.
- Assess climate change adaptation and mitigation policies and actions, and take opportunities for improving food and nutrition security.

Index

Page numbers in **bold** type refer to figures, tables and boxed text.

Appendix: Presentation of the Publication
Combating Micronutrient Deficiencies: Food-based Approaches

Brian Thompson and Leslie Amoroso*

*Nutrition and Consumer Protection Division (AGN), Agriculture and Consumer
Protection Department (AG), Food and Agriculture Organization of the United
Nations, Rome, Italy*

Distinguished guests, dear colleagues, ladies and gentlemen.

Good afternoon everybody.

Welcome

It our great pleasure and pride to present to you the first edition of the publication *Combating Micronutrient Deficiencies: Food-based Approaches*. The release of the book during this international symposium is timely and demonstrates the commitment of the Food and Agriculture Organization (FAO) from a food and agriculture perspective to improve diets and raise levels of nutrition and, in so doing, prevent and control micronutrient deficiencies.

Micronutrient deficiencies affect more than two billion people in the world today – about a third of the world's population. With long-ranging effects on health, learning ability and productivity, they contribute to the vicious cycle of malnutrition, underdevelopment and poverty. Inadequate attention has so far been paid to food-based approaches in achieving sustainable improvements in the micronutrient status of vulnerable populations. The Nutrition and Consumer Protection Division therefore undertook the preparation of this publication to provide more emphasis, importance and investment to these strategies. For the first time in one volume, *Combating Micronutrient Deficiencies: Food-based Approaches* brings together available knowledge, case studies on country-level activities, lessons learned and success stories showing that food-based approaches are viable, sustainable and long-term solutions to overcome micronutrient malnutrition.

Food-based Approaches

The book aims at documenting the benefits of food-based approaches, particularly of dietary improvement and diversification interventions, in controlling and preventing micronutrient deficiencies. The focus of the publication is on practical actions for overcoming micronutrient malnutrition in a sustainable manner through increasing access to and availability and consumption of adequate quantities and varieties of safe, good-quality food.

---

*Contacts: brian.thompson@fao.org; leslie.amoroso@fao.org

Food-based approaches promote the diversity of food systems and supplies and thus of the consumption of foods that are naturally good sources of or rich in micronutrients, or that are enriched through fortification or biofortification. Food-based strategies have been overlooked in recent decades as governments, researchers, the donor community, and health-oriented international agencies, have sought approaches for overcoming micronutrient malnutrition that have rapid start-up times and produce quick, measurable results. For example, much of the effort to control the three major deficiencies of greatest public health concern – vitamin A, iron and iodine – have focused on supplementation. Although many lives have been saved and much suffering has been avoided as a result of these efforts, there is wider recognition that food-based strategies are a viable, cost-effective and sustainable solution for controlling and preventing micronutrient malnutrition.

Idea for the Book

The idea for this peer-reviewed publication originated during the First International Meeting of the Micronutrient Forum held in Istanbul, Turkey, in April 2007. With little attention given to food or to diets, the meeting highlighted the lack of attention to and information on this important aspect of the fight against micronutrient malnutrition.

A 'call for papers' was prepared and widely circulated through different Internet sites and web fora, inviting experts from around the world to submit articles. The publication has benefited from the contribution of 100 authors from diverse disciplines, including nutrition, agriculture, horticulture, education, communication and development, to capture a rich collection of knowledge and experience. A booklet about the publication has been prepared which contains the abstracts for each chapter.

The Chapters

The publication has 19 chapters, each of which shows the benefits – and in some cases

the limitations – of food-based approaches for preventing and controlling micronutrient malnutrition.

The first two chapters present an overview of current developments in food-based approaches and examine some of the studies and programmes applying these strategies.

While agricultural approaches have the potential to have significant impact on nutritional outcomes in a sustainable way, the third chapter notes that there is insufficient understanding of the evidence base on how best to achieve this potential. Looking at the available evidence linking agricultural interventions to nutrition outcomes, the chapter describes the pathways through which agricultural interventions have an impact on nutrition and reviews the types of studies that have provided insights on the links between agriculture and nutrition.

The next two chapters show how multisectoral programmes with food-based approach components can alleviate undernutrition and micronutrient malnutrition. Increased intake of animal source foods improves nutritional status in populations with high levels of nutrient deficiencies. However, the identification of effective strategies to increase access to and consumption of animal source foods by vulnerable populations has proven challenging.

The benefits of animal source foods in combating micronutrient deficiencies are discussed from the sixth to the eighth chapters.

Fruits and vegetables are a fundamental part of a balanced diet and a good source of vitamins and minerals. Chapters 9 to 13 describe the benefits of vegetables and fruits in preventing and combating micronutrient malnutrition.

The next two chapters illustrate the benefits of food-based approaches for overcoming single specific micronutrient deficiencies (zinc and iron).

Chapters 16 to 18 discuss food fortification.

In conclusion, the last chapter describes how the disability-adjusted life years (DALYs) methodology can be a useful approach for economically assessing cost-effectiveness in terms of the nutritional impact of interventions.

Progress in promoting and implementing food-based strategies to achieve sustainable improvements in micronutrient status has been slow. We hope that this publication convinces readers that food-based approaches can tackle the root causes of micronutrient malnutrition and can assist communities and households to feed and nourish themselves adequately, thereby providing overall long-term benefits.

We hope you enjoy the book.

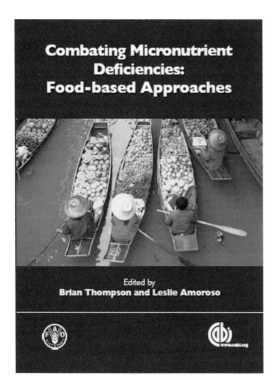

Combating Micronutrient Deficiencies: Food-based Approaches

Edited by Brian Thompson and Leslie Amoroso

Published in 2011 by the Food and Agriculture Organization of the United Nations (FAO), Rome and CAB International, Wallingford, UK, 2011, 397 pp.

ISBN-13: 978 92 5 106546 4 (FAO)

ISBN-13: 978 1 84593 714 0 (CABI)

The publication and a booklet providing a summary and chapter abstracts are available electronically on FAO's website: http://www.fao.org
Copies of the print book can be ordered from the CABI bookshop at: http://www.cabi.org/bookshop